Respiratory Medicine

Series Editor:
Sharon I.S. Rounds

More information about this series at http://www.springer.com/series/7665

James R. Klinger • Robert P. Frantz
Editors

Diagnosis and Management of Pulmonary Hypertension

Humana Press

ATS
We help the world breathe®
PULMONARY • CRITICAL CARE • SLEEP

Editors
James R. Klinger, MD
Division of Pulmonary,
Sleep and Critical Care Medicine
Rhode Island Hospital
Alpert Medical School of Brown University
Providence, RI, USA

Robert P. Frantz, MD
Department of Medicine
Mayo Clinic College of Medicine
Rochester, MN, USA

ISSN 2197-7372 ISSN 2197-7380 (electronic)
Respiratory Medicine
ISBN 978-1-4939-2635-0 ISBN 978-1-4939-2636-7 (eBook)
DOI 10.1007/978-1-4939-2636-7

Library of Congress Control Number: 2015938155

Springer New York Heidelberg Dordrecht London

Printed on acid-free paper

Humana Press is a brand of Springer
Springer Science+Business Media LLC New York is part of Springer Science+Business Media (www.springer.com)

Preface

Over the last few decades, the study of pulmonary arterial hypertension (PAH) has become one of the most rapidly developing fields of cardiopulmonary medicine. This may seem surprising considering the relatively small number of patients who carry this diagnosis, but like many rare diseases that were once untreatable, interest in PAH has been spurred on by an intense desire to improve the outcome of those who are affected. At the same time, numerous discoveries in the field of pulmonary vascular biology have led to a marked shift in how we view the pulmonary circulation. Many of these discoveries have led directly to the development and licensing of over a dozen drugs in the last 20 years.

When we began our training in pulmonary and cardiac medicine, primary pulmonary hypertension, as the disease was known then, had no approved treatment and less than 50 % of patients survived more than three years after diagnosis. Nitric oxide and endothelin had not yet been discovered and there were no genetic defects that were known to be associated with familial pulmonary hypertension. In less than 30 years, a staggering number of cell signaling pathways vital to the maintenance of normal pulmonary vascular tone and remodeling have been found to be impaired or deregulated in PAH and point mutations in a single gene have been found to be responsible for nearly 80 % of patients with heritable PAH and up to 25 % of those with no known family history. Although no cure has been found yet, four distinct classes of drugs are available for treatment and recent registries from the USA, China, and Europe suggest that five-year survival now exceeds 60 %. Many of the therapies that are presently available for the treatment of PAH were newly discovered agents that we tested in animals with experimental models of pulmonary hypertension in the lab not so long ago. The rapid increase in our understanding of the disease and the rapid development of effective therapy are very much a part of the intense interest that PAH has generated.

Today, the diagnosis and treatment of pulmonary vascular disease has become an important part of cardiopulmonary medicine. Most major medical centers have faculty and staff who have received specialized training in this area or who have devoted a major part of their practice to this disease. Many institutions have developed pulmonary hypertension centers that specialize in the evaluation and care of patients with pulmonary hypertensive disease. Recently, the Pulmonary Hypertension Association (PHA), a nonprofit organization created by patients and their families for the advancement of research and treatment of PAH, has embarked on an accreditation initiative that aims to identify centers with special expertise in PAH. Pulmonary hypertension programs across the nation will be designated as Centers of Comprehensive Care or Regional Clinical Programs. This program aims to improve the overall quality of care by ensuring that PAH patients are able to find experienced medical care close to home and establish referral patterns that can provide rapid access to more invasive testing and aggressive treatment options when needed.

Presently, health care providers face several major challenges in the field of pulmonary vascular disease. The first is the need for earlier diagnosis. Despite the marked increase in awareness of PAH that has been brought about by advances in its understanding and treatment, the delay in diagnosis has not improved. In fact, the median time between symptom onset and diagnosis of PAH remains greater than two years and has not decreased since the initial NIH registry reported this data in the 1980s. Delay in diagnosis is due to the rarity of the disease, its nonspecific symptoms, and lack of readily available and highly sensitive screening tools. To improve the time to diagnosis and ultimately response to treatment, practitioners must have a high level of suspicion and stay alert to the possibility of PAH in any patient with unexplained dyspnea. The second challenge is proper clinical classification. Although PAH is rare, pulmonary hypertension is not. From 1980 through 2002, the estimated number of hospitalizations with pulmonary hypertension as any-listed diagnosis tripled for the total US population from 87,000 to 260,000. However, epidemiologic studies suggest that less than 3 % of patients with elevated pulmonary arterial pressure have PAH. In one well-known study, three-quarters of cases of elevated pulmonary artery pressure on echocardiogram were found to be due to left-sided heart disease and another 20 % were attributed to chronic lung disease. Less than 3 % had PAH. The most recent disease classification system developed during a series of meetings sponsored by the World Health Organization divides pulmonary hypertension into five distinct groups. Proper identification of which type of pulmonary hypertension a patient has is absolutely essential to proper management. Some patients have complex phenotypes with what appear to be multiple contributors to their pulmonary hypertension. It is our hope that future research will further elucidate the pathophysiology and best management of these challenging cases. Finally, health care providers may struggle with the large number of options that are rapidly becoming available for the treatment of PAH. This is an issue complicated by the high cost of most medications and recent data suggesting that combinations of PAH-specific medications may be more effective than single-drug therapy.

In *Diagnosis and Management of Pulmonary Hypertension*, we have tried to provide the reader with an overview of the pulmonary hypertensive diseases, the current understanding of their pathobiology, and a contemporary approach to diagnosis and treatment. Chapters 1 and 2 discuss the definition and classification of the pulmonary hypertensive diseases and the epidemiology of PAH. Chapters 3 through 11 review the approach to diagnosis and evaluation and discuss the considerable body of data that has stemmed from the broad use of echocardiography, right-heart catheterization, and, more recently, cardiopulmonary exercise testing to diagnose and monitor the progression of PAH. Each of the major drug classes used to treat PAH and the cell signaling pathways that they target are described in Chaps. 12 through 15. Adjunct treatments and investigative therapies that are likely to herald the next generation of PAH medications are explored in Chaps. 16 and 17. Finally, the book concludes with several chapters that discuss special situations that have been particularly challenging in the management of PAH including perioperative evaluation and treatment of the critically ill patient with PAH. Each of the chapters is written by experts in their respective fields, many of whom have helped to shape the face of the modern-day approach to the diagnosis and treatment of PAH. We are indebted to the authors for their outstanding contributions and hope that you will find their chapters as helpful and as insightful as we have.

Providence, RI, USA — James R. Klinger, MD
Rochester, MN, USA — Robert P. Frantz, MD

Contents

1 **The Pulmonary Circulation** 1
Victor F. Tapson

2 **Epidemiology and Disease Classification of Pulmonary Hypertension** 21
Rogerio Souza, Carlos Jardim, and Marc Humbert

3 **Pathogenesis of Pulmonary Arterial Hypertension** 37
Aaron W. Trammell and Anna R. Hemnes

4 **Hypoxic Pulmonary Hypertension** 67
Kara Goss and Tim Lahm

5 **Pulmonary Hypertension in Chronic Heart and Lung Disease** 93
Robert P. Frantz

6 **Chronic Thromboembolic Pulmonary Hypertension** 115
William R. Auger and Peter F. Fedullo

7 **Schistosomiasis-Associated Pulmonary Arterial Hypertension** 143
Rita de Cassia dos Santos Ferreira, Angela Pontes Bandeira, and Ana Lúcia Coutinho Domingues

8 **Approach to the Patient with Elevated Pulmonary Arterial Pressure** 165
Jason S. Fritz and Harold I. Palevsky

9 **Echocardiography** 203
Paul Forfia

10 **Pulmonary Hemodynamics and Right Heart Catheterization** 225
Saurabh Rajpal, Yonatan Buber, and Michael J. Landzberg

11 **Cardiopulmonary Exercise Testing in Pulmonary Hypertension** 265
David M. Systrom and Aaron B. Waxman

12 Adjunct Therapy and Calcium Channel Blockers ... 303
Terence K. Trow

13 Prostacyclin Therapy for Pulmonary Arterial Hypertension ... 323
Ioana R. Preston

14 Endothelin Receptor Antagonists ... 341
Josanna Rodriguez-Lopez and Richard N. Channick

15 Modulation of cGMP Synthesis and Metabolism ... 355
Kristen J. Bubb, Adrian J. Hobbs, and James R. Klinger

16 Combination Therapy for the Treatment of Pulmonary Arterial Hypertension ... 377
Andrew T. Levinson and James R. Klinger

17 Investigative Therapies in Pulmonary Arterial Hypertension ... 397
Karen A. Fagan

18 Pulmonary Hypertension in Critically Ill Patients ... 413
Hooman D. Poor, Corey E. Ventetuolo, and Todd M. Bull

19 Perioperative Management of Pulmonary Hypertension ... 437
Yuliya B. Goldsmith, Natalia Ivascu, Dana McGlothlin, Paul M. Heerdt, and Evelyn M. Horn

Erratum to ... E1

Index ... 465

Contributors

William R. Auger, MD Division of Pulmonary and Critical Care Medicine, University of California, San Diego, La Jolla, CA, USA

Angela Pontes Bandeira, MD University of Pernambuco, Recife, Brazil

Kristen J. Bubb William Harvey Research Institute, Barts and The London Medical School, London, UK

Yonatan Buber, MD Boston Adult Congenital Heart (BACH) and Pulmonary Hypertension Group, Brigham and Women's Hospital and Children's Hospital, Harvard Medical School, Boston, MA, USA

Sheba Medical Center, Sackler School of Medicine, Tel Aviv, Israel

Todd M. Bull, MD Division of Pulmonary Sciences and Critical Care Medicine and Cardiology, University of Colorado, Denver, CO, USA

Richard N. Channick, MD Pulmonary and Critical Care Division, Massachusetts General Hospital, Harvard Medical School, Boston, MA, USA

Ana Lúcia Coutinho Domingues, PhD Health Sciences Centre, Federal University of Pernambuco, Recife, Brazil

Karen A. Fagan, MD Pulmonary Diseases and Critical Care Medicine, Division of Pulmonary and Critical Care, Pulmonary Hypertension Center, University of South Alabama, Mobile, AL, USA

Peter F. Fedullo, MD Division of Pulmonary and Critical Care Medicine, University of California, San Diego, La Jolla, CA, USA

Rita de Cassia dos Santos Ferreira, PhD Department of Pneumology, Hospital das Clínicas - Universidade Federal de Pernambuco, Cidade Universitária, Recife, Brazil

Paul Forfia, MD Section of Cardiology, Department of Medicine, Temple University, Philadelphia, PA, USA

Robert P. Frantz, MD Department of Medicine, Mayo Clinic College of Medicine, Rochester, MN, USA

Jason S. Fritz, MD Pulmonary Vascular Disease Program, Pulmonary, Allergy, and Critical Care Division, Department of Medicine, Penn Presbyterian Medical Center, Perelman School of Medicine at the University of Pennsylvania, Philadelphia, PA, USA

Yuliya B. Goldsmith Department of Medicine, Weill Cornell Medical College, New York, NY, USA

Perkin Heart Failure Center, Division of Cardiology, Weill Cornell Medical Center, New York, NY, USA

Kara Goss, MD Division of Pulmonary, Allergy, Critical Care, Occupational and Sleep Medicine, Department of Medicine, Indiana University School of Medicine, Indianapolis, IN, USA

Paul M. Heerdt Department of Anesthesiology, Weill Cornell Medical College, New York, NY, USA

Department of Pharmacology, Weill Cornell Medical College, New York, NY, USA

Anna R. Hemnes, MD Department of Medicine, Allergy, Pulmonary, and Critical Care Medicine, Vanderbilt University Medical Center, Nashville, TN, USA

Adrian J. Hobbs William Harvey Research Institute, Barts and The London Medical School, London, UK

Evelyn M. Horn, MD Department of Medicine, Weill Cornell Medical College, New York, NY, USA

Perkin Heart Failure Center, Division of Cardiology, Weill Cornell Medical Center, New York, NY, USA

Marc Humbert, MD Service de Pneumologie, Hopital Bicetre, Université Paris-Sud, Paris, France

Natalia Ivascu Department of Anesthesiology, Weill Cornell Medical College, New York, NY, USA

Carlos Jardim, MD Pulmonary Department, Heart Institute, University of Sao Paulo Medical School, Sao Paulo, Brazil

James R. Klinger, MD Division of Pulmonary, Sleep and Critical Care Medicine, Rhode Island Hospital, Alpert Medical School of Brown University, Providence, RI, USA

Tim Lahm, MD Division of Pulmonary, Allergy, Critical Care, Occupational and Sleep Medicine, Department of Medicine, Richard L. Roudebush VA Medical Center, Indiana University School of Medicine, Indianapolis, IN, USA

Michael J. Landzberg, MD Boston Adult Congenital Heart (BACH) and Pulmonary Hypertension Group, Brigham and Women's Hospital and Children's Hospital, Harvard Medical School, Boston, MA, USA

Andrew T. Levinson, MD, MPH Division of Pulmonary, Sleep and Critical Care Medicine, Rhode Island Hospital, Alpert Medical School of Brown University, Providence, RI, USA

Dana McGlothlin, MD Department of Cardiology, Kaiser San Francisco Medical Center, San Francisco, CA, USA

Harold I. Palevsky, MD Pulmonary Vascular Disease Program, Pulmonary, Allergy, and Critical Care Division, Department of Medicine, Penn Presbyterian Medical Center, Perelman School of Medicine at the University of Pennsylvania, Philadelphia, PA, USA

Hooman D. Poor, MD Division of Pulmonary, Critical Care and Sleep, Mount Sinai Hospital, New York, NY, USA

Ioana R. Preston, MD Pulmonary, Critical Care and Sleep Division, Tufts Medical Center, Boston, MA, USA

Saurabh Rajpal, MD Louisiana State University School of Medicine, Shreveport, LA, USA

Boston Adult Congenital Heart (BACH) and Pulmonary Hypertension Group, Brigham and Women's Hospital and Children's Hospital, Harvard Medical School, Boston, MA, USA

Josanna Rodriguez-Lopez, MD Pulmonary and Critical Care Division, Massachusetts General Hospital, Harvard Medical School, Boston, MA, USA

Rogerio Souza, M.D. Pulmonary Department, Heart Institute, University of Sao Paulo Medical School, Sao Paulo, Brazil

David M. Systrom, MD Pulmonary and Critical Care Medicine, Pulmonary Vascular Disease Program Director, Dyspnea and Performance Evaluation Program, Brigham and Women's Hospital Heart and Vascular, Center Assistant Professor of Medicine/Harvard Medical School, Boston, MA, USA

Victor F. Tapson, MD Department of Pulmonary and Critical Care Medicine, Cedars-Sinai Medical Center, Los Angeles, CA, USA

Pulmonary Hypertension Clinic, Beverly Hills, CA, USA

Aaron W. Trammell, MD Department of Medicine, Allergy, Pulmonary, and Critical Care Medicine, Vanderbilt University Medical Center, Nashville, TN, USA

Terence K. Trow, MD Yale Pulmonary Vascular Disease Program, Section of Pulmonary, Critical Care, and Sleep Medicine, Department of Internal Medicine, Yale University School of Medicine, New Haven, CT, USA

Corey E. Ventetuolo, MD, MS Division of Pulmonary, Sleep and Critical Care Medicine, Rhode Island Hospital, Alpert Medical School of Brown University, Providence, RI, USA

Aaron B. Waxman, MD, PhD Pulmonary Vascular Disease Program, Pulmonary Critical Care Medicine and Cardiovascular Medicine, Brigham and Women's Hospital, Harvard Medical School, Boston, MA, USA

Chapter 1
The Pulmonary Circulation

Victor F. Tapson

Abstract The pulmonary circulation carries oxygen-depleted blood from the right heart to the lungs and returns oxygenated blood to the left heart for delivery to the systemic circulation while serving as a source of humoral mediator production and a barrier to the exchange of fluid and solutes. This chapter discusses several aspects of this unique circulation, including a brief history of its discovery and the tools used to explore it; an overview of pulmonary hemodynamics and how they affect right ventricular function; structure and mechanical properties of the pulmonary circulation; and neural/humoral regulation of the pulmonary vascular tone and barrier properties that prevent leakage of fluid and solutes into the alveolar space. The chapter is written to highlight those unique properties of the pulmonary circulation that are involved with the pathogenesis of pulmonary hypertension and the response of the right ventricle and pulmonary blood vessels to disease development. The overall aim is to prepare the reader for an in-depth discussion of pulmonary hypertensive diseases that follows in the subsequent chapters.

Keywords Pulmonary circulation • Right ventricle • Pulmonary vascular disease • Pulmonary hypertension

Abbreviations

ACE	Angiotensin-converting enzyme
CO	Cardiac output
LA	Left atrium
LAP	Left atrial pressure
MDCT	Multidetector row computed tomography
mPAP	Mean pulmonary artery pressure

V.F. Tapson, M.D. (✉)
Department of Pulmonary and Critical Care Medicine,
Cedars-Sinai Medical Center, Los Angeles, CA, USA

Pulmonary Hypertension Clinic, 8536 Wilshire Blvd., Suite 201,
Beverly Hills, CA 90211, USA
e-mail: Victor.Tapson@cshs.org

J.R. Klinger, R.P. Frantz (eds.), *Diagnosis and Management of Pulmonary Hypertension*, Respiratory Medicine 12, DOI 10.1007/978-1-4939-2636-7_1

PA	Pulmonary artery
PAH	Pulmonary arterial hypertension
PCWP	Pulmonary capillary wedge pressure
PH	Pulmonary hypertension
PVR	Pulmonary vascular resistance
RV	Right ventricle
VCO_2	Carbon dioxide output
VO_2	Oxygen uptake

Introduction

The pulmonary circulation carries oxygen-depleted blood from the heart to the lungs and returns oxygenated blood back to the heart to be delivered to the systemic circulation. Specifically, the pulmonary arteries carry *venous* blood to the capillaries so that carbon dioxide can diffuse out of the blood cell into the alveoli, and oxygen can diffuse out of the alveoli into the blood. Blood leaves the capillaries and enters the pulmonary veins, which carry *arterial* (oxygen-rich) blood to the left atrium, left ventricle, and then aorta.

In addition to delivering the entire cardiac output, the pulmonary circulation also serves as a source of humoral mediator production and processing. Finally, this vasculature serves as a barrier to the exchange of fluid and solutes, thus maintaining pulmonary fluid balance.

The pulmonary circulation is not the only blood supply to the lungs; the bronchial circulation supplies systemic arterial blood to ensure nutrition to the airways [1]. While the bronchial arterial supply is only a small percentage of the cardiac output, it is capable of extensive proliferation when pulmonary blood flow is compromised or in the setting of chronic pulmonary inflammation [2].

The pulmonary vasculature can be profoundly affected in certain disease states. Our goal is to discuss certain aspects of this unique circulation, particularly as they relate to pulmonary hypertensive disease. A number of topics in this textbook potentially overlap with this chapter, including pathogenesis of PAH, hypoxemic PH, pulmonary vascular remodeling from chronic lung and heart disease, and pulmonary hemodynamics and right heart catheterization. Our focus is a historic overview, followed by a description of the normal pulmonary circulation, but also includes some pathogenetic concepts as they relate to PH and certain aspects of its evolution.

Historical Aspects

The discovery and characterization of the pulmonary circulation is a fascinating story. The Greek anatomist Erasistratus, in the mid-200's B.C., was credited with discovering that the heart was a pump and described the valves of the heart [3].

However, he believed that the arteries and the left side of the heart were empty, and functioned to convey the "spirit of life" to the body. This concept remained until Galen proved that blood emanated from any living mammal when an artery was pierced [4]. His theory was that blood from the right side of the heart passed to the left side through invisible pores in the cardiac septum. There, it mixed with air to "create spirit" and was distributed to the body. He indicated that a small portion of the blood passed back from the left side into the lungs to be cleansed of its "soot." He did believe that a small portion of the blood on the right side passed through the *vena arteriosa* to the *arteria venosa*, and on to the left side. Thus, Galen understood certain basic principles of the pulmonary circulation (Fig. 1.1).

For at least the next 1,000 years, there were no apparent major discoveries involving the pulmonary circulation. Michael Servetus, the Spanish physician and theologist, was credited with the first description of the pulmonary circulation in his book "Christianismi Restitutio," published in 1553 [5]. "The vital spirit has its origin in the left ventricle of the heart, the lungs especially helping towards its perfection. It is generated through the commingling which is effected in the lungs of the inspired air with the elaborated subtle blood communicated from the right ventricle to the left [5]." Servetus trained in Paris with Vesalius and was considered an exceptionally skilled dissector [4–7]. Sadly, he was regarded as a heretic and was ultimately tried in Geneva and burned at the stake [8]. His contributions were substantial. Only three surviving copies of the original document are known, although it was translated into a number of languages.

In 1924, an Egyptian physician, Muhyo Al-Deen Altawi, studying the history of medicine discovered a treatise by a physician, Ibn al-Nafis, entitled "Commentary on the Anatomy of Canon of Avicenna" in the Prussian State Library in Berlin [9]. These writings covered human anatomy, physiology, and pathology [9]. They were translated by two Syrian physicians, and it was learned that al-Nafis had made essentially the same observations as Servetus, in the thirteenth century, prior to several hundred years [9–11]. This work of Ibn al-Nafis was believed to be the earliest description of the pulmonary circulation.

Al-Nafis, a Syrian physician, trained in Damascus and ultimately practiced and researched in Egypt in the thirteenth century. He became the Sultan's personal physician. Al-Nafis was credited as the first person to challenge the long-held belief of Galen that blood could pass through the cardiac interventricular septum; he was emphatic that all the blood that reached the left ventricle passed through the lungs [9–11]. He also stated that there must be small communications or pores between the pulmonary artery and vein (this concept preceded Marcello Malpighi's discovery of the pulmonary capillaries by four centuries). Al-Nafis also postulated that nutrients for the heart are extracted from the coronary arteries [9–11]. Thus, Ibn al-Nafis and another prominent physiologist of the period, Avicenna (approximately 1000 A.D.), were among very few physician researchers to link the Galenic period in the second century to the European scientific Renaissance in the sixteenth century. The Haddad translation published in the Annals of Surgery in 1936 offers detailed descriptions of Al-Nafis' discoveries [9]. In summary, Ibn al-Nafis should be regarded as a major influence and as the primary forerunner of Servetus, Vesalius, Colombo, and Harvey in the description of the pulmonary circulation as we now know it.

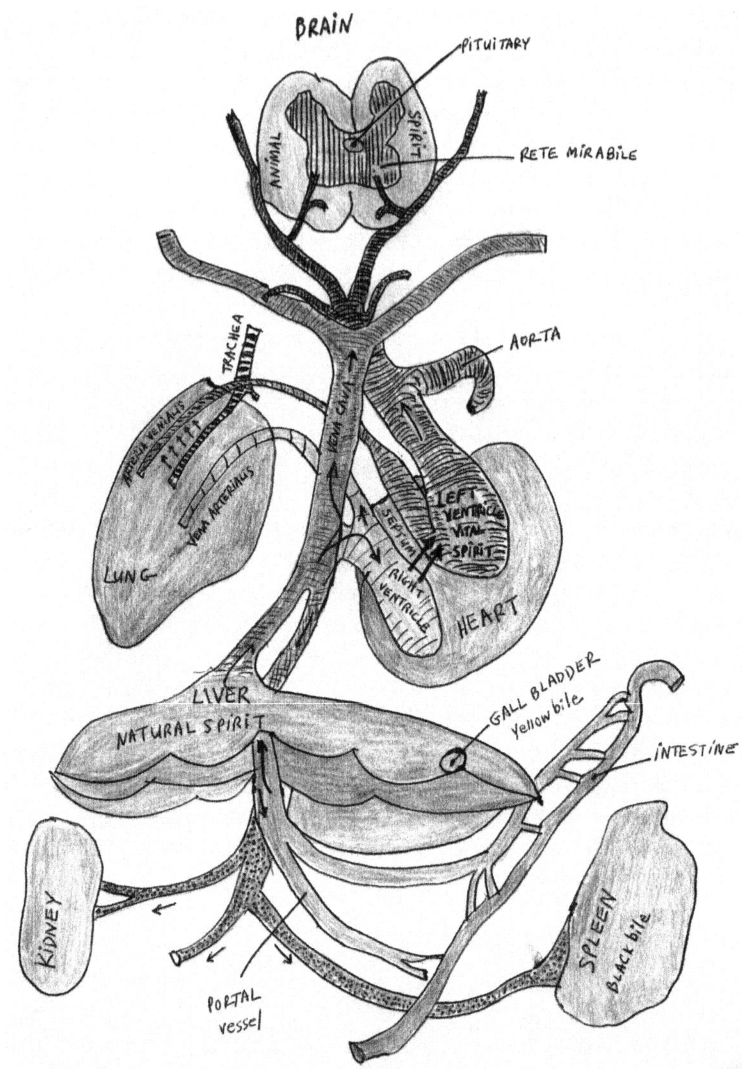

Fig. 1.1 A reproduction of Galen's scheme. In Galen's schema, the venous, arterial, and nervous systems, with the liver, heart, and brain as their respective centers, were separate, and each distributed through the body one of the three pneumata: respectively, the natural, vital, and animal spirits. Blood was carried both within the venous system and the arterial system. The heart and lungs worked together, with some of the blood passing through the pulmonary artery into the lungs; there it nourished the lungs and also mixed with the air breathed in. Some of the blood in the heart passed from right to left through "pores" in the interventricular septum. It was bright red because it had the vital spirit infused within it; from the left heart, it went out via the aorta to warm up the body

In the sixteenth century, in his book, "De Fabrica," Vesalius described the pulmonary circulation in a way that very much resembled the description of Ibn al-Nafis [12]. In the first edition of his book in 1543, Vesalius agreed with Galen that the blood "... soaks plentifully through the septum from the right ventricle into the left ..." [12, 13]. When he published his second edition in 1555, he omitted the above statement and wrote instead "... I still do not see how even the smallest quantity of blood can be transfused through the substance of the septum from the right ventricle to the left ..." [12, 13]. Colombo, who studied under Vesalius at Padua, ultimately queried this concept, and determined through vivisection and dissection of human cadavers that "almost everyone assumes that the blood passes from the right ventricle to the left ventricle across this wall ... But they are completely wrong. For the blood is conducted to the lungs by the pulmonary artery, where it is diluted and together with air is led to the left ventricle by the pulmonary veins, which no one has noticed until now, nor described in writing ..." [12].

The work by Ibn al-Nafis, Servetus, and subsequently Vesalius and Colombo, paved the way for Harvey's elegant description of the pulmonary circulation. "*Exercitatio Anatomica de Motu Cordis et Sanguinis in Animalibus*" (An Anatomical Exercise on the Motion of the Heart and Blood in Living Beings) is the best known work of William Harvey [14–17]. The book was first published in Latin in Frankfurt in 1628 and remains one of the most important works establishing concepts of the circulation of the blood. Harvey's methods combined observations and experimental methods; among them were the examination of the effect of ligatures on blood flow. The book taught that blood was pumped around the body in a "double circulation," so that after being returned to the heart, it was recirculated in a closed system to the lungs and back to the heart, where it was returned to the main circulation [14–17]. There was, however, one portion of the circulation which Harvey could not characterize, although he did postulate it, i.e., the way in which the veins and arteries subdivide into a capillary network. As alluded to above, it was in 1660, 3 years after Harvey's death, that Marcello Malpighi of Bologna saw the blood moving in the capillaries of the frog's lung, and thus the missing link that Harvey needed to fully characterize the circulation of the blood [18]. The period of the Islamic Golden Age, the long influence of the teachings of the Galen School, and the European Renaissance are shown on a timeline in Fig. 1.2.

Subsequent relevant discoveries included the demonstration by Boyle with his air-pump experiments in 1666 that air was essential to life [7]. The next year, Hooke demonstrated that it was the supply of air *to the blood* that was crucial to respiration [19]. In 1669, Lower found that the difference between arterial and venous blood was the change in color and that this change took place in the lungs and not the heart. In 1668, Mayow discovered that only part of the air, the "spiritus nitro-aereus," was necessary for life [19]. Priestley, in 1774, called oxygen "dephlogisticated air." In 1777, Lavoisier further clarified these concepts, demonstrating for the first time that during respiration, the air that was breathed in lost oxygen and gained "fixed air of Black." (Black had discovered carbon dioxide 20 years prior.) Spallanzini subsequently characterized concepts involving tissue respiration [19].

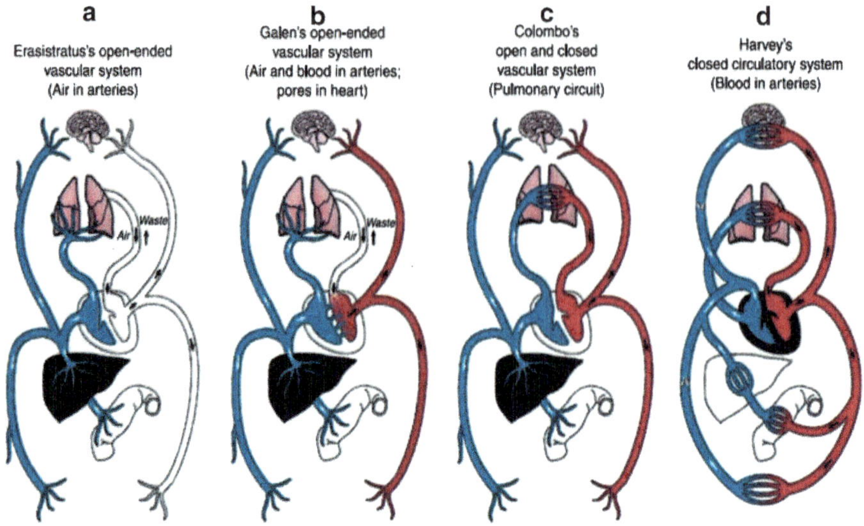

Fig. 1.2 Cardiovascular models over the course of time. (**a**) Erasistratus' model, (**b**) Galen's model, (**c**) Colombo's model, (**d**) Harvey's model. Reference: Arid WC. Discovery of the cardiovascular system: from Galen to William Harvey

Steven Hales deduced and published that the thinner walls of the right ventricle indicated that it had less work to do to force blood through the pulmonary circulation than the left ventricle did to maintain the systemic circulation [20]. In the early nineteenth century, Hope also studied the physics of the failing heart and described the symptoms and signs of heart failure, differentiating the effects of failure of the right ventricle from those of the left. By 1847, the work of Poiseuille together with Ludwig enabled blood pressure measurement [21].

Over the ensuing decades, pioneers in cardiopulmonary disease improved the means through which to access the pulmonary circulation and further characterize it. Werner Forssmann performed right-heart catheterization on himself in 1929, and thus demonstrated its feasibility in humans [22]. The catheter, however, was only advanced into the right atrium. Andre Cournand and Dickinson Richards developed catheters that could be advanced into the pulmonary arteries for pathophysiological studies of various congenital and acquired cardiac disorders [23, 24]. Drs. Forssmann, Cournand, and Richards received the Nobel Prize in Medicine in 1956 for their work [24]. Subsequent investigations advanced the field of right-heart catheterization and in 1970, balloon flotation flow-directed catheters that could be used at the bedside, without fluoroscopy, were introduced by Drs. Swan and Ganz [25–28]. These balloon flotation catheters were developed further for measuring all right-sided pressures, cardiac output (by thermodilution), and pulmonary capillary wedge pressure (PCWP), and for right atrial and right ventricular pacing [29, 30]. This technique evolved into, and still remains, the standard of care for diagnosing PH and characterizing its severity (Fig. 1.3).

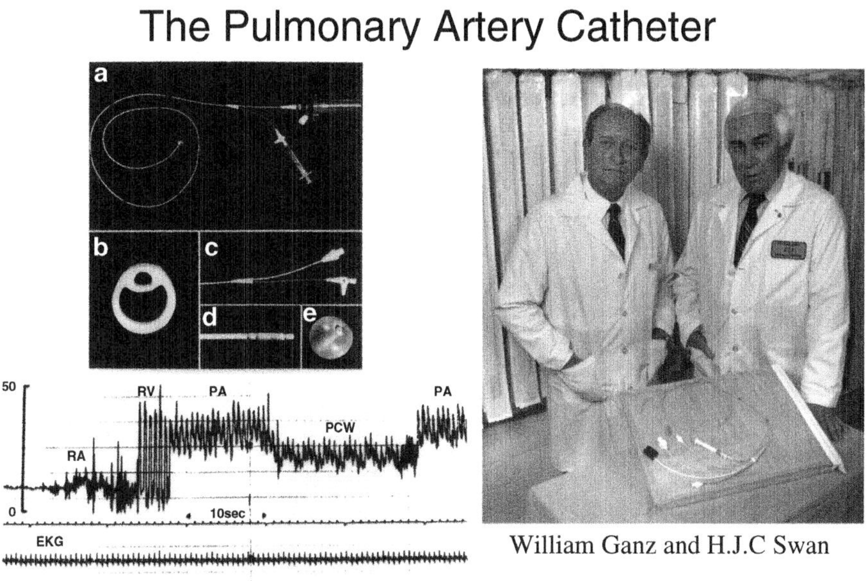

Fig. 1.3 In 1970, balloon flotation flow-directed catheters that could be used for right-heart catheterization at the bedside without fluoroscopy were introduced by Drs. Swan and Ganz (reproduced with permission from the American Heart Association)

The world's first scientific conference dedicated to the pulmonary circulation was organized by the Chicago Heart Association and held in Chicago in 1958. This progress has been outlined in detail in a treatise arising from the Chicago conference [31].

Interest in the pulmonary circulation was furthered by the PAH epidemic in Europe caused by the diet drug aminorex [32]. As interest in PH evolved, international conferences organized by the World Health Organization (WHO) have taken place during which experts in the field have gathered to review the science and available literature as well as clinical practice experience in PH. Twenty-five years after the first meeting in Geneva, Switzerland, in 1973, a second WHO meeting on PH took place in Evian, France, in 1998 [33, 34]. Since that time, these international consensus conferences have taken place every 5 years, with the most recent meeting in Nice, France, in 2013. At these meetings, the classification, risk factors, and diagnostic and therapeutic approaches to PH have been progressively scrutinized and updated based upon international research efforts. Consensus statements/guidelines have been published based upon this work [35–37]. Modern-day PAH is rich with discoveries in both basic science and clinic research that have led to the development of at least four new drug classes of pulmonary vasodilators over the last 25 years that are now available to treat patients with PAH and other pulmonary vascular disease.

Structure and Function of the Pulmonary Circulation

The genes, molecules, cells, and tissues of the pulmonary circulation work in synchrony to determine function, with the primary function of the pulmonary circulation being to optimize the exposure of blood to alveolar air while maintaining a low enough resistance to accommodate passage of the full cardiac output. The lungs receive the entire cardiac output, with the normal cardiac index being approximately 3.5 L/min/m^2. The lungs contain approximately 300 billion capillaries which supply approximately 300 million alveoli. The surface area of capillaries interfacing with alveoli for gas exchange is between 50 and 100 m^2; this contact occurs at the 1–2 μm thick alveolar capillary membrane [38–40].

Importantly, at rest, in the absence of pulmonary vascular disease, the thin-walled right ventricle functions at a very low energy level; that is, the right ventricular (RV) afterload is such that this chamber is often described as merely a conduit. When an individual exercises, oxygen uptake (VO_2) and carbon dioxide output (VCO_2) increase by as much as 20-fold above resting values, and this increased gas exchange is matched by a substantial increase in cardiac output as emphasized above. In normal exercising individuals without left or right ventricular failure, the entire cardiac output is handled by the pulmonary circulation with neither pulmonary edema nor RV failure. Disease of structural components of the lung affecting blood flow through the pulmonary vessels at any level can lead to PH, and in turn result in RV dysfunction and failure. While both the pulmonary and the systemic circulations transport the same amount of blood, the pulmonary circulation is characterized by high flow and low pressure, with the average pulmonary vascular resistance (PVR) in the range of 1 mmHg × min/L (1 Wood unit) in healthy young adults. With normal aging, the PVR eventually increases to approximately 2–3 Wood units, and to 5–10 times higher with significant PH.

The calculation of total PVR is based upon Ohm's law, and is calculated as the difference between mean pulmonary arterial (PA) and mean left atrial (LA) pressure, divided by the cardiac output (where LA pressure is approximated by PCWP); that is,

$$\mathrm{PVR} = \frac{\mathrm{mPAP} - \mathrm{mLAP}}{\mathrm{CO}}$$

where mPAP = mean pulmonary artery pressure, mLAP = mean left atrial pressure, and CO = cardiac output.

The diameters of small pulmonary arteries and capillaries account for the greater part of pressure drop across the pulmonary vascular bed. With exercise, significant elevation of PA pressure is prevented by recruitment of unopened capillaries and, to a smaller extent, distension of the elastic vessels [41]. Thus, at rest, a substantial portion of the capillary bed is unrecruited; some or all of these capillaries open when cardiac output increases in order to increase the total cross-sectional area of capillary bed, and decrease the PVR [42]. Because of this, when a healthy person exercises and the cardiac output is enhanced sixfold, the PA pressure increases only moderately [43]. The normally low pressure in the lung circulation prevents fluid from moving out from the vasculature into the interstitial/alveolar space. In pathologic states, when left-sided pressures are significantly elevated, this transudation can occur. With progressive elevation of the PA pressure in PAH, there is elevation of the RV pressure and for a period, the cardiac output is maintained. When the pressure rises too high, particularly over a relatively short period of time, compensation becomes impossible and RV failure ensures.

Modeling analyses have demonstrated the interface between vascular geometry and elasticity to pressure-flow relationships and PVR [44, 45]. Recruitment and distension mechanisms become markedly abnormal in PAH. Even early in PAH, when resting PA pressure is normal, these mechanisms impact upon exercise tolerance, and over time the inability to compensate even at rest results in marked dyspnea, that is, functional class IV symptoms. In PAH, the elevated pressure results from progressive vascular remodeling, vasoconstriction, and thrombosis of small pulmonary arteries and thus from the resistance increase.

Clinicians generally define RV afterload in terms of PVR and this measure has been used as a primary or secondary end-point in clinical trials. However, PVR reflects only the non-pulsatile component of blood flow, and neglects the significant contribution of compliance [44, 45]. Compliance takes into account the pulsatile components of the arterial load. Thus, compliance (or stiffness; the reciprocal of compliance) is an important factor contributing to systolic and diastolic pressure in the pulmonary circulation. In turn, systolic pressure determines systolic wall stress which represents the true ventricular afterload. In the early stages of PAH, a small increase in PVR will be accompanied by a relatively large drop in compliance. Later as the vascular disease progresses, the increase in PVR will continue but the decrease in compliance will be limited as vessel wall stiffness reaches a maximum.

The PVR can also be characterized by Poiseuille's equation. Here, for laminar flow, the relationship of the resistance of a tube to the tube's physical characteristics and viscosity of the perfusing fluid is described:

$$R = \frac{8L\eta}{\pi r^4}$$

where R = resistance, L = tube length, r = tube radius, and η = viscosity of perfusion fluid.

Thus, based upon this equation, the crucial determinant of PVR is the vessel's radius, since resistance is proportional to L/r^4. In the body, however, flow does not conform precisely to this relationship because it assumes long, straight blood vessels, a Newtonian fluid (e.g., water; blood is non-Newtonian), and steady, laminar flow. Nonetheless, the relationship clarifies the dominant influence of vessel radius on resistance and flow and thus relates how physiological vascular tone and pathological vascular stenosis dramatically affect pressure and flow.

To better conceptualize the hemodynamics of the pulmonary circulation in PAH, studies have investigated the measurement of PVR and compliance in healthy subjects and PH patients [46, 47]. Resistance and compliance in the pulmonary circulation have proven inversely related by a "hyperbola" [46]. It appears that PVR and compliance *together* describe RV afterload better than either of them alone. These concepts are discussed in more depth in Chaps. 3 and 5.

Biophysically based computational models offer the potential for integrating and analyzing experimental observations of the pulmonary circulation. These tools have evolved to sophisticated models that predict integrated structure-function relationships. In order to facilitate a more detailed analysis of structure-function relationships in the pulmonary circulation Burrowes and colleagues developed an anatomically based finite element model of the pulmonary vasculature. This model represents the complex geometry found in the pulmonary circulatory system for application in future, more detailed structure-functional investigations [45]. Multidetector row computed tomography (MDCT) imaging was utilized together with a volume-filling branching algorithm and an empirically based algorithm to generate the supernumerary vessel geometry. Analysis of branching properties and geometric parameters demonstrated close correlation between the model geometry and anatomical measures of human pulmonary arteries and veins. A review of mathematical and computational models of the pulmonary circulation has recently been published [48].

The Distribution of Blood Flow in the Lung

In the 1960s, experimental studies in isolated lung models indicated that blood flow distribution in the zonal model was gravitationally dependent, with lung tissue in the nondependent apical upright lung receiving proportionately less cardiac output than the dependent lung bases [49]. Perfusion is defined by the arterial-venous gradient. In zone 1, where mPAP is essentially zero, the alveolar pressure is greater than either the arterial and venous pressures and so there is collapse of the blood vessels, preventing perfusion. In zone 2, the mPAP is greater than alveolar pressure and perfusion is defined by the arterial-alveolar gradient. In zone 3, both mPAP and pulmonary venous pressure are greater than alveolar pressure. This zonal concept had been the accepted model for decades. More recent studies however have emphasized irreversibility of the flow gradient with reversal of posture [50] and "isogravitational heterogeneity of flow" [51]. These results do not suggest a theory of flow distribution that is *purely* gravitational. These findings together with other investigations imply that the hydrostatic effects of gravity are not the only factors determining the distribution of pulmonary blood flow [50–52]. Furthermore, imaging studies have suggested that gravitational effects on the regional distribution of pulmonary blood flow occur primarily via deformation of parenchymal tissue rather than by the balance of microcirculatory pressures, as dictated by the classic zonal model [50–52]. The potential contribution of each of these mechanisms remains unclear [53, 54], but modern studies in large animals suggest that the effect of gravity on regional blood flow in the lung is relatively low and that the primary determinant of flow is vascular resistance.

Hemodynamic Comparisons with the Systemic Circulation

In contrast to the distribution of compliance in the pulmonary circulation, the number of arterioles in the systemic circulation is approximately ten times less, with resistance ten times higher and compliance ten times lower. Thus, in the systemic circulation resistance is mainly located in the distal small arteries and arterioles, with compliance mainly located in the aorta [46, 55]. In the pulmonary circulation, arterial compliance is distributed over the entire arterial tree. This means that occlusion of a whole lung or lobe or segment not only increases resistance but also decreases compliance.

The ranges of pressures in systemic hypertension are relatively small compared to the very large range of pressures in PH. As patients age with *systemic* hypertension, resistance increases by only about 20 % whereas compliance can decrease by threefold. In PH, however, resistance can increase and compliance can decrease by a factor of 20.

The concept of oscillatory power fraction (ratio of oscillatory to mean power) has been used to characterize reactive circulatory beds. The oscillatory power fraction of the left ventricle is only about 10–15 % and increases in the setting of systemic hypertension [46, 56]. Oscillations play a more important role, however, in the pulmonary vascular bed so that the RV oscillatory power fraction is twice that of the systemic vascular bed. However, in contrast to systemic hypertension oscillatory power *fraction* remains constant in PH [57]. A more exhaustive discussion of components of the arterial load on the RV in terms of resistance and arterial compliance, and the consequences of load changes for RV work and function, has been published [46].

Thus, the pulmonary circulation is a low-resistance, highly compliant vascular bed that is markedly influenced by pressures generated by the heart and the thorax. Based on the intrinsic properties of the pulmonary circulation and its relatively insignificant potential for vasomotor control, relatively modest external forces can exert relatively large hemodynamic effects, making attempts to distinguish between active and passive changes in vessel size difficult. Detection and characterization of such vasomotor activity require substantial attention to the effects of respiration and cardiac activity on vascular pressures [58, 59].

Neural and Humoral and Regulation of the Pulmonary Vasculature

Adrenergic and cholinergic efferent nerves innervate the pulmonary circulation. The concentration of nerve fibers is greatest in larger vessels and at vascular bifurcations and is less influential in smaller vessels. Stimulation of α-adrenergic receptors mediates vasoconstriction, while β-adrenergic receptors mediate vasodilation [60]. α-Adrenergic mechanisms appear to contribute little to normal pulmonary vasomotor tone;

blockade of these receptors modifies neither baseline pulmonary vasomotor tone nor the hypoxic response. Because pulmonary vessels are normally in a dilated state, β-adrenergic responses are not evident. However, β-adrenergic blockade does enhance the vasoconstrictor response to catecholamines, which stimulate both α- and β-receptors, and increases in vascular tone enhance responses to β-adrenergic agents [60]. In summary, the pulmonary vascular bed is quite richly innervated and yet stimulation of these nerves produces relatively small changes in vasomotor tone. Perhaps the influence of vasodilators such as nitric oxide (NO) and prostacyclin normally predominate, minimizing the vasoconstrictor effect of the sympathetic nerve stimulation [61].

A number of mediators have the potential to affect the pulmonary circulation [62]. Vasoconstrictors include endothelin, serotonin, histamine, thromboxane, leukotrienes C_4 and D_4, angiotensin II, norepinephrine, and platelet-activating factor. These mediators bind to specific receptors on pulmonary vascular smooth muscle cells and induce smooth muscle contraction via activation of second messenger pathways. Key pulmonary vasodilators include NO, prostacyclin, acetylcholine, and bradykinin [62]. NO plays a key role in regulating the changes in pulmonary vasomotor tone induced by these vasoconstrictors [61]. The NO, endothelin, and prostanoid pathways have been by far the most influential mediators in the evolution of PAH therapy.

PAH is associated with impaired production of NO [63]. NO is produced by many cell types in the lung and plays an important physiologic role in the regulation of pulmonary vasomotor tone by several known mechanisms. NO stimulates soluble guanylyl cyclase, resulting in increased levels of cyclic GMP in pulmonary vascular smooth muscle cells leading to increased activation of cGMP-dependent protein kinase resulting in pulmonary vasodilation [64, 65]. In addition to regulating vascular tone, NO and cGMP signaling can also inhibit proliferation and induce apoptosis in vascular smooth muscle cells [66, 67]. Based upon the NO pathway, drug therapy in PAH continues to be explored with phosphodiesterase-5 inhibitors such as sildenafil and tadalafil that inhibit the metabolism of cGMP and soluble guanine cyclase stimulators such as riociguat that increase cGMP synthesis, and more recently, with nitric oxide itself [68–70].

The endothelin system has been extensively studied since its discovery by Yanagisawa and colleagues in 1988. Endothelin-1 (ET-1) is a powerful vasoconstrictor and proliferative cytokine, serving as a key mediator in pulmonary vascular biology, and an important mediator of PAH. Plasma ET-1 levels are elevated in patients with PH [71]. Expression of ET-1 mRNA and protein is increased in the endothelial cells found in vascular lesions in idiopathic PAH [72]. ET_A receptors are found in smooth muscle cells and ET_B receptors are located in both endothelial cells and smooth muscle cells. ET-1 is released from endothelial cells and acts primarily on underlying smooth muscle cells. Several ET-driven processes appear involved in lung vascular and structural remodeling. These include smooth muscle vasoconstriction and proliferation, an effect on fibroblasts resulting in contraction, proliferation and fibrosis, and finally an effect upon the endothelium itself causing proliferation, vasodilation (mediated through NO and prostacyclin), and vasoconstriction (via thromboxane A_2) [73]. Evidence suggests a role for autocrine/paracrine signaling in the ET system and PAH pathway [74]. ET receptor antagonists have clearly proven beneficial in PAH [68].

Prostanoids are implicated in the regulation of pulmonary vascular tone under physiological as well as pathological conditions. PAH patients have been shown to have reduced levels of endogenous prostacyclin and reduced expression of prostacyclin synthase in the lung [75, 76]. Prostacyclin and prostanoids with vasodilator properties are believed to contribute to the maintenance of normal, low pulmonary vascular tone. Prostacyclin stimulates the prostaglandin I2 (IP) receptor, leading to increased cyclic adenosine monophosphate and resulting in vasodilator and antiproliferative effects [77]. The impact of prostacyclin therapy on PAH has been quite substantial [78].

Several growth factors have been implicated in the abnormal proliferation and migration of SMCs, including platelet-derived growth factor (PDGF), basic fibroblast growth factor, and epidermal growth factor [79]. In vitro studies have established that PDGF acts as a potent mitogen and chemoattractant for smooth muscle cells [80]. Tyrosine kinase inhibitors such as imatinib have been shown to reverse pulmonary vascular remodeling in preclinical models of pulmonary hypertension by inducing apoptosis and blocking proliferation and have shown some success in the clinical studies of PAH as well [81].

The pulmonary endothelium serves as a major source of angiotensin-converting enzyme (ACE) expression and angiotensin II production [82]. Angiotensin type I and type II receptors are both expressed in normal lung. Recent data, involving the administration of a lentiviral vector containing angiotensin-converting enzyme 2, suggest that overexpression of this enzyme prevents and reverses increased RV systolic pressure in monocrotaline-induced PH. Inhibition of proinflammatory cytokines was also documented [83].

Systemic and pulmonary renin-angiotensin-aldosterone activities have been shown to be increased in patients with idiopathic PAH and appear to be associated with increased pulmonary vascular remodeling [84]. Chronic inhibition with losartan was shown to decrease RV afterload and pulmonary vascular remodeling, and restored RV-arterial coupling in rats with PAH [84]. In spite of these data, no large-scale clinical trials support the use of ACE inhibitors in PAH at this time. While other humoral mediators may be important in pulmonary vascular physiology, most of these have not been explored as potential therapy for PAH.

Mechanical Effects on the Pulmonary Vasculature

Blood vessels respond to variations in mechanical load from circulating blood in the form of shear stress and mechanical strain. The pulsatile nature of PA pressure and flow subjects the pulmonary arterial bed to continuous hemodynamic stresses in the form of shear stress and cyclic strain or "stretch." The endothelium converts these mechanical forces into intracellular signals that affect cellular functions including proliferation, migration, remodeling, apoptosis, and permeability, and finally gene expression [85]. Clinical studies in PAH have focused primarily on the contribution of PVR in the distal vasculature to the underlying disease. However, it is clear that biomechanical factors such as sheer stress throughout the vasculature affect endothelial function.

Laminar blood flow produces fluid shear stress from the friction of the blood against the endothelial cell wall. At physiological levels of sheer stress, the endothelial cell responds with a variety of critical regulatory functions. These include vasomotor changes through the release of vasodilators and vasoconstrictors, vascular remodeling encouraged by the production of growth factors and growth inhibitors, and modulation of hemostasis and thrombosis via secretion of substances with procoagulant, anticoagulant, and fibrinolytic properties. Finally, inflammatory changes may evolve through the expression of chemokines and adhesion molecules [85].

Endothelial cells sense sheer stress via membrane receptors, interacting with each other and transactivating multiple signaling pathways leading to differential gene expression [86]. The development of flow-directed reorientation of the endothelium serves as evidence of rapid actin cytoskeletal rearrangement [87, 88]. Shear stress can reduce endothelial cell turnover through inhibition of cell proliferation and suppression of apoptosis. This process may be beneficial, offering a protective role for the vasculature [89]. The pulsatile nature of blood flow results in temporal and spatial variations of shear stress on the vessel surface. However, flow patterns in curved and bifurcating sections of the vasculature are distressed by variable and accelerated peak shear rates. Thus, the effect of blood flow on the endothelium depends on differing and changing aspects of the particular vascular microenvironment.

A recent small study of five PAH patients and five controls used the combination of magnetic resonance imaging and computational fluid dynamics and determined that PA wall sheer stress was significantly lower in the proximal pulmonary arteries of PAH patients compared to controls. It was suggested that this reduced shear stress may contribute to pulmonary endothelial cell dysfunction and as a result PAH progression [90].

Cyclic stretch is another critically important mechanical force in the pulmonary vasculature generated either from blood flow (which results in pulsatile distension of the arterial wall), or from tidal breathing; arterial wall stretch is primarily determined by intravascular pressure [91, 92]. As with sheer stress, cyclic stretch leads to reshaping of the endothelium. Chronic cyclic stretch occurs in the setting of chronically increased PA pressure, increasing the level of signaling and contractile proteins; activating vascular cell proliferation, collagen, and fibronectin synthesis; and resulting in thickening of the vascular wall leading to pulmonary vascular remodeling. These effects may in turn influence cellular responses to mechanical stress via increased inflammatory cytokine production, and macrophage activation [91]. Recent evidence indicates that endothelial cells discriminate between steady and cyclic, and low- and high-amplitude mechanical strain. The specific pattern of mechanical stimulation appears to determine how vascular remodeling evolves into pathological states such as PAH [93]. Thus, vascular cells can sense changes in mechanical forces and transduce the mechanical signal into a biological response. Mechanisms of this "mechanotransduction" that have been proposed include stretch-activated ion channels, integrins, receptor tyrosine kinases, cytoskeletal meshwork, and signaling by reactive oxygen species [93–97]. More detailed insight into molecular mechanisms of vascular remodeling are beyond our scope and are offered in separate chapters (Chaps. 4 and 5).

Fluid and Solute Exchange in the Lung

The normal, healthy lung consists of about 80 % water. An important function of the pulmonary circulation is to serve as a barrier to the exchange of fluid and solutes, thus maintaining pulmonary fluid balance. The balance of Starling forces in the lung favors reabsorption to facilitate gas exchange. A variety of mechanisms are involved in the development of fluid accumulation in the lung. Increases in left-sided pressures or in vessel wall permeability occur in the setting of various pathologic states. In the setting of PH, it is crucial to exclude left ventricular dysfunction, which is sometimes present, but often not accompanied by obvious clinical or radiographic evidence of pulmonary edema. The regulation of fluid exchange between the pulmonary vasculature and the interstitium has been described in detail and are beyond the scope of this chapter [98–100].

Clinical Assessment of the Pulmonary Circulation

In spite of tremendous insights and discoveries into the pathophysiology, molecular biology, and genetics of PAH, the gold standard approach to clinical evaluation of suspected or proven PH remains the relatively simple approach of right-heart catheterization. Pulmonary artery pressures are measured most accurately via a balloon-tipped flotation catheter introduced into the pulmonary artery [27–29]. In addition to measuring the pulmonary artery pressure directly (definition of PH = mean PA pressure of ≥25 mmHg), the right atrial, RV, and PCWP can be determined. The latter is determined by advancing the catheter with the balloon inflated until it "wedges" and occludes a peripheral pulmonary artery. The mean pressure measured at end expiration (normally 5–10 mmHg) is an estimate of the vascular pressure at the point of confluence of the pulmonary veins, and thus reflects left atrial pressure. The cardiac output is measured by either the Fick method or thermodilution. PVR is subsequently calculated. These measurements play a key role in the assessment, and often the follow-up of the patient with PH. A detailed overview of right-heart catheterization and the appropriate approach to suspected or proven PH is discussed in other chapters.

Conclusions

The pulmonary circulation performs the vital function of carrying oxygen-depleted blood from the heart to the lungs and returns oxygenated blood back to the heart to be delivered to the systemic circulation. The pulmonary vasculature can be profoundly affected in certain disease states. Normally, the entire cardiac output is accommodated by the pulmonary circulation with neither pulmonary edema nor RV failure. Disease of structural components of the lung affecting blood flow through the pulmonary vessels at any level can lead to PH, and in turn result in RV dysfunction and failure. Tremendous progress in basic and clinical research has led to a better understanding of this circulation. Based upon this science, there have been substantial inroads into the diagnosis and therapy of pulmonary vascular diseases such as PH.

References

1. Osiro S, Wear C, Hudson R, et al. A friend to the airways: a review of the emerging clinical importance of the bronchial arterial circulation. Surg Radiol Anat. 2012;34:791–8.
2. McCullagh A, Rosenthal M, Wanner A, et al. The bronchial circulation–worth a closer look: a review of the relationship between the bronchial vasculature and airway inflammation. Pediatr Pulmonol. 2012;45:1–13.
3. Lonie IM. Erasistratus, the Erasistrateans, and Aristotle. Bull Hist Med. 1964;38:426–43.
4. Persaud TV. Historical development of the concept of a pulmonary circulation. Can J Cardiol. 1989;5:12–6.
5. Christianismi Restitutio 1553 Vienna "Las ideas teológicas de Miguel Servet acerca de la circulación de la sangre". Ed. Instituto de Estudios Sijenenses "Miguel Servet" (Michael Servetus Institute). 2010.
6. West JB. Ibn al-Nafis, the pulmonary circulation, and the Islamic Golden Age. J Appl Physiol. 2008;105(6):1877–80.
7. Young RA. The pulmonary circulation—before and after Harvey. Part 1. Br Med J. 1940;1(4122):1–5.
8. Owen RD. The debatable land between this world and the next. New York, NY: G.W. Carleton & Co.; 1872. p. 69. notes.
9. Haddad SI, Khairallah AA. A forgotten chapter in the history of the circulation of the blood. Ann Surg. 1936;104(1):1–8.
10. Qatayyah S. The Arabic physician Ibn Nafis (in Arabic). 1st ed. Beirut: Arabic Corporation for Studies and Publication; 1984. p. 37–43.
11. Al-Dabbagh SA. Ibn Al-Nafis and the pulmonary circulation. Lancet. 1978;1:1148.
12. Coppola ED. The discovery of the pulmonary circulation: a new approach. Bull Hist Med. 1957;31:44–77.
13. Cushing H. A bio-bibliography of Andreas Vesalius. New York, NY: Schuman's; 1943. Anatomy Bibliog A12.V3.
14. Willis, R. (translator) (1847). The works of William Harvey, MD. London: 1847 The Sydenham Soc. Level 5 Main Lib Medicine Z313.H27 1847-W.
15. Franklin, K. J. (translator) The circulation of the blood and other writings by Harvey. 1963 London: Dent. Level 5 Main Lib Physiology L8 1963-H.
16. Keynes, G. (translator) (1928) The anatomical exercises of Dr. William Harvey De motu cordis 1628: The first English text of 1653 (by Harvey). London: Nonesuch. Level 12 Spec Coll 113.

17. Gordon EJ. William Harvey and the circulation of the blood. South Med J. 1991;84: 1439–44.
18. Pearce JMS. Malpighi and the discovery of capillaries. Eur Neurol. 2007;58:253–5.
19. Keilin D. The history of cell respiration and cytochrome. Cambridge: Cambridge University Press; 1966. p. 17–23.
20. Hales S. Statistical essays. Containing haemosticks. Vol ii W. Innys and R Manby London 1933; p. 1.
21. Poiseuille JLM. Recherches sur la force du couer aortique. J Physiol Exp. 1828;8:272.
22. Forssmann W. Die Sondierung des rechten Herzens. Klin Wochenschr. 1929;8:2085.
23. Cournand A. Cardiac catheterization: development of the technique, its contributions to experimental medicine, and its initial application in man. Acta Med Scand Suppl. 1975; 579:1–32.
24. Cournand AF. Nobel lecture, December 11, 1956. In: Nobel lectures, physiology and medicine 1942–1962. Amsterdam, The Netherlands: Elsevier Publishing Co; 1964. p. 529.
25. Bradley RD. Diagnostic right-heart catheterization with miniature catheters in severely ill patients. Lancet. 1964;2:941.
26. Fife WP, Lees BS. Construction and use of self guiding right heart and pulmonary artery catheter. J Appl Physiol. 1965;20:148.
27. Scheinman MM, Abbot JA, Rapaport E. Clinical uses of a flow-directed right heart catheter. Arch Intern Med. 1969;124:19.
28. Swan HJ, Ganz W, Forrester J, Marcus H, Diamond G, Chonette D. Catheterization of the heart in man with the use of a flow-directed balloon-tipped catheter. N Engl J Med. 1970;283:447.
29. Forrester JS, Ganz W, Diamond G, McHugh T, Chonette DW, Swan HJ. Thermodilution cardiac output determination with a single flow directed catheter for cardiac monitoring. Am Heart J. 1972;83:306.
30. Chatterjee K, Swan HJC, Ganz W, Gray R, Loebel H, Forrester JS, Chonette D. Use of a balloon-tipped flotation electrode catheter for cardiac monitoring. Am J Cardiol. 1975; 36:56–61.
31. Adams W, Veith I. Pulmonary circulation. New York, NY: Grune & Stratton; 1959.
32. Kay JM, Smith P, Heath D. Aminorex and the pulmonary circulation. Thorax. 1971;26: 262–70.
33. Hatano E, Toma S. Primary pulmonary hypertension: report on a WHO meeting. Geneva: World Health Organization; 1973.
34. Rich S. Executive summary from the World Symposium on Primary pulmonary hypertension 1998, Evian, France. Geneva: World Health Organization; 1998.
35. McGoon M, Gutterman D, Steen V, et al. Screening, early detection, and diagnosis of pulmonary arterial hypertension: ACCP evidence-based clinical practice guidelines. Chest. 2004;126:14S–34.
36. ACCF/AHA. Expert consensus document on pulmonary hypertension: a report of the American College of Cardiology Foundation Task Force on Expert Consensus Documents and the American Heart Association: developed in Collaboration with the American College of Chest Physicians, American Thoracic Society, Inc., and the Pulmonary Hypertension Association. Circulation. 2009;119(16):2250–94.
37. Galie N, Hoeper MM, Humbert M, et al. Guidelines for the diagnosis and treatment of pulmonary hypertension: The Task Force for the Diagnosis and Treatment of Pulmonary Hypertension of the European Society of Cardiology (ESC) and the European Respiratory Society (ERS), endorsed by the International Society of Heart and Lung Transplantation (ISHLT). Eur Heart J. 2009;30:2493–537.
38. Bates DV, Varvis CJ, Dowevan RE, Christie RV. Variations in the pulmonary capillary blood volume and membrane diffusion component in health and disease. J Clin Invest. 1960;39: 1401–12.
39. Singhal S, Henderson R, Horsfeld K, et al. Morphometry of the human pulmonary arterial tree. Circ Res. 1973;33:190–7.

40. Butler J, Paley HW. Lung volume and pulmonary circulation. Med Thorac. 1962;19:261–7.
41. Maseri A, Caldini P, Harward P, Joshi RC, Permutt S, Zierler KL. Determinants of pulmonary vascular volume: recruitment versus distensibility. Circ Res. 1972;31:218–28.
42. Godbey PS, Graham JA, Presson Jr RG, Wagner Jr WW, Lloyd Jr TC. Effect of capillary pressure and lung distension on capillary recruitment. J Appl Physiol. 1995;79:1142–7.
43. Fletcher GF, Balady GJ, Amsterdam EA, Chaitman B, Eckel R, Fleg J, et al. Exercise standards for testing and training: a statement for healthcare professionals from the American Heart Association. Circulation. 2001;104:1694–740.
44. Tawhai MH, Hunter PJ, Tschirren J, Reinhardt JM, McLennan G, Hoffman EA. CT-based geometry analysis and finite element models of the human and ovine bronchial tree. J Appl Physiol. 2004;97:2310–21.
45. Burrowes KS, Hunter PJ, Tawhai MH. Anatomically-based finite element models of the human pulmonary arterial and venous trees including supernumerary vessels. J Appl Physiol. 2005;99:731–8.
46. Saouti N, Westerhof N, Postmus PE, Vonk-Noordegraaf A. The arterial load in pulmonary hypertension. Eur Respir Rev. 2010;117:197–203.
47. Lankhaar JW, Westerhof N, Faes TJ. Pulmonary vascular resistance and compliance stay inversely related during treatment of pulmonary hypertension. Eur Heart J. 2008;29:1688–95.
48. Tawhai MH, Clark AR, Burrowes KS. Computational models of the pulmonary circulation: insights and the move towards clinically directed studies. Pulm Circ. 2011;1:224–38.
49. West JB, Dollery CT, Naimark A. Distribution of blood flow in isolated lung: relation to vascular and alveolar pressures. J Appl Physiol. 1964;19:713–24.
50. Glenny RW, Bernard S, Robertson HT, Hlastala MP. Gravity is an important but secondary determinant of regional pulmonary blood flow in upright primates. J Appl Physiol. 1999;86:623–32.
51. Glenny RW, Lamm WJ, Albert RK, Robertson HT. Gravity is a minor determinant of pulmonary blood flow distribution. J Appl Physiol. 1991;71:620–9.
52. Hopkins SR, Henderson AC, et al. Vertical gradients in regional lung density and perfusion in the supine human lung: the Slinky effect. J Appl Physiol. 2007;103:240–8.
53. Petersson J, Rohdin M, Sánchez-Crespo A, Nyrén S, Jacobsson H, Larsson SA, et al. Posture primarily affects lung tissue distribution with minor effect on blood flow and ventilation. Respir Physiol Neurobiol. 2007;156:293–303.
54. Hlastala MP, Glenny RW. Vascular structure determines pulmonary blood flow distribution. News Physiol Sci. 1999;14:182–6.
55. Westerhof N, Bosman F, DeVries CJ, et al. Analog studies of the human arterial tree. J Biomech. 1969;2:121–43.
56. O'Rourke MF. Steady and pulsatile energy losses in the systemic circulation under normal conditions and in simulated arterial disease. Cardiovasc Res. 1967;1:313–26.
57. Saouti N, Westerhof N, Helderman F, et al. Right ventricular oscillatory power is a constant fraction of total power irrespective of pulmonary artery pressure. Am J Respir Crit Care Med. 2010;182:1315–20.
58. Fishman AP. Dynamics of the pulmonary circulation. In: Hamilton WF, editor. Handbook of physiology. Bethesda, MD: Am Physiol Soc; 1963. sect. 2, vol. II, chapter 48.
59. Hughes JMB. Pulmonary circulation and fluid balance. In: Widdicombe JG, editor. Respiratory physiology II, vol. 14. Baltimore, MD: University Park; 1977. p. 135–83.
60. Hyman AL, Kadowitz PJ. Enhancement of alpha- and beta-adrenoceptor responses by elevations in vascular tone in pulmonary circulation. Am J Physiol. 1986;250(6 Pt 2):H1109–16.
61. Vanhoutte PM, Rubanyi GM, Miller VM, et al. Modulation of vascular smooth muscle contraction by the endothelium. Annu Rev Physiol. 1986;48:307–20.
62. Barnes PJ, Liu SF. Regulation of pulmonary vascular tone. Pharmacol Rev. 1995;47:87–131.
63. McLaughlin VV, McGoon MD. Pulmonary arterial hypertension. Circulation. 2006;114:1417–31.

64. Michelakis ED. The role of the NO axis and its therapeutic implications in pulmonary arterial hypertension. Heart Fail Rev. 2003;8:5–21.
65. Chiche JD, Schlutsmeyer SM, Bloch DB, de la Monte SM, Roberts J, Filippov G, Janssens SP, Rosenzweig A, Bloch KD. Adenovirus-mediated gene transfer of cGMP-dependent protein kinase increases the sensitivity of cultured vascular smooth muscle cells to the antiproliferative and pro-apoptotic effects of nitric oxide/cGMP. J Biol Chem. 1998;273:34263–71.
66. Garg UC, Hassid A. Nitric oxide-generating vasodilators and 8-bromo-cyclic guanosine monophosphate inhibit mitogenesis and proliferation of cultured rat vascular smooth muscle cells. J Clin Invest. 1989;83:1774–7.
67. Pollman MJ, Yamada T, Horiuchi M, Gibbons GH. Vasoactive substances regulate vascular smooth muscle cell apoptosis: countervailing influences of nitric oxide and angiotensin II. Circ Res. 1996;79:748–56.
68. Galie N, Manes A, Negro L, et al. A meta-analysis of randomized controlled trials in pulmonary arterial hypertension. Eur Heart J. 2009;30:394–403.
69. Grimminger F, Weimann G, Frey R, et al. First acute haemodynamic study of soluble guanylate cyclase stimulator riociguat in pulmonary hypertension. Eur Respir J. 2009;33:785–92.
70. Inhaled Nitric Oxide/INOpulse DS for Pulmonary Arterial Hypertension (PAH) ClinicalTrials.gov Identifier: NCT01457781.
71. Giaid A, Yanagisawa M, Langleben D, et al. Expression of endothelin-1 in the lungs of patients with pulmonary hypertension. N Engl J Med. 1993;328:1732–9.
72. Stewart DJ, Levy RD, Cernacek P, et al. Increased plasma endothelin-1 in pulmonary hypertension: marker or mediator of disease. Ann Intern Med. 1991;114:464–9.
73. Dupuis J, Hoeper MM. Endothelin receptor antagonists in pulmonary arterial hypertension. Eur J Respir. 2008;31:407–15.
74. Iglarz M, Clozel M. At the heart of tissue: endothelin system and end-organ damage. Clin Sci (Lond). 2010;119:453–63.
75. Christman BW, McPherson CD, Newman JH, et al. An imbalance between the excretion of thromboxane and prostacyclin metabolites in pulmonary hypertension. N Engl J Med. 1992;327:70–5.
76. Tuder RM, Cool CD, Geraci MW, et al. Prostacyclin synthase expression is decreased in lungs from patients with severe pulmonary hypertension. Am J Respir Crit Care Med. 1999;159:1925–32.
77. Mubarak KK. A review of prostaglandin analogs in the management of patients with pulmonary arterial hypertension. Respir Med. 2010;104:9–21.
78. Barst RJ, Rubin LJ, Long WA, et al. Continuous intravenous prostacyclin versus conventional therapy in primary pulmonary hypertension: results of a 12-week randomized trial in 81 patients. N Engl J Med. 1996;334:296–301.
79. Balasubramaniam V, Le Cras TD, Ivy DD, et al. Role of platelet-derived growth factor in vascular remodeling during pulmonary hypertension in the ovine fetus. Am J Physiol Lung Cell Mol Physiol. 2003;284:L826–33.
80. Yu Y, Sweeney M, Zhang S, et al. PDGF stimulates pulmonary vascular smooth muscle cell proliferation by upregulating TRPC6 expression. Am J Physiol Cell Physiol. 2003;284: C316–30.
81. Grimminger F, Schermuly RT. PDGF receptor and its antagonists: role in treatment of PAH. Adv Exp Med Biol. 2010;661:435–46.
82. Studdy PR, Lapworth R, Bird R. Angiotensin-converting enzyme and its clinical significance—a review. J Clin Pathol. 1983;36:938–47.
83. Yamazato Y, Ferreira AJ, Hong KH, et al. Prevention of pulmonary hypertension by Angiotensin-converting enzyme 2 gene transfer. Hypertension. 2009;54:365–71.
84. de Man FS, Tu L, Handoko ML, et al. Dysregulated renin-angiotensin-aldosterone system contributes to pulmonary arterial hypertension. Am J Respir Crit Care Med. 2012;186(8):780–9.
85. Li YS, Haga JH, Chien S. Molecular basis of the effects of shear stress on vascular endothelial cells. J Biomech. 2005;38:1949–71.

86. Chen KD, Li YS, Kim M, et al. Mechanotransduction in response to shear stress: roles of receptor tyrosine kinases, integrins, and Shc. J Biol Chem. 1999;274:18393–400.
87. Lehoux S, Castier Y, Tedgui A. Molecular mechanisms of the vascular responses to haemodynamic forces. J Intern Med. 2006;259:381–92.
88. Malek AM, Izumo S. Mechanism of endothelial cell shape change and cytoskeletal remodeling in response to fluid shear stress. J Cell Sci. 1996;109(Pt 4):713–26.
89. Nerem RM, Alexander RW, Chappell DC, et al. The study of the influence of flow on vascular endothelial biology. Am J Med Sci. 1998;316:169–75.
90. Tang BT, Pickard SS, Chan FP, et al. Wall shear stress is decreased in the pulmonary arteries of patients with pulmonary arterial hypertension: an image-based, computational fluid dynamics study. Pulm Circ. 2012;2:470–6.
91. Birukov KG, Jacobson JR, Flores AA, et al. Magnitude-dependent regulation of pulmonary endothelial cell barrier function by cyclic stretch. Am J Physiol Lung Cell Mol Physiol. 2003;285:L785–97.
92. Reinhart-King CA, Fujiwara K, Berk BC. Physiologic stress-mediated signaling in the endothelium. Methods Enzymol. 2008;443:25–44.
93. Birukov KG. Cyclic stretch, reactive oxygen species, and vascular remodeling. Antioxid Redox Signal. 2009;11:1651–67.
94. Davies PF. Flow-mediated endothelial mechanotransduction. Physiol Rev. 1995;75:519–60.
95. Haga JH, Li YS, Chien S. Molecular basis of the effects of mechanical stretch on vascular smooth muscle cells. J Biomech. 2007;40:947–60.
96. Ali MH, Schumacker PT. Endothelial responses to mechanical stress: where is the mechanosensor? Crit Care Med. 2002;30:S198–206.
97. Paravicini TM, Touyz RM. Redox signaling in hypertension. Cardiovasc Res. 2006;71: 247–58.
98. Staub NC. Pulmonary edema. Physiol Rev. 1974;54:678–811.
99. Dudek SM, Garcia JG. Cytoskeletal regulation of pulmonary vascular permeability. J Appl Physiol. 2001;91:1487–500.
100. Mehta D, Malik AB. Signaling mechanisms regulating endothelial permeability. Physiol Rev. 2006;86:279–367.

Chapter 2
Epidemiology and Disease Classification of Pulmonary Hypertension

Rogerio Souza, Carlos Jardim, and Marc Humbert

Abstract Numerous conditions lead to a sustained increase in pulmonary arterial pressure. Pulmonary hypertension is defined as an elevation of mean pulmonary arterial pressure to 25 mmHg or greater. Currently, the pulmonary hypertensive diseases are organized into five groups that include (1) pulmonary arterial hypertension, (2) pulmonary hypertension owing to left-sided heart disease, (3) pulmonary hypertension owing to chronic lung disease, (4) chronic thromboembolic pulmonary hypertension, and (5) miscellaneous causes. Group 2 and 3 represent the most common causes of pulmonary hypertension. Group 1 (PAH) is exceedingly rare but normally progresses to severe pulmonary hypertension and right ventricular failure. PAH is seen more frequently in patients with connective tissue disease, HIV infection, portal hypertension, congenital cardiac shunts, and those who have used amphetamine-like drugs. This chapter provides an in-depth description of the various pulmonary hypertensive diseases and an overview of their epidemiology, including demographics, risk factors, and distinguishing characteristics.

Keywords Pulmonary hypertension • Pulmonary arterial hypertension • Pulmonary venous hypertension • Pulmonary vascular disease • Chronic thromboembolic pulmonary hypertension • Aminorexfumarate • Fenfluramine • Schistosomiasis

Abbreviations

BMPR2	Bone morphogenic protein receptor-2
CHD	Congenital heart disease
CTD	Connective tissue disease

R. Souza, M.D. • C. Jardim, M.D.
Pulmonary Department, Heart Institute, University of Sao Paulo Medical School, Sao Paulo, Brazil

M. Humbert, M.D. (✉)
Service de Pneumologie, Hopital Bicetre, Université Paris-Sud, 78 rue du Général Leclerc, Le Kremlin-Bicetre, 94270 Paris, France
e-mail: Marc.humbert@bct.aphp.fr

J.R. Klinger, R.P. Frantz (eds.), *Diagnosis and Management of Pulmonary Hypertension*, Respiratory Medicine 12, DOI 10.1007/978-1-4939-2636-7_2

IPAH	Idiopathic pulmonary arterial hypertension
mPAP	Mean pulmonary artery pressure
NIH	National Institutes of Health
PA	Pulmonary artery
PAH	Pulmonary arterial hypertension
PAOP	Pulmonary artery occlusion pressure
PAP	Pulmonary artery pressure
RHC	Right heart catheterization
Sch-PAH	Schistosomiasis associated pulmonary arterial hypertension
TGF-β	Transforming growth factor beta
WHO	World Health Organization

Definitions

Pulmonary hypertension (PH) defines a group of chronic conditions presenting as high pressure in the pulmonary circulation [1]. During the last decades, the understanding of these diseases has significantly improved [2]. The last world symposium on pulmonary hypertension, held in 2013, highlighted the advances made in the last 40 years since the first international conference was sponsored by the World Health Organization (WHO) in 1973 after the sudden increase in cases of PH associated with the use of aminorexfumarate to lose weight [3].

Pulmonary hypertension is defined as a mean pulmonary artery pressure (mPAP) of ≥25 mmHg at rest as assessed by right heart catheterization (RHC) [1]. Although this value is slightly greater than the upper level of normal for resting mPAP (defined as 2 standard definitions above the mean or about 21 mmHg [4]), it has been utilized for selecting patients in nearly all randomized controlled trials on PAH and in PAH registries. It is currently unclear how to consider the values of mPAP between 21 and 24 mmHg, since this level of PA pressure elevation does not necessarily reflect the presence of a pathological state. It is possible that in some patients, the borderline level of elevated PAP represents an early phase of the disease. Specifically in patients within the scleroderma spectrum of disease, this mild increase in mPAP has been associated with a higher risk of developing PAH in the near future [5].

The need for an accurate determination of mPAP requires that right heart catheterization (RHC) be performed to ensure proper diagnosis, since noninvasive estimates are not reliable enough. Moreover, RHC allows the measurement of cardiac function, by means of cardiac output, as well as the determination of right- and left-sided filling pressures (right atrial and pulmonary artery occlusion pressures) [6].

Two distinct hemodynamic profiles are seen in PH and are defined according to the left-sided filling pressures. Precapillary PH, referred to as pulmonary arterial hypertension (PAH), is defined by the presence of elevated mPAP with normal left-sided filling pressures defined as pulmonary artery occlusion pressure (PAOP), left

Table 2.1 Hemodynamic patterns in PH

Definition	Hemodynamic characteristics
Pulmonary hypertension	mPAP ≥ 25 mmHg
Pre-capillary PH	mPAP ≥ 25 mmHg PAOP ≤ 15 mmHg CO normal or reduced
Post-capillary PH	mPAP ≥ 25 mmHg PAOP > 15 mmHg
Combined post-capillary and pre-capillary PH	mPAP ≥ 25 mmHg PAOP > 15 mmHg Diastolic PAP—PAOP > 7 mmHg

PH pulmonary hypertension, *mPAP* mean pulmonary arterial pressure, *PAOP* pulmonary artery occlusion pressure, *CO* cardiac output

atrial pressure, or left ventricular filling pressure less than 15 mmHg whilst postcapillary PH or pulmonary venous hypertension is defined by left-sided filling pressures greater than 15 mmHg. The current classification of PH hypertension is based on the combination of the hemodynamic profile and of baseline clinical conditions that could be associated with the genesis of pulmonary hypertension (Table 2.1). These baseline conditions are determined after extensive investigation of the potential causes of PH. Although diagnostic investigation is not the focus of this chapter, the suggested algorithm derived from the fifth World Symposium on pulmonary hypertension is shown in Fig. 2.1.

Classification

The first classification of PH was described in 1973 and categorized patients as having "primary" or "secondary" pulmonary hypertension according to the presence or absence of an identifiable cause for the disease. During the second world symposium on PH, in 1998, the basis for the classification system currently used was proposed. This system groups patients with similar pathological findings, similar hemodynamic profiles, as well as similar management strategies into a single category. Five different categories were proposed: (1) pulmonary arterial hypertension; (2) pulmonary hypertension due to left heart disease; (3) pulmonary hypertension due to chronic lung disease and/or hypoxia; (4) chronic thromboembolic pulmonary hypertension; and (5) pulmonary hypertension due to unclear multifactorial mechanisms (previously called "miscellanea") [8]. Although small modifications have been made during the last decade, the concept of the current classification remains the same. The updated classification for pulmonary hypertension, derived from the last world symposium on PH, is presented in Table 2.2 [9].

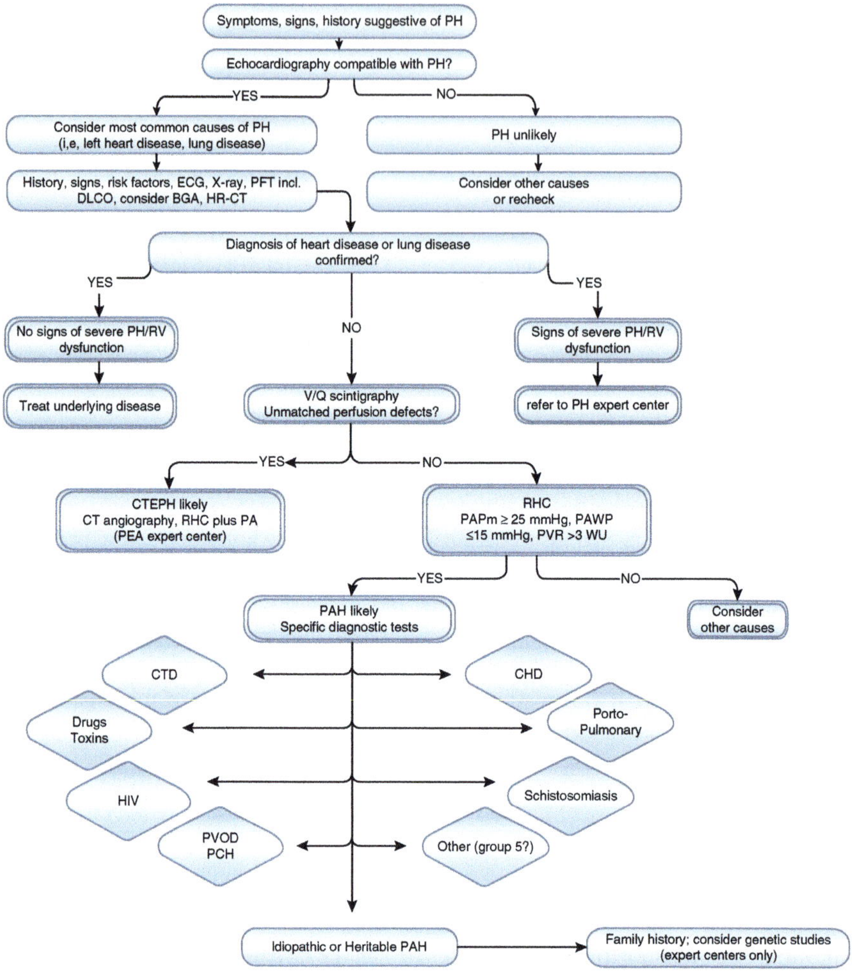

Fig. 2.1 Diagnostic approach to PH (from [7])

Pulmonary Arterial Hypertension

Pulmonary arterial hypertension (PAH) encompasses a group of clinical conditions that result in precapillary PH and share similar pathological and/or clinical findings. Idiopathic PAH corresponds to sporadic disease in which no family history of PAH or an identified risk factor is present [8]. IPAH is only diagnosed after alternative diagnoses are ruled out according to current guidelines [1]. Up to 70 % of familial cases of PAH have been linked to germline mutations in the gene coding for the bone morphogenetic protein receptor 2 (*BMPR2*), a member of the transforming growth factor beta (TGF-β) signaling family [10]. *BMPR2* mutations have also been

Table 2.2 Clinical classification of pulmonary hypertension 9

1. Pulmonary arterial hypertension (PAH)
1.1. Idiopathic PAH
1.2. Heritable
• 1.2.1. BMPR2
• 1.2.2. ALK1, ENG, SMAD9, CAV1, KCNK3
• 1.2.3. Unknown
1.3. Drug- and toxin-induced
1.4. Associated with
• 1.4.1. Connective tissue diseases
• 1.4.2. HIV infection
• 1.4.3. Portal hypertension
• 1.4.4. Congenital heart diseases
• 1.4.5. Schistosomiasis
1′ Pulmonary veno-occlusive disease and/or pulmonary capillary hemangiomatosis
1″ Persistent pulmonary hypertension of the newborn
2. Pulmonary hypertension owing to left heart disease
• 2.1. Left ventricular systolic dysfunction
• 2.2. Left ventricular diastolic dysfunction
• 2.3. Valvular disease
• 2.4. Congenital/acquired left heart inflow/outflow tract obstruction and congenital cardiomyopathies
3. Pulmonary hypertension owing to lung diseases and/or hypoxia
• 3.1. Chronic obstructive pulmonary disease
• 3.2. Interstitial lung disease
• 3.3. Other pulmonary diseases with mixed restrictive and obstructive pattern
• 3.4. Sleep-disordered breathing
• 3.5. Alveolar hypoventilation disorders
• 3.6. Chronic exposure to high altitude
• 3.7. Developmental lung diseases
4. Chronic thromboembolic pulmonary hypertension (CTEPH)
5. Pulmonary hypertension with unclear multifactorial mechanisms
• 5.1. Hematologic disorders: chronic hemolytic anemia, myeloproliferative disorders, splenectomy
• 5.2. Systemic disorders: sarcoidosis, pulmonary Langerhans cell histiocytosis: lymphangioleiomyomatosis, neurofibromatosis, vasculitis
• 5.3. Metabolic disorders: glycogen storage disease, Gaucher disease, thyroid disorders
• 5.4. Others: tumoral obstruction, fibrosing mediastinitis, chronic renal failure, segmental PH

detected in a significant proportion of apparently idiopathic cases without familial history [11]. Indeed, the distinction between idiopathic and familial PAH with *BMPR2* mutations is artificial, as all patients with a *BMPR2* mutation have heritable disease. Thus, it was decided to abandon the term "familial PAH" in favor of the term "heritable PAH" [8]. Heritable forms of PAH include those with identified mutations (mainly *BMPR2* but also *ACVRL1* or endoglin and more recently SMAD9,

KCNK3, and CAV1) and familial cases without identified mutations. Idiopathic and heritable PAH are more common in women than in men with a gender ratio around 2:1 [12] and as high as 3.2 in the REVEAL registry [13].

PAH patients carrying a *BMPR2* mutation are prone to be younger at diagnosis and present with more severe disease than IPAH patients without a *BMPR2* mutation [14]. As a result, genetic testing and counseling have played an increasingly important role in the comprehensive assessment of patients with newly diagnosed PAH [15–17].

Besides genetic predisposition, there are a number of risk factors that are associated with the development of PAH. The use of aminorexfumarate, a potent appetite suppressant, in the 1960s led to an outbreak of rapidly progressive PAH in Switzerland, Austria, and Germany. The incidence of PAH in patients who had used aminorex was shown to be about 0.2 % with a median exposure-to-onset time of 8 months, as first described in a Swiss medical clinic. The incidence was proportional to the amount of drug taken and if discontinued early enough, a regression of PAH could be seen. Subsequently, aminorex was withdrawn from the market in 1968 [18]. More than 20 years later, fenfluramine and dexfenfluramine were marketed as appetite suppressants with another outbreak of drug-induced PAH associated with these two agents in the 1980s–1990s. PAH cases in patients exposed to fenfluramine derivatives share clinical, functional, hemodynamic, and genetic features with IPAH. This suggests that fenfluramine exposure represents a potential trigger for PAH without influencing its clinical course [19]. The association of fenfluramine and dexfenfluramine with the development of PAH was confirmed by a registry that enrolled 1,335 subjects at tertiary PH centers in the United States between 1998 and 2001. Of note, these agents have also been associated with an increased risk of valvular heart diseases, presumably because of their serotoninergic properties. As a result, fenfluramine and dexfenfluramine were withdrawn from the market in the late 1990s [20].

More recently, Benfluorex, a benzoate ester that shares structural and pharmacologic characteristics with dexfenfluramine and fenfluramine, has also been associated with the development of PAH. The active and common metabolite of each of these molecules is norfenfluramine, which itself has a chemical structure similar to that of the amphetamines. Given its pharmacological properties, benfluorex would be expected to have similar toxic effects to the fenfluramine derivatives [21, 22]. An outbreak of valvular heart disease and/or PAH induced by benfluorex use was identified by the French PH network from June 1999 to March 2011 and included 85 cases of PAH. The analysis of these cases led to the withdrawal of benfluorex from the French market in 2009 [23].

Other classes of drugs have also been linked to the development of PAH. Cases of precapillary PH fulfilling the criteria of drug-induced PAH have been reported in chronic myelogenous leukemia patients treated with the tyrosine kinase inhibitor dasatinib. At diagnosis, patients had moderate to severe precapillary PH with functional and hemodynamic impairment. Clinical, functional, and hemodynamic improvements were observed within a few months of dasatinib discontinuation in most patients. However, after a median follow-up of 9 months (range 3–36 months),

Table 2.3 Updated classification for drug- and toxin-induced PAH[a]

Definite	Possible
Aminorex	Cocaine
Fenfluramine	Phenylpropanolamine
Dexfluramine	St. John's wort
Toxic rapeseed oil	Chemotherapeutic agents
Benfluorex	**Interferon α and β**
SSRIs[b]	**Amphetamine-like drugs**
Likely	Unlikely
Amphetamines	Oral contraceptives
Tryptophan	Estrogen
Methamphetamines	Cigarette smoking
Dasatinib	

From [9]

[a]Nice 2013

[b]Selective serotonin reuptake inhibitors (SSRIs) have been demonstrated as a risk factor for the development of persistent pulmonary hypertension in the newborn (PPHN) in pregnant women exposed to SSRIs (especially after 20 weeks of gestation). PPHN does not strictly belong to Group 1 (pulmonary arterial hypertension[PAH]) but to a separated Group 1. Main modification to the previous Danapoint classification is in bold

the majority of patients failed to demonstrate complete clinical and hemodynamic recovery and no patients reached a normal value of mPAH (≤20 mmHg). The lowest estimate of incident PH occurring in patients exposed to dasatinib in France was 0.45 %. Thus, dasatinib may induce severe PAH, suggesting a direct and specific effect of dasatinib on pulmonary vessels [24].

The potential association of PAH and the use of interferon alfa or beta has also been reported. Fifty-three PAH patients in the French registry had a history of interferon use, raising the question about whether or not a causal relation could be present.

The presence of genetic abnormalities and risk factors (such as specific drug exposures) reinforces the "multiple hit" concept for the development of pulmonary hypertension [25]. The list of the recognized risk factors potentially associated with the development of pulmonary hypertension is presented in Table 2.3.

One of the most important forms of PAH is the one associated with connective tissue diseases, not only due to its clinical course but also because of its prevalence. Connective tissue diseases (CTD) represented about 15 % of all PAH cases in the French registry, with systemic sclerosis and systemic lupus erythematosus as the leading causes (76 and 15 % of all CTD-PAH, respectively) [26]. CTD represented about 25 % of cases in the REVEAL registry from the United States [46]. The prognosis of these patients is worse than other forms of PAH, reaching a 1-year mortality of about 30 % as compared to about 15 % in IPAH [27, 28]. Recently, it has been suggested that implementation of a systematic screening program that allows the

Table 2.4 Updated clinical classification of pulmonary arterial hypertension associated with congenital heart disease[a]

1. Eisenmenger syndrome
Includes all large intra- and extracardiac defects which begin as systemic-to-pulmonary shunts and progress with time to severe elevation of pulmonary vascular resistance (PVR) and to reversal (pulmonary-to-systemic) or bidirectional shunting; cyanosis, secondary erythrocytosis, and multiple organ involvement are usually present.
2. Left-to-right shunts
• Correctable[b]
• Noncorrectable
Include moderate to large defects; PVR is mildly to moderately increased, systemic-to-pulmonary shunting is still prevalent, whereas cyanosis is not a feature.
3. Pulmonary arterial hypertension (PAH) with coincidental congenital heart disease. Marked elevation in PVR in the presence of small cardiac defects, which themselves do not account for the development of elevated PVR; the clinical picture is very similar to idiopathic PAH. To close the defects is contraindicated.
4. Postoperative PAH
Congenital heart disease is repaired but PAH either persists immediately after surgery or recurs/develops months or years after surgery in the absence of significant postoperative hemodynamic lesions. The clinical phenotype is often aggressive.

From [9]

use of specific therapies in a less symptomatic phase of the disease might result in better long-term outcome for this subgroup of PAH patients [29].

Patients with HIV infection also have a greater risk of developing PAH. The prevalence of PAH in this group is estimated to be 0.5 %, with clinical and hemodynamic presentation very similar to IPAH [30, 31]. Prognosis of this particular subgroup of PAH has improved in recent years. In the REVEAL registry, the mortality of HIV-PAH patients was 7 and 25 % at 1 and 3 years, respectively [32].

Another group at risk for PAH is patients with portal hypertension. About 6 % of these patients develop PAH [33] independent of the severity of their liver disease, although the long-term prognosis of these patients is related to the severity of both liver and pulmonary vascular diseases [34]. Portopulmonary hypertension represents an important problem for liver transplantation programs since its presence is related to increased mortality during the procedure [35]. The prognosis in POPH is worse than in IPAH. Recent data suggest a 3-year survival of 40 % [36].

About 10 % of children with congenital heart disease (CHD) develop PAH. Since more of these children now survive to adulthood, PAH associated with CHD is a significant subgroup of PH seen in many referral centers [37]. According to the last world symposium, patients with CHD-PAH (except those with more complex congenital heart defects) should be subclassified into four different subgroups (Table 2.4). The concept of this subclassification is to provide guidance on the management of the disease. For instance, patients with small cardiac defects and PAH are considered as having IPAH and coincidental congenital heart disease and should be managed as any other patient with idiopathic disease. On the other hand, patients with CHD and persistent left-to-right shunts should be considered for possible correction of the defect causing the shunt, although criteria for the definition of operability is still a matter of debate [9].

Schistosomiasis is an infectious disease caused by parasitic trematode worms that is strongly linked to poor sanitary conditions and poverty. Nevertheless, due to migratory practices, the prevalence of schistosomiasis is increasing in nonendemic regions. Pulmonary hypertension represents one of the most severe complications of chronic schistosomiasis [38]. A screening program for pulmonary hypertension in a tertiary center in Brazil identified a 4.6 % prevalence of PAH among patients diagnosed with hepatosplenic Schistosomiasis mansoni [39]. When this prevalence rate is considered in the context of the high prevalence of schistosomal infection globally, schistosomiasis associated PAH (Sch-PAH) is one of the leading causes of PH in the world. Indeed, it is estimated that up to 30 % of all pulmonary hypertension patients followed at referral centers in Brazil have Sch-PAH [40]. A subsequent study showed that although Sch-PAH has a clinical profile similar to IPAH at the time of diagnosis, the clinical course appears to be more benign with a 3-year mortality of about 15 % [41].

Epidemiology

Our knowledge of the epidemiology of PAH has changed dramatically over the last 30 years. The earlier clinical picture of IPAH was mainly derived from the landmark study conducted by the National Institutes of Health (NIH) in the 1980s [42, 43]. By that time, IPAH was described as a disease affecting young patients (mean age of 36 yo), with a female to male ratio of 1.7:1. Time from the first symptom to the appropriate diagnosis exceeded 2 years and the mortality rate at 1 year was about 32 %. Since then, the development of target therapies has not only led to improved survival but has also increased disease awareness. Several multicenter registries have been published in recent years, evidencing a changing epidemiology of PAH (Tables 2.5 and 2.6). The first of these multicenter registries was the French national registry. A total of 674 patients were enrolled by 17 different referral centers [26]. The French Registry confirmed the female predominance, but described a mean age at diagnosis of 50 years, with older patients presenting worse prognosis [27, 45]. Concomitantly, data from the multicenter US registry REVEAL, that included more than 2,000 patients from 54 reference centers, also demonstrated this older age at diagnosis (53 yo) as well as a worse prognosis in male patients presenting at older age [46, 47]. Both registries also demonstrated disturbing data concerning PAH diagnosis. Although an increase in disease awareness is believed to have occurred during the last decade, the appropriate diagnosis still takes about 2 years with most of the patients being diagnosed in functional class III and IV. This is particularly alarming if one takes into consideration that the worse the functional class at the diagnosis, the worse the survival despite all available medical treatments. Therefore,

Table 2.5 Pulmonary arterial hypertension registries from different countries and time periods [44]

General information of PAH registries from different countries and time periods						
Registry (ref. #)	Study cohort	Study design and time period	No. of centers	No. of patients	Incidence/prevalence	Predominant etiologies of PAH
U.S. NIH	IPAH	Prospective, 1981–1985	32	187	NA	NA
U.S. PHC	Group 1 PH, age >18 years	Retrospective, 1982–2004; prospective, 2004–2006	3	578	NA	IPAH, 48 %; CTD-PAH, 30 %; CHD-PAH, 11 %
Scottish-SMR	Group 1 PH (IPAH, CHD-PAH, and CTD-PAH), age 16–65 years	Retrospective, 1986–2001	N/A	374	PAH, 7.6/26 cases/MAI; IPAH, 2.6/9 cases/MAI	IPAH, 47 %; CTD-PAH, 30 %; CHD-PAH, 23 %
French	Group 1 PH, age >18 years	Prospective, 2002–2003	17	674	PAH, 2.4/15 cases/MAI; IPAH, 1.0/5.9 cases/MAI	IPAH, 38 %; CTD-PAH, 15 % (SSc, 76 %); CHD-PAH, 11 %
Chinese	IPAH and HPAH	Prospective, 1999–2004	1	72	NA	NA
U.S. REVEAL	Group 1 PH	Prospective, 2006–2009	55	3,515 (age >3 months)	PAH, 2.0/10.6 cases/MAI IPAH, 0.9 cases/MAI	IPAH, 46 %; CTD-PAH, 25 % (SSc, 62 %); CHD-PAH, 10 %
Spanish	Group 1 PH and CTEPH, age >14 years	Retrospective, 1998–2006; prospective, 2007–2008	31	PAH, 866; CTEPH, 162	PAH, 3.2/16 cases/MAI; IPAH, 1.2/4.6 cases/MAI	IPAH, 30 %, CTD-PAH, 15 % (SSc 61 %); CHD-PAH, 16 %
UK	IPAH, HPAH, and anorexigen-associated PAH	Prospective, 2001–2009	8	482	1.1/6.6 cases/MI	NA
New Chinese Registry	Group 1 PH, age >18 years	Prospective, 2008–2011	9	956	NA	CHD-PAH, 43 %; IPAH, 35 %; CTD-PAH, 19 % (SLE, 51 %; SSc, 9 %)
Mayo	Group 1 PH	Prospective, 1995–2004	1	484	NA	IPAH, HPAH 56 %; CTD-PAH, 24 %, other, 20 %
Compera	IPAH, age >18 years	Prospective, 2007–2011	28	587	NA	IPAH, 100 %

CHD congenial heart disease, *CTD* connective tissue disease, *CTEPH* chronic thromboembolic pulmonary hypertension, *HPAH* heritable pulmonary arterial hypertension, *IPAH* idiopathic pulmonary arterial hypertension, *MAI* million adult inhabitants, *MI* million inhabitants, *NA* not available, *NIH* National Institutes of Health, *PAH* pulmonary arterial hypertension, *PHC* pulmonary hypertension connection, *SMR* Scottish morbidity record, *SSc* systemic sclerosis

Table 2.6 Demographic, clinical, and hemodynamic characteristics of PAH registries from different countries and time periods [44]

	Age (years)		Female (%)		WHO III/IV (%)		6MWD (m)		RAP (mmHg)		mPAP (mmHg)		PVRI (U m^2)	
Registry (ref. #)	PAH	IPAH	PAH	IPAH	PAH	IPAH	PAH	IPAH	PAH	IPAH	PAH	IPAH	PAH	IPAH
U.S. NIH	NA	36 ± 15	NA	63	NA	75	NA	NA	NA	10 ± 6	NA	60 ± 18	NA	26 ± 14
U.S. PHC	48 ± 14	45 ± 14	77	75	80	80	NA	NA	11 ± 7	11 ± 7	52 ± 14	56 ± 13	NA	NA
Scottish-SMR	52 ± 12	49 ± 11	70	62	NA	NA	NA	NA	NA	NA	NA	NA	NA	NA
French	50 ± 15	52 ± 15	65	62	75	81	329 ± 109	328 ± 112	8 ± 5	9 ± 5	55 ± 15	56 ± 14	21 ± 10	23 ± 10
Chinese	NA	36 ± 12	NA	71	NA	61	NA	NA	NA	13 ± 6	NA	69 ± 19	NA	NA
U.S. REVEAL	50 ± 14	50 ± 15	80	83	56	55	366 ± 126	374 ± 129	9 ± 6	10 ± 6	51 ± 14	52 ± 13	21 ± 13	23 ± 11
Spanish	45 ± 17	46 ± 18	71	73	69	70	363 ± 120	382 ± 117	9 ± 5	8 ± 5	54 ± 16	55 ± 15	NA	NA
UK	NA	50 ± 17	NA	70	NA	84	NA	292 ± 123	NA	10 ± 6	NA	54 ± 14	NA	23 ± 10
New Chinese Registry	36 ± 13	38 ± 13	70	70	54	66	378 ± 125	353 ± 127	8 ± 5	8 ± 6	63 ± 20	63 ± 15	25 ± 14	27 ± 12
Mayo	52 ± 15	52 ± 15	75	76	55	56	329 ± 125	344 ± 125	13 ± 6	13 ± 6	53 ± 13	55 ± 12	NA	NA
Compera	NA	65 ± 15	NA	60	NA	91	NA	293 ± 126	NA	8 ± 5	NA	44 ± 12	NA	NA

Values are frequency (female, WHO functional class) and men ± SD (age, 6MWD, and hemodynamic variables)

6MWD 6-min walking distance, *mPAP* mean pulmonary arterial pressure, *PVRI* pulmonary vascular resistance index, *RAP* mean right atrial pressure, *SMR* Scottish morbidity record, *WHO* World Health Organization, other abbreviations as in Table 2.4

late diagnosis is a true problem, more specifically for IPAH, and might be one of the scenarios to be changed in the near future, in order to better improve survival.

The French registry estimated the incidence and prevalence of PAH as 2.4 cases per million inhabitants per year and 15 cases per million inhabitants, respectively [26]. Data from a more recent registry, developed in the United Kingdom and Ireland, enrolling almost 500 patients with idiopathic, familial, or anorexigen-induced PAH evidenced incidence and prevalence rates of 1.1 cases per million inhabitants per year and 6.6 cases per million inhabitants, respectively (in agreement with the IPAH prevalence found in the French Registry of 5.9 cases per million inhabitants) [48]. This registry also confirmed that nowadays, newly diagnosed patients have older age (50 yo) and still present a female predominance. More interestingly, the UK and Ireland registry recognized two different phenotypes when stratifying patients according to the mean age. Patients older than 50 years at the diagnosis had a greater delay between first symptom and diagnosis and also presented more comorbidities such as diabetes, systemic hypertension, and ischemic heart disease [48, 49]. Thus, there has been a clear change in phenotype and the complexity of the disease has increased. The current reality of PAH obligates physicians to deal with more drug-drug interactions and also a more complex process for diagnosis. For example, older patients with the aforementioned comorbidities are also prone to develop heart failure with preserved ejection fraction, a particularly challenging differential diagnosis in PH [50, 51].

The prognosis of IPAH, in the absence of specific treatment, is poor. Data from the NIH registry demonstrated survival rates of 68 %, 48 %, and 34 % at 1, 3, and 5 years, respectively [43]. Different studies have demonstrated beneficial survival effects of different drugs when comparing patients receiving active treatment in extension phases of clinical trials or from retrospective cohorts to the predicted survival estimated by the NIH equation [41, 52]. This approach, although valid for exploratory analysis, implies a major bias [53]. Patients enrolled in clinical trials are stable by definition; this excludes patients with rapidly progressive disease, for instance. The resulting cohort for the long-term analysis will be then composed mainly of prevalent cases with less progressive disease, resulting in overestimation of survival. Fortunately, recent prospective registries composed of newly diagnosed patients allow a view of the real-life picture on PAH management. The UK and Ireland registry described a 1-, 3-, and 5-year survival of 92.7 %, 73.3 %, and 61.1 %, respectively, supporting the impact of the available treatments and strategies on PAH survival, but also highlighting the unacceptable mortality rate of almost 40 % in 5 years [48].

In summary, there is a changing picture on the PAH scenario. New epidemiological data provided further insights on the pathophysiology of the disease and also demonstrated the growing complexity of diagnosis and clinical management. Nonetheless, the classification of pulmonary hypertension patients constitutes a landmark for determining prognosis and appropriate therapeutical management.

References

1. Galie N, Hoeper MM, Humbert M, Torbicki A, Vachiery JL, Barbera JA, et al. Guidelines for the diagnosis and treatment of pulmonary hypertension: the Task Force for the Diagnosis and Treatment of Pulmonary Hypertension of the European Society of Cardiology (ESC) and the European Respiratory Society (ERS), endorsed by the International Society of Heart and Lung Transplantation (ISHLT). Eur Heart J. 2009;30:2493–537.
2. Souza R, Jardim C. Trends in pulmonary arterial hypertension. Eur Respir Rev. 2009;18: 7–12.
3. Humbert M. The fifth world symposium on pulmonary hypertension will REVEAL the impact of registries. Eur Respir Rev. 2012;21:4–5.
4. Kovacs G, Berghold A, Scheidl S, Olschewski H. Pulmonary arterial pressure during rest and exercise in healthy subjects: a systematic review. Eur Respir J. 2009;34:888–94.
5. Bae S, Saggar R, Bolster MB, Chung L, Csuka ME, Derk C, et al. Baseline characteristics and follow-up in patients with normal haemodynamics versus borderline mean pulmonary arterial pressure in systemic sclerosis: results from the PHAROS registry. Ann Rheum Dis. 2012; 71:1335–42.
6. Badesch DB, Champion HC, Sanchez MA, Hoeper MM, Loyd JE, Manes A, et al. Diagnosis and assessment of pulmonary arterial hypertension. J Am Coll Cardiol. 2009;54:S55–66.
7. Hoeper MM, Bogaard HJ, Condliffe R, Frantz R, Khanna D, Kurzyna M, et al. Definitions and diagnosis of pulmonary hypertension. J Am Coll Cardiol. 2013;62:D42–50.
8. Simonneau G, Robbins IM, Beghetti M, Channick RN, Delcroix M, Denton CP, et al. Updated clinical classification of pulmonary hypertension. J Am Coll Cardiol. 2009;54:S43–54.
9. Simonneau G, Gatzoulis MA, Adatia I, Celermajer D, Denton C, Ghofrani A, et al. Updated clinical classification of pulmonary hypertension. J Am Coll Cardiol. 2013;62:D34–41.
10. Cogan JD, Pauciulo MW, Batchman AP, Prince MA, Robbins IM, Hedges LK, et al. High frequency of BMPR2 exonic deletions/duplications in familial pulmonary arterial hypertension. Am J Respir Crit Care Med. 2006;174:590–8.
11. Thomson JR, Machado RD, Pauciulo MW, Morgan NV, Humbert M, Elliott GC, et al. Sporadic primary pulmonary hypertension is associated with germline mutations of the gene encoding BMPR-II, a receptor member of the TGF-beta family. J Med Genet. 2000;37:741–5.
12. Machado RD, Eickelberg O, Elliott CG, Geraci MW, Hanaoka M, Loyd JE, et al. Genetics and genomics of pulmonary arterial hypertension. J Am Coll Cardiol. 2009;54:S32–42.
13. Frost AE, Badesch DB, Barst RJ, Benza RL, Elliott CG, Farber HW, Krichman A, Liou TG, Raskob GE, Wason P, Feldkircher K, Turner M, McGoon MD. The changing picture of patients with pulmonary arterial hypertension in the United States:how REVEAL differs from historic and non-US Contemporary Registries. Chest. 2011;139(1):128–37.
14. Sztrymf B, Coulet F, Girerd B, Yaici A, Jais X, Sitbon O, et al. Clinical outcomes of pulmonary arterial hypertension in carriers of BMPR2 mutation. Am J Respir Crit Care Med. 2008; 177:1377–83.
15. Germain M, Eyries M, Montani D, Poirier O, Girerd B, Dorfmuller P, et al. Genome-wide association analysis identifies a susceptibility locus for pulmonary arterial hypertension. Nat Genet. 2013;45:518–21.
16. Girerd B, Montani D, Coulet F, Sztrymf B, Yaici A, Jais X, et al. Clinical outcomes of pulmonary arterial hypertension in patients carrying an ACVRL1 (ALK1) mutation. Am J Respir Crit Care Med. 2010;181:851–61.
17. Girerd B, Montani D, Eyries M, Yaici A, Sztrymf B, Coulet F, et al. Absence of influence of gender and BMPR2 mutation type on clinical phenotypes of pulmonary arterial hypertension. Respir Res. 2010;11:73.
18. Gurtner HP. Aminorex and pulmonary hypertension. A review. Cor Vasa. 1985;27:160–71.

19. Souza R, Humbert M, Sztrymf B, Jais X, Yaici A, Le Pavec J, et al. Pulmonary arterial hypertension associated with fenfluramine exposure: report of 109 cases. Eur Respir J. 2008;31:343–8.
20. Walker AM, Langleben D, Korelitz JJ, Rich S, Rubin LJ, Strom BL, et al. Temporal trends and drug exposures in pulmonary hypertension: an American experience. Am Heart J. 2006;152:521–6.
21. Boutet K, Frachon I, Jobic Y, Gut-Gobert C, Leroyer C, Carlhant-Kowalski D, et al. Fenfluramine-like cardiovascular side-effects of benfluorex. Eur Respir J. 2009;33:684–8.
22. Frachon I, Etienne Y, Jobic Y, Le Gal G, Humbert M, Leroyer C. Benfluorex and unexplained valvular heart disease: a case-control study. PLoS One. 2010;5:e10128.
23. Savale L, Chaumais MC, Cottin V, Bergot E, Frachon I, Prevot G, et al. Pulmonary hypertension associated with benfluorex exposure. Eur Respir J. 2012;40:1164–72.
24. Montani D, Bergot E, Gunther S, Savale L, Bergeron A, Bourdin A, et al. Pulmonary arterial hypertension in patients treated by dasatinib. Circulation. 2012;125:2128–37.
25. Yuan JX, Rubin LJ. Pathogenesis of pulmonary arterial hypertension: the need for multiple hits. Circulation. 2005;111:534–8.
26. Humbert M, Sitbon O, Chaouat A, Bertocchi M, Habib G, Gressin V, et al. Pulmonary arterial hypertension in France: results from a national registry. Am J Respir Crit Care Med. 2006;173:1023–30.
27. Humbert M, Sitbon O, Chaouat A, Bertocchi M, Habib G, Gressin V, et al. Survival in patients with idiopathic, familial, and anorexigen-associated pulmonary arterial hypertension in the modern management era. Circulation. 2010;122:156–63.
28. Tyndall AJ, Bannert B, Vonk M, Airo P, Cozzi F, Carreira PE, et al. Causes and risk factors for death in systemic sclerosis: a study from the EULAR Scleroderma Trials and Research (EUSTAR) database. Ann Rheum Dis. 2010;69:1809–15.
29. Humbert M, Yaici A, de Groote P, Montani D, Sitbon O, Launay D, et al. Screening for pulmonary arterial hypertension in patients with systemic sclerosis: clinical characteristics at diagnosis and long-term survival. Arthritis Rheum. 2011;63:3522–30.
30. Degano B, Sitbon O, Simonneau G. Pulmonary arterial hypertension and HIV infection. Semin Respir Crit Care Med. 2009;30:440–7.
31. Sitbon O, Lascoux-Combe C, Delfraissy JF, Yeni PG, Raffi F, De Zuttere D, et al. Prevalence of HIV-related pulmonary arterial hypertension in the current antiretroviral therapy era. Am J Respir Crit Care Med. 2008;177:108–13.
32. Benza RL, Miller DP, Barst RJ, Badesch DB, Frost AE, McGoon MD. An evaluation of long-term survival from time of diagnosis in pulmonary arterial hypertension from the REVEAL Registry. Chest. 2012;142:448–56.
33. Souza R, Fernandes CJ, Jardim CV. Other causes of PAH (schistosomiasis, porto-pulmonary hypertension and hemolysis-associated pulmonary hypertension). Semin Respir Crit Care Med. 2009;30:448–57.
34. Le Pavec J, Souza R, Herve P, Lebrec D, Savale L, Tcherakian C, et al. Portopulmonary hypertension: survival and prognostic factors. Am J Respir Crit Care Med. 2008;178:637–43.
35. Krowka MJ. Portopulmonary hypertension. Semin Respir Crit Care Med. 2012;33:17–25.
36. Krowka MJ, Miller DP, Barst RJ, Taichman D, Dweik RA, Badesch DB, et al. Portopulmonary hypertension: a report from the US-based REVEAL Registry. Chest. 2012;141:906–15.
37. Engelfriet PM, Duffels MG, Moller T, Boersma E, Tijssen JG, Thaulow E, et al. Pulmonary arterial hypertension in adults born with a heart septal defect: the Euro Heart Survey on adult congenital heart disease. Heart. 2007;93:682–7.
38. Fernandes CJ, Jardim CV, Hovnanian A, Hoette S, Morinaga LK, Souza R. Schistosomiasis and pulmonary hypertension. Expert Rev Respir Med. 2011;5:675–81.
39. Lapa M, Dias B, Jardim C, Fernandes CJ, Dourado PM, Figueiredo M, et al. Cardiopulmonary manifestations of hepatosplenic schistosomiasis. Circulation. 2009;119:1518–23.

40. Lapa MS, Ferreira EV, Jardim C, Martins Bdo C, Arakaki JS, Souza R. Clinical characteristics of pulmonary hypertension patients in two reference centers in the city of Sao Paulo. Rev Assoc Med Bras. 2006;52:139–43.
41. dos Santos Fernandes CJ, Jardim CV, Hovnanian A, Hoette S, Dias BA, Souza S, et al. Survival in schistosomiasis-associated pulmonary arterial hypertension. J Am Coll Cardiol. 2010;56:715–20.
42. Rich S, Dantzker DR, Ayres SM, Bergofsky EH, Brundage BH, Detre KM, et al. Primary pulmonary hypertension. A national prospective study. Ann Intern Med. 1987;107:216–23.
43. D'Alonzo GE, Barst RJ, Ayres SM, Bergofsky EH, Brundage BH, Detre KM, et al. Survival in patients with primary pulmonary hypertension. Results from a national prospective registry. Ann Intern Med. 1991;115:343–9.
44. McGoon MD, Benza RL, Escribano-Subias P, Jiang X, Miller DP, Peacock AJ, et al. Pulmonary arterial hypertension: epidemiology and registries. J Am Coll Cardiol. 2013;62:D51–9.
45. Humbert M, Sitbon O, Yaici A, Montani D, O'Callaghan DS, Jais X, et al. Survival in incident and prevalent cohorts of patients with pulmonary arterial hypertension. Eur Respir J. 2010;36:549–55.
46. Badesch DB, Raskob GE, Elliott CG, Krichman AM, Farber HW, Frost AE, et al. Pulmonary arterial hypertension: baseline characteristics from the REVEAL Registry. Chest. 2010;137:376–87.
47. Benza RL, Miller DP, Gomberg-Maitland M, Frantz RP, Foreman AJ, Coffey CS, et al. Predicting survival in pulmonary arterial hypertension: insights from the Registry to Evaluate Early and Long-Term Pulmonary Arterial Hypertension Disease Management (REVEAL). Circulation. 2010;122:164–72.
48. Ling Y, Johnson MK, Kiely DG, Condliffe R, Elliot CA, Gibbs JS, et al. Changing demographics, epidemiology, and survival of incident pulmonary arterial hypertension: results from the pulmonary hypertension registry of the United Kingdom and Ireland. Am J Respir Crit Care Med. 2012;186:790–6.
49. Lee WT, Ling Y, Sheares KK, Pepke-Zaba J, Peacock AJ, Johnson MK. Predicting survival in pulmonary arterial hypertension in the UK. Eur Respir J. 2012;40:604–11.
50. Naeije R, Vachiery JL, Yerly P, Vanderpool R. The transpulmonary pressure gradient for the diagnosis of pulmonary vascular disease. Eur Respir J. 2013;41:217–23.
51. Vachiery JL, Gaine S. Challenges in the diagnosis and treatment of pulmonary arterial hypertension. Eur Respir Rev. 2012;21:313–20.
52. Sitbon O, McLaughlin VV, Badesch DB, Barst RJ, Black C, Galie N, et al. Survival in patients with class III idiopathic pulmonary arterial hypertension treated with first line oral bosentan compared with an historical cohort of patients started on intravenous epoprostenol. Thorax. 2005;60:1025–30.
53. O'Callaghan DS, Humbert M. A critical analysis of survival in pulmonary arterial hypertension. Eur Respir Rev. 2012;21:218–22.

Chapter 3
Pathogenesis of Pulmonary Arterial Hypertension

Aaron W. Trammell and Anna R. Hemnes

Abstract Pulmonary arterial hypertension (PAH) is a rare disease of the pulmonary vasculature characterized by progressive vascular obliteration, right heart failure, and ultimately death. Basic science has focused for the past several decades on identification of underlying molecular causes of this disease, and multiple potential derangements have been identified and some have led to development of drugs to treat PAH. Unfortunately, however, there is no cure for PAH and research continues to identify common mechanisms of development of pulmonary vascular disease and to develop new, more effective therapies. This chapter highlights much of our understanding of the basic pathobiology underlying PAH including genetic underpinnings, vasoactive substances, alterations in cell proliferation and apoptosis, inflammation, thrombosis, and endocrine factors.

Keywords Pulmonary arterial hypertension • Pathogenesis • Etiology • Vasoconstriction • Thrombosis • Proliferation • Plexiform lesion • Nitric oxide • BMPR2

Abbreviations

5-HT	5-Hydroxytryptamine or serotonin
5-HTT	5-Hydroxytryptamine (serotonin) transporter
ADMA	Asymmetric dimethylarginine
ALK	Activin receptor-like kinase
AVM	Arteriovenous malformation
bFGF	Basic fibroblast growth factor
BMP	Bone morphogenic protein
BMPR2	Bone morphogenic protein receptor type 2
Cav-1	Caveolin-1

A.W. Trammell, M.D. • A.R. Hemnes, M.D. (✉)
Department of Medicine, Allergy, Pulmonary, and Critical Care Medicine, Vanderbilt University Medical Center, T1218 MCN, 1161 21st Avenue South, Nashville, TN 37205, USA
e-mail: aaron.trammell@vanderbilt.edu; anna.r.hemnes@vanderbilt.edu

J.R. Klinger, R.P. Frantz (eds.), *Diagnosis and Management of Pulmonary Hypertension*, Respiratory Medicine 12, DOI 10.1007/978-1-4939-2636-7_3

cGMP	Cyclic guanosine monophosphate
COPD	Chronic obstructive pulmonary disease
CTD	Connective tissue disease
CTEPH	Chronic thromboembolic pulmonary hypertension
DDAH	Dimethylarginine dimethyaminohydrolase
EC	Endothelial cell
EGF	Epidermal growth factor
EGFR	Epidermal growth factor receptor
ENG	Endoglin
ET	Endothelin
GDF	Growth/differentiation factor
HHT	Hereditary hemorrhagic telangiectasia
HHV-8	Human herpesvirus 8
HIF	Hypoxia-inducible factor
HIV	Human immunodeficiency virus
HPAH	Heritable pulmonary arterial hypertension
IPAH	Idiopathic pulmonary arterial hypertension
IV	Intravenous
K_V	Voltage-gated potassium channel
NO	Nitric oxide
NOS	Nitric oxide synthase
PA	Pulmonary artery
PAH	Pulmonary arterial hypertension
PAP	Pulmonary arterial pressure
PASMC	Pulmonary artery smooth muscle cell
PDE5	Phosphodiesterase type 5
PDGF	Platelet-derived growth factor
PH	Pulmonary hypertension
PPARγ	Peroxisome proliferator-activator receptor gamma
PVR	Pulmonary vascular resistance
RV	Right ventricle
siRNA	Small interfering RNA
SIV	Simian immunodeficiency virus
SMC	Smooth muscle cell
SSRI	Selective serotonin reuptake inhibitors
TFG-α	Transforming growth factor α
TGF-β	Transforming growth factor β
VEGF	Vascular endothelial growth factor
VEGFR	Vascular endothelial growth factor receptor
vSMC	Vascular smooth muscle cell
vWF	von Willebrand factor
WHO	World Health Organization

Genetic Background

No single mechanism has been shown to be sufficient to cause PAH in man. Rather, a combination of factors likely contributes to disease development and risk. While most PAH develops sporadically, registry data show that ≥6 % of subjects with PAH have a first-degree relative with the disease (familial or heritable PAH, HPAH) and these subjects are clinically indistinguishable from those without a family history (sporadic or idiopathic PAH) [1]. Females are disproportionately affected at a 3:1 ratio [2, 3]. An autosomal dominant inheritance pattern with reduced penetrance (10–20 %) was demonstrated prior to discovery of a genetic locus. Early registry data also suggested genetic anticipation, but later reanalysis with more families and longer follow-up intervals suggest that genetic anticipation is not a feature of familial PAH [4]. Early study of HPAH carried hopes of elucidating the underlying genetic and pathobiologic basis of the disease [5, 6].

Through genetic linkage analysis, the locus for inheritance of HPAH was found to be on the long arm of chromosome 2 [7, 8], and later narrowed to a segment of 2q33 [9, 10]. In 2000, using information from the Human Genome Project, candidate genes in this chromosomal region were sequenced in multiple kindreds of HPAH by two independent groups. Heterogeneous mutations in the gene for bone morphogenic protein receptor type II (BMPR2) were discovered including frameshift, missense, and nonsense mutations which span the *BMPR2* gene and resultant TGF-β family protein [11–13]. Given that patients with familial and sporadic PAH are clinically indistinguishable [5, 6], genotyping was undertaken in patients with sporadic disease. Fifty patients with sporadic PAH (defined as having no family history suggestive of PAH) were genotyped. *BMPR2* mutations were found in 13 of 50 patients including 11 different mutations [14]. With parental genetic analysis, some mutations were de novo while others were demonstrated in a parent despite exclusion of family history of clinical disease by detailed pedigrees. We now know that *BMPR2* mutations are present in up to 80 % of subjects with familial PAH and 15 % of those with sporadic PAH [1, 15–17].

BMPR2 is a member of the TGF-β receptor superfamily which is split into type I and type II receptors; BMPR2 is a type II receptor. All type II receptors are constitutively active serine/threonine kinases. BMPR2 is distinguished from other type II receptors by a long cytoplasmic tail following the kinase domain. There are more than a dozen extracellular ligands which typically have high affinity for the type I receptor and lower affinity for BMPR2. In the presence of extracellular ligand, the type I receptor dimerizes and recruits a type II receptor, forming a functional heterotetrameric receptor complex. The type I receptor is phosphorylated by the constitutively active kinase domain of BMPR2 (or other type II receptor). This signaling family exhibits tissue specificity likely mediated by the specific extracellular ligand and the other receptor proteins present within the heterotetramer as well as multiple known BMP receptor inhibitors (e.g., Noggin, Chordin, Smurf 1). The canonical pathway of downstream signaling involves phosphorylation of Smad1, -5, and -8 by the activated type I receptor. These Smads activate Smad4, a transcription factor.

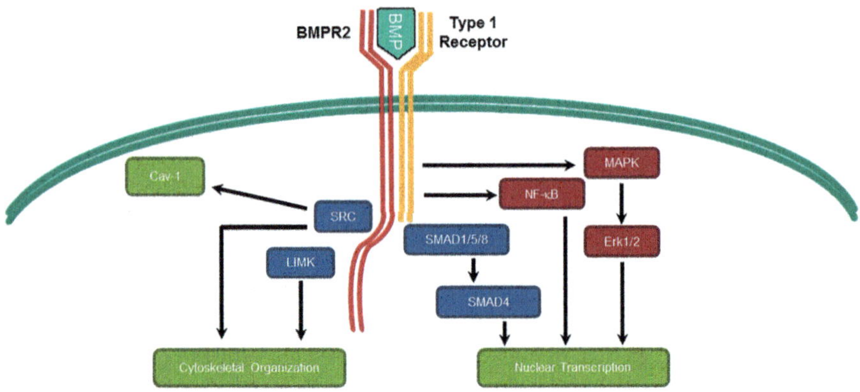

Fig. 3.1 Signaling pathways downstream of BMPR2

While this is the most ubiquitous description of BMP signaling in the literature, other pathways have been reported and, thus, BMP signaling is much more complex than the canonical pathway alone. BMP signaling also involves mitogen-activated protein kinases ($p38^{MAPK}$, $p42/44^{MAPK}$ also known as Erk1/2) which activate other nuclear transcription factors, and LIMK which regulates actin polymerization and therefore the cytoskeleton, Tetex-type I, NF-κB, and Src among others [18–21] (Fig. 3.1).

Interestingly, it is clear that not all persons with *BMPR2* mutation develop PAH and within the same family there is variation in age of onset and disease severity. This variability suggests a "second hit," perhaps an environmental exposure or additional genetic factor modulating risk of disease development [22]. Recent work has suggested that alterations in expression of the estrogen-metabolizing enzyme CYP1B1 favoring 16-hydroxyestrone over 2-methoxyestradiol may underlie development of PAH in many patients with *BMPR2* mutation [23]. Alternative splicing of the normal BMPR2 allele in heterozygous mutation carriers may affect pulmonary vascular disease development [24].

Although *BMPR2* mutation is found in many cases of HPAH and some sporadic PAH, we now know that BMPR2 expression is depressed in many forms of PAH including IPAH not associated with mutation [25]. Despite over a decade of research on BMPR2, the exact mechanism through which altered BMPR2 signaling results in the clinical phenotype of pulmonary vascular disease is unknown. Recent work has highlighted the potentially important role that cytoskeletal abnormalities as a function of rac1 defects and metabolic derangements regulated by BMPR2 signaling may play in PAH development [26]. Work continues to explore these and other hypotheses in the development of pulmonary vascular disease related to *BMPR2* mutation and signaling depression. Downstream effects of BMPR2 signaling will follow later in this section.

Hereditary hemorrhagic telangiectasia (HHT) is another heritable vascular disorder linked to the TGF-β signaling pathway. Prior to discovery of *BMPR2*-associated

Table 3.1 Evidence for abnormal signaling pathways in PAH

Proposed signaling pathway	Evidence in cell culture	Evidence in animal models	Abnormal in human subjects	Therapeutic targets readily available
BMPR2	Yes	Yes (genetic models)	Yes	No
Smad	Yes	Yes	Yes	No
MAPKK/MAPK	Yes	Yes	Yes	No
LIMK	Yes	Yes	Lack of evidence	No
Src	Yes	Yes	Limited data	No
Nitric oxide	Yes	Yes	Yes	Yes, FDA approved
Prostacyclin	Yes	Yes	Yes	Yes, FDA approved
Endothelin-1	Yes	Yes	Yes	Yes, FDA approved
Serotonin	–	Yes	Yes (conflicting data)	Yes
VEGF	Yes	Yes	Yes (conflicting data)	Yes
PDGF	Yes		Yes	Yes (kinase inhibitors)
bFGF	Yes	No	Yes	Yes (kinase inhibitors)
EGF	Yes	Yes	No	Yes (kinase inhibitors)

PAH, mutations in two TGF-β signaling proteins (ALK-1 and endoglin) were demonstrated as the genetic basis of HHT [27–29]. Unlike its more common phenotype, a minority of subjects with HHT have PAH that is clinically indistinguishable and pathologically similar to those with IPAH [30, 31]. Mutations of endoglin or ALK-1 have been identified in those families affected by HHT and PAH [29, 31, 32]. PAH in children is often secondary to congenital heart disease, but when this is excluded, they may be more likely to carry an identifiable genetic mutation in BMPR2, endoglin, or ALK-1, reconfirming that different mutations in the TGF-β signaling pathway are often indistinguishable from one another and are frequently found in patients with idiopathic disease [33] (Table 3.1).

Most recently, whole-exome sequencing was used in a family with multiple PAH-affected members in whom no identifiable mutation had been found. All affected family members, and some unaffected members, carried a mutation in the gene encoding caveolin-1 (*cav-1*), a protein important in formation of caveolae which are cell surface invaginations that modulate cell surface protein endocytosis and recycling. An additional sporadic case of IPAH secondary to *cav-1* mutation was also discovered [34]. This study suggests that mutations in *cav-1* are a rare cause of PAH and is the first mutation known that does not involve TGF-β signaling directly. Caveolin-1 is known to be important in vascular biology and physiology because it is a crucial negative regulator of eNOS activity [35, 36]. Recent studies using cav-1 and eNOS knockout mice suggest that the lack of cav-1 results in excessive eNOS activity associated with generation of ROS and inactivation of

PKG (the major downstream target of NO-generated cGMP) by nitrosylation [37]. Cav-1 knockout mice develop cardiovascular disease including spontaneous PAH and RV failure when exposed to chronic hypoxia [38–40].

Vasoactive Substances and Imbalance

The hallmarks of pulmonary hypertension are elevated pulmonary arterial pressure (PAP) and vascular resistance (PVR). Patients with what is now categorized as IPAH were described early on in biopsy and autopsy series as those with normal lung parenchyma and pathologic findings limited to the small muscular arteries [41]. A logical area of investigation was the balance of vasoactive substances.

Vascular smooth muscle (SMCs) and endothelial cells (ECs) participate in regulation of blood flow in both the systemic and pulmonary vascular bed. The regulation of pulmonary circulation is unique to that of the systemic circulation especially in regard to hypoxic pulmonary vasoconstriction (see Chap. 4). While hypoxic pulmonary vasoconstriction is effective and necessary to maintain homeostasis in health and disease, chronic lung diseases featuring hypoxemia are a common cause of PH (WHO Group 3). While there is still debate as to the mechanism of hypoxic pulmonary vasoconstriction, research in this area has led to a better understanding of pulmonary physiology and a wealth of knowledge that has been adapted to the study of pulmonary vascular disease broadly.

It has long been known that histologic specimens from patients with PAH show normal lung parenchyma but intimal and medial thickening of the vascular wall and intraluminal findings of cellular proliferation and often thrombotic material [41–43]. In addition to pathologic findings limited to pulmonary vessels, an early observation was an acute response to administration of pulmonary vasodilators leading to the theory that the underlying pathobiologic mechanism was a "vasoconstrictive factor" [44–46].

Nitric Oxide

In the 1950s Paul Wood developed a classification scheme for PH not dissimilar to our current WHO classification. He was interested in vasoconstriction as a possible cause of elevated PAP and PVR. In a subject with mitral stenosis and PH, he administered acetylcholine, a known vasodilator. He noted that PAP and PVR fell and systemic pressure increased, presumably from increased cardiac output. This was shown to be reproducible in patients with PAH and PH secondary to mitral stenosis or COPD, but not in Eisenmenger's syndrome [46]. Through elegant experiments in several labs over the ensuing three decades, acetylcholine's effect was demonstrated to be via an endothelial dependent mechanism with the effector compound being nitric oxide (NO) from ECs and the target being the vascular SMC [47, 48].

Subsequently it was shown that strips of excised but still endothelialized PA from patients with Eisenmenger's syndrome and chronic lung disease with secondary PH had blunted vasodilatory responses to acetylcholine, but preserved response to nitroprusside (an NO donor) [49, 50]. Endothelial dysfunction was proposed as the mechanism.

Nitric oxide is a short-lived powerful vasodilator produced from metabolism of L-arginine by the enzyme nitric oxide synthase (NOS). In the lung, endothelial NOS (eNOS) is the predominant isoform. Nitric oxide exerts its effect by increasing cyclic guanosine monophosphate (cGMP) within PASMCs which causes relaxation by activating cGMP-dependent protein kinase (PKG) that then acts on a variety of downstream targets to decrease intracellular calcium concentration. Inhaled NO reduces PAP and PVR in some subjects with PH [51]. Lung specimens from subjects with PAH show reduced or absent eNOS expression. Also, eNOS and endothelin-1 (a vasoconstrictor discussed below) have inverse staining patterns in the endothelium of PAH subjects compared with controls [52]. Subjects with PAH also have higher levels of ADMA (an eNOS inhibitor) and reduced expression of DDAH2 (an enzyme which metabolizes ADMA) in lung specimens compared to controls [53]. Taken together, these findings suggest that endothelial derived NO is reduced in PAH. Whether reduced NO availability is a cause or effect of pulmonary vascular disease is uncertain, but it has led to development of pharmacologic agents designed to increase pulmonary vascular cGMP levels. A family of phosphodiesterases (PDE) degrade cGMP and cAMP. PDE5 is the predominant isoform in pulmonary vascular smooth muscle and PDE5-specific inhibitors such as sildenafil and tadalafil have been shown to reduce PAP in animal models of pulmonary hypertension and in humans with PAH [54–56]. L-arginine has been used with limited success in the treatment of PAH and has been shown to reduce PAP and PVR in some subjects [57, 58]. Recently, soluble guanylate cyclase stimulators that act synergistically with NO to increase cGMP synthesis have also been approved for the treatment of PAH (see Chap. 15 for more discussion on cGMP modifiers for the treatment of PAH).

Prostacyclin

Prostacyclin is also produced by ECs and relaxes pulmonary and systemic smooth muscle [56]. Rubin administered prostacyclin to subjects with PAH and reported favorable acute hemodynamic changes [59] and later a favorable randomized trial of continuous IV prostacyclin therapy [60]. Despite the efficacious effects of prostacyclin (see Chap. 13), it was not known at that time whether abnormalities of prostacyclin synthesis contributed to the pathophysiology of PAH. Further studies found that thromboxane, that is derived from the same synthetic pathway as prostacyclin, but is a known procoagulant and vasoconstrictor, is increased in subjects with PH, whereas prostacyclin metabolites are decreased. The ratio of thromboxane:prostacyclin is increased in subjects with PH of any cause relative to controls [61]. This suggests increased platelet activation and lends further support to the presence of endothelial dysfunction in subjects with PH.

Endothelin-1

Endothelins (ET-1, ET-2, and ET-3) are another potent mediator of pulmonary vasoconstriction and are also SMC mitogens. Endothelin receptors ET_A and ET_B are both present in the pulmonary vasculature, although their relative expression varies depending on vessel size [62]. The action of ET-1 on ET_A receptor on PASMCs causes vasoconstriction and mitogenesis. The ET_B receptor has a less clear role in vascular tone, but plays an important role in clearance of ET-1. ET_A receptor blockade in experimental conditions reliably attenuates endothelin-induced vascular SMC mitogenesis [62–66] and improves symptoms, exercise tolerance, and hemodynamic parameters in patients [67–71].

In vivo, plasma levels of ET-1 are higher in subjects with PAH or secondary PH compared to controls and are higher in the arterial than venous circulation [72, 73] suggesting increased production or reduced clearance within the pulmonary bed. Compared to controls, PAH subjects have increased ET-1 gene and protein expression in lung tissue which is concentrated in areas of vascular remodeling, especially plexiform lesions [74, 75]. Endothelin effects clearly contribute to pulmonary vascular disease but whether ET-1 overexpression initiates or only propagates pulmonary vascular disease is unknown. Likely, initial endothelial injury results in maladaptive ET-1 release which promotes mitogenesis of vascular SMCs and fibroblasts in patients already prone to uncontrolled cellular proliferation (i.e., those with *BMPR2* mutation) or in those in whom endothelial injury is constantly present (i.e., congenital cardiac shunt). Regardless of mechanism, inhibition of the endothelin system has offered another attractive therapeutic target in the treatment of pulmonary hypertension (see Chap. 14).

Serotonin

The "serotonin hypothesis" of PAH was borne out of the observation that certain serotonergic medications are associated with PAH development [76–79]. Serotonin or 5-hydroxytryptamine (5-HT) causes intense vasoconstriction of systemic and pulmonary vessels and also acts as a mitogen for vascular SMCs [80, 81]. Within the circulation 5-HT exists almost exclusively within platelets for release "on demand," and plasma levels are normally very low. After release from activated platelets, 5-HT is transported into cells including ECs and SMCs via the 5-HT transporter (SERT or 5-HTT) and metabolized by monoamine oxidase. 5-HT_{1B} is the receptor most important for pulmonary vasoconstriction [82, 83].

Experimental disruptions of the 5-HT system have yielded some understanding of its role in human PAH but have not resulted in any therapeutic breakthroughs. Some studies have shown subjects with PAH to have higher concentrations of 5-HT in plasma and within platelets compared to controls which persist after lung transplantation [84]. Polymorphisms of the 5-HTT (the "LL" variant) are likely not associated with PAH in the largest and most recent studies [85–87]. PASMCs from subjects with PAH have higher expression of 5-HTT and are more susceptible to 5-HT-mediated mitogenesis which is reduced by 5-HTT inhibition [85]. Experimental overexpression of 5-HTT causes worsened PH phenotype in animals [88], and 5-HTT knockout mice are protected from pulmonary vascular disease [89]. There are various medications which target the 5-HTT with varying affinities, these being the selective serotonin reuptake inhibitors (SSRIs) commonly employed in the treatment of depression and anxiety. Proliferation of vascular SMCs in response to 5-HT in vitro is inhibited by SSRIs [85, 90]. SSRIs protect against PH in the chronic hypoxia mouse model [91]. In terms of receptors, it is known that the 5-HT_{1B} receptor is involved in pulmonary vasoconstriction and sumatriptan, an FDA-approved medication for treatment of migraine and 5-$HT_{1B/D}$ receptor agonist, causes acute rise in PA pressure [83, 92]. Knockout of the 5-HT_{2B} receptor and knockout or antagonism of the 5-HT_{1B} receptor protect rodents from PH [93, 94]. Further study of the serotonin system and its role in pulmonary vascular disease is ongoing.

Solute Channels

Potassium channels regulate resting membrane potential and voltage-gated Ca^{2+} influx. Calcium is essential for both vascular SMC contraction and proliferation and higher cytosolic Ca^{2+} concentration leads to both. Subjects with IPAH have reduced PASMC expression and activity of voltage-gated K_V channels [95, 96] which promotes membrane depolarization and Ca^{2+} influx. Resting and stimulated cytosolic Ca^{2+} concentrations are known to be higher in PASMCs from subjects with IPAH than controls [95, 97] and this is likely due to both the K_V channel defect and upregulation of several Ca^{2+} channels and regulators [97–100].

Multiple circulating and autocrine vasoactive substances, some having mitogenic potential, are altered in subjects with PAH. The nitric oxide, endothelin, and prostacyclin systems have met realization of clinically useful pharmacologic targets. Further study of other vasoactive mediators may lead to additional treatment options which are sorely needed. There is substantial interaction of vasoconstriction and cellular proliferation which is discussed in the next section.

Cellular Proliferation and Vascular Remodeling

In addition to vasoconstriction, cellular proliferation is one of the major underlying commonalities of PAH pathogenesis. Pulmonary vascular remodeling and proliferation are manifested in all components of the vessel wall: media thickening with vascular smooth muscle cell (SMC) hypertrophy and proliferation, intimal thickening and fibrosis, and intraluminal obstruction of proliferative endothelial cells (ECs) and plexiform lesions. Regulation of the growth and differentiation of ECs and vascular SMCs has been studied extensively in health and disease. Multiple mediators are known, some affecting both ECs and SMCs. Several of these with a focus on their specific role in pulmonary vascular disease will be reviewed herein. Some small molecules, such as 5-HT and ET-1, with prominent pulmonary vasoconstriction properties which have already been discussed also modulate growth and differentiation.

Vascular Endothelial Growth Factor

Vascular remodeling with cellular proliferation is most apparent at plexiform lesions. These histologic lesions are unique to PAH (WHO Group 1). They are composed of proliferating and apoptosis-resistant ECs and other cellular components which have been debated to be myofibroblasts, SMCs, or undifferentiated mesenchymal cells [98]. Within plexiform lesions expression of vascular endothelial growth factor (VEGF), its receptor (VEGFR), HIF-1α, and other remodeling genes are increased [101–103]. VEGF is also increased in plasma samples from subjects with IPAH compared to controls [104]. While VEGF and VEGFR are required for normal angiogenesis, they are also an exploited pathway of malignant-transformed cells. Given increased expression of VEGF and VEGFR within plexiform lesions a cancer paradigm of PAH developed, suggesting that excessive angiogenesis due to a molecular defect within a clone of cells leads to the clinically manifest disease. Preclinical research on VEGF signaling and PH has given conflicting data and has not yet arrived at a therapeutic modality. Experimental overexpression of VEGF is protective in some PH models [105, 106]. Consistent with this, VEGFR inhibition via receptor blockade (with SU5416) in the chronic hypoxia model results in worsened PH and increased EC proliferation [107]. A different VEGF signaling inhibitor, the multikinase inhibitor sorafenib, reduces progression of established PH in monocrotaline-treated rats [108] and prevents PH development in rats exposed to chronic hypoxia and SU5416 [109]. Taken together, this indicates that VEGF signaling is important in vascular maintenance and interrupting the pathway can worsen pulmonary vascular disease phenotype. However, some downstream effects of VEGF signaling may ultimately be maladaptive. The complex relationship of VEGF signaling in pulmonary vascular disease animal models and varying results of treatment approaches has recently been reviewed [110]. Further study is needed in this intriguing area before clinical application can be developed for treatment of PAH.

Mitogens

Several mitogens have been evaluated in PAH including platelet-derived growth factor (PDGF), basic fibroblast growth factor (bFGF), and epidermal growth factor (EGF). While the precise function of PDGF in vivo is still somewhat of a question, it is known as a potent vascular SMC mitogen in vitro which also causes SMC and fibroblast migration. It has been implicated in the pathogenesis of multiple vascular and fibroproliferative diseases [111]. PDGF and its receptor (PDGFR) are increased in vessels of lung specimens from subjects with PAH [112, 113]. bFGF is another mitogen for ECs and vascular SMCs and has been found to be increased in patient samples [114] and overexpressed in patient-derived PA ECs. Interference of bFGF signaling via siRNA for bFGF reduces PASMC proliferation in vivo and in vitro [115]. EGF and TGF-α both activate EGFR and cause growth and vascular remodeling, a pathway exploited in some tumors and targeted pharmacologically. Overexpression of TGF-α leads to pulmonary vascular disease in mice through EGFR signaling [116], and EGFR is overexpressed in the monocrotaline PH model. Inhibition of this pathway is effective in vitro [117] and prevents development of monocrotaline-induced PH in rats, but is ineffective in a chronic hypoxia model [118]. In addition, EGFR expression is no different in clinical specimens of PAH patients versus controls [118]. EGF inhibition therefore has limited therapeutic promise.

Tyrosine Kinases

Many of the above substrates and receptors signal through tyrosine-kinase mechanisms. Multiple tyrosine-kinase inhibitors exist. One of the earliest, imatinib (Gleevec), has been studied in basic and clinical studies of PAH. Imatinib blocks PDGF-mediated PASMC proliferation. However, it does not mitigate the effects of many other known growth factors (VEGF, EGF, bFGF). In monocrotaline-treated or chronic hypoxic rats, imatinib improves pulmonary vascular disease via reduced downstream signaling of PDGF [113]. There are several clinical case reports of beneficial effect of treatment with imatinib (Gleevec) [119–121]. A small phase II study in PAH demonstrated a decline in PVR with imatinib compared to placebo [122]. A subsequent phase III study in PAH patients already on combination PAH therapy demonstrated improvement in 6-min walk distance and in PVR, but there was a greater incidence of hospitalization in the imatinib group and increased risk of cerebral hemorrhage in imatinib-treated patients who also were receiving warfarin therapy [123]. Other multi-targeted tyrosine kinase inhibitors have been considered in PAH, but predicting their clinical effects and avoiding off-target effects remain of concern. The importance of such considerations is exemplified by the finding that dasatinib can cause pulmonary hypertension and pleural effusions in patients being treated for malignancy [124]. These issues are discussed further in Chap. 17.

TGF-β Signaling

As discussed previously, mutations in the gene encoding BMPR2 are the genetic basis of disease in most cases of familial and many cases of sporadic PAH [1, 11, 12]. The TGF-β family of receptors including BMPR2 is highly evolutionarily conserved.

BMPR2 is required for embryogenesis and alteration of signals downstream of BMPR2 result in defects in angiogenesis [125]. BMP signaling has been studied extensively since the discovery of a link between *BMPR2* mutation and PAH. The major downstream pathways of BMPR2 include (1) Smad1/5/8 which signals through the common Smad2 transcription factor, (2) $p38^{MAPK}$ and Erk1/2, (3) Src, and (4) LIMK, among others. Smad 1/5/8 signaling is facilitated by cGMP activation of PKG. Activated PKGI binds to and phosphorylates BMPR2. In response to ligand binding, PKG1 detaches from BMPR2 and associates with activated Smads and then translocates to the nucleus where it regulates transcription as a nuclear cofactor for Smads [126]. Recent studies demonstrate that Smad signaling is impaired in mice with reduced PKG expression and activation of PKG by cGMP improves Smad signaling in a rat model of PAH [127].

The cellular effects of BMP stimulation and its disruption are dependent on cell type. It is helpful to review the effects of normal and abnormal BMP signaling in SMCs and ECs separately.

In proximal PASMCs, BMP inhibits proliferation, and promotes apoptosis and SMC phenotype differentiation [128–130]. Peripheral PASMCs may have a different response to BMP stimulation, responding with proliferation [130]. BMP's effect on control of proliferation is mediated through Smad signaling [128, 130]. Subjects with IPAH have less Smad1 activation than controls and unchanged $p38^{MAPK}$/Erk activation, resulting in an unopposed proliferative stimulus [128, 130].

In contrast to the predominant effect on PASMCs, BMPR2 activation in endothelial cells promotes survival, proliferation, and migration [131, 132]. This effect is also mediated through Smad signaling. *BMPR2* gene silencing results in EC apoptosis and makes the endothelium susceptible to damage. In vivo, this loss of endothelial integrity may allow PASMCs to be exposed to serum growth factors and proliferate in the absence of BMPR2-mediated growth regulation. In addition, increased endothelial apoptosis may select for apoptosis-resistant clones which have been demonstrated in plexiform lesions of PAH subjects [98].

Notch Signaling

The Notch family of receptors are single transmembrane proteins which bind to ligands on the surface of adjacent cells. Upon this stimulus, the intracellular portion of Notch is cleaved and translocates to the nucleus where it acts as a transcription factor. Notch ligands are primarily expressed on ECs and the receptors allow cell-cell communication affecting vascular development [133]. There are four known Notch receptors (Notch1–4). Notch3 is expressed only in arterial vascular SMCs and is crucial for development of normal arterial morphology, as evidenced by the study of Notch3-null mice which lack a normal arterial muscular layer [134, 135]. Notch3 overexpression results in vascular SMC proliferation that continues post-confluence in vitro [136]. Li et al. [137] have studied the association of Notch3 and PAH in both humans and animal models, finding increased expression at an mRNA and protein level as well as increased HES-5, a downstream effector. Inhibition of this pathway is protective in the chronic hypoxic PH model. Notch is also known to interact with other pertinent signaling pathways including Smad1, HIF-1α, and VEGF [133, 138].

The components of the vessel wall are under constant stress and appropriate regulation of proliferation, migration, and apoptosis are required to maintain homeostasis in health and under insults of disease. Cellular regulation of these processes is complex and varies not only by cell type, but also by tissue bed. VEGF, VEGFR, BMPR2, and Notch are required for formation of normal vessels during development. When injury to the vascular wall occurs, autocrine and paracrine signals such as VEGF, ET-1, PDGF, EGF, 5-HT, and BMP (and likely many others) respond to direct cellular response. Dysregulation of these adaptive signals in PAH subjects leads to abnormal PASMC and EC proliferation. The number of PAH therapies that target these pathways is minimal. A greater molecular understanding of the intricate balance of this proproliferative/antiproliferative balance has been attained in the last two decades, but research is ongoing and translation to clinical care is still needed.

Inflammation and Infection

Within WHO Group 1, there is a subset of patients with associated inflammatory, immune, or infectious conditions known to result in pulmonary vascular disease [139]. The most common of these are the connective diseases (CTD) and infectious diseases HIV and schistosomiasis. The study of pulmonary vascular disease associated with these diseases has uncovered links with inflammation and immunity. At the same time, study of patients with IPAH and HPAH has also revealed elements of dysregulated inflammation. Thus, there appears to be a strong influence of the immune system on pulmonary vascular disease onset and progression.

Pulmonary hypertension is a frequent manifestation of multiple autoimmune conditions [139] with systemic sclerosis being the most common. Up to 12–40 % of patients with systemic sclerosis will develop PAH and this complication portends a poor prognosis [140, 141]. Systemic sclerosis and other CTDs are characterized by circulating autoantibodies, and clinical evaluation for these conditions is indicated in a patient with newly diagnosed PAH. Study of patients with IPAH has also revealed the presence of autoantibodies, primarily anti-Ku, which in one study was found in 23 % of presumed IPAH patients. Raynaud's phenomenon, a common feature of systemic sclerosis, was frequently seen (39 %) in the same study [142].

Inflammation is a prominent feature of the pathology of pulmonary vascular disease. Pathologic review of several cohorts has demonstrated B- and T-lymphocytes (CD8+ and CD4+), macrophages, mast cells, and dendritic cells concentrated near areas of vascular remodeling [143–145]. Subjects with IPAH have increased circulating regulatory T-cells compared with subjects with CTEPH or normal controls but lower numbers of them in lung specimens [144–146]. There may also be alterations in natural killer (NK) cell population and function [147]. Any of these changes in circulating immune cell populations may result in altered cytokine response and inadequate control of immune activation manifested in the pulmonary vascular bed. In fact, multiple cytokines are known to be increased in PAH [148–150]. IL-6 levels are increased, correlate with clinical outcome, and do so better than hemodynamics or 6-min walk distance in some studies [149, 150]. Injection of IL-6 [151] or IL-6 overexpression [152] in mice results in PH, and knockout of IL-6 is protective against chronic hypoxic PH [153]. CX_3CL1 (also known as fractalkine) and its soluble receptor (CX_3CR1) are increased in the plasma and pulmonary endothelium of subjects with IPAH. CX_3CL1 and CCL2 expression are elevated in plasma and in pulmonary ECs of PAH patients compared to controls. These chemokines increase leukocyte adhesion to ECs, further propagating perivascular inflammation. Increased cytokine production may be a central component of PAH but its temporal relation to disease development is uncertain.

Some infectious diseases are causally related to PAH development. In the USA, HIV is the most common, whereas schistosomiasis may be the most common cause of PAH worldwide. Up to 1 in 200 AIDS patients will develop PAH, meaning that HIV patients have up to a 600-fold higher incidence of PAH than the general population; [154, 155]. These patients have plexiform lesions indistinguishable from those seen in IPAH. However, the HIV virus has not itself been identified in pulmonary vessels [156, 157]. Indirect effects of HIV infection, either mediated by immune dysregulation or viral proteins, are proposed as mechanisms of pulmonary vascular disease. Several pertinent HIV proteins have been implicated, the most studied being the protein Nef. The predominant animal model of HIV, simian immunodeficiency virus (SIV)-infected macaques, has a low penetrance of pulmonary vascular disease. When infected with a chimeric HIV-SIV virus containing HIV Nef, they develop plexiform lesions containing Nef [158]. Nef, which has a soluble form, can enter non-HIV-infected cells via the chemokine receptor, CXCR4. In addition to lymphocytes, CXCR4 is present on ECs and may allow entry of Nef without direct infection of ECs by HIV virus [159]. Indeed, Nef has been demonstrated in pulmonary ECs of HIV-associated PAH subjects [150]. Nef increases IL-6 expression and multiple proproliferative signals including $p38^{MAPK}$ [155] which could promote PH development. More recently, study of the HIV envelope protein (Env) using SHIV-*env* in macaques also showed increased pulmonary vascular lesions in those animals compared to SIV-infected animals [160]. Exogenous Env protein has been shown to induce endothelial cell ET-1 expression. It is uncertain if this or another mechanism may underlie its role in HIV-associated PAH development. HIV proteins gp120 and Tat affect pulmonary ECs in vitro and could play a role, but data is preliminary [161, 162].

HHV-8 is a gamma-herpesvirus associated with Kaposi's sarcoma which is a proliferative vascular lesion seen in patients with HIV infection. HHV-8 encodes a protein similar to IL-6 which induces VEGF expression explaining its disease manifestation. One group reported HHV-8 detected in lung specimens of 10 of 16 patients with IPAH and none of a matched secondary PAH cohort [163]. Since this study, multiple groups have failed to identify HHV-8 infection in various PAH cohorts [164–168]. As it stands, HHV-8 is felt to be unlikely to cause pulmonary vascular disease on its own.

Schistosomiasis is rare in the USA, but probably the most common cause of PAH worldwide. In chronic infections, endemic *Schistosoma* blood flukes reside in the mesenteric venous system and shed eggs and antigens causing an intense granulomatous reaction. This results in periportal fibrosis and portal hypertension, a syndrome known as hepatosplenic schistosomiasis [169, 170]. Hepatosplenic schistosomiasis precedes pulmonary vascular disease development, but the stepwise progression is uncertain. Regardless of cause, the histology is similar to that of other forms of PAH [171]. Mechanistic studies of PAH secondary to schistosomiasis are limited. One study of lung specimens from subjects with schistosomiasis and PAH failed to demonstrate the presence of egg antigens in pulmonary vessels, but it is uncertain whether antihelmenthic treatments may have eliminated their parasite burden [169, 171, 172]. Intense inflammation in this disorder may result in early pulmonary vascular changes and with continued immune activation, progression to an irreversible vasculopathy of the pulmonary bed. IL-13 has recently been implicated as a mediator of pulmonary vascular disease in schistosomiasis-associated PAH [173]. Schistosomiasis-associated PH is further discussed in Chap. 7.

Thrombosis and Hypercoagulability

Thrombosis has been a proposed central mediator or pulmonary vascular disease for decades. Pulmonary vascular thrombosis and thrombotic arteriopathy are common pathologic findings of PAH, found in 30–56 % of specimens [43, 174–176]. While incomplete evaluation for CTEPH in some studies may reduce the true incidence of thrombotic lesions, it is clear that many subjects with IPAH have some degree of pulmonary vascular thrombosis. Similar thrombotic lesions have been demonstrated in patients with congenital heart disease complicated by PAH, portopulmonary hypertension, and aminorex use [177]. These lesions are described as eccentric with post-thrombotic intimal fibrosis and recanalization. These changes are felt to be the same whether the cause was embolus or in situ thrombus formation [42, 178]. Much debate exists as to whether these real pathologic findings are an epiphenomenon of pulmonary vascular disease or rather a true contributor to disease development and/or progression.

In addition to circulating coagulation factors, the endothelium and its interaction with platelets are integral components of both prothrombotic and antithrombotic pathways [177]. While characterized inherited hypercoagulable states are no more common in patients with PAH or CTEPH than the general population [179], multiple studies demonstrate abnormalities in the prothrombotic and antithrombotic systems. In general, the pro/antithrombotic balance is tipped in favor of coagulation. Circulating von Willebrand factor (vWF) is increased in all forms of PAH [180], but its function may be reduced due to alterations of vWF multimer distribution [177, 180–182]. High shear stress in the pulmonary vasculature may contribute to depletion of high-molecular-weight multimers of vWF in PAH, akin to what occurs in the setting of left ventricular assist devices. vWF abnormalities due to endothelial dysfunction may promote platelet dysfunction and release of multiple mediators. For example, patients with IPAH have higher urinary thromboxane metabolites [61] and plasma 5-HT [83, 84]. Markers of thrombin action and fibrin formation (d-dimers, fibrinopeptide A, fibrin degradation products) are also elevated, but so are the anticoagulant/fibrinolytic factors such as thrombomodulin, tissue factor pathway inhibitor, and PAI-1, a fibrinolytic inhibitor [180, 183, 184].

Control of hemostasis is a complex, highly regulated system. The endothelium is a central component of this system and must balance both constant free-flowing blood and the possibility of endothelial disruption. Multiple lines of evidence suggest that pulmonary vascular disease, especially IPAH or HPAH, demonstrate multiple abnormalities of these systems which may lead to a procoagulant phenotype. Circumstantial evidence that anticoagulation may be beneficial in patients with PAH [185, 186] suggests that a procoagulant phenotype may at least play a role in continued or worsening pulmonary vascular disease.

Endocrine Factors

Rising rates of obesity and metabolic disease in the developed world coupled with recent registry data showing high rates of obesity in PAH [187] has brought intense interest into how endocrine factors may affect the pulmonary vasculature. The first observations were of high incidence of insulin resistance and glucose intolerance in subjects with PAH [188, 189], but other data has recently suggested that dyslipidemia may also play a role [190]. Animal models of PAH have been used to help define if these endocrine factors may play a role in disease promotion. Animal models of obesity, such as adiponectin-deficient mice and ApoE knockout mice, spontaneously develop PH [191, 192]. Moreover, pulmonary vascular disease is reversed by peroxisome proliferator activator receptor gamma (PPARγ) activation with rosiglitazone. BMPR2 signaling has been shown to be a key downregulator of PPARγ-mediated transcription and likely plays a role in promotion of insulin resistance in PAH [193]. Recently, we have demonstrated that in a model of HPAH using transgenic overexpression of mutant BMPR2, insulin resistance is present and worsened insulin resistance through a high-fat diet results in increased pulmonary vascular disease [194]. How insulin signaling is modified by *BMPR2* mutation is currently under investigation, and it is presently unknown if reversing insulin resistance in humans with PAH may be a therapeutic option for this disease.

Other endocrine factors, such as estrogen signaling, are also implicated in PAH. The impressive female predominance in PAH has led to the hypothesis that estrogen may promote PAH development [2, 3, 195]. While there is extensive data in chronic hypoxic and monocrotaline models that estrogen and its metabolite 2-methoxyestradiol attenuate PH [196–200], these findings have not been replicated in human specimens or transgenic models of PAH. Indeed, there is growing evidence that estrogen may worsen pulmonary vascular disease in certain animal models that may more closely recapitulate human disease [80, 201–203]. At the same time, recent studies suggest that in patients with PAH, female sex is associated with better right ventricular ejection fraction, cardiac index, and pulmonary hemodynamics than male sex [204–206] and that estrogen and its metabolites may improve right ventricular function in healthy patients and those with cardiovascular diseases [207]. These findings may explain the better overall survival in women than in men with PAH [208]. Further study is needed to reconcile the potentially beneficial effects of estrogens in some animal models with detrimental effects in others and the female predominance of PAH in human disease.

Conclusion

In summary, there are many signaling cascades, exposures, and molecules implicated in PAH development and promotion. While advances have been made in developing successful drug therapy for this disease, none has resulted in a cure. Unfortunately, we do not understand the critical initiating event in PAH, nor how to interrupt it. Another unknown is whether human pulmonary vascular disease is reversible once established. These fundamental questions will need to be answered before curative or disease-altering therapy is available to patients with this devastating disease.

References

1. Fessel JP, Loyd JE, Austin ED. The genetics of pulmonary arterial hypertension in the post-BMPR2 era. Pulm Circ. 2011;1(3):305–19. PubMed PMID: 22140620, Pubmed Central PMCID: PMC3224422.
2. Humbert M, Sitbon O, Chaouat A, Bertocchi M, Habib G, Gressin V, et al. Pulmonary arterial hypertension in France: results from a national registry. Am J Respir Crit Care Med. 2006;173(9):1023–30. PubMed PMID: 16456139.
3. Badesch DB, Raskob GE, Elliott CG, Krichman AM, Farber HW, Frost AE, et al. Pulmonary arterial hypertension: baseline characteristics from the REVEAL Registry. Chest. 2010; 137(2):376–87. PubMed PMID: 19837821.
4. Larkin EK, Newman JH, Austin ED, Hemnes AR, Wheeler L, Robbins IM, et al. Longitudinal analysis casts doubt on the presence of genetic anticipation in heritable pulmonary arterial hypertension. Am J Respir Crit Care Med. 2012;186:892. PubMed PMID: 22923661.
5. Rich S, Dantzker DR, Ayres SM, Bergofsky EH, Brundage BH, Detre KM, et al. Primary pulmonary hypertension. A national prospective study. Ann Intern Med. 1987;107(2):216–23. PubMed PMID: 3605900.
6. Loyd JE, Primm RK, Newman JH. Familial primary pulmonary hypertension: clinical patterns. Am Rev Respir Dis. 1984;129(1):194–7. PubMed PMID: 6703480.
7. Morse JH, Jones AC, Barst RJ, Hodge SE, Wilhelmsen KC, Nygaard TG. Mapping of familial primary pulmonary hypertension locus (PPH1) to chromosome 2q31-q32. Circulation. 1997;95(12):2603–6. PubMed PMID: 9193425.

8. Nichols WC, Koller DL, Slovis B, Foroud T, Terry VH, Arnold ND, et al. Localization of the gene for familial primary pulmonary hypertension to chromosome 2q31-32. Nat Genet. 1997;15(3):277–80. PubMed PMID: 9054941.
9. Machado RD, Pauciulo MW, Fretwell N, Veal C, Thomson JR, Vilarino Guell C, et al. A physical and transcript map based upon refinement of the critical interval for PPH1, a gene for familial primary pulmonary hypertension. The International PPH Consortium. Genomics. 2000;68(2):220–8. PubMed PMID: 10964520.
10. Deng Z, Haghighi F, Helleby L, Vanterpool K, Horn EM, Barst RJ, et al. Fine mapping of PPH1, a gene for familial primary pulmonary hypertension, to a 3-cM region on chromosome 2q33. Am J Respir Crit Care Med. 2000;161(3 Pt 1):1055–9. PubMed PMID: 10712363.
11. Lane KB, Machado RD, Pauciulo MW, Thomson JR, Phillips 3rd JA, Loyd JE, et al. Heterozygous germline mutations in BMPR2, encoding a TGF-beta receptor, cause familial primary pulmonary hypertension. Nat Genet. 2000;26(1):81–4. PubMed PMID: 10973254.
12. Deng Z, Morse JH, Slager SL, Cuervo N, Moore KJ, Venetos G, et al. Familial primary pulmonary hypertension (gene PPH1) is caused by mutations in the bone morphogenetic protein receptor-II gene. Am J Hum Genet. 2000;67(3):737–44. PubMed PMID: 10903931, Pubmed Central PMCID: PMC1287532.
13. Newman JH, Wheeler L, Lane KB, Loyd E, Gaddipati R, Phillips 3rd JA, et al. Mutation in the gene for bone morphogenetic protein receptor II as a cause of primary pulmonary hypertension in a large kindred. N Engl J Med. 2001;345(5):319–24. PubMed PMID: 11484688.
14. Thomson JR, Machado RD, Pauciulo MW, Morgan NV, Humbert M, Elliott GC, et al. Sporadic primary pulmonary hypertension is associated with germline mutations of the gene encoding BMPR-II, a receptor member of the TGF-beta family. J Med Genet. 2000;37(10):741–5. PubMed PMID: 11015450, Pubmed Central PMCID: PMC1757155.
15. Machado RD, Aldred MA, James V, Harrison RE, Patel B, Schwalbe EC, et al. Mutations of the TGF-beta type II receptor BMPR2 in pulmonary arterial hypertension. Hum Mutat. 2006;27(2):121–32. PubMed PMID: 16429395.
16. Aldred MA, Vijayakrishnan J, James V, Soubrier F, Gomez-Sanchez MA, Martensson G, et al. BMPR2 gene rearrangements account for a significant proportion of mutations in familial and idiopathic pulmonary arterial hypertension. Hum Mutat. 2006;27(2):212–3. PubMed PMID: 16429403.
17. Cogan JD, Pauciulo MW, Batchman AP, Prince MA, Robbins IM, Hedges LK, et al. High frequency of BMPR2 exonic deletions/duplications in familial pulmonary arterial hypertension. Am J Respir Crit Care Med. 2006;174(5):590–8. PubMed PMID: 16728714, Pubmed Central PMCID: 2648061.
18. Zeng S, Chen J, Shen H. Controlling of bone morphogenetic protein signaling. Cell Signal. 2010;22(6):888–93. PubMed PMID: 20060893.
19. Machado RD, Eickelberg O, Elliott CG, Geraci MW, Hanaoka M, Loyd JE, et al. Genetics and genomics of pulmonary arterial hypertension. J Am Coll Cardiol. 2009;54(1 Suppl): S32–42. PubMed PMID: 19555857.
20. West J. Cross talk between Smad, MAPK, and actin in the etiology of pulmonary arterial hypertension. Adv Exp Med Biol. 2010;661:265–78. PubMed PMID: 20204735.
21. Morrell NW. Role of bone morphogenetic protein receptors in the development of pulmonary arterial hypertension. Adv Exp Med Biol. 2010;661:251–64. PubMed PMID: 20204735.
22. Machado RD, Pauciulo MW, Thomson JR, Lane KB, Morgan NV, Wheeler L, et al. BMPR2 haploinsufficiency as the inherited molecular mechanism for primary pulmonary hypertension. Am J Hum Genet. 2001;68(1):92–102. PubMed PMID: 11115378, Pubmed Central PMCID: PMC1234937.
23. Austin ED, Cogan JD, West JD, Hedges LK, Hamid R, Dawson EP, et al. Alterations in oestrogen metabolism: implications for higher penetrance of familial pulmonary arterial hypertension in females. Eur Respir J. 2009;34(5):1093–9. PubMed PMID: 19357154.
24. Cogan J, Austin E, Hedges L, Womack B, West J, Loyd J, et al. Role of BMPR2 alternative splicing in HPAH penetrance. Circulation. 2012;126:1907. PubMed PMID: 22923426.

25. Atkinson C, Stewart S, Upton PD, Machado R, Thomson JR, Trembath RC, et al. Primary pulmonary hypertension is associated with reduced pulmonary vascular expression of type II bone morphogenetic protein receptor. Circulation. 2002;105(14):1672–8. PubMed PMID: 11940546.
26. Johnson JA, Hemnes AR, Perrien DS, Schuster M, Robinson LJ, Gladson S, et al. Cytoskeletal defects in Bmpr2-associated pulmonary arterial hypertension. Am J Physiol Lung Cell Mol Physiol. 2012;302(5):L474–84. PubMed PMID: 22180660, Pubmed Central PMCID: PMC3311512.
27. Johnson DW, Berg JN, Baldwin MA, Gallione CJ, Marondel I, Yoon SJ, et al. Mutations in the activin receptor-like kinase 1 gene in hereditary haemorrhagic telangiectasia type 2. Nat Genet. 1996;13(2):189–95. PubMed PMID: 8640225.
28. McAllister KA, Grogg KM, Johnson DW, Gallione CJ, Baldwin MA, Jackson CE, et al. Endoglin, a TGF-beta binding protein of endothelial cells, is the gene for hereditary haemorrhagic telangiectasia type 1. Nat Genet. 1994;8(4):345–51. PubMed PMID: 7894484.
29. Harrison RE, Flanagan JA, Sankelo M, Abdalla SA, Rowell J, Machado RD, et al. Molecular and functional analysis identifies ALK-1 as the predominant cause of pulmonary hypertension related to hereditary haemorrhagic telangiectasia. J Med Genet. 2003;40(12):865–71. PubMed PMID: 14684682, Pubmed Central PMCID: PMC1735342.
30. Trell E, Johansson BW, Linell F, Ripa J. Familial pulmonary hypertension and multiple abnormalities of large systemic arteries in Osler's disease. Am J Med. 1972;53(1):50–63. PubMed PMID: 5037289.
31. Trembath RC, Thomson JR, Machado RD, Morgan NV, Atkinson C, Winship I, et al. Clinical and molecular genetic features of pulmonary hypertension in patients with hereditary hemorrhagic telangiectasia. N Engl J Med. 2001;345(5):325–34. PubMed PMID: 11484689.
32. Chaouat A, Coulet F, Favre C, Simonneau G, Weitzenblum E, Soubrier F, et al. Endoglin germline mutation in a patient with hereditary haemorrhagic telangiectasia and dexfenfluramine associated pulmonary arterial hypertension. Thorax. 2004;59(5):446–8. PubMed PMID: 15115879, Pubmed Central PMCID: PMC1746994.
33. Harrison RE, Berger R, Haworth SG, Tulloh R, Mache CJ, Morrell NW, et al. Transforming growth factor-beta receptor mutations and pulmonary arterial hypertension in childhood. Circulation. 2005;111(4):435–41. PubMed PMID: 15687131.
34. Austin ED, Ma L, LeDuc C, Berman Rosenzweig E, Borczuk A, Phillips 3rd JA, et al. Whole exome sequencing to identify a novel gene (caveolin-1) associated with human pulmonary arterial hypertension. Circ Cardiovasc Genet. 2012;5(3):336–43. PubMed PMID: 22474227, Pubmed Central PMCID: PMC3380156.
35. Bucci M, et al. In vivo delivery of the caveolin-1 scaffolding domain inhibits nitric oxide synthesis and reduces inflammation. Nat Med. 2000;6:1362–7.
36. Michel JB, Feron O, Sacks D, Michel T. Reciprocal regulation of endothelial nitric oxide synthase by Ca2+-calmodulin and caveolin. J Biol Chem. 1997;272:15583–6.
37. Zhao YY, Zhao YD, Mirza MK, Huang JH, Potula HH, Vogel SM, Brovkovych V, Yuan JX, Wharton J, Malik AB. Persistent eNOS activation secondary to caveolin-1 deficiency induces pulmonary hypertension in mice and humans through PKG nitration. J Clin Invest. 2009; 119(7):2009–18.
38. Cruz JA, Bauer EM, Rodriguez AI, Gangopadhyay A, Zeineh NS, Wang Y, et al. Chronic hypoxia induces right heart failure in caveolin-1-/- mice. Am J Physiol Heart Circ Physiol. 2012;302(12):H2518–27. PubMed PMID: 22505641, Pubmed Central PMCID: PMC3378264.
39. Wertz JW, Bauer PM. Caveolin-1 regulates BMPRII localization and signaling in vascular smooth muscle cells. Biochem Biophys Res Commun. 2008;375(4):557–61. PubMed PMID: 18725205.
40. Zhao YY, Liu Y, Stan RV, Fan L, Gu Y, Dalton N, et al. Defects in caveolin-1 cause dilated cardiomyopathy and pulmonary hypertension in knockout mice. Proc Natl Acad Sci U S A. 2002;99(17):11375–80. PubMed PMID: 12177436, Pubmed Central PMCID: PMC123264.

41. Newman JH, Ross JC. Primary pulmonary hypertension: a look at the future. J Am Coll Cardiol. 1989;14(3):551–5. PubMed PMID: 2671094.
42. Heath D, Edwards JE. The pathology of hypertensive pulmonary vascular disease; a description of six grades of structural changes in the pulmonary arteries with special reference to congenital cardiac septal defects. Circulation. 1958;18(4 Part 1):533–47. PubMed PMID: 13573570.
43. Pietra GG, Edwards WD, Kay JM, Rich S, Kernis J, Schloo B, et al. Histopathology of primary pulmonary hypertension. A qualitative and quantitative study of pulmonary blood vessels from 58 patients in the National Heart, Lung, and Blood Institute, Primary Pulmonary Hypertension Registry. Circulation. 1989;80(5):1198–206. PubMed PMID: 2805258.
44. Harris P. Influence of acetylcholine on the pulmonary arterial pressure. Br Heart J. 1957;19(2):272–8. PubMed PMID: 13413015, Pubmed Central PMCID: 479625.
45. Wood P, Besterman EM, Towers MK, McIlroy MB. The effect of acetylcholine on pulmonary vascular resistance and left atrial pressure in mitral stenosis. Br Heart J. 1957;19(2):279–86. PubMed PMID: 13413016, Pubmed Central PMCID: 479626.
46. Wood P. Pulmonary hypertension with special reference to the vasoconstrictive factor. Br Heart J. 1958;20(4):557–70. PubMed PMID: 13584643, Pubmed Central PMCID: 491807.
47. Palmer RM, Ferrige AG, Moncada S. Nitric oxide release accounts for the biological activity of endothelium-derived relaxing factor. Nature. 1987;327(6122):524–6. PubMed PMID: 3495737.
48. Furchgott RF, Zawadzki JV. The obligatory role of endothelial cells in the relaxation of arterial smooth muscle by acetylcholine. Nature. 1980;288(5789):373–6. PubMed PMID: 6253831.
49. Dinh-Xuan AT, Higenbottam TW, Clelland CA, Pepke-Zaba J, Cremona G, Butt AY, et al. Impairment of endothelium-dependent pulmonary-artery relaxation in chronic obstructive lung disease. N Engl J Med. 1991;324(22):1539–47. PubMed PMID: 2027358.
50. Dinh Xuan AT, Higenbottam TW, Clelland C, Pepke-Zaba J, Cremona G, Wallwork J. Impairment of pulmonary endothelium-dependent relaxation in patients with Eisenmenger's syndrome. Br J Pharmacol. 1990;99(1):9–10. PubMed PMID: 2331577, Pubmed Central PMCID: 1917494.
51. Pepke-Zaba J, Higenbottam TW, Dinh-Xuan AT, Stone D, Wallwork J. Inhaled nitric oxide as a cause of selective pulmonary vasodilatation in pulmonary hypertension. Lancet. 1991; 338(8776):1173–4. PubMed PMID: 1682593.
52. Giaid A, Saleh D. Reduced expression of endothelial nitric oxide synthase in the lungs of patients with pulmonary hypertension. N Engl J Med. 1995;333(4):214–21. PubMed PMID: 7540722.
53. Pullamsetti S, Kiss L, Ghofrani HA, Voswinckel R, Haredza P, Klepetko W, et al. Increased levels and reduced catabolism of asymmetric and symmetric dimethylarginines in pulmonary hypertension. FASEB J. 2005;19(9):1175–7. PubMed PMID: 15827267.
54. Weimann J, Ullrich R, Hromi J, Fujino Y, Clark MW, Bloch KD, et al. Sildenafil is a pulmonary vasodilator in awake lambs with acute pulmonary hypertension. Anesthesiology. 2000;92(6):1702–12. PubMed PMID: 10839922.
55. Prasad S, Wilkinson J, Gatzoulis MA. Sildenafil in primary pulmonary hypertension. N Engl J Med. 2000;343(18):1342. PubMed PMID: 11183578.
56. Wilkens H, Guth A, Konig J, Forestier N, Cremers B, Hennen B, et al. Effect of inhaled iloprost plus oral sildenafil in patients with primary pulmonary hypertension. Circulation. 2001;104(11):1218–22. PubMed PMID: 11551870.
57. Nagaya N, Uematsu M, Oya H, Sato N, Sakamaki F, Kyotani S, et al. Short-term oral administration of L-arginine improves hemodynamics and exercise capacity in patients with precapillary pulmonary hypertension. Am J Respir Crit Care Med. 2001;163(4):887–91. PubMed PMID: 11282761.
58. Mehta S, Stewart DJ, Langleben D, Levy RD. Short-term pulmonary vasodilation with L-arginine in pulmonary hypertension. Circulation. 1995;92(6):1539–45. PubMed PMID: 7664438.

59. Rubin LJ, Groves BM, Reeves JT, Frosolono M, Handel F, Cato AE. Prostacyclin-induced acute pulmonary vasodilation in primary pulmonary hypertension. Circulation. 1982; 66(2):334–8. PubMed PMID: 7046988.
60. Rubin LJ, Mendoza J, Hood M, McGoon M, Barst R, Williams WB, et al. Treatment of primary pulmonary hypertension with continuous intravenous prostacyclin (epoprostenol). Results of a randomized trial. Ann Intern Med. 1990;112(7):485–91. PubMed PMID: 2107780.
61. Christman BW, McPherson CD, Newman JH, King GA, Bernard GR, Groves BM, et al. An imbalance between the excretion of thromboxane and prostacyclin metabolites in pulmonary hypertension. N Engl J Med. 1992;327(2):70–5. PubMed PMID: 1603138.
62. Davie N, Haleen SJ, Upton PD, Polak JM, Yacoub MH, Morrell NW, et al. ET(A) and ET(B) receptors modulate the proliferation of human pulmonary artery smooth muscle cells. Am J Respir Crit Care Med. 2002;165(3):398–405. PubMed PMID: 11818328.
63. Yanagisawa M, Kurihara H, Kimura S, Tomobe Y, Kobayashi M, Mitsui Y, et al. A novel potent vasoconstrictor peptide produced by vascular endothelial cells. Nature. 1988; 332(6163):411–5. PubMed PMID: 2451132.
64. Ryan US, Glassberg MK, Nolop KB. Endothelin-1 from pulmonary artery and microvessels acts on vascular and airway smooth muscle. J Cardiovasc Pharmacol. 1989;13 Suppl 5:S57–62. discussion S74, PubMed PMID: 2473329.
65. Lippton HL, Hauth TA, Summer WR, Hyman AL. Endothelin produces pulmonary vasoconstriction and systemic vasodilation. J Appl Physiol. 1989;66(2):1008–12. PubMed PMID: 2565328.
66. Zamora MA, Dempsey EC, Walchak SJ, Stelzner TJ. BQ123, an ETA receptor antagonist, inhibits endothelin-1-mediated proliferation of human pulmonary artery smooth muscle cells. Am J Respir Cell Mol Biol. 1993;9(4):429–33. PubMed PMID: 8398181.
67. Sitbon O, Badesch DB, Channick RN, Frost A, Robbins IM, Simonneau G, et al. Effects of the dual endothelin receptor antagonist bosentan in patients with pulmonary arterial hypertension: a 1-year follow-up study. Chest. 2003;124(1):247–54. PubMed PMID: 12853530.
68. McLaughlin VV, Sitbon O, Badesch DB, Barst RJ, Black C, Galie N, et al. Survival with first-line bosentan in patients with primary pulmonary hypertension. Eur Respir J. 2005; 25(2):244–9. PubMed PMID: 15684287.
69. Rubin LJ, Badesch DB, Barst RJ, Galie N, Black CM, Keogh A, et al. Bosentan therapy for pulmonary arterial hypertension. N Engl J Med. 2002;346(12):896–903. PubMed PMID: 11907289.
70. Channick RN, Simonneau G, Sitbon O, Robbins IM, Frost A, Tapson VF, et al. Effects of the dual endothelin-receptor antagonist bosentan in patients with pulmonary hypertension: a randomised placebo-controlled study. Lancet. 2001;358(9288):1119–23. PubMed PMID: 11597664.
71. Liu C, Chen J. Endothelin receptor antagonists for pulmonary arterial hypertension. Cochrane Database Syst Rev. 2006;(3):CD004434. PubMed PMID: 16856046
72. Cacoub P, Dorent R, Maistre G, Nataf P, Carayon A, Piette C, et al. Endothelin-1 in primary pulmonary hypertension and the Eisenmenger syndrome. Am J Cardiol. 1993;71(5):448–50. PubMed PMID: 8430638.
73. Stewart DJ, Levy RD, Cernacek P, Langleben D. Increased plasma endothelin-1 in pulmonary hypertension: marker or mediator of disease? Ann Intern Med. 1991;114(6):464–9. PubMed PMID: 1994793.
74. Cacoub P, Dorent R, Nataf P, Carayon A. Endothelin-1 in pulmonary hypertension. N Engl J Med. 1993;329(26):1967–8. PubMed PMID: 8247067.
75. Giaid A, Yanagisawa M, Langleben D, Michel RP, Levy R, Shennib H, et al. Expression of endothelin-1 in the lungs of patients with pulmonary hypertension. N Engl J Med. 1993;328(24):1732–9. PubMed PMID: 8497283.
76. Abenhaim L, Moride Y, Brenot F, Rich S, Benichou J, Kurz X, et al. Appetite-suppressant drugs and the risk of primary pulmonary hypertension. International Primary Pulmonary Hypertension Study Group. N Engl J Med. 1996;335(9):609–16. PubMed PMID: 8692238.

77. Douglas JG, Munro JF, Kitchin AH, Muir AL, Proudfoot AT. Pulmonary hypertension and fenfluramine. Br Med J (Clin Res Ed). 1981;283(6296):881–3. PubMed PMID: 6793158, Pubmed Central PMCID: PMC1507127.
78. Kay JM, Smith P, Heath D. Aminorex and the pulmonary circulation. Thorax. 1971;26(3): 262–70. PubMed PMID: 5089490, Pubmed Central PMCID: PMC1019080.
79. Fishman AP. Aminorex to fen/phen: an epidemic foretold. Circulation. 1999;99(1):156–61. PubMed PMID: 9884392.
80. McGoon MD, Vanhoutte PM. Aggregating platelets contract isolated canine pulmonary arteries by releasing 5-hydroxytryptamine. J Clin Invest. 1984;74(3):828–33. PubMed PMID: 6470141, Pubmed Central PMCID: PMC425237.
81. Nemecek GM, Coughlin SR, Handley DA, Moskowitz MA. Stimulation of aortic smooth muscle cell mitogenesis by serotonin. Proc Natl Acad Sci U S A. 1986;83(3):674–8. PubMed PMID: 3456163, Pubmed Central PMCID: PMC322926.
82. Eddahibi S, Adnot S. Anorexigen-induced pulmonary hypertension and the serotonin (5-HT) hypothesis: lessons for the future in pathogenesis. Respir Res. 2002;3:9. PubMed PMID: 11806844, Pubmed Central PMCID: PMC64820.
83. Maclean MR, Dempsie Y. The serotonin hypothesis of pulmonary hypertension revisited. Adv Exp Med Biol. 2010;661:309–22. PubMed PMID: 20204739.
84. Herve P, Launay JM, Scrobohaci ML, Brenot F, Simonneau G, Petitpretz P, et al. Increased plasma serotonin in primary pulmonary hypertension. Am J Med. 1995;99(3):249–54. PubMed PMID: 7653484.
85. Eddahibi S, Humbert M, Fadel E, Raffestin B, Darmon M, Capron F, et al. Serotonin transporter overexpression is responsible for pulmonary artery smooth muscle hyperplasia in primary pulmonary hypertension. J Clin Invest. 2001;108(8):1141–50. PubMed PMID: 11602621, Pubmed Central PMCID: 209526.
86. Willers ED, Newman JH, Loyd JE, Robbins IM, Wheeler LA, Prince MA, et al. Serotonin transporter polymorphisms in familial and idiopathic pulmonary arterial hypertension. Am J Respir Crit Care Med. 2006;173(7):798–802. PubMed PMID: 16339917, Pubmed Central PMCID: 2662954.
87. Machado RD, Koehler R, Glissmeyer E, Veal C, Suntharalingam J, Kim M, et al. Genetic association of the serotonin transporter in pulmonary arterial hypertension. Am J Respir Crit Care Med. 2006;173(7):793–7. PubMed PMID: 16399993.
88. MacLean MR, Deuchar GA, Hicks MN, Morecroft I, Shen S, Sheward J, et al. Overexpression of the 5-hydroxytryptamine transporter gene: effect on pulmonary hemodynamics and hypoxia-induced pulmonary hypertension. Circulation. 2004;109(17):2150–5. PubMed PMID: 15078799.
89. Eddahibi S, Hanoun N, Lanfumey L, Lesch KP, Raffestin B, Hamon M, et al. Attenuated hypoxic pulmonary hypertension in mice lacking the 5-hydroxytryptamine transporter gene. J Clin Invest. 2000;105(11):1555–62. PubMed PMID: 10841514, Pubmed Central PMCID: PMC300850.
90. Marcos E, Fadel E, Sanchez O, Humbert M, Dartevelle P, Simonneau G, et al. Serotonin-induced smooth muscle hyperplasia in various forms of human pulmonary hypertension. Circ Res. 2004;94(9):1263–70. PubMed PMID: 15059929.
91. Marcos E, Adnot S, Pham MH, Nosjean A, Raffestin B, Hamon M, et al. Serotonin transporter inhibitors protect against hypoxic pulmonary hypertension. Am J Respir Crit Care Med. 2003;168(4):487–93. PubMed PMID: 12773327.
92. MacIntyre PD, Bhargava B, Hogg KJ, Gemmill JD, Hillis WS. Effect of subcutaneous sumatriptan, a selective 5HT1 agonist, on the systemic, pulmonary, and coronary circulation. Circulation. 1993;87(2):401–5. PubMed PMID: 8381056.
93. Launay JM, Herve P, Peoc'h K, Tournois C, Callebert J, Nebigil CG, et al. Function of the serotonin 5-hydroxytryptamine 2B receptor in pulmonary hypertension. Nat Med. 2002;8(10):1129–35. PubMed PMID: 12244304.

94. Keegan A, Morecroft I, Smillie D, Hicks MN, MacLean MR. Contribution of the 5-HT(1B) receptor to hypoxia-induced pulmonary hypertension: converging evidence using 5-HT(1B)-receptor knockout mice and the 5-HT(1B/1D)-receptor antagonist GR127935. Circ Res. 2001;89(12):1231–9. PubMed PMID: 11739290.
95. Yuan JX, Aldinger AM, Juhaszova M, Wang J, Conte Jr JV, Gaine SP, et al. Dysfunctional voltage-gated K+ channels in pulmonary artery smooth muscle cells of patients with primary pulmonary hypertension. Circulation. 1998;98(14):1400–6. PubMed PMID: 9760294.
96. Yuan XJ, Wang J, Juhaszova M, Gaine SP, Rubin LJ. Attenuated K+ channel gene transcription in primary pulmonary hypertension. Lancet. 1998;351(9104):726–7. PubMed PMID: 9504523.
97. Yu Y, Fantozzi I, Remillard CV, Landsberg JW, Kunichika N, Platoshyn O, et al. Enhanced expression of transient receptor potential channels in idiopathic pulmonary arterial hypertension. Proc Natl Acad Sci U S A. 2004;101(38):13861–6. PubMed PMID: 15358862, Pubmed Central PMCID: PMC518765.
98. Song MY, Makino A, Yuan JX. STIM2 contributes to enhanced store-operated Ca entry in pulmonary artery smooth muscle cells from patients with idiopathic pulmonary arterial hypertension. Pulm Circ. 2011;1(1):84–94. PubMed PMID: 21709766, Pubmed Central PMCID: PMC3121304.
99. Golovina VA, Platoshyn O, Bailey CL, Wang J, Limsuwan A, Sweeney M, et al. Upregulated TRP and enhanced capacitative Ca(2+) entry in human pulmonary artery myocytes during proliferation. Am J Physiol Heart Circ Physiol. 2001;280(2):H746–55. PubMed PMID: 11158974.
100. Kuhr FK, Smith KA, Song MY, Levitan I, Yuan JX. New mechanisms of pulmonary arterial hypertension: role of Ca(2)(+) signaling. Am J Physiol Heart Circ Physiol. 2012;302(8):H1546–62. PubMed PMID: 22245772, Pubmed Central PMCID: PMC3330808.
101. Jonigk D, Golpon H, Bockmeyer CL, Maegel L, Hoeper MM, Gottlieb J, et al. Plexiform lesions in pulmonary arterial hypertension composition, architecture, and microenvironment. Am J Pathol. 2011;179(1):167–79. PubMed PMID: 21703400, Pubmed Central PMCID: 3123793.
102. Geiger R, Berger RM, Hess J, Bogers AJ, Sharma HS, Mooi WJ. Enhanced expression of vascular endothelial growth factor in pulmonary plexogenic arteriopathy due to congenital heart disease. J Pathol. 2000;191(2):202–7. PubMed PMID: 10861582.
103. Tuder RM, Chacon M, Alger L, Wang J, Taraseviciene-Stewart L, Kasahara Y, et al. Expression of angiogenesis-related molecules in plexiform lesions in severe pulmonary hypertension: evidence for a process of disordered angiogenesis. J Pathol. 2001;195(3):367–74. PubMed PMID: 11673836.
104. Kumpers P, Nickel N, Lukasz A, Golpon H, Westerkamp V, Olsson KM, et al. Circulating angiopoietins in idiopathic pulmonary arterial hypertension. Eur Heart J. 2010;31(18): 2291–300. PubMed PMID: 20601390.
105. Partovian C, Adnot S, Raffestin B, Louzier V, Levame M, Mavier IM, et al. Adenovirus-mediated lung vascular endothelial growth factor overexpression protects against hypoxic pulmonary hypertension in rats. Am J Respir Cell Mol Biol. 2000;23(6):762–71. PubMed PMID: 11104729.
106. Campbell AI, Zhao Y, Sandhu R, Stewart DJ. Cell-based gene transfer of vascular endothelial growth factor attenuates monocrotaline-induced pulmonary hypertension. Circulation. 2001;104(18):2242–8. PubMed PMID: 11684638.
107. Taraseviciene-Stewart L, Kasahara Y, Alger L, Hirth P, Mc Mahon G, Waltenberger J, et al. Inhibition of the VEGF receptor 2 combined with chronic hypoxia causes cell death-dependent pulmonary endothelial cell proliferation and severe pulmonary hypertension. FASEB J. 2001;15(2):427–38. PubMed PMID: 11156958.
108. Klein M, Schermuly RT, Ellinghaus P, Milting H, Riedl B, Nikolova S, et al. Combined tyrosine and serine/threonine kinase inhibition by sorafenib prevents progression of experimental pulmonary hypertension and myocardial remodeling. Circulation. 2008;118(20):2081–90. PubMed PMID: 18955668.

109. Moreno-Vinasco L, Gomberg-Maitland M, Maitland ML, Desai AA, Singleton PA, Sammani S, et al. Genomic assessment of a multikinase inhibitor, sorafenib, in a rodent model of pulmonary hypertension. Physiol Genomics. 2008;33(2):278–91. PubMed PMID: 18303084.
110. Voelkel NF, Gomez-Arroyo J. The role of vascular endothelial growth factor in pulmonary arterial hypertension: the angiogenesis paradox. Am J Respir Cell Mol Biol. 2014;51:474.
111. Grimminger F, Schermuly RT. PDGF receptor and its antagonists: role in treatment of PAH. Adv Exp Med Biol. 2010;661:435–46. PubMed PMID: 20204747.
112. Perros F, Montani D, Dorfmuller P, Durand-Gasselin I, Tcherakian C, Le Pavec J, et al. Platelet-derived growth factor expression and function in idiopathic pulmonary arterial hypertension. Am J Respir Crit Care Med. 2008;178(1):81–8. PubMed PMID: 18420966.
113. Schermuly RT, Dony E, Ghofrani HA, Pullamsetti S, Savai R, Roth M, et al. Reversal of experimental pulmonary hypertension by PDGF inhibition. J Clin Invest. 2005;115(10): 2811–21. PubMed PMID: 16200212, Pubmed Central PMCID: PMC1236676.
114. Benisty JI, McLaughlin VV, Landzberg MJ, Rich JD, Newburger JW, Rich S, et al. Elevated basic fibroblast growth factor levels in patients with pulmonary arterial hypertension. Chest. 2004;126(4):1255–61. PubMed PMID: 15486390.
115. Izikki M, Guignabert C, Fadel E, Humbert M, Tu L, Zadigue P, et al. Endothelial-derived FGF2 contributes to the progression of pulmonary hypertension in humans and rodents. J Clin Invest. 2009;119(3):512–23. PubMed PMID: 19197140, Pubmed Central PMCID: PMC2648677.
116. Le Cras TD, Hardie WD, Fagan K, Whitsett JA, Korfhagen TR. Disrupted pulmonary vascular development and pulmonary hypertension in transgenic mice overexpressing transforming growth factor-alpha. Am J Physiol Lung Cell Mol Physiol. 2003;285(5):L1046–54. PubMed PMID: 12896876.
117. Merklinger SL, Jones PL, Martinez EC, Rabinovitch M. Epidermal growth factor receptor blockade mediates smooth muscle cell apoptosis and improves survival in rats with pulmonary hypertension. Circulation. 2005;112(3):423–31. PubMed PMID: 16027270.
118. Dahal BK, Cornitescu T, Tretyn A, Pullamsetti SS, Kosanovic D, Dumitrascu R, et al. Role of epidermal growth factor inhibition in experimental pulmonary hypertension. Am J Respir Crit Care Med. 2010;181(2):158–67. PubMed PMID: 19850946.
119. Souza R, Sitbon O, Parent F, Simonneau G, Humbert M. Long term imatinib treatment in pulmonary arterial hypertension. Thorax. 2006;61(8):736. PubMed PMID: 16877696, Pubmed Central PMCID: PMC2104679.
120. Patterson KC, Weissmann A, Ahmadi T, Farber HW. Imatinib mesylate in the treatment of refractory idiopathic pulmonary arterial hypertension. Ann Intern Med. 2006;145(2):152–3. PubMed PMID: 16847299.
121. Ghofrani HA, Seeger W, Grimminger F. Imatinib for the treatment of pulmonary arterial hypertension. N Engl J Med. 2005;353(13):1412–3. PubMed PMID: 16192491.
122. Ghofrani HA, Morrell NW, Hoeper MM, Olschewski H, Peacock AJ, Barst RJ, et al. Imatinib in pulmonary arterial hypertension patients with inadequate response to established therapy. Am J Respir Crit Care Med. 2010;182(9):1171–7. PubMed PMID: 20581169, Pubmed Central PMCID: PMC3001259.
123. Hoeper MM, Barst RJ, Bourge RC, Feldman J, Frost AE, Galié N, Gómez-Sánchez MA, Grimminger F, Grünig E, Hassoun PM, Morrell NW, Peacock AJ, Satoh T, Simonneau G, Tapson VF, Torres F, Lawrence D, Quinn DA, Ghofrani HA. Imatinib mesylate as add-on therapy for pulmonary arterial hypertension: results of the randomized IMPRES study. Circulation. 2013;127(10):1128–38.
124. Montani D, Bergot E, Günther S, Savale L, Bergeron A, Bourdin A, Bouvaist H, Canuet M, Pison C, Macro M, Poubeau P, Girerd B, Natali D, Guignabert C, Perros F, O'Callaghan DS, Jaïs X, Tubert-Bitter P, Zalcman G, Sitbon O, Simonneau G, Humbert M. Pulmonary arterial hypertension in patients treated by dasatinib. Circulation. 2012;125(17):2128–37.
125. Humbert M, Morrell NW, Archer SL, Stenmark KR, MacLean MR, Lang IM, et al. Cellular and molecular pathobiology of pulmonary arterial hypertension. J Am Coll Cardiol. 2004;43(12 Suppl S):13S–24. PubMed PMID: 15194174.

126. Schwappacher R, Weiske J, Heining E, Ezerski V, Marom B, Henis YI, Huber O, Knaus P. Novel crosstalk to BMP signalling: cGMP-dependent kinase I modulates BMP receptor and Smad activity. EMBO J. 2009;28(11):1537–50.
127. Schwappacher R, Kilic A, Kojonazarov B, Lang M, Diep T, Zhuang S, Gawlowski T, Schermuly RT, Pfeifer A, Boss GR, Pilz RB. A molecular mechanism for therapeutic effects of cGMP-elevating agents in pulmonary arterial hypertension. J Biol Chem. 2013; 288(23):16557–66.
128. Morrell NW, Yang X, Upton PD, Jourdan KB, Morgan N, Sheares KK, et al. Altered growth responses of pulmonary artery smooth muscle cells from patients with primary pulmonary hypertension to transforming growth factor-beta(1) and bone morphogenetic proteins. Circulation. 2001;104(7):790–5. PubMed PMID: 11502704.
129. Hautmann MB, Madsen CS, Owens GK. A transforming growth factor beta (TGFbeta) control element drives TGFbeta-induced stimulation of smooth muscle alpha-actin gene expression in concert with two CArG elements. J Biol Chem. 1997;272(16):10948–56. PubMed PMID: 9099754.
130. Yang X, Long L, Southwood M, Rudarakanchana N, Upton PD, Jeffery TK, et al. Dysfunctional Smad signaling contributes to abnormal smooth muscle cell proliferation in familial pulmonary arterial hypertension. Circ Res. 2005;96(10):1053–63. PubMed PMID: 15845886.
131. Valdimarsdottir G, Goumans MJ, Rosendahl A, Brugman M, Itoh S, Lebrin F, et al. Stimulation of Id1 expression by bone morphogenetic protein is sufficient and necessary for bone morphogenetic protein-induced activation of endothelial cells. Circulation. 2002; 106(17):2263–70. PubMed PMID: 12390958.
132. Teichert-Kuliszewska K, Kutryk MJ, Kuliszewski MA, Karoubi G, Courtman DW, Zucco L, et al. Bone morphogenetic protein receptor-2 signaling promotes pulmonary arterial endothelial cell survival: implications for loss-of-function mutations in the pathogenesis of pulmonary hypertension. Circ Res. 2006;98(2):209–17. PubMed PMID: 16357305.
133. Thistlethwaite PA, Li X, Zhang X. Notch signaling in pulmonary hypertension. Adv Exp Med Biol. 2010;661:279–98. PubMed PMID: 20204737.
134. Domenga V, Fardoux P, Lacombe P, Monet M, Maciazek J, Krebs LT, et al. Notch3 is required for arterial identity and maturation of vascular smooth muscle cells. Genes Dev. 2004;18(22):2730–5. PubMed PMID: 15545631, Pubmed Central PMCID: PMC528893.
135. Villa N, Walker L, Lindsell CE, Gasson J, Iruela-Arispe ML, Weinmaster G. Vascular expression of Notch pathway receptors and ligands is restricted to arterial vessels. Mech Dev. 2001;108(1–2):161–4. PubMed PMID: 11578869.
136. Campos AH, Wang W, Pollman MJ, Gibbons GH. Determinants of Notch-3 receptor expression and signaling in vascular smooth muscle cells: implications in cell-cycle regulation. Circ Res. 2002;91(11):999–1006. PubMed PMID: 12456485.
137. Li X, Zhang X, Leathers R, Makino A, Huang C, Parsa P, et al. Notch3 signaling promotes the development of pulmonary arterial hypertension. Nat Med. 2009;15(11):1289–97. PubMed PMID: 19855400, Pubmed Central PMCID: PMC2780347.
138. Benedito R, Rocha SF, Woeste M, Zamykal M, Radtke F, Casanovas O, et al. Notch-dependent VEGFR3 upregulation allows angiogenesis without VEGF-VEGFR2 signalling. Nature. 2012;484(7392):110–4. PubMed PMID: 22426001.
139. Simonneau G, Robbins IM, Beghetti M, Channick RN, Delcroix M, Denton CP, et al. Updated clinical classification of pulmonary hypertension. J Am Coll Cardiol. 2009;54(1 Suppl):S43–54. PubMed PMID: 19555858.
140. Mukerjee D, St George D, Coleiro B, Knight C, Denton CP, Davar J, et al. Prevalence and outcome in systemic sclerosis associated pulmonary arterial hypertension: application of a registry approach. Ann Rheum Dis. 2003;62(11):1088–93. PubMed PMID: 14583573, Pubmed Central PMCID: PMC1754353.
141. de Azevedo AB, Sampaio-Barros PD, Torres RM, Moreira C. Prevalence of pulmonary hypertension in systemic sclerosis. Clin Exp Rheumatol. 2005;23(4):447–54. PubMed PMID: 16095111.

142. Isern RA, Yaneva M, Weiner E, Parke A, Rothfield N, Dantzker D, et al. Autoantibodies in patients with primary pulmonary hypertension: association with anti-Ku. Am J Med. 1992;93(3):307–12. PubMed PMID: 1524083.
143. Tuder RM, Groves B, Badesch DB, Voelkel NF. Exuberant endothelial cell growth and elements of inflammation are present in plexiform lesions of pulmonary hypertension. Am J Pathol. 1994;144(2):275–85. PubMed PMID: 7508683, Pubmed Central PMCID: PMC1887146.
144. Savai R, Pullamsetti SS, Kolbe J, Bieniek E, Voswinckel R, Fink L, et al. Immune/inflammatory cell involvement in the pathology of idiopathic pulmonary arterial hypertension. Am J Respir Crit Care Med. 2012;186:897. PubMed PMID: 22955318.
145. Austin ED, Rock MT, Mosse CA, Vnencak-Jones CL, Yoder SM, Robbins IM, et al. T lymphocyte subset abnormalities in the blood and lung in pulmonary arterial hypertension. Respir Med. 2010;104(3):454–62. PubMed PMID: 19880300, Pubmed Central PMCID: PMC2826574.
146. Ulrich S, Nicolls MR, Taraseviciene L, Speich R, Voelkel N. Increased regulatory and decreased CD8+ cytotoxic T cells in the blood of patients with idiopathic pulmonary arterial hypertension. Respiration. 2008;75(3):272–80. PubMed PMID: 18025812, Pubmed Central PMCID: PMC3030245.
147. Ormiston ML, Chang C, Long LL, Soon E, Jones D, Machado R, et al. Impaired natural killer cell phenotype and function in idiopathic and heritable pulmonary arterial hypertension. Circulation. 2012;126(9):1099–109. PubMed PMID: 22832786.
148. Humbert M, Monti G, Brenot F, Sitbon O, Portier A, Grangeot-Keros L, et al. Increased interleukin-1 and interleukin-6 serum concentrations in severe primary pulmonary hypertension. Am J Respir Crit Care Med. 1995;151(5):1628–31. PubMed PMID: 7735624.
149. Soon E, Holmes AM, Treacy CM, Doughty NJ, Southgate L, Machado RD, et al. Elevated levels of inflammatory cytokines predict survival in idiopathic and familial pulmonary arterial hypertension. Circulation. 2010;122(9):920–7. PubMed PMID: 20713898.
150. Montani D, Humbert M, Souza R. Letter by Montani et al. regarding article, "Elevated levels of inflammatory cytokines predict survival in idiopathic and familial pulmonary arterial hypertension". Circulation. 2011;123(21):e614. author reply e5. PubMed PMID: 21632514.
151. Golembeski SM, West J, Tada Y, Fagan KA. Interleukin-6 causes mild pulmonary hypertension and augments hypoxia-induced pulmonary hypertension in mice. Chest. 2005;128(6 Suppl):572S–3. PubMed PMID: 16373831.
152. Steiner MK, Syrkina OL, Kolliputi N, Mark EJ, Hales CA, Waxman AB. Interleukin-6 overexpression induces pulmonary hypertension. Circ Res. 2009;104(2):236–44. 28p following 44. PubMed PMID: 19074475.
153. Savale L, Tu L, Rideau D, Izziki M, Maitre B, Adnot S, et al. Impact of interleukin-6 on hypoxia-induced pulmonary hypertension and lung inflammation in mice. Respir Res. 2009;10:6. PubMed PMID: 19173740, Pubmed Central PMCID: PMC2644669.
154. Speich R, Jenni R, Opravil M, Pfab M, Russi EW. Primary pulmonary hypertension in HIV infection. Chest. 1991;100(5):1268–71. PubMed PMID: 1935280.
155. Cool CD, Voelkel NF, Bull T. Viral infection and pulmonary hypertension: is there an association? Expert Rev Respir Med. 2011;5(2):207–16. PubMed PMID: 21510731.
156. Humbert M, Monti G, Fartoukh M, Magnan A, Brenot F, Rain B, et al. Platelet-derived growth factor expression in primary pulmonary hypertension: comparison of HIV seropositive and HIV seronegative patients. Eur Respir J. 1998;11(3):554–9. PubMed PMID: 9596101.
157. Mette SA, Palevsky HI, Pietra GG, Williams TM, Bruder E, Prestipino AJ, et al. Primary pulmonary hypertension in association with human immunodeficiency virus infection. A possible viral etiology for some forms of hypertensive pulmonary arteriopathy. Am Rev Respir Dis. 1992;145(5):1196–200. PubMed PMID: 1586065.
158. Marecki JC, Cool CD, Parr JE, Beckey VE, Luciw PA, Tarantal AF, et al. HIV-1 Nef is associated with complex pulmonary vascular lesions in SHIV-nef-infected macaques. Am J

Respir Crit Care Med. 2006;174(4):437–45. PubMed PMID: 16728715, Pubmed Central PMCID: PMC2648120.

159. James CO, Huang MB, Khan M, Garcia-Barrio M, Powell MD, Bond VC. Extracellular Nef protein targets CD4+ T cells for apoptosis by interacting with CXCR4 surface receptors. J Virol. 2004;78(6):3099–109. PubMed PMID: 14990729, Pubmed Central PMCID: PMC353732.
160. George MP, Brower A, Kling H, Shipley T, Kristoff J, Reinhart TA, et al. Pulmonary vascular lesions are common in SIV- and SHIV-env-infected macaques. AIDS Res Hum Retroviruses. 2011;27(2):103–11. PubMed PMID: 20961277, Pubmed Central PMCID: PMC3043941.
161. Hofman FM, Wright AD, Dohadwala MM, Wong-Staal F, Walker SM. Exogenous tat protein activates human endothelial cells. Blood. 1993;82(9):2774–80. PubMed PMID: 7693046.
162. Kanmogne GD, Primeaux C, Grammas P. Induction of apoptosis and endothelin-1 secretion in primary human lung endothelial cells by HIV-1 gp120 proteins. Biochem Biophys Res Commun. 2005;333(4):1107–15. PubMed PMID: 15979050.
163. Cool CD, Rai PR, Yeager ME, Hernandez-Saavedra D, Serls AE, Bull TM, et al. Expression of human herpesvirus 8 in primary pulmonary hypertension. N Engl J Med. 2003;349(12): 1113–22. PubMed PMID: 13679525.
164. Laney AS, De Marco T, Peters JS, Malloy M, Teehankee C, Moore PS, et al. Kaposi sarcoma-associated herpesvirus and primary and secondary pulmonary hypertension. Chest. 2005; 127(3):762–7. PubMed PMID: 15764755.
165. Henke-Gendo C, Mengel M, Hoeper MM, Alkharsah K, Schulz TF. Absence of Kaposi's sarcoma-associated herpesvirus in patients with pulmonary arterial hypertension. Am J Respir Crit Care Med. 2005;172(12):1581–5. PubMed PMID: 16192453.
166. Bresser P, Cornelissen MI, van der Bij W, van Noesel CJ, Timens W. Idiopathic pulmonary arterial hypertension in Dutch Caucasian patients is not associated with human herpes virus-8 infection. Respir Med. 2007;101(4):854–6. PubMed PMID: 17011770.
167. Bendayan D, Sarid R, Cohen A, Shitrit D, Shechtman I, Kramer MR. Absence of human herpesvirus 8 DNA sequences in lung biopsies from Israeli patients with pulmonary arterial hypertension. Respiration. 2008;75(2):155–7. PubMed PMID: 17124380.
168. Valmary S, Dorfmuller P, Montani D, Humbert M, Brousset P, Degano B. Human gamma-herpesviruses Epstein-Barr virus and human herpesvirus-8 are not detected in the lungs of patients with severe pulmonary arterial hypertension. Chest. 2011;139(6):1310–6. PubMed PMID: 21051388.
169. Bica I, Hamer DH, Stadecker MJ. Hepatic schistosomiasis. Infect Dis Clin North Am. 2000;14(3):583–604. viii, PubMed PMID: 10987111.
170. Kolosionek E, Graham BB, Tuder RM, Butrous G. Pulmonary vascular disease associated with parasitic infection–the role of schistosomiasis. Clin Microbiol Infect. 2011;17(1):15–24. PubMed PMID: 20636425.
171. Graham BB, Chabon J, Bandeira A, Espinheira L, Butrous G, Tuder RM. Significant intrapulmonary Schistosoma egg antigens are not present in schistosomiasis-associated pulmonary hypertension. Pulm Circ. 2011;1(4):456–61. PubMed PMID: 22530100, Pubmed Central PMCID: PMC3329075.
172. Richter J. The impact of chemotherapy on morbidity due to schistosomiasis. Acta Trop. 2003;86(2–3):161–83. PubMed PMID: 12745135.
173. Graham BB, Mentink-Kane MM, El-Haddad H, Purnell S, Zhang L, Zaiman A, et al. Schistosomiasis-induced experimental pulmonary hypertension: role of interleukin-13 signaling. Am J Pathol. 2010;177(3):1549–61. PubMed PMID: 20671265, Pubmed Central PMCID: PMC2928984.
174. Wagenvoort CA. Lung biopsy specimens in the evaluation of pulmonary vascular disease. Chest. 1980;77(5):614–25. PubMed PMID: 7363679.
175. Bjornsson J, Edwards WD. Primary pulmonary hypertension: a histopathologic study of 80 cases. Mayo Clin Proc. 1985;60(1):16–25. PubMed PMID: 3965821.
176. Wagenvoort CA, Wagenvoort N. Primary pulmonary hypertension. Circulation. 1970; 42(6):1163–84.

177. Johnson SR, Granton JT, Mehta S. Thrombotic arteriopathy and anticoagulation in pulmonary hypertension. Chest. 2006;130(2):545–52. PubMed PMID: 16899857.
178. Wagenvoort CA. Morphological substrate for the reversibility and irreversibility of pulmonary hypertension. Eur Heart J. 1988;9(Suppl J):7–12. PubMed PMID: 3053185.
179. Wolf M, Boyer-Neumann C, Parent F, Eschwege V, Jaillet H, Meyer D, et al. Thrombotic risk factors in pulmonary hypertension. Eur Respir J. 2000;15(2):395–9. PubMed PMID: 10706510.
180. Hoeper MM, Sosada M, Fabel H. Plasma coagulation profiles in patients with severe primary pulmonary hypertension. Eur Respir J. 1998;12(6):1446–9. PubMed PMID: 9877507.
181. Veyradier A, Nishikubo T, Humbert M, Wolf M, Sitbon O, Simonneau G, et al. Improvement of von Willebrand factor proteolysis after prostacyclin infusion in severe pulmonary arterial hypertension. Circulation. 2000;102(20):2460–2. PubMed PMID: 11076816.
182. Lopes AA, Maeda NY. Circulating von Willebrand factor antigen as a predictor of short-term prognosis in pulmonary hypertension. Chest. 1998;114(5):1276–82. PubMed PMID: 9824001.
183. Eisenberg PR, Lucore C, Kaufman L, Sobel BE, Jaffe AS, Rich S. Fibrinopeptide A levels indicative of pulmonary vascular thrombosis in patients with primary pulmonary hypertension. Circulation. 1990;82(3):841–7. PubMed PMID: 2394005.
184. Tournier A, Wahl D, Chaouat A, Max JP, Regnault V, Lecompte T, et al. Calibrated automated thrombography demonstrates hypercoagulability in patients with idiopathic pulmonary arterial hypertension. Thromb Res. 2010;126(6):e418–22. PubMed PMID: 20888030.
185. Fuster V, Steele PM, Edwards WD, Gersh BJ, McGoon MD, Frye RL. Primary pulmonary hypertension: natural history and the importance of thrombosis. Circulation. 1984;70(4):580–7. PubMed PMID: 6148159.
186. Kawut SM, Horn EM, Berekashvili KK, Garofano RP, Goldsmith RL, Widlitz AC, et al. New predictors of outcome in idiopathic pulmonary arterial hypertension. Am J Cardiol. 2005;95(2):199–203. PubMed PMID: 15642552.
187. Burger CD, Foreman AJ, Miller DP, Safford RE, McGoon MD, Badesch DB. Comparison of body habitus in patients with pulmonary arterial hypertension enrolled in the Registry to Evaluate Early and Long-term PAH Disease Management with normative values from the National Health and Nutrition Examination Survey. Mayo Clin Proc. 2011;86(2):105–12. PubMed PMID: 21282484, Pubmed Central PMCID: PMC3031434.
188. Zamanian RT, Hansmann G, Snook S, Lilienfeld D, Rappaport KM, Reaven GM, et al. Insulin resistance in pulmonary arterial hypertension. Eur Respir J. 2009;33(2):318–24. PubMed PMID: 19047320, Pubmed Central PMCID: PMC2785883.
189. Pugh ME, Robbins IM, Rice TW, West J, Newman JH, Hemnes AR. Unrecognized glucose intolerance is common in pulmonary arterial hypertension. J Heart Lung Transplant. 2011;30(8):904–11. PubMed PMID: 21493097, Pubmed Central PMCID: PMC3129440.
190. Heresi GA, Aytekin M, Newman J, DiDonato J, Dweik RA. Plasma levels of high-density lipoprotein cholesterol and outcomes in pulmonary arterial hypertension. Am J Respir Crit Care Med. 2010;182(5):661–8. PubMed PMID: 20448092, Pubmed Central PMCID: PMC2937236.
191. Hansmann G, Wagner RA, Schellong S, Perez VA, Urashima T, Wang L, et al. Pulmonary arterial hypertension is linked to insulin resistance and reversed by peroxisome proliferator-activated receptor-gamma activation. Circulation. 2007;115(10):1275–84. PubMed PMID: 17339547.
192. Summer R, Fiack CA, Ikeda Y, Sato K, Dwyer D, Ouchi N, et al. Adiponectin deficiency: a model of pulmonary hypertension associated with pulmonary vascular disease. Am J Physiol Lung Cell Mol Physiol. 2009;297(3):L432–8. PubMed PMID: 19561137, Pubmed Central PMCID: PMC2739777.
193. Hansmann G, de Jesus Perez VA, Alastalo TP, Alvira CM, Guignabert C, Bekker JM, et al. An antiproliferative BMP-2/PPARgamma/apoE axis in human and murine SMCs and its role in pulmonary hypertension. J Clin Invest. 2008;118(5):1846–57. PubMed PMID: 18382765, Pubmed Central PMCID: PMC2276393.

194. West J, Niswender KD, Johnson JA, Pugh ME, Gleaves L, Fessel JP, et al. A potential role for Insulin resistance in experimental pulmonary hypertension. Eur Respir J. 2013;41:861. PubMed PMID: 22936709.
195. Pugh ME, Hemnes AR. Development of pulmonary arterial hypertension in women: interplay of sex hormones and pulmonary vascular disease. Womens Health (Lond Engl). 2010;6(2):285–96. PubMed PMID: 20187732, Pubmed Central PMCID: PMC2853883.
196. Tofovic SP, Zhang X, Jackson EK, Dacic S, Petrusevska G. 2-Methoxyestradiol mediates the protective effects of estradiol in monocrotaline-induced pulmonary hypertension. Vascul Pharmacol. 2006;45(6):358–67. PubMed PMID: 16872912.
197. Tofovic SP, Zhang X, Jackson EK, Zhu H, Petrusevska G. 2-methoxyestradiol attenuates bleomycin-induced pulmonary hypertension and fibrosis in estrogen-deficient rats. Vascul Pharmacol. 2009;51(2–3):190–7. PubMed PMID: 19540933, Pubmed Central PMCID: PMC2760300.
198. Lahm T, Patel KM, Crisostomo PR, Markel TA, Wang M, Herring C, et al. Endogenous estrogen attenuates pulmonary artery vasoreactivity and acute hypoxic pulmonary vasoconstriction: the effects of sex and menstrual cycle. Am J Physiol Endocrinol Metab. 2007;293(3):E865–71. PubMed PMID: 17595218.
199. Lahm T, Crisostomo PR, Markel TA, Wang M, Weil BR, Novotny NM, et al. The effects of estrogen on pulmonary artery vasoreactivity and hypoxic pulmonary vasoconstriction: potential new clinical implications for an old hormone. Crit Care Med. 2008;36(7):2174–83. PubMed PMID: 18552699.
200. Lahm T, Crisostomo PR, Markel TA, Wang M, Wang Y, Tan J, et al. Selective estrogen receptor-alpha and estrogen receptor-beta agonists rapidly decrease pulmonary artery vasoconstriction by a nitric oxide-dependent mechanism. Am J Physiol Regul Integr Comp Physiol. 2008;295(5):R1486–93. PubMed PMID: 18832085, Pubmed Central PMCID: PMC2584849.
201. White K, Loughlin L, Maqbool Z, Nilsen M, McClure J, Dempsie Y, et al. Serotonin transporter, sex, and hypoxia: microarray analysis in the pulmonary arteries of mice identifies genes with relevance to human PAH. Physiol Genomics. 2011;43(8):417–37. PubMed PMID: 21303932, Pubmed Central PMCID: PMC3092337.
202. Dempsie Y, Nilsen M, White K, Mair KM, Loughlin L, Ambartsumian N, et al. Development of pulmonary arterial hypertension in mice over-expressing S100A4/Mts1 is specific to females. Respir Res. 2011;12:159. PubMed PMID: 22185646, Pubmed Central PMCID: PMC3276452.
203. West J, Harral J, Lane K, Deng Y, Ickes B, Crona D, et al. Mice expressing BMPR2R899X transgene in smooth muscle develop pulmonary vascular lesions. Am J Physiol Lung Cell Mol Physiol. 2008;295(5):L744–55. PubMed PMID: 18723761, Pubmed Central PMCID: PMC2584890.
204. Kawut SM, Al-Naamani N, Agerstrand C, et al. Determinants of right ventricular ejection fraction in pulmonary arterial hypertension. Chest. 2009;135:752–9.
205. Shapiro S, Traiger GL, Turner M, et al. Sex differences in the diagnosis, treatment, and outcome of patients with pulmonary arterial hypertension enrolled in the Registry To Evaluate Early And Long-Term Pulmonary Arterial Hypertension Disease Management. Chest. 2012;141:363–73.
206. Ventetuolo CE, Praestgaard A, Palevsky HI, Klinger JR, Halpern SD, Kawut SM. Sex and haemodynamics in pulmonary arterial hypertension. Eur Respir J. 2014;43(2):523–30.
207. Ventetuolo CE, Ouyang P, Bluemke DA, Tandri H, Barr RG, Bagiella E, Cappola AR, Bristow MR, Johnson C, Kronmal RA, Kizer JR, Lima JA, Kawut SM. Sex hormones are associated with right ventricular structure and function: the MESA-right ventricle study. Am J Respir Crit Care Med. 2011;183(5):659–67.
208. Humbert M, Sitbon O, Chaouat A, et al. Survival in patients with idiopathic, familial, and anorexigen-associated pulmonary arterial hypertension in the modern management era. Circulation. 2010;122:156–63.

Chapter 4
Hypoxic Pulmonary Hypertension

Kara Goss and Tim Lahm

Abstract Elevation in pulmonary arterial pressure is a common occurrence in patients with chronic lung disease. Hypoxic pulmonary vasoconstriction, parenchymal lung disease, and inflammation contribute to increased pulmonary vascular tone and remodeling. Diagnosis of pulmonary vascular disease in patients with lung disease may be especially challenging due to the lack of specificity of common complaints of dyspnea and inaccuracy of echocardiographic estimates such as pulmonary arterial pressure in this group of patients. The presence of pulmonary hypertension (PH) in chronic lung disease is associated with increased morbidity and mortality, but the efficacy of pharmacologic treatment of PH in this population has not been established. This chapter will review the epidemiology and pathogenesis of PH associated with chronic lung disease and provide an approach to evaluation and management including the identification and selection of some patients who may benefit from currently available pulmonary vasodilator therapies.

Keywords WHO group 3 pulmonary hypertension • Cor pulmonale • Hypoxic pulmonary vasoconstriction • Hypoxic pulmonary vascular remodeling • COPD • Pulmonary fibrosis • Sleep-disordered breathing • High-altitude exposure

Introduction

The World Health Organization defines group 3 pulmonary hypertension (PH) as a mean pulmonary artery pressure (PAP) of ≥25 mmHg at rest (though some studies use a mean PAP ≥ 20 mmHg) and a mean pulmonary capillary wedge pressure of <15 mmHg in the setting of chronic lung disease, sleep-disordered breathing, or high altitude, all of which can induce chronic or intermittent hypoxia (see Table 4.1) [1, 2]. Group 3 PH, frequently referred to as hypoxic pulmonary hypertension or hypoxia-induced pulmonary hypertension (HPH), has a strikingly different pathophysiology

K. Goss, M.D. • T. Lahm, M.D. (✉)
Division of Pulmonary, Allergy, Critical Care, Occupational and Sleep Medicine, Department of Medicine, Indiana University School of Medicine and Richard L. Roudebush VA Medical Center, 980 W. Walnut Street, Room C-400, Indianapolis, IN 46202, USA
e-mail: tlahm@iupui.edu

J.R. Klinger, R.P. Frantz (eds.), *Diagnosis and Management of Pulmonary Hypertension*, Respiratory Medicine 12, DOI 10.1007/978-1-4939-2636-7_4

Table 4.1 Classification of group 3 pulmonary hypertension (from [1])

3.1	Chronic obstructive pulmonary disease
3.2	Interstitial lung disease
3.3	Other pulmonary diseases with mixed restrictive and obstructive pattern
3.4	Sleep-disordered breathing
3.5	Alveolar hypoventilation disorders
3.6	Chronic exposure to high altitude
3.7	Developmental abnormalities

compared with group 1 pulmonary arterial hypertension (PAH), leading to variable responses to PAH therapies [3, 4]. The epidemiology, pathophysiology, clinical presentation, diagnosis, and treatment of group 3 PH will be reviewed here.

Epidemiology

PH owing to chronic lung disease is the second most common cause of PH in the Western world [5]. Exact determinations of the prevalence of PH in chronic lung disease are difficult due to differences in methodology and definitions employed across the various studies. Recent studies suggest that PH is present in up to 50 % of hospitalized patients with chronic obstructive pulmonary disease (COPD), but in as many as 70–90 % of patients with severe emphysema evaluated for lung volume reduction surgery or lung transplant [6–8]. Similarly, estimates among patients with idiopathic pulmonary fibrosis (IPF) range from 10 to 84 %, with at least 45 % of patients listed for lung transplant being affected [4, 9–11]. The incidence of PH appears even higher at initial diagnosis among patients with combined pulmonary fibrosis and emphysema (CPFE) at 47 %, increasing to 55 % of patients during follow-up [12]. Among patients with obstructive sleep apnea (OSA), 27–42 % of patients have a mean PAP>20 mmHg, with an even higher prevalence noted in obesity hypoventilation syndrome [13, 14]. High-altitude pulmonary edema (HAPE), a condition characterized by exaggerated hypoxic vasoconstriction and acute PH, is seen in 0.01–0.1 % of visitors of ski resorts in the Rocky Mountains, and in 0.2 % of a general alpine mountaineering population [15, 16]. However, its prevalence can reach up to 7 % in regular mountaineers reaching high altitudes (>4,500 m) within a short period of time, and up to 62 % in predisposed mountaineers [17]. The incidence of PH in patients living at high altitude is not well known. In a Kyrgyz population living at >3,000 m, 20 % of dyspneic patients had hemodynamically confirmed PH [18]. Other studies have shown a prevalence of high-altitude PH between 5 and 18 % in a population living at >3,200 m in South America [19].

Although the mean PAP in group 3 PH is typically between 20 and 35 mmHg, a minority of patients present with a mean PAP greater than 35–40 mmHg, some with relatively preserved lung function [6]. Some experts have labeled this entity PH "out of proportion" to lung disease. For example, this group of patients comprises about 5 % of patients with COPD, and some studies have estimated the prevalence of out of proportion PH in COPD to be similar to the prevalence of idiopathic PAH [6, 20]. Although it is not clear if patients with lung disease and out of proportion PH represent a more permissive phenotype characterized by genetic polymorphisms such as those seen in the serotonin transporter or IL-6 genes [21, 22], or if they represent true group 1 PAH that is superimposed on chronic lung disease, at least epidemiologically true idiopathic PAH may coexist with chronic lung disease.

Pathogenesis

Group 3 PH is pathologically distinct from PAH. The hallmark of PAH is a severe progressive pulmonary hypertensive arteriopathy characterized by plexiform lesions, in situ thrombosis, and extensive arterial wall remodeling and fibrosis [4, 23]. In contrast, the vascular remodeling in group 3 PH is characterized by media hypertrophy, muscularization of small normally nonmuscular arteries, and fibrosis and stiffening of large proximal pulmonary arteries, with notable absence of plexiform lesions (see Fig. 4.1 and Table 4.2). There is also significant vascular inflammation that intensifies the perivascular remodeling [4, 24]. These changes can occur

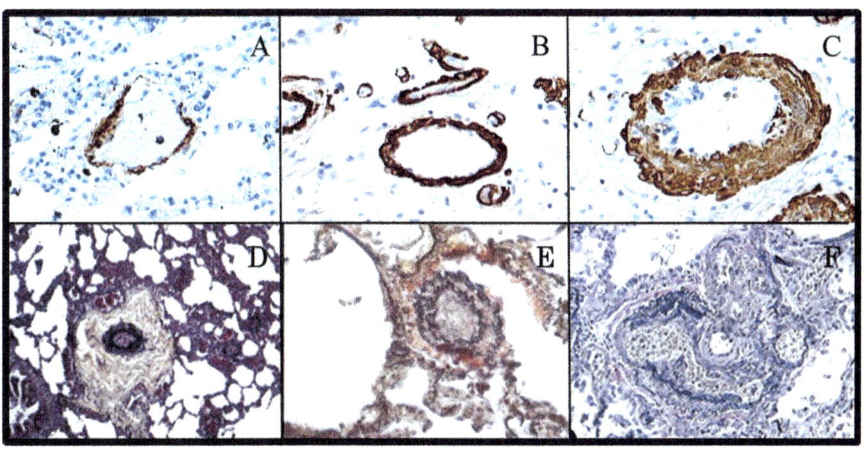

Fig. 4.1 Distinct pulmonary vascular remodeling in group 3 and group 1 pulmonary hypertension. (**a**) Normal small pulmonary artery. Note thin wall and open lumen. (**b**, **c**) Pulmonary arteries from patients with COPD-PH (group 3 PH). Note thickened vascular walls with significant media hypertrophy, especially in (**c**). However, in both patients, vessel lumens are widely patent. (**d–f**) Pulmonary vascular remodeling in patients with PAH (group 1 PH). Note significant remodeling of the intima, media, and adventitia (**d**), with vessel occlusion (**e**) and plexiform lesions (**f**). Such massive remodeling is not observed in patients with group 3 PH. (**a–c**) Reproduced with permission from [21]; D-F reproduced with permission from [4]

Table 4.2 Histologic features of group 3 pulmonary hypertension (modified from [4])

Muscularization of previously nonmuscularized arterioles
Medial hypertrophy of muscularized arteries (particularly in smaller branches)
Longitudinally oriented intimal smooth muscle cells
Mild medial hypertrophy of veins
Perivascular inflammatory infiltrates
In patients with interstitial lung disease: Eccentric intimal fibrosis of arteries (and to a lesser degree of veins)

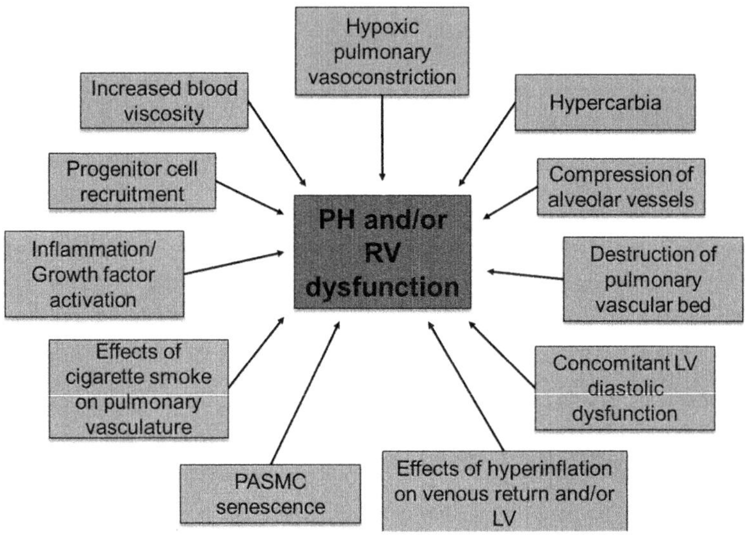

Fig. 4.2 Mechanisms of PH and RV dysfunction in HPH. Note multifactorial mechanism of PH development and/or RV dysfunction (cor pulmonale). Contribution of the listed factors may vary depending on type and severity of the underlying lung disease, disease stage (early vs. late), comorbidities, ongoing exposures, and genetic predisposition. *LV* left ventricle, *PASMC* pulmonary artery smooth muscle cells, *PH* pulmonary hypertension, *RV* right ventricle

in the presence or absence of hypoxia; in the latter case, factors such as cigarette smoke or mechanical alterations may be the inciting factors (see Fig. 4.2). Technically speaking, the term "hypoxic pulmonary hypertension" is therefore a misnomer; however, since most lung diseases are characterized at least in part by hypoxemia, the term is commonly used.

The Effects of Hypoxia on the Pulmonary Vasculature

Hypoxia has an immediate effect on PAP via hypoxic pulmonary vasoconstriction (HPV). In the setting of sustained exposure, there is also a delayed effect via hypoxia-induced pulmonary vascular remodeling.

Hypoxic Pulmonary Vasoconstriction (HPV)

HPV refers to a process in which the pulmonary vasculature responds to a hypoxic stimulus with a vasoconstrictor response. This process, which is unique to the pulmonary vasculature (systemic vessels dilate upon hypoxia exposure), is thought to be a protective reflex in order to maintain ventilation and perfusion matching in the setting of focal lung disease such as consolidation [25, 26]. However, if the entire pulmonary vasculature constricts due to global hypoxia exposure, a significant increase in pulmonary vascular resistance (PVR) and thus right ventricular (RV) afterload ensues.

Excessive HPV is also the culprit of high-altitude pulmonary edema (HAPE), a potentially lethal complication in susceptible individuals visiting altitudes >2,500 m [17]. HAPE is characterized by exaggerated vasoconstriction, increased PA pressures, excessive shear stress, and subsequent stress fracture of the pulmonary vascular endothelium [27–30]. The latter appears to occur as the result of perfusion heterogeneity within the lung caused by uneven distribution of the severity of the HPV response [31]. This results in areas of the lung in which blood flow is severely diminished and redirected to areas where HPV is less intense. These high flow areas are prone to capillary failure leading to the patchy distribution of pulmonary edema formation that is characteristic of HAPE (Fig. 4.3) [32]. Rapid ascent and exercise at high altitude are risk factors, as are conditions causing a restricted pulmonary vascular bed (e.g., unilateral absence of a pulmonary artery) [33, 34].

Even though first described many years ago, the exact mechanisms of HPV are still incompletely understood [33]. Recent research implicates mitochondria in pulmonary artery smooth muscle cells as sensors of hypoxia and effectors of HPV, with hypoxia-induced changes in mitochondrial concentration of reactive

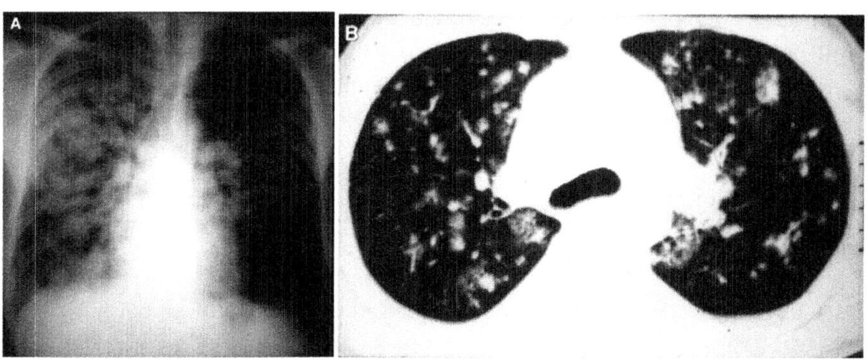

Fig. 4.3 High-altitude pulmonary edema. (**a**) Predominant right-sided patchy airspace disease in a 37-year-old mountaineer with high-altitude pulmonary edema (HAPE). (**b**) Chest CT of a 27-year-old mountaineer with history of recurrent HAPE demonstrating nondependent, patchy airspace disease. Note areas of normal lung adjacent to areas of dense infiltrate (with permission from reference 30b)

oxygen species (ROS) leading to inhibition of membrane potassium channels (e.g., Kv1.5, Kv2.1), depolarization of membrane potential, opening of voltage-dependent calcium channels, increases in intracellular calcium concentration, and subsequent vasoconstriction [25, 26, 35–39].

Hypoxic Pulmonary Vascular Remodeling

Chronic hypoxia induces significant structural remodeling characterized by the hallmark appearance of smooth muscle-like cells in previously nonmuscularized pulmonary vessels. This is demonstrated even in otherwise healthy persons chronically living at altitude, who have an increased number of muscularized peripheral pulmonary arterial branches associated with increased PAP at rest and with exertion [40, 41]. In humans, after as little as 6 weeks of chronic hypoxia exposure, changes in PVR are not immediately reversible with administration of oxygen, suggesting significant remodeling has already taken place [42]. Importantly, and in striking contrast to PAH, the hypoxia-induced pulmonary artery remodeling is partially to fully reversible upon cessation of the hypoxic stimulus (e.g., moving to a lower altitude) [41, 43].

All portions of the pulmonary arterial wall are involved in hypoxic pulmonary vascular remodeling. Major contributors to the development of HPH are the hypoxia-inducible factors (HIFs), in particular HIF-1α and HIF-2α [44, 45]. HIFs function as transcription factors that bind to specific hypoxia-responsive elements of their target genes (e.g., erythropoietin, vascular endothelial growth factor, Glut-1, endothelin-1, angiopoietin-2), thus regulating almost every single process affected by hypoxia. In the pulmonary vasculature, HIF-1α appears to play a more predominant role in smooth muscle cells, while HIF-2α is primary located in pulmonary artery endothelial cells [44, 45]. The critical role of HIFs in the development of HPH was demonstrated by an elegant animal study, in which mice partially deficient in HIF-1α had an attenuated response to hypoxia and were largely protected from HPH [46]. Interestingly, genetic variations in the HIF system are associated with better adaptation to high altitude. For example, several studies have recently demonstrated that Tibetan highlanders, a population that has previously been shown to exhibit better adaptation to high altitude than other populations living at similar altitude, exhibit single nucleotide polymorphisms (SNPs) in the gene encoding for HIF-2α, as well as in genes encoding for regulators of HIF-1α signaling [47–49].

On a cellular level, hypoxic pulmonary vascular remodeling is characterized by activation and involvement of all cell types of the pulmonary vasculature. In particular, the hypoxic pulmonary vasculature is characterized by endothelial cell activation, smooth muscle cell proliferation, de-differentiation of adventitial fibroblasts into myofibroblasts, activation and recruitment of inflammatory cells and progenitor cells, and increased collagen production [3, 4, 50].

Fibroblasts within the adventitia are among the first cells to be activated by hypoxia and vascular stress, resulting in increased expression of proinflammatory cytokines (e.g., IL-1β, IL-6, CCL2, CXCL12, VCAM-1) and cellular proliferation and differentiation into myofibroblasts, with increased matrix protein production and deposition of collagen and elastin, as well as migration of cells into the media and even intima [3, 24]. An influx of macrophages, fibroblasts, and myofibroblasts, as well as resident and circulating progenitor cells, contributes to the intimal hyperplasia found in HPH. Medial hypertrophy and muscularization of previously non-muscularized arterioles are driven by the same processes, as well as by smooth muscle cell hypertrophy and proliferation.

Endothelial cells, while not significantly proliferating after exposure to low oxygen levels, contribute to hypoxic pulmonary vascular remodeling through cell surface activation and secretion of paracrine factors, thus resulting in smooth muscle cell proliferation, as well as recruitment of progenitor and proinflammatory cells. In particular, hypoxic endothelial cell activation results in increased production of vasoconstrictors and growth factors (PDGF-β, IGF, VEGF, bFGF, serotonin), adhesion molecules (P-selectin, ICAM, VCAM), cytokines (IL-1, IL-8), procoagulants (tissue factor, PAI-1), and matrix molecules (laminin, fibronectin) [3, 21, 50].

In addition to external and paracrine factors, smooth muscle cells within the media are also stimulated to proliferate by various intracellular signaling mechanisms. For example, changes in mitochondrial redox potential lead to inhibition of potassium channels, activation of voltage-dependent calcium channels, and calcium influx, resulting in both vasoconstriction and smooth muscle cell proliferation [25, 26, 35–39, 51]. Together, the cells of the pulmonary artery wall serve to recruit and activate circulating inflammatory cells such as monocytes and fibrocytes (predominantly via the vasa vasorum), as well as resident and circulating progenitor cells, thus further contributing to ongoing chronic inflammation, vasoconstriction, and structural remodeling [3, 24, 52]. In this context, it is important to note that upon chronic hypoxia exposure, alveolar inflammation seems to precede pulmonary vascular inflammation, and amelioration of the inflammatory process in the alveolar space is associated with decreased pulmonary vascular remodeling and HPH [53, 54].

Hypoxia-Independent Mechanisms of Pulmonary Vascular Remodeling

Pulmonary vasoconstriction and activation of the pulmonary vascular remodeling process may also occur independently of hypoxia. For example, hypoxia-independent factors implicated in PH pathogenesis in chronic lung disease include vasoconstrictive effects of hypercarbia [55], compression and destruction of alveolar vessels from structural alterations and fibrotic lung disease [56–58], concomitant left ventricular systolic or diastolic dysfunction [59, 60], hemodynamic effects of hyperinflation on pulmonary vascular filling and RV or left ventricular function [61, 62], as well as pulmonary artery smooth muscle cell senescence [63, 64] and toxic effects of cigarette smoke (see Fig. 4.2) [65–68].

Pulmonary artery wall cell senescence has recently been identified as a potential contributor to PH in COPD [63, 64]. This paradigm encompasses a scenario where senescent pulmonary artery smooth muscle cells from COPD patients (characterized by increased p16, p21 and β-galactosidase expression, fewer cell population doublings, and shorter telomeres than cells from controls) stimulate growth and migration of adjacent normal smooth muscle cells through the production and release of paracrine factors such as IL-6, IL-8, TNF-α, MCP-1, and TGF-β [63]. This notion is supported by the fact that the senescent cells are almost exclusively confined to the media, thus being adjacent to areas of marked cell proliferation [63]. Interestingly, this paradigm of telomere shortening, premature senescence, and pro-inflammatory signaling has also been described for pulmonary artery endothelial cells in COPD patients [64]. However, even though there is an association between senescence and pulmonary vascular remodeling, as well as an inverse relationship between telomere length and mean PAP and PVR [63], it currently remains unknown if senescence is a cause or a consequence of the pulmonary vascular remodeling observed in COPD. In addition, the potential triggers for pulmonary artery smooth muscle cell and endothelial cell senescence (e.g., age, hypoxia, inflammation, oxidative stress) have not yet been identified [69].

Importantly, recent studies implicated chronic exposure to cigarette smoke as a major contributor to PH development. In particular, cigarette smoke has been shown to result in endothelial cell dysfunction with a subsequent vasodilator-vasoconstrictor imbalance due to decreased nitric oxide and prostacyclin and increased ET-1. This is associated with smooth muscle cell proliferation, progenitor and inflammatory cell recruitment, and distortion of the normal pulmonary wall architecture [65–68]. Oxidative stress, reactive nitrogen species, and inflammation have been implicated as major mediators of cigarette smoke-induced vascular damage [65, 68, 70–72]. Such changes may be seen even in smokers without overt emphysema. For example, an intriguing recent study demonstrated that in the setting of chronic cigarette smoke exposure, pulmonary vascular dysfunction and PH can precede alveolar destruction and emphysema [70]. The authors showed that cigarette smoke causes endothelial dysfunction with increased inducible nitric oxide synthase (iNOS), inflammation, and smooth muscle cell proliferation, clinically resulting in RV hypertrophy and PH [67]. Interestingly, development of PH in this model was dependent on iNOS from bone marrow-derived cells [70].

Right Ventricular Dysfunction in Chronic Lung Disease (Cor Pulmonale)

The vascular remodeling and inflammation in HPH ultimately lead to pressure overload of the RV, complicated by RV hypertrophy, remodeling, and ultimately death. Elevated RV afterload is reflected by a steady increase in the resistance of the pulmonary vascular bed, by increased blood viscosity from elevated red blood cell mass, and by decreased dynamic compliance and stiffening of the large proximal pulmonary arteries [4, 73]. The initial response of the RV is an adaptive remodeling, characterized by increased capillarization and cardiac myocyte hypertrophy, with absence of apoptosis and fibrosis [74]. RV contractility is relatively preserved, but the RV is prone to dysfunction during episodes of further hypoxemia or air trapping, which may occur during pulmonary exacerbations, exercise, or nocturnal desaturations [75].

While RV dysfunction in these settings most likely is due to increases in afterload, thoracic hyperinflation (as seen in emphysema or bullous lung disease) may further decrease RV stroke volume by decreasing cardiac preload [61].

Importantly in HPH, the degree of RV hypertrophy correlates with the severity of hypoxemia. Hypoxia-induced RV hypertrophy occurs in conjunction with increases in gene expression of mRNA encoding for proinflammatory and chemotactic cytokines (e.g., IL-1β, S100A4, MCP-1, and SDF-1) [76]. The end result is cor pulmonale, characterized by RV hypertrophy, dilatation, and dysfunction in the setting of chronic lung disease and HPH.

Systemic factors such as neurohormonal activation further contribute to RV dysfunction and fluid retention. Neurohormonal activation is particularly pronounced in the setting of hypercarbic states, as can be seen in end-stage COPD, severe restrictive lung disease, and obesity hypoventilation syndrome [77]. In these conditions, the combination of hypercarbia and hypoxia results in decreased effective renal plasma flow, increased activation of the renin-aldosterone system, and increased production of vasopressin [78]. The result is excessive sodium and water retention, leading to edema and further increases in preload and afterload, ultimately further exacerbating RV dysfunction [75, 77].

Clinical Presentation, Relevance, and Prognostic Implications

Pathologic pulmonary vascular abnormalities precede the development of clinically apparent HPH. Initially, elevated PAP may only be seen during exercise, exacerbations, or nocturnal desaturations, and the presence of exercise-induced PH is a strong predictor for later development of resting PH [79]. The clinical presentation of HPH may be difficult to distinguish from the associated pulmonary disease, as dyspnea, fatigue, cough, chest pain, and edema may all be due to the underlying lung disease. Thus, a high index of suspicion is required. One notable difference is the presentation of "out of proportion" PH. Although most patients with group 3 PH have mild-to-moderate increases in PAP with mean PAP typically not exceeding 35–40 mmHg, a small percentage (<5 % of COPD patients) present with mean PAP greater than 40 mmHg [6]. These patients often exhibit only mild-to-moderate airflow obstruction but significant impairments in diffusing capacity, as well as more severe hypoxemia and hypocarbia [6]. The extent of pulmonary arterial lesions in explanted lungs after transplantation correlates with the severity of pulmonary hypertension in COPD, with progressively severe medial hypertrophy and intimal fibrosis [80].

Similar to the COPD-PH population, PH in the setting of pulmonary fibrosis usually falls into the mild-to-moderate range. For example, in a study of IPF patients evaluated for lung transplantation, median mean PAP was 31 mmHg, with an interquartile range of 28–38 mmHg [81]. PH appears to be more pronounced, however, in the syndrome of CPFE. In a series of 40 patients with CPFE and PH, mean PAP was 40 ± 9 mmHg, cardiac index was 2.5 ± 0.7 L/min/m^2, and PVR was 521 ± 205 dyn s cm^{-5} [82].

Finally, among patients with sleep-disordered breathing, mean PAP was found to be 28 ± 6 mmHg, and cardiac output was maintained, again indicating that group 3 is usually mild to moderate [13]. Higher body mass index, higher daytime carbon dioxide tension, and lower daytime oxygen tension are strongly correlated with the development of PH in this setting [13]. Among 26 patients with obesity hypoventilation syndrome undergoing evaluation for bariatric surgery, mean PAP was 36 ± 14 mmHg, compared to 18 ± 6 mmHg in 20 obese patients without hypoventilation. The higher elevations in PAP in this study may be in part due to a high incidence of diastolic dysfunction, which was frequently identified in this study [83].

Regardless of the cause, even mild PH in the setting of chronic lung disease is associated with poorer clinical outcomes. For example, there are significant increases in the frequency of pulmonary exacerbations and hospitalizations in COPD patients with mean PAP above 18 mmHg [84]. Furthermore, patients with COPD or IPF and concomitant PH have poorer exercise capacity [58]. A recent study of COPD patients with mild, moderate, or severe PH further investigated this phenomenon and demonstrated that COPD patients with mild or moderate PH exhibit ventilatory limitations during exercise, while patients with severe PH are characterized by circulatory limitations, as evidenced by decreased cardiac output and central venous oxygen saturation [85]. Lastly, for those patients who require lung transplant, there is an increased risk of primary graft dysfunction, with a 1.6-fold increased risk for every 10 mmHg increase in mean PAP [86].

Importantly, PH and RV dysfunction in the setting of chronic lung disease are associated with worse survival, with increasing mortality correlating with the severity of elevation in mean PAP [11, 56, 73, 82, 87, 88]. In fact, the best prognostic factor in COPD patients requiring long-term home oxygen therapy was not the forced expiratory volume, hypoxemia, or hypercapnia but the degree of PH [89]. Similar findings were observed in a recent study of IPF patients referred for lung transplantation. In this cohort, echocardiographically determined RV size and RV dysfunction, as well as higher PVR, were independent predictors of mortality [88].

Diagnosis

Diagnostic tools for the detection of group 3 PH do not differ substantially from those used in group 1 PH, but there are some special considerations in patients with chronic lung disease. Unfortunately, clinical examination is insensitive in diagnosing group 3 PH. A loud second heart sound or tricuspid regurgitation may be obscured by hyperinflation or adventitious lung sounds, and edema, though indicating the presence of cor pulmonale, is a late finding in HPH.

Routine pulmonary diagnostics such as electrocardiogram, pulmonary function testing, 6 min walk testing, and brain natriuretic peptide level determination may provide important clues for the diagnosis. Although an electrocardiogram showing right atrial and RV hypertrophy and RV strain is fairly specific for PH, the absence of these findings does not preclude a diagnosis of PH. On pulmonary function testing, diffusing capacity is frequently decreased out of proportion to the decrease in the forced expiratory volume or forced vital capacity, particularly in patients with PH out of proportion to their underlying disease or in CPFE [82]. Significant desaturations during 6 min walk testing suggest an inadequate cardiopulmonary reserve and point towards PH [6]. Similarly, profound hypoxemia at rest may be a sign of significant PH. Brain natriuretic peptide levels, when elevated in the absence of left heart disease, renal insufficiency, or pulmonary embolism, may serve as an indicator of RV strain and as a prognostic marker for mortality [90].

Standard CT imaging may show evidence of RV dysfunction, such as an enlarged RV with a right ventricle-to-left ventricle ratio greater than one, a dilated pulmonary artery, or reflux of intravenous contrast into the inferior vena cava and hepatic veins indicative of tricuspid regurgitation (see Fig. 4.4). The presence of an increased pulmonary artery diameter on routine chest CT imaging has recently been identified

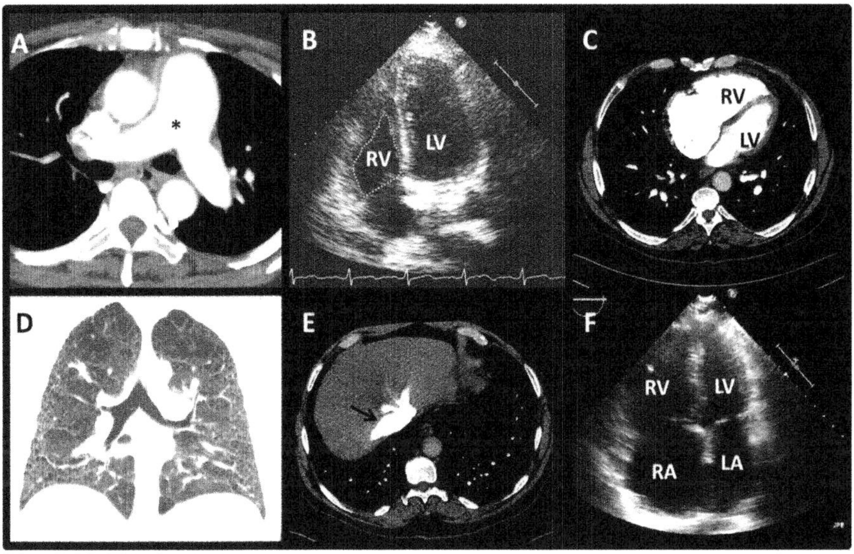

Fig. 4.4 Distinct PH phenotypes in group 3 PH. (**a**, **b**) Radiographic and echocardiographic imaging studies in a 51-year-old female with obesity and obstructive sleep apnea. Note enlarged PA diameter in (**a**; *asterisk*). Echocardiogram shows preserved RV and LV size and function (**b**). Right heart catheterization revealed an RA pressure of 3 mmHg, PA pressure of 41/17 (mean 26) mmHg, and a pulmonary capillary wedge pressure of 4 mmHg. This patient was treated with continuous positive airway pressure and weight loss; no pulmonary vasodilators were used. (**c**–**f**) Radiographic and echocardiographic imaging studies in a 60-year-old male with combined pulmonary fibrosis and emphysema. In addition to an enlarged PA (not shown), CT shows evidence of an elevated RV to LV ratio (**c**), severe parenchymal lung disease (**d**), and reflux of contrast media into the inferior vena cava and hepatic veins (**e**; *arrow*). Echocardiogram revealed RA and RV dilation and leftward septal shift, consistent with right heart failure (**f**). Right heart catheterization revealed a RA pressure of 9 mmHg, PA pressure of 73/24 (mean 41) mmHg, and a pulmonary capillary wedge pressure of 8 mmHg. Due to significant hypoxemia, functional limitations, and the severity of the hemodynamic alterations with severe RV dysfunction, PAH-specific therapy was initiated at a PAH center under close monitoring of oxygenation parameters. *LA* left atrium, *LV* left ventricle, *PA* pulmonary artery, *RA* right atrium, *RV* right ventricle

as a predictor of exacerbations in patients with COPD [91]. However, pulmonary artery enlargement (especially if mild to moderate) is not specific for the presence of group 3 PH and may indicate PAP increases from volume overload, left heart disease, pulmonary embolism, or sleep apnea [92].

Echocardiography is an important screening tool in patients with lung disease and is critical for detecting RV structural abnormalities. Unfortunately, echocardiography is less accurate for the estimation of PAP in patients with chronic lung disease. A cohort study of 374 lung transplant candidates showed a sensitivity and specificity of only 85 % and 55 %, respectively, for diagnosis of PH, with 52 % of RV systolic pressure measurements being inaccurate by >10 mmHg [93]. This inaccuracy is due at least in part to poor echocardiographic windows and inadequate visualization of the tricuspid regurgitant jet due to lung hyperinflation. Consequentially, PH should be suspected if there is echocardiographic evidence of right heart chamber enlargement, leftward septal shift, and/or RV hypokinesis, even if the RV systolic pressure is not significantly elevated or not measurable. The role of newer echocardiographic methods such as tissue Doppler or speckle tracking for assessment of cor pulmonale and group 3 PH has not been assessed in detail, but studies in patients with PAH suggest that these are sensitive methods for the assessment of RV function [94–97]. However, limitations with regard to lung hyperinflation may apply to these techniques as well.

Cardiac MRI, though limited by availability and cost, is increasingly being used for determination of RV form and function [98, 99]. While there is no role for routine MRI scanning of the RV in chronic lung disease at this point, cardiac MRI should be considered if an accurate assessment of RV form and function is required and the RV cannot be visualized adequately on echocardiography.

As with other forms of PH, right heart catheterization (RHC) remains the gold standard for diagnosis of HPH. RHC should be considered in patients with significant PH risk factors, such as otherwise unexplained dyspnea, significant hypoxemia, desaturations during 6 min walk testing, elevated brain natriuretic peptide levels, or isolated decreases in DLCO. Similarly, RHC is indicated if there is echocardiographic evidence of significant PH. Since the presence of PH increases the risk of COPD exacerbations, RHC should also be considered in patients with recurrent admissions for COPD exacerbation and/or cor pulmonale [84]. However, it is important to emphasize that other etiologies of dyspnea and exacerbations commonly encountered in chronic lung disease need to be ruled out before proceeding with RHC, including venous thromboembolism, coronary artery disease, ongoing tobacco abuse, medical nonadherence, or infection with nontuberculous mycobacteria. Similarly, treatment for the underlying lung disease and/or hypoxemia should be optimized as much as possible before RHC is considered. Lastly, RHC in the setting of an acute exacerbation of the underlying lung disease yields little information about the patient's chronic state, as PA pressures may be temporarily elevated due to hypoxemia, hypercarbia, or volume overload.

In addition to quantifying the severity of PH, RHC may help exclude other causes of PH. Hemodynamic assessment during RHC should reveal a mean PAP $\geq$ 25 mmHg and a pulmonary capillary wedge pressure $\leq$15 mmHg to confirm group 3 PH. Borderline or elevated pulmonary capillary wedge pressures may suggest concomitant systolic or diastolic heart disease, and can be further assessed by measuring a concomitant left ventricular end-diastolic pressure or by reassessing hemodynamics after a saline bolus or exercise challenge [100]. Typically, PVR and transpulmonary pressure gradient (mPAP-PCWP) are low ($\leq$3 Wood units and $\leq$12 mmHg, respectively). However, in the setting of out of proportion PH, or in the presence of other comorbidities known to cause PH (e.g., sleep-disordered breathing, pulmonary emboli, or left heart disease), both parameters may be markedly elevated.

Of note, patients with severe dyspnea or obesity may exhibit significant intrathoracic pressure changes due to increased respiratory efforts [101]. This may lead to artifactual decreases in hemodynamic parameters if software-generated pressure readings are used, as those values simply represent an automated mean of the pressure readings [102]. It is therefore important to emphasize that all pressures should be determined at end-expiration with the patient breathing comfortably [101]. One exception to this paradigm applies to patients with significant dynamic hyperinflation and air trapping, in whom end-expiratory pressures may be falsely elevated, and thus in these patients pressures should be determined as the mean over several respiratory cycles.

Treatment

General Treatment Strategies

Therapeutic strategies for group 3 PH focus on aggressively treating the underlying condition causing the elevated PAP. In hypoxemic patients with severe COPD, continuous long-term oxygen therapy is associated with improvement in survival irrespective of the presence of PH [103]. However, among patients with concomitant PH, oxygen therapy for greater than 18 h per day was shown to decrease resting PAP by 3 mmHg and exercise PAP by 6 mmHg. On the other hand, the same study showed that nocturnal oxygen therapy alone was not sufficient to improve mortality [103]. It is currently recommended that hypoxemia during exercise be corrected with the use of oxygen supplementation, even though the evidence supporting this approach is less robust.

Smoking cessation is critical to attenuating the ongoing endothelial dysfunction and inflammation that promote pulmonary vascular remodeling and PH development from tobacco exposure. Recent studies show that cigarette smoke can induce PH though iNOS activation, even before the parenchymal changes of emphysema develop [70]. Similarly, smoking cessation also prevents further parenchymal damage as a contributor to PH development.

Pulmonary rehabilitation may be beneficial in HPH, though special considerations are required. Symptoms can help determine a safe level of submaximal exercise, and patients should avoid activities that cause symptoms such as dizziness, presyncope, and chest pain. Exercises such as heavy lifting, valsalva maneuvers, or interval training should be avoided due to potential rapid changes in cardiopulmonary hemodynamics [104].

Due to the high incidence of sleep-disordered breathing among patients with HPH, polysomnography should be considered in all patients with sleep-disordered breathing symptoms, including morning headaches, excessive fatigue, or witnessed apneas. Patients with both COPD and OSA have significantly higher mortality and risk of hospitalization than patients with either COPD or OSA alone, and both hospitalizations and mortality are ameliorated by the use of positive airway pressure [105]. In OSA, the use of continuous positive airway pressure begins improving RV end-diastolic diameter and RV systolic pressure in as little as 3 months, with continued cardiac remodeling with long-term use [106]. Patients with obesity hypoventilation syndrome benefit from noninvasive positive pressure ventilation and weight loss, including bariatric surgery [83].

Even though there is a general lack of published and evidence-based strategies, clinical experience suggests that diuretics are indicated if there is clinical, echocardiographic, or hemodynamic evidence of elevated right atrial pressures. Loop diuretics such as furosemide are generally preferred. Although aldosterone antagonists are conceptually appealing due to inhibition of the renin-aldosterone system, there are no studies in HPH to guide therapy. Significant diuresis is frequently required, though caution must be taken to avoid over diuresis [75]. When indicated, the use of continuous positive airway pressure or noninvasive positive pressure ventilation may help with fluid mobilization.

Lastly, given the reversibility of hypoxia-induced pulmonary vascular remodeling upon exposure to higher alveolar oxygen pressures, patients with HPH living at high altitude are recommended to move to lower altitudes [4]. If such an approach is not feasible, an alternative but technically much more challenging strategy encompasses oxygen enrichment of the ambient air [41]. HAPE is treated with descent to lower altitudes, oxygen, and nifedipine [41].

Pulmonary Vasodilators

Given the development of several new drugs in PAH over the past decade, there has been significant excitement to translate these medications into use within group 3 PH. Unfortunately, this excitement has been met largely with disappointment, likely because pulmonary vasodilators may inhibit HPV, resulting in increased ventilation-perfusion mismatch and impaired gas exchange. As such, a clear role for pulmonary vasodilators in group 3 PH has not yet been established, and the general use of PAH-specific therapies in this patient population is currently not recommended. Studies of pulmonary vasodilator use in group 3 PH are reviewed in detail below and in Table 4.3.

Pulmonary Vasodilators in COPD

Several studies have assessed the role of pulmonary vasodilators in COPD. A single dose of the phosphodiesterase type 5 (PDE5) inhibitor sildenafil was shown to improve pulmonary hemodynamics, but at the expense of inhibiting HPV and

Table 4.3 Overview of studies of PAH-specific therapies in WHO group 3 PH

Study	Design	Patient population	Study size	Study duration	Medication	Outcome
Stolz, *ERJ* (2008)	2:1 Randomized double blind placebo controlled	Severe to very severe COPD and mild PH by ECHO	30	12 weeks	Bosentan 62.5 mg bid orally, increased to 125 mg bid after 2 weeks	No change in exercise capacity, ↓ oxygenation, ↓QOL
Dernaika, *Respiration* (2010)	Cohort single treatment	Severe COPD and mild-to-moderate PH by ECHO	10	1 visit	Iloprost 2.5–5 μg inhaled once	↑ 6MWD, no change in oxygenation, improved V/Q matching
Lederer, *COPD* (2012)	Randomized double blind crossover	Severe COPD without PH	10	9 weeks	Sildenafil 75 mg orally tid	No change in exercise capacity, ↓ oxygenation, ↓QOL, ↑ symptoms
Boeck, *PLoS One* (2012)	Randomized double blind crossover	Moderate-to-severe COPD and mild-to-moderate PH	16	3 visits	Iloprost 10 and 20 μg inhaled once on separate visits	No change in 6MWD, ↓ oxygenation, ↓ peak oxygen consumption
Blanco, *AJRCCM* (2013)	Randomized double blind placebo controlled	Severe COPD and mild-to-moderate PH	63	12 weeks	Sildenafil 20 mg orally tid	No change in exercise capacity, adverse events, or oxygenation
Olschewski *AJRCCM* (1999)	Randomized drug challenge during RHC	Moderate-to-severe pulmonary fibrosis (multiple etiologies) and moderate-to-severe PH	8	1 visit	iNO 15–80 ppm; epoprostenol IV 5–16 ng/kg/min; aerosolized epoprostenol 54–68 μg	iNO and aerosolized prostaglandin cause selective pulmonary vasodilation and improve pulmonary hemodynamics without worsening oxygenation; IV prostaglandin worsened V/Q mismatch
Ghofrani, *Lancet* (2002)	Randomized open-label	Moderate pulmonary fibrosis (multiple etiologies) and moderate PH	16	1 visit	Sildenafil 50 mg orally once or intravenous epoprostenol	Sildenafil ↑ oxygenation and maintained V/Q matching; epoprostenol ↑ V/Q mismatch and ↓ oxygenation

(continued)

Table 4.3 (continued)

Study	Design	Patient population	Study size	Study duration	Medication	Outcome
Zisman, *NEJM* (2010)	Randomized double blind placebo controlled	Moderate-to-severe IPF	180	24 weeks	Sildenafil 20 mg orally tid	No change in 6MWD but ↑ QOL and ↓ dyspnea
Han, *Chest* (2013)	Subgroup analysis of Zisman (above)		119	12 weeks	Sildenafil 20 mg orally tid	Sildenafil preserved exercise capacity, ↑ QOL and ↓ dyspnea in patients with IPF and RV dysfunction
Blanco, *J Appl Physiol* (2011)	Open-label uncontrolled pilot study	Moderate IPF and mild PH	7	1 visit	iNO 40 ppm	iNO ↓ PAP at rest and with exertion without altering V/Q matching
King, *AJRCCM* (2011)	2:1 Randomized double blind placebo controlled	Moderate IPF	616	20 months	Bosentan 62.5 mg orally bid, increased to 125 mg bid after 4 weeks	No change in time to IPF worsening, death, QOL, or dyspnea
Raghu. *Ann Int Med* (2013)	2:1 Randomized double blind placebo controlled	IPF; PH present only in 11 % of study patients	492	34 weeks	Ambrisentan 5 or 10 mg orally daily	Ambrisentan ↑ hospitalizations and shortened time to IPF progression; study terminated prematurely
Hoeper, *ERJ* (2013)	Open-label uncontrolled pilot study	Moderate pulmonary fibrosis and moderate-to-severe PH	22	12 weeks; 12 month extension	Riociguat 1.0–2.5 mg orally tid (up-titrated)	Riociguat improved cardiac output and PVR but mean PAP was unchanged

6MWD 6 min walk distance, *COPD* chronic obstructive pulmonary disease, *ECHO* echocardiogram, *iNO* inhaled nitric oxide, *IPF* idiopathic pulmonary fibrosis, *PAP* pulmonary artery pressure, *PH* pulmonary hypertension, *PVR* pulmonary vascular resistance, *QOL* quality of life, *RHC* right heart catheterization, *RV* right ventricle, *V/Q* ventilation-perfusion

worsening hypoxemia [107]. Based on the rationale that sildenafil may increase exercise capacity during altitude-induced hypoxia [108], a study of 63 patients with severe COPD and mild-to-moderate PH (mean PAP 27–32 mmHg) investigated the effects of sildenafil during 3 months of pulmonary rehabilitation. Sildenafil at 20 mg three times daily caused no significant adverse events, but also no difference in oxygenation or exercise tolerance [109]. A second crossover exercise study in ten patients with COPD *without* PH showed no effect on exercise capacity, but worsening oxygenation, poorer quality of life, and increased symptoms [110]. Finally, the endothelial receptor antagonist bosentan was found to have no effect on exercise capacity, and to worsen oxygenation and quality of life in patients with severe COPD and mild PH [111].

The above studies suggest no benefit to oral pulmonary vasodilators in COPD with the potential to cause harm. Consequently, additional studies have evaluated the role of *inhaled* pulmonary vasodilators, with the intention to deliver drug preferentially to well-ventilated areas of the lung and thus avoid worsening ventilation-perfusion mismatching. Two studies have evaluated the acute effect of iloprost, a short-acting inhaled prostacyclin, in COPD patients with PH, but with conflicting effects on exercise capacity and oxygenation [112, 113]. Thus the potential benefit of inhaled vasodilators in COPD-related PH remains undefined.

Pulmonary Vasodilators in Pulmonary Fibrosis

Small studies in patients with pulmonary fibrosis and PH demonstrated that inhaled pulmonary vasodilators including iloprost and nitric oxide can improve PAP and PVR without worsening ventilation-perfusion mismatching [114, 115]. In contrast, intravenous epoprostenol was shown to worsen ventilation-perfusion mismatch and cause increased hypoxia and hypotension [114, 116].

Interestingly, a single dose of sildenafil was shown to improve oxygenation and maintain ventilation-perfusion matching in a small group of pulmonary fibrosis patients [116]. Longer term oral administration of sildenafil (20 mg three times daily) slightly improved quality of life and dyspnea in patients with advanced IPF (DLCO <35 %), with an attenuated decline in exercise tolerance specifically amongst patients with RV dysfunction [117, 118]. On the other hand, endothelin receptor antagonists have not shown any benefit in IPF, though these studies have not focused specifically on patients with PH and/or RV dysfunction in the setting of pulmonary fibrosis [119–121]. Finally, a small pilot study of riociguat, a soluble guanylate cyclase stimulator, in patients with moderate pulmonary fibrosis and moderate-to-severe PH showed improvement in PVR and cardiac output, although there was no change in PAP and a relatively large number of patients exhibited adverse events [122]. Small decreases in oxygenation were offset by increases in mixed venous oxygen saturation (likely from increased cardiac output); however, this did not translate into significant increases in exercise capacity.

Pulmonary Vasodilators in Other Conditions

No prospective studies exist investigating the use of pulmonary vasodilators in CPFE or sleep-disordered breathing. In the series by Cottin et al., 60 % of CPFE patients were treated with pulmonary vasodilators. No significant effect of treatment was observed on NHYA class, 6MWD, or estimated systolic PAP at echocardiography [82]. PDE5 inhibitors may be beneficial for the prevention or treatment of HAPE, but their role at this point is unclear. While one study showed that tadalafil decreased systolic PAP and reduced the incidence of HAPE in adults with a history of HAPE [123], in a more recent study, sildenafil did not affect systolic PAP in healthy lowlanders at 5,200 m [124].

Treatment of Out of Proportion Pulmonary Hypertension

In general, the above-mentioned studies demonstrate that treatment of all-comers with group 3 PH is not associated with significant merit. However, when focusing on patients with more pronounced PH and/or RV dysfunction, treatment effects seem to be more pronounced. In general, the signal for beneficial treatment effects appears to be strongest in patients with pulmonary fibrosis with significant PH and/or RV dysfunction being treated with a PDE5 inhibitor [118]. Inhaled prostacyclins or soluble guanylate cyclase stimulators may be beneficial in this population as well [114, 116, 122].

Thus it currently remains unclear if selected patients with preserved lung function and significantly increased PAP and/or evidence of RV dysfunction (so-called out of proportion PH) would benefit from pulmonary vasodilators. In theory, such patients would be less likely to exhibit clinically significant ventilation-perfusion mismatch yet have more hemodynamic effects, and thus would be more likely to derive significant clinical benefit (see Fig. 4.4). Case reports suggest this may be true [125]. For example, the use of subcutaneous treprostinil to treat patients with advanced interstitial lung disease suffering from severe right ventricular failure has been reported in a recent case series [122]. These patients appeared to have hemodynamic and clinical improvement, raising the possibility of this approach as a bridge to transplantation. However, randomized placebo controlled trials in this population have not been performed and are clearly needed.

In summary, the general treatment of group 3 PH with pulmonary vasodilators clearly is discouraged. Rather, a strategy of aggressive treatment of the underlying disease with a thorough evaluation for potential other contributors to PH development (e.g., hypoxemia, sleep-disordered breathing, volume overload, ongoing tobacco abuse, pulmonary embolism, and left heart disease) should be pursued. Correction of these factors is of utmost importance. Once all potential contributors to PH development have been adequately addressed, treatment of *selected* patients with severe hemodynamic alterations and RV dysfunction may be pursued on a case-by-case basis, but should only be performed by providers with experience in PAH treatment, ideally in the framework of a clinical study

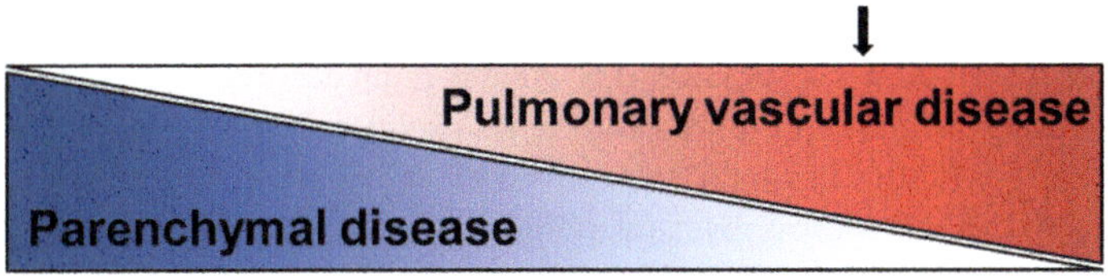

Fig. 4.5 Paradigm for treatment of patients with group 3 PH. Treatment of all patients with group 3 PH aims at optimizing the treatment of the underlying lung disease and contributing comorbidities. Evidence-based treatments with known attenuating effects on PA pressure elevations (e.g., oxygen supplementation, treatment of sleep-disordered breathing, diuresis) should be employed whenever indicated. In patients that exhibit signs and symptoms of PH despite these interventions, pulmonary vasodilators may be of merit in the subpopulation of patients with presence of significant pulmonary vascular disease and/or RV dysfunction, and lack of severe parenchymal abnormalities (*arrow*). If used, pulmonary vasodilators should only be administered at a PAH center and under close monitoring of oxygenation parameters, ideally in the framework of a clinical study

(see Fig. 4.5). Close follow-up with measurement of oxygenation and a low threshold to discontinue treatment in case of adverse events or lack of benefit are mandatory. Patients with advanced lung disease, with or without PH, should also be considered for lung transplantation.

Potential Novel Treatment Strategies for Group 3 PH

With improved understanding of the pathogenesis of HPH, there is growing interest in new treatment options. First, with the discovery of HIF as a key regulator of hypoxic vasoconstriction and remodeling, there has been increased interest in iron metabolism. This is based on the rationale that iron is a key coenzyme for the proteasomal degradation of HIF. Thus iron deficiency states can lead to upregulation of HIF pathways, hypoxic pulmonary vascular remodeling, and HPV [126]. Recent studies demonstrate that acute HPV can be attenuated by administration of intravenous iron, while chronic hypoxic vasoconstriction such as is seen in chronic mountain sickness is exacerbated by iron depletion [127]. In fact, iron deficiency has now been shown to be an independent predictor of mortality in patients with idiopathic PAH [128].

Direct inhibition of HIF is also under investigation. Cardiac glycosides such as digoxin have demonstrated in vitro inhibitory effects on HIF-1 dependent gene transcription [129]. A recent study of digoxin in mice exposed to chronic hypoxia demonstrated that daily digoxin therapy attenuated the development of RV hypertrophy and PH, whereas therapy initiated after HPH was established led to less severe hypoxia-induced elevations in PAP [130].

Investigations are also under way to inhibit the inflammatory response that accompanies HPH. Multiple studies demonstrated that activation of alveolar macrophages precedes and precipitates the activation of other cell types leading to subsequent vascular inflammation and remodeling [53, 54]. A recent study in mice injected with exosome preparations from mesenchymal stem cells prior to hypoxia exposure demonstrated suppression of hypoxia-induced influx of macrophages in bronchoalveolar lavage fluid. Furthermore, two sequential injections of mesenchymal stem cell exosomes during a 3-week course of hypoxia ameliorated the development of PH, RV hypertrophy, and pulmonary vascular remodeling by further attenuating the inflammatory response to hypoxia [53].

Given the inhibitory effects of sex hormones on HPV and hypoxic vascular remodeling, hormonal therapies or nonhormonal strategies targeting signaling pathways employed by sex hormones may be able to attenuate HPH [72, 131, 132]. In particular, 17β-estradiol, as well as specific activators of the estrogen receptor, has been shown to attenuate HPV, HPH, and hypoxia-induced RV dysfunction without increasing ventilation/perfusion mismatch in rodent models [72, 131, 132].

Finally, research continues in the role of cigarette smoke in the development of HPH, with interest in blocking cigarette smoke-induced pulmonary vascular dysfunction. Given the identification that iNOS-deficient mice are protected from the development of both emphysema and PH, pharmacologic iNOS inhibition represents a new potential target in PH associated with tobacco smoke exposure and emphysema [70]. Further studies assessing the role of treatment with iNOS inhibitors are under way.

Unfortunately, treatment options for patients with lung disease who develop HPH are relatively limited at this time. As our understanding of the pathogenesis of HPH improves, new treatment targets will likely be identified. The above-mentioned molecular targets are promising, but rigorous further study is required.

References

1. Simonneau G, Robbins IM, Beghetti M, et al. Updated clinical classification of pulmonary hypertension. J Am Coll Cardiol. 2009;54(1 Suppl):S43–54.
2. Hoeper MM, Barbera JA, Channick RN, et al. Diagnosis, assessment, and treatment of non-pulmonary arterial hypertension pulmonary hypertension. J Am Coll Cardiol. 2009;54(1 Suppl):S85–96.
3. Stenmark KR, Fagan KA, Frid MG. Hypoxia-induced pulmonary vascular remodeling: cellular and molecular mechanisms. Circ Res. 2006;99(7):675–91.
4. Stenmark KR, Meyrick B, Galie N, Mooi WJ, McMurtry IF. Animal models of pulmonary arterial hypertension: the hope for etiological discovery and pharmacological cure. Am J Physiol. 2009;297(6):L1013–32.
5. Strange G, Playford D, Stewart S, et al. Pulmonary hypertension: prevalence and mortality in the Armadale echocardiography cohort. Heart. 2012;98(24):1805–11.
6. Chaouat A, Naeije R, Weitzenblum E. Pulmonary hypertension in COPD. Eur Respir J. 2008;32(5):1371–85.
7. Andersen KH, Iversen M, Kjaergaard J, et al. Prevalence, predictors, and survival in pulmonary hypertension related to end-stage chronic obstructive pulmonary disease. J Heart Lung Transplant. 2012;31(4):373–80.
8. Thabut G, Dauriat G, Stern JB, et al. Pulmonary hemodynamics in advanced COPD candidates for lung volume reduction surgery or lung transplantation. Chest. 2005;127(5):1531–6.

9. Shorr AF, Wainright JL, Cors CS, Lettieri CJ, Nathan SD. Pulmonary hypertension in patients with pulmonary fibrosis awaiting lung transplant. Eur Respir J. 2007;30(4):715–21.
10. Lettieri CJ, Nathan SD, Barnett SD, Ahmad S, Shorr AF. Prevalence and outcomes of pulmonary arterial hypertension in advanced idiopathic pulmonary fibrosis. Chest. 2006;129(3): 746–52.
11. Nathan SD, Shlobin OA, Ahmad S, et al. Serial development of pulmonary hypertension in patients with idiopathic pulmonary fibrosis. Respiration. 2008;76(3):288–94.
12. Cottin V, Nunes H, Brillet PY, et al. Combined pulmonary fibrosis and emphysema: a distinct underrecognised entity. Eur Respir J. 2005;26(4):586–93.
13. Bady E, Achkar A, Pascal S, Orvoen-Frija E, Laaban JP. Pulmonary arterial hypertension in patients with sleep apnoea syndrome. Thorax. 2000;55(11):934–9.
14. Laks L, Lehrhaft B, Grunstein RR, Sullivan CE. Pulmonary hypertension in obstructive sleep apnoea. Eur Respir J. 1995;8(4):537–41.
15. Sophocles Jr AM. High-altitude pulmonary edema in Vail, Colorado, 1975-1982. West J Med. 1986;144(5):569–73.
16. Hochstrasser J, Nanzer A, Oelz O. [Altitude edema in the Swiss Alps. Observations on the incidence and clinical course in 50 patients 1980–1984]. Schweiz Med Wochenschr. 1986;116(26):866–73.
17. Maggiorini M. High altitude-induced pulmonary oedema. Cardiovasc Res. 2006;72(1): 41–50.
18. Aldashev AA, Sarybaev AS, Sydykov AS, et al. Characterization of high-altitude pulmonary hypertension in the Kyrgyz: association with angiotensin-converting enzyme genotype. Am J Respir Crit Care Med. 2002;166(10):1396–402.
19. Xu XQ, Jing ZC. High-altitude pulmonary hypertension. Eur Respir Rev. 2009;18(111): 13–7.
20. Chaouat A, Bugnet AS, Kadaoui N, et al. Severe pulmonary hypertension and chronic obstructive pulmonary disease. Am J Respir Crit Care Med. 2005;172(2):189–94.
21. Eddahibi S, Chaouat A, Morrell N, et al. Polymorphism of the serotonin transporter gene and pulmonary hypertension in chronic obstructive pulmonary disease. Circulation. 2003;108(15): 1839–44.
22. Chaouat A, Savale L, Chouaid C, et al. Role for interleukin-6 in COPD-related pulmonary hypertension. Chest. 2009;136(3):678–87.
23. Tuder RM, Abman SH, Braun T, et al. Development and pathology of pulmonary hypertension. J Am Coll Cardiol. 2009;54(1 Suppl):S3–9.
24. Li M, Riddle SR, Frid MG, et al. Emergence of fibroblasts with a proinflammatory epigenetically altered phenotype in severe hypoxic pulmonary hypertension. J Immunol. 2011;187(5): 2711–22.
25. Sylvester JT, Shimoda LA, Aaronson PI, Ward JP. Hypoxic pulmonary vasoconstriction. Physiol Rev. 2012;92(1):367–520.
26. Sommer N, Dietrich A, Schermuly RT, et al. Regulation of hypoxic pulmonary vasoconstriction: basic mechanisms. Eur Respir J. 2008;32(6):1639–51.
27. Hultgren HN, Lopez CE, Lundberg E, Miller H. Physiologic studies of pulmonary edema at high altitude. Circulation. 1964;29:393–408.
28. Hultgren HN, Grover RF, Hartley LH. Abnormal circulatory responses to high altitude in subjects with a previous history of high-altitude pulmonary edema. Circulation. 1971;44(5):759–70.
29. Tsukimoto K, Mathieu-Costello O, Prediletto R, Elliott AR, West JB. Ultrastructural appearances of pulmonary capillaries at high transmural pressures. J Appl Physiol. 1991;71(2): 573–82.
30. West JB, Tsukimoto K, Mathieu-Costello O, Prediletto R. Stress failure in pulmonary capillaries. J Appl Physiol. 1991;70(4):1731–42.
31. Hultgren HN. High-altitude pulmonary edema: current concepts. Annu Rev Med. 1996;47: 267–84.

32. Bärtsch P, Mairbäurl H, Maggiorini M, Swenson ER. Physiological aspects of high-altitude pulmonary edema. J Appl Physiol. 2005;98:1101–10.
33. Houston CS. Acute pulmonary edema of high altitude. N Engl J Med. 1960;263:478–80.
34. Hackett PH, Creagh CE, Grover RF, et al. High-altitude pulmonary edema in persons without the right pulmonary artery. N Engl J Med. 1980;302(19):1070–3.
35. Schumacker PT. Lung cell hypoxia: role of mitochondrial reactive oxygen species signaling in triggering responses. Proc Am Thorac Soc. 2011;8(6):477–84.
36. Archer SL, Huang J, Henry T, Peterson D, Weir EK. A redox-based O_2 sensor in rat pulmonary vasculature. Circ Res. 1993;73(6):1100–12.
37. Waypa GB, Chandel NS, Schumacker PT. Model for hypoxic pulmonary vasoconstriction involving mitochondrial oxygen sensing. Circ Res. 2001;88(12):1259–66.
38. Moudgil R, Michelakis ED, Archer SL. Hypoxic pulmonary vasoconstriction. J Appl Physiol. 2005;98(1):390–403.
39. Pozeg ZI, Michelakis ED, McMurtry MS, et al. In vivo gene transfer of the O_2-sensitive potassium channel Kv1.5 reduces pulmonary hypertension and restores hypoxic pulmonary vasoconstriction in chronically hypoxic rats. Circulation. 2003;107(15):2037–44.
40. Arias-Stella J, Saldana M. The terminal portion of the pulmonary arterial tree in people native to high altitudes. Circulation. 1963;28:915–25.
41. West JB. High-altitude medicine. Am J Respir Crit Care Med. 2012;186(12):1229–37.
42. Groves BM, Reeves JT, Sutton JR, et al. Operation Everest II: elevated high-altitude pulmonary resistance unresponsive to oxygen. J Appl Physiol. 1987;63(2):521–30.
43. Maggiorini M, Leon-Velarde F. High-altitude pulmonary hypertension: a pathophysiological entity to different diseases. Eur Respir J. 2003;22(6):1019–25.
44. Shimoda LA, Semenza GL. HIF and the lung: role of hypoxia-inducible factors in pulmonary development and disease. Am J Respir Crit Care Med. 2011;183(2):152–6.
45. Semenza GL. Hypoxia-inducible factors in physiology and medicine. Cell. 2012;148(3): 399–408.
46. Yu AY, Shimoda LA, Iyer NV, et al. Impaired physiological responses to chronic hypoxia in mice partially deficient for hypoxia-inducible factor 1alpha. J Clin Invest. 1999;103(5): 691–6.
47. Beall CM, Cavalleri GL, Deng L, et al. Natural selection on EPAS1 (HIF2alpha) associated with low hemoglobin concentration in Tibetan highlanders. Proc Natl Acad Sci U S A. 2010;107(25):11459–64.
48. Bigham A, Bauchet M, Pinto D, et al. Identifying signatures of natural selection in Tibetan and Andean populations using dense genome scan data. PLoS Genet. 2010;6(9):e1001116.
49. Peng Y, Yang Z, Zhang H, et al. Genetic variations in Tibetan populations and high-altitude adaptation at the Himalayas. Mol Biol Evol. 2011;28(2):1075–81.
50. Pak O, Aldashev A, Welsh D, Peacock A. The effects of hypoxia on the cells of the pulmonary vasculature. Eur Respir J. 2007;30(2):364–72.
51. Platoshyn O, Golovina VA, Bailey CL, et al. Sustained membrane depolarization and pulmonary artery smooth muscle cell proliferation. Am J Physiol. 2000;279(5):C1540–9.
52. Frid MG, Brunetti JA, Burke DL, et al. Hypoxia-induced pulmonary vascular remodeling requires recruitment of circulating mesenchymal precursors of a monocyte/macrophage lineage. Am J Pathol. 2006;168(2):659–69.
53. Lee C, Mitsialis SA, Aslam M, et al. Exosomes mediate the cytoprotective action of mesenchymal stromal cells on hypoxia-induced pulmonary hypertension. Circulation. 2012; 126(22):2601–11.
54. Vergadi E, Chang MS, Lee C, et al. Early macrophage recruitment and alternative activation are critical for the later development of hypoxia-induced pulmonary hypertension. Circulation. 2011;123(18):1986–95.
55. Balanos GM, Talbot NP, Dorrington KL, Robbins PA. Human pulmonary vascular response to 4 h of hypercapnia and hypocapnia measured using Doppler echocardiography. J Appl Physiol. 2003;94(4):1543–51.
56. Thannickal VJ, Toews GB, White ES, Lynch 3rd JP, Martinez FJ. Mechanisms of pulmonary fibrosis. Annu Rev Med. 2004;55:395–417.

57. Corte TJ, Wort SJ, Wells AU. Pulmonary hypertension in idiopathic pulmonary fibrosis: a review. Sarcoidosis Vasc Diffuse Lung Dis. 2009;26(1):7–19.
58. Patel NM, Lederer DJ, Borczuk AC, Kawut SM. Pulmonary hypertension in idiopathic pulmonary fibrosis. Chest. 2007;132(3):998–1006.
59. Guazzi M, Galie N. Pulmonary hypertension in left heart disease. Eur Respir Rev. 2012;21(126):338–46.
60. Segers VF, Brutsaert DL, De Keulenaer GW. Pulmonary hypertension and right heart failure in heart failure with preserved left ventricular ejection fraction: pathophysiology and natural history. Curr Opin Cardiol. 2012;27(3):273–80.
61. Grau M, Barr RG, Lima JA, et al. Percent emphysema and right ventricular structure and function: the MESA lung and MESA-RV studies. Chest. 2013;144(1):136–44.
62. Barr RG, Bluemke DA, Ahmed FS, et al. Percent emphysema, airflow obstruction, and impaired left ventricular filling. N Engl J Med. 2010;362(3):217–27.
63. Noureddine H, Gary-Bobo G, Alifano M, et al. Pulmonary artery smooth muscle cell senescence is a pathogenic mechanism for pulmonary hypertension in chronic lung disease. Circ Res. 2011;109(5):543–53.
64. Amsellem V, Gary-Bobo G, Marcos E, et al. Telomere dysfunction causes sustained inflammation in chronic obstructive pulmonary disease. Am J Respir Crit Care Med. 2011;184(12):1358–66.
65. Wright JL, Churg A. Animal models of cigarette smoke-induced chronic obstructive pulmonary disease. Exp Rev Respir Med. 2010;4(6):723–34.
66. Voelkel NF, Gomez-Arroyo J, Mizuno S. COPD/emphysema: the vascular story. Pulm Circ. 2011;1(3):320–6.
67. Peinado VI, Pizarro S, Barbera JA. Pulmonary vascular involvement in COPD. Chest. 2008;134(4):808–14.
68. Barbera J. Mechanisms of development of chronic obstructive pulmonary disease-associated pulmonary hypertension. Pulm Circ. 2013;3(1):160–4.
69. Ryan JJ, Rehman J, Archer SL. Paracrine proliferative signaling by senescent cells in world health organization group 3 pulmonary hypertension: age corrupting youth? Circ Res. 2011;109(5):476–9.
70. Seimetz M, Parajuli N, Pichl A, et al. Inducible NOS inhibition reverses tobacco-smoke-induced emphysema and pulmonary hypertension in mice. Cell. 2011;147(2):293–305.
71. Churg A, Zhou S, Wright JL. Series "matrix metalloproteinases in lung health and disease": matrix metalloproteinases in COPD. Eur Respir J. 2012;39(1):197–209.
72. Wright JL, Zhou S, Churg A. Pulmonary hypertension and vascular oxidative damage in cigarette smoke exposed eNOS(−/−) mice and human smokers. Inhal Toxicol. 2012;24(11):732–40.
73. Mahapatra S, Nishimura RA, Sorajja P, Cha S, McGoon MD. Relationship of pulmonary arterial capacitance and mortality in idiopathic pulmonary arterial hypertension. J Am Coll Cardiol. 2006;47(4):799–803.
74. Lahm T, Albrecht M, Fisher AJ, et al. 17beta-Estradiol attenuates hypoxic pulmonary hypertension via estrogen receptor-mediated effects. Am J Respir Crit Care Med. 2012;185(9):965–80.
75. Macnee W. Right heart function in COPD. Semin Respir Crit Care Med. 2010;31(3):295–312.
76. Brown RD, Ambler SK, Li M, et al. MAP kinase kinase kinase-2 (MEKK2) regulates hypertrophic remodeling of the right ventricle in hypoxia-induced pulmonary hypertension. Am J Physiol Heart Circ Physiol. 2013;304(2):H269–81.
77. MacNee W, Skwarski K. The pathogenesis of peripheral edema in chronic obstructive pulmonary disease. Clin Pulm Med. 1997;4(6):309–15.
78. Skwarski KM, Morrison D, Barratt A, Lee M, MacNee W. Effects of hypoxia on renal hormonal balance in normal subjects and in patients with COPD. Respir Med. 1998;92:1331–6.
79. Kessler R, Faller M, Weitzenblum E, et al. "Natural history" of pulmonary hypertension in a series of 131 patients with chronic obstructive lung disease. Am J Respir Crit Care Med. 2001;164(2):219–24.

80. Carlsen J, Andersen HK, Boesgaard S, et al. Pulmonary arterial lesions in explanted lungs after transplantation correlate with severity of pulmonary hypertension in chronic obstructive pulmonary disease. J Heart Lung Transplant. 2013;32:347–54.
81. Lederer DJ, Arcasoy SM, Wilt JS, D'Ovidio F, Sonett JR, Kawut SM. Six-minute-walk distance predicts waiting list survival in idiopathic pulmonary fibrosis. Am J Respir Crit Care Med. 2006;174(6):659–64.
82. Cottin V, Le Pavec J, Prevot G, et al. Pulmonary hypertension in patients with combined pulmonary fibrosis and emphysema syndrome. Eur Respir J. 2010;35(1):105–11.
83. Sugerman HJ, Baron PL, Fairman RP, Evans CR, Vetrovec GW. Hemodynamic dysfunction in obesity hypoventilation syndrome and the effects of treatment with surgically induced weight loss. Ann Surg. 1988;207(5):604–13.
84. Kessler R, Faller M, Fourgaut G, Mennecier B, Weitzenblum E. Predictive factors of hospitalization for acute exacerbation in a series of 64 patients with chronic obstructive pulmonary disease. Am J Respir Crit Care Med. 1999;159(1):158–64.
85. Boerrigter BG, Bogaard HJ, Trip P, et al. Ventilatory and cardiocirculatory exercise profiles in COPD: the role of pulmonary hypertension. Chest. 2012;142(5):1166–74.
86. Fang A, Studer S, Kawut SM, et al. Elevated pulmonary artery pressure is a risk factor for primary graft dysfunction following lung transplantation for idiopathic pulmonary fibrosis. Chest. 2011;139(4):782–7.
87. Diamond JM, Lee JC, Kawut SM, et al. Clinical risk factors for primary graft dysfunction after lung transplantation. Am J Respir Crit Care Med. 2013;187(5):527–34.
88. Rivera-Lebron BN, Forfia PR, Kreider M, Lee J, Holmes JH, Kawut SM. Echocardiographic and hemodynamic predictors of mortality in idiopathic pulmonary fibrosis. Chest. 2013;144(2):564–70.
89. Oswald-Mammosser M, Weitzenblum E, Quoix E, et al. Prognostic factors in COPD patients receiving long-term oxygen therapy. Importance of pulmonary artery pressure. Chest. 1995;107(5):1193–8.
90. Leuchte HH, Baumgartner RA, Nounou ME, et al. Brain natriuretic peptide is a prognostic parameter in chronic lung disease. Am J Respir Crit Care Med. 2006;173(7):744–50.
91. Wells JM, Washko GR, Han MK, et al. Pulmonary arterial enlargement and acute exacerbations of COPD. N Engl J Med. 2012;367(10):913–21.
92. Stanbrook MB. The pulmonary artery in COPD—does size matter? N Engl J Med. 2012;367(10):946–8.
93. Arcasoy SM, Christie JD, Ferrari VA, et al. Echocardiographic assessment of pulmonary hypertension in patients with advanced lung disease. Am J Respir Crit Care Med. 2003;167(5):735–40.
94. Forfia PR, Vachiery JL. Echocardiography in pulmonary arterial hypertension. Am J Cardiol. 2012;110(6 Suppl):16S–24.
95. Pirat B, McCulloch ML, Zoghbi WA. Evaluation of global and regional right ventricular systolic function in patients with pulmonary hypertension using a novel speckle tracking method. Am J Cardiol. 2006;98(5):699–704.
96. Matias C, Isla LP, Vasconcelos M, et al. Speckle-tracking-derived strain and strain-rate analysis: a technique for the evaluation of early alterations in right ventricle systolic function in patients with systemic sclerosis and normal pulmonary artery pressure. J Cardiovasc Med (Hagerstown). 2009;10(2):129–34.
97. Hardegree EL, Sachdev A, Villarraga HR, et al. Role of serial quantitative assessment of right ventricular function by strain in pulmonary arterial hypertension. Am J Cardiol. 2013; 111(1):143–8.
98. Vonk-Noordegraaf A, Souza R. Cardiac magnetic resonance imaging: what can it add to our knowledge of the right ventricle in pulmonary arterial hypertension? Am J Cardiol. 2012;110(6 Suppl):25S–31.
99. Sanz J, Conroy J, Narula J. Imaging of the right ventricle. Cardiol Clin. 2012;30(2): 189–203.

100. Halpern SD, Taichman DB. Misclassification of pulmonary hypertension due to reliance on pulmonary capillary wedge pressure rather than left ventricular end-diastolic pressure. Chest. 2009;136(1):37–43.
101. Champion HC, Michelakis ED, Hassoun PM. Comprehensive invasive and noninvasive approach to the right ventricle-pulmonary circulation unit: state of the art and clinical and research implications. Circulation. 2009;120(11):992–1007.
102. Ryan JJ, Rich JD, Thiruvoipati T, Swamy R, Kim GH, Rich S. Current practice for determining pulmonary capillary wedge pressure predisposes to serious errors in the classification of patients with pulmonary hypertension. Am Heart J. 2012;163(4):589–94.
103. Nocturnal Oxygen Therapy Trial Group. Continuous or nocturnal oxygen therapy in hypoxemic chronic obstructive lung disease: a clinical trial. Ann Intern Med. 1980;93(3):391–8.
104. Garvey C. Interstitial lung disease and pulmonary rehabilitation. J Cardiopulm Rehabil Prev. 2010;30(3):141–6.
105. Marin JM, Soriano JB, Carrizo SJ, Boldova A, Celli BR. Outcomes in patients with chronic obstructive pulmonary disease and obstructive sleep apnea: the overlap syndrome. Am J Respir Crit Care Med. 2010;182(3):325–31.
106. Colish J, Walker JR, Elmayergi N, et al. Obstructive sleep apnea: effects of continuous positive airway pressure on cardiac remodeling as assessed by cardiac biomarkers, echocardiography, and cardiac MRI. Chest. 2012;141(3):674–81.
107. Blanco I, Gimeno E, Munoz PA, et al. Hemodynamic and gas exchange effects of sildenafil in patients with chronic obstructive pulmonary disease and pulmonary hypertension. Am J Respir Crit Care Med. 2010;181(3):270–8.
108. Ghofrani HA, Reichenberger F, Kohstall MG, et al. Sildenafil increased exercise capacity during hypoxia at low altitudes and at Mount Everest base camp: a randomized, double-blind, placebo-controlled crossover trial. Ann Intern Med. 2004;141(3):169–77.
109. Blanco I, Santos S, Gea J, et al. Sildenafil to improve respiratory rehabilitation outcomes in COPD: a controlled trial. Eur Respir J. 2013;42(4):982–92.
110. Lederer DJ, Bartels MN, Schluger NW, et al. Sildenafil for chronic obstructive pulmonary disease: a randomized crossover trial. COPD. 2012;9(3):268–75.
111. Stolz D, Rasch H, Linka A, et al. A randomised, controlled trial of bosentan in severe COPD. Eur Respir J. 2008;32(3):619–28.
112. Dernaika TA, Beavin M, Kinasewitz GT. Iloprost improves gas exchange and exercise tolerance in patients with pulmonary hypertension and chronic obstructive pulmonary disease. Respiration. 2010;79(5):377–82.
113. Boeck L, Tamm M, Grendelmeier P, Stolz D. Acute effects of aerosolized iloprost in COPD related pulmonary hypertension—a randomized controlled crossover trial. PLoS One. 2012;7(12):e52248.
114. Olschewski H, Ghofrani HA, Walmrath D, et al. Inhaled prostacyclin and iloprost in severe pulmonary hypertension secondary to lung fibrosis. Am J Respir Crit Care Med. 1999;160(2):600–7.
115. Blanco I, Ribas J, Xaubet A, et al. Effects of inhaled nitric oxide at rest and during exercise in idiopathic pulmonary fibrosis. J Appl Physiol. 2011;110(3):638–45.
116. Ghofrani HA, Wiedemann R, Rose F, et al. Sildenafil for treatment of lung fibrosis and pulmonary hypertension: a randomised controlled trial. Lancet. 2002;360(9337):895–900.
117. Zisman DA, Schwarz M, Anstrom KJ, Collard HR, Flaherty KR, Hunninghake GW. A controlled trial of sildenafil in advanced idiopathic pulmonary fibrosis. N Engl J Med. 2010;363(7):620–8.
118. Han MK, Bach DS, Hagan P, et al. Sildenafil preserves exercise capacity in IPF patients with right ventricular dysfunction. Chest. 2013;143(6):1699–708.
119. King Jr TE, Brown KK, Raghu G, et al. BUILD-3: a randomized, controlled trial of bosentan in idiopathic pulmonary fibrosis. Am J Respir Crit Care Med. 2011;184(1):92–9.
120. Raghu G, Behr J, Brown KK, et al. Treatment of idiopathic pulmonary fibrosis with ambrisentan: a parallel, randomized trial. Ann Intern Med. 2013;158(9):641–9.

121. Raghu G, Million-Rousseau R, Marganti A, et al. Macitentan for the treatment of idiopathic pulmonary fibrosis: the randomised controlled MUSIC trial. Eur Respir J. 2013; 42(6): 1622–32.
122. Hoeper MM, Halank M, Wilkens H, et al. Riociguat for interstitial lung disease and pulmonary hypertension: a pilot trial. Eur Respir J. 2013;41(4):853–60.
123. Maggiorini M, Brunner-La Rocca HP, Peth S, et al. Both tadalafil and dexamethasone may reduce the incidence of high-altitude pulmonary edema: a randomized trial. Ann Intern Med. 2006;145(7):497–506.
124. Bates MG, Thompson AA, Baillie JK, et al. Sildenafil citrate for the prevention of high altitude hypoxic pulmonary hypertension: double blind, randomized, placebo-controlled trial. High Alt Med Biol. 2011;12(3):207–14.
125. Hegewald MJ, Elliott CG. Sustained improvement with iloprost in a COPD patient with severe pulmonary hypertension. Chest. 2009;135(2):536–7.
126. Wang GL, Semenza GL. Desferrioxamine induces erythropoietin gene expression and hypoxia-inducible factor 1 DNA-binding activity: implications for models of hypoxia signal transduction. Blood. 1993;82(12):3610–5.
127. Smith TG, Talbot NP, Privat C, et al. Effects of iron supplementation and depletion on hypoxic pulmonary hypertension: two randomized controlled trials. JAMA. 2009;302(13): 1444–50.
128. Rhodes CJ, Howard LS, Busbridge M, et al. Iron deficiency and raised hepcidin in idiopathic pulmonary arterial hypertension: clinical prevalence, outcomes, and mechanistic insights. J Am Coll Cardiol. 2011;58(3):300–9.
129. Zhang H, Qian DZ, Tan YS, et al. Digoxin and other cardiac glycosides inhibit HIF-1alpha synthesis and block tumor growth. Proc Natl Acad Sci U S A. 2008;105(50):19579–86.
130. Abud EM, Maylor J, Undem C, et al. Digoxin inhibits development of hypoxic pulmonary hypertension in mice. Proc Natl Acad Sci U S A. 2012;109(4):1239–44.
131. Lahm T, Crisostomo PR, Markel TA, et al. Selective estrogen receptor-alpha and estrogen receptor-beta agonists rapidly decrease pulmonary artery vasoconstriction by a nitric oxide-dependent mechanism. Am J Physiol. 2008;295(5):R1486–93.
132. Resta TC, Kanagy NL, Walker BR. Estradiol-induced attenuation of pulmonary hypertension is not associated with altered eNOS expression. Am J Physiol. 2001;280(1):L88–97.

Chapter 5
Pulmonary Hypertension in Chronic Heart and Lung Disease

Robert P. Frantz

Abstract Pulmonary hypertension commonly accompanies left heart disease (Group 2 Pulmonary Hypertension in the Dana Point classification scheme), and often accompanies hypoxic/parenchymal lung disease (Group 3). The phenotypic and hemodynamic spectrum of pulmonary hypertension in these settings is enormous, and the clinician is often left with uncertainty regarding the appropriate evaluation and management of these patients. A comprehensive understanding of the prognostic significance of pulmonary hypertension, and appropriate strategies for its evaluation and management, is critical for practitioners caring for these challenging patients. Management of pulmonary hypertension in the setting of left heart disease focuses primarily on identification and management of factors such as hypoxemia or pulmonary emboli that may be superimposed on left heart disease, and on optimization of conventional heart failure therapy. An evolving role for pulmonary vasoactive therapy is foreseen. In parenchymal lung disease, pulmonary hypertension often portends a poor prognosis, but whether there is a role for pulmonary vasoactive therapy beyond correction of hypoxemia is a matter of much debate. This chapter provides a comprehensive review of the current understanding of these important issues.

Keywords Pulmonary hypertension • Heart failure with preserved ejection fraction • Congestive heart failure • Lung transplantation • Chronic obstructive pulmonary disease • Interstitial lung disease • Cystic fibrosis

Abbreviations

CO	Cardiac output
COPD	Chronic obstructive pulmonary disease
HFpEF	Heart failure with preserved left ventricular ejection fraction
HFrEF	Heart failure with reduced left ventricular ejection fraction

R.P. Frantz, M.D. (✉)
Department of Medicine, Mayo Clinic College of Medicine,
200 First Street, SW, Rochester, MN 55905, USA
e-mail: frantz.robert@mayo.edu

J.R. Klinger, R.P. Frantz (eds.), *Diagnosis and Management of Pulmonary Hypertension*, Respiratory Medicine 12, DOI 10.1007/978-1-4939-2636-7_5

LV	Left ventricle
MPAP	Mean pulmonary artery pressure
NYHA	New York Heart Association
PA	Pulmonary artery
PAH	Pulmonary arterial hypertension
PCWP	Pulmonary capillary wedge pressure
PDE5i	Phosphodiesterase type 5 inhibition
PHHFrEF	Pulmonary hypertension with heart failure with reduced left ventricular ejection fraction
PVR	Pulmonary vascular resistance
RV	Right ventricle
TPG	Transpulmonary gradient
WHO	World Health Organization

Introduction

Pulmonary hypertension commonly accompanies many forms of chronic heart and lung disease, and usually is associated with worse prognosis than is the case for patients with those diseases occurring in the absence of coexistent pulmonary hypertension. This fact presents both an opportunity and a challenge for the clinician. The extent to which the pulmonary hypertension is due to the underlying heart or lung disease or reflects a superimposed condition with differing source and differing needs for treatment is often unclear. For example, a patient with left heart failure may have pulmonary hypertension with right heart failure that is ascribed to the underlying heart condition, but could in fact represent occult pulmonary emboli which, if unrecognized, could result in serious complications or death. In addition, the range of severity of the pulmonary hypertension vis-à-vis the heart and lung disease can vary tremendously, rendering broad generalizations about significance and management difficult. Furthermore, the simple association of pulmonary hypertension with worse prognosis does not necessarily mean that treating the pulmonary hypertension per se will improve symptoms or outcome. In this chapter we will address the epidemiology of pulmonary hypertension in chronic heart and lung disease, discuss approaches to understanding of the complex and varied clinical and hemodynamic presentations, review current understanding of the therapeutic approach to these challenging patients, and describe areas ripe for future investigation.

Pulmonary Hypertension Accompanying Left Heart Disease

Group 2 pulmonary hypertension comprises patients with pulmonary hypertension related to left ventricular systolic failure, heart failure with preserved ejection fraction, and left-sided valvular disease (Fig. 5.1) [1]. The nomenclature regarding pulmonary hypertension accompanying left heart disease has recently been reviewed and is nicely outlined in the accompanying table (Table 5.1) from Fang et al. [1].

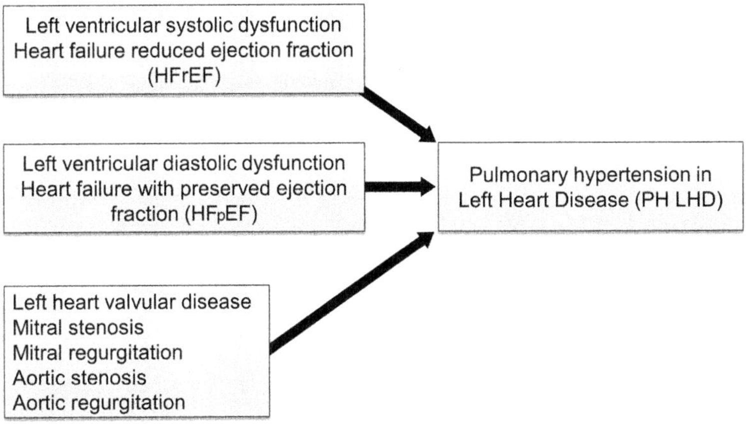

Fig. 5.1 Group 2 pulmonary hypertension subcategories (left heart disease). Reproduced with permission [1]

Heart Failure with Reduced Ejection Fraction

Left ventricular systolic failure in the Western world is most commonly due to coronary artery disease or dilated cardiomyopathy due to systemic hypertension. A range of other heritable and acquired diseases and toxins can result in systolic failure. Presence of left ventricular systolic failure may result in exertional dyspnea, orthopnea, paroxysmal nocturnal dyspnea, cough which may be frothy in the setting of frank pulmonary edema, and development of concomitant right heart failure with corresponding signs and symptoms. Presence of pulmonary hypertension heralds a worse prognosis in patients with left ventricular (LV) systolic failure [2]. A study of patients with LV systolic failure who had ambulatory right ventricular pressure monitors implanted demonstrated that those patients who had subsequent clinical events had higher pulmonary artery systolic pressures, estimated pulmonary artery diastolic pressures, and right ventricular end-diastolic pressures than those who did not have such events [3]. For convenience, LV systolic failure is often abbreviated as HFrEF (heart failure with reduced ejection fraction), while HFrEF accompanied by pulmonary hypertension may be referred to as PHHFrEF (pulmonary hypertension with heart failure with reduced left ventricular ejection fraction).

Mechanisms of pulmonary hypertension in HFrEF include simple passive elevation in pulmonary artery pressure as a consequence of elevated left heart filling pressures. Presence of left heart filling pressure elevation may also induce vasoconstriction of the pulmonary vasculature, contributing a "reactive" component, further elevating the pulmonary artery pressure. This is described as "mixed" pulmonary hypertension. In such circumstances, acute administration of a vasodilator such as nitroprusside will often both correct the elevation in left heart filling pressure and dilate the pulmonary vasculature, ideally resulting in full normalization of the pulmonary artery pressure and pulmonary vascular resistance. In advanced LV systolic

Table 5.1 Definitions used in the description of pulmonary hypertension

Nomenclature	Description	Physiologic definition	Hemodynamic criteria in literature
Pulmonary hypertension (PH)	Sustained elevation of PAP at rest	Pre-capillary, post-capillary, mixed, high flow state	Mean PAP ≥ 25 mmHg (2 SD above normal)
Pulmonary arterial hypertension (PAH)	PH with "normal" left-sided filling pressure	Pre-capillary vasoconstriction, remodeling, thrombosis-in-situ	Mean PAP ≥ 25 mmHg PCW, LAP, LVEDP ≤ 15 mmHg PVR > 3 WU
Pulmonary venous hypertension (PVH)	PH with elevated left-sided filling pressure	Post-capillary passive congestion	Mean PAP ≥ 25 mmHg PCW, LAP, LVEDP > 15 mmHg TPG ≤ 12–15 mmHg PVR ≤ 2.5–3.0 WU
Mixed PH or PH out-of-proportion to left-sided filling pressure	PH with elevated left-sided filling pressure and elevated pulmonary vascular resistance (PVH + PAH)	Pre- and post-capillary (passive congestion with excessive arterial vasoconstriction ± vascular remodeling)	Mean PAP ≥ 25 mmHg PCW, LAP, LVEDP > 15 mmHg TPG > 12–15 mmHg PVR > 2.5–3.0 WU
Reversible, reactive, or vasoreactive PH	Component of mixed PH that is acutely or chronically responsive to pharmacologic (diuretics, vasodilators, inodilators) and/or mechanical circulatory support device therapies		With vasodilators/inodilators: TPG ≤ 12–15 mmHg PVR ≤ 2.5–3.0 WU
Irreversible, fixed, refractory, or persistent PH	Component of mixed PH that is not responsive to above strategies		Despite vasodilators/inodilators: TPG > 12-15 mmHg PVR > 2.5–3.0 WU
High-flow PH	PH with high cardiac output state or high pulmonary flow	Pre-, post-, or mixed depending on etiology (e.g., AV shunt, chronic anemia, thyrotoxicosis, nutritional or obesity, cardiomyopathies, congenital heart disease)	Mean PAP ≥ 25 mmHg PCWP, LAP, LVEDP variable TPG variable PVR variable High cardiac output

AV arteriovenous, *LAP* left atrial pressure, *LVEDP* left ventricular end diastolic pressure, *PAP* pulmonary arterial pressure, *PCWP* pulmonary capillary wedge pressure, *PVR* pulmonary vascular resistance, *SD* standard deviation, *TPG* transpulmonary gradient (mean PAP–PAWP). Reproduced with permission [1]

failure, particularly if volume overload is present, acute vasodilator challenge will often improve, but not normalize LV filling pressures; in such a situation, continued diuresis and potentially a period of inotropic support in the ICU will often further improve the hemodynamics. These techniques are routinely employed in assessing suitability of patients for cardiac transplantation, since irreversible elevation in pulmonary vascular resistance is a risk factor for right ventricular (RV) failure and impaired survival following transplantation [4]. Longstanding elevation in pulmonary venous pressure may result in remodeling of the pulmonary vasculature. In this situation, correction of the elevation in left heart filling pressure will not immediately fully correct the pulmonary artery pressure. The *sine qua non* of this situation is that seen in mitral stenosis, where very longstanding and severe pulmonary venous pressure elevation can result in pulmonary artery systolic pressures over 100 mmHg. Correction of the mitral stenosis will result in some immediate improvement in pulmonary artery pressure, but further improvement usually occurs with passage of time, apparently reflecting reverse remodeling of the pulmonary vasculature [5, 6]. The same phenomenon has been observed in patients undergoing left ventricular assist device implantation for refractory cardiac failure. For many of these patients, the pulmonary artery pressures approach normal values within days of device implant, while in some patients, continued fall will occur over additional months, thereby facilitating subsequent cardiac transplantation (Fig. 5.2) [7]. In occasional patients, device implantation does not result in resolution of the pulmonary hypertension, presumably either because of failure of reverse remodeling of the pulmonary vasculature, or because causes other than the prior elevation in venous pressure are driving the presence of the pulmonary hypertension and vasculopathy.

Pulmonary hypertension accompanying HFrEF can be analyzed based on a variety of hemodynamic parameters, including pulmonary artery (PA) systolic pressure,

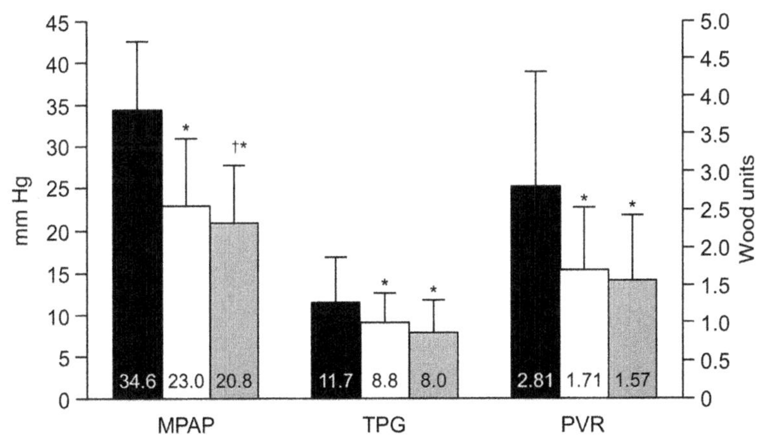

Fig. 5.2 Pulmonary hemodynamics in 58 patients at baseline and after left ventricular assist device (LVAD) support. Early improvements in hemodynamics were sustained during late support. The *black, white*, and *striped bars* represent *baseline* (median 1 day pre-implant), early (median 1 day post-implant) and late (median 75 days post-implant) LVAD support, respectively. Values are mean ± standard deviation. *MPAP* mean pulmonary artery pressure (mmHg), *TPG* transpulmonary gradient (mmHg), *PVR* pulmonary vascular resistance (Wood units); $^{*}p<0.001$ compared with baseline; $^{\dagger}p=0.028$ compared with early LVAD support. Nair PK JHLT 2010:29. Reproduced with permission [7]

mean pulmonary artery pressure (MPAP), transpulmonary gradient (TPG) (defined as the difference between mean PA pressure and pulmonary capillary occlusion pressure), and pulmonary vascular resistance (PVR) (defined as transpulmonary gradient divided by cardiac output, and expressed in Wood units (mmHg × min/L), or TPG divided by cardiac index and then expressed in Wood units × m^2. Multiplying by 80 converts the resistance parameter to dynes × s/cm^5. A transpulmonary gradient of 12 mmHg or less is often used as a definition of purely passive pulmonary hypertension, while a TPG ≥ 12 mmHg refers to mixed pulmonary hypertension. Of course the significance of TPG is dependent on the accompanying cardiac output (CO); if the CO is high, an elevated TPG can occur in the presence of normal PVR. The higher the transpulmonary gradient in the setting of HFrEF, the worse the prognosis; a TPG greater than 18 mmHg has recently been associated with particularly increased risk [2]. Gradients in risk are also seen with mean pulmonary artery pressure (MPAP), pulmonary capillary wedge pressure (PCWP), PVR, and pulmonary artery compliance defined as stroke volume divided by pulmonary artery pulse pressure, with a PA compliance ≤2 mL/mmHg demonstrating particularly increased risk (Figs. 5.3 and 5.4).

The difficult conundrum of biventricular failure has resulted in a search for approaches to treatment that includes consideration of pulmonary vasodilators. Currently such an approach must be considered unproven, and not without risk. In addition, the attractiveness of such an approach may interfere with recognition of the tremendous value of optimization of conventional heart failure therapies in such patients. Table 5.2 shows hemodynamic measurements before and after nitroprusside administration in the catheterization laboratory in a patient with idiopathic dilated cardiomyopathy who was referred for discussion regarding management of pulmonary hypertension in the context of what was felt to be optimally managed heart failure including ACE inhibition, beta-blockade, digoxin and diuretics. The dramatic hemodynamic response to nitroprusside demonstrated the potential for additional systemic vasodilator therapy. The patient responded very favorably to gradual up titration of the ACE inhibitor and adjustment of diuretic dose.

Elevation of the pulmonary capillary wedge pressure in patients with left heart failure also has adverse effects on pulmonary arterial compliance. PA compliance reflects the ability of the pulmonary vasculature to accept an incoming bolus of volume from the ejecting right ventricle during systole. Ordinarily, there is a tight hyperbolic inverse relationship between pulmonary arterial compliance and resistance. However, for any given pulmonary vascular resistance, a rise in the pulmonary capillary wedge pressure will reduce the pulmonary arterial compliance, making it more difficult for the RV to eject into the pulmonary bed (Fig. 5.5) [8].

The tendency to underutilize conventional heart failure therapy may in part explain the heralded success of pulmonary artery pressure monitoring in improving pulmonary hypertension and reducing heart failure hospitalizations in New York Heart Association (NYHA) Class III patients with LV systolic failure demonstrated in the CardioMEMS Heart Sensor Allows Monitoring of Pressure to Improve Outcomes in NYHA Class III Heart Failure Patients (CHAMPION)

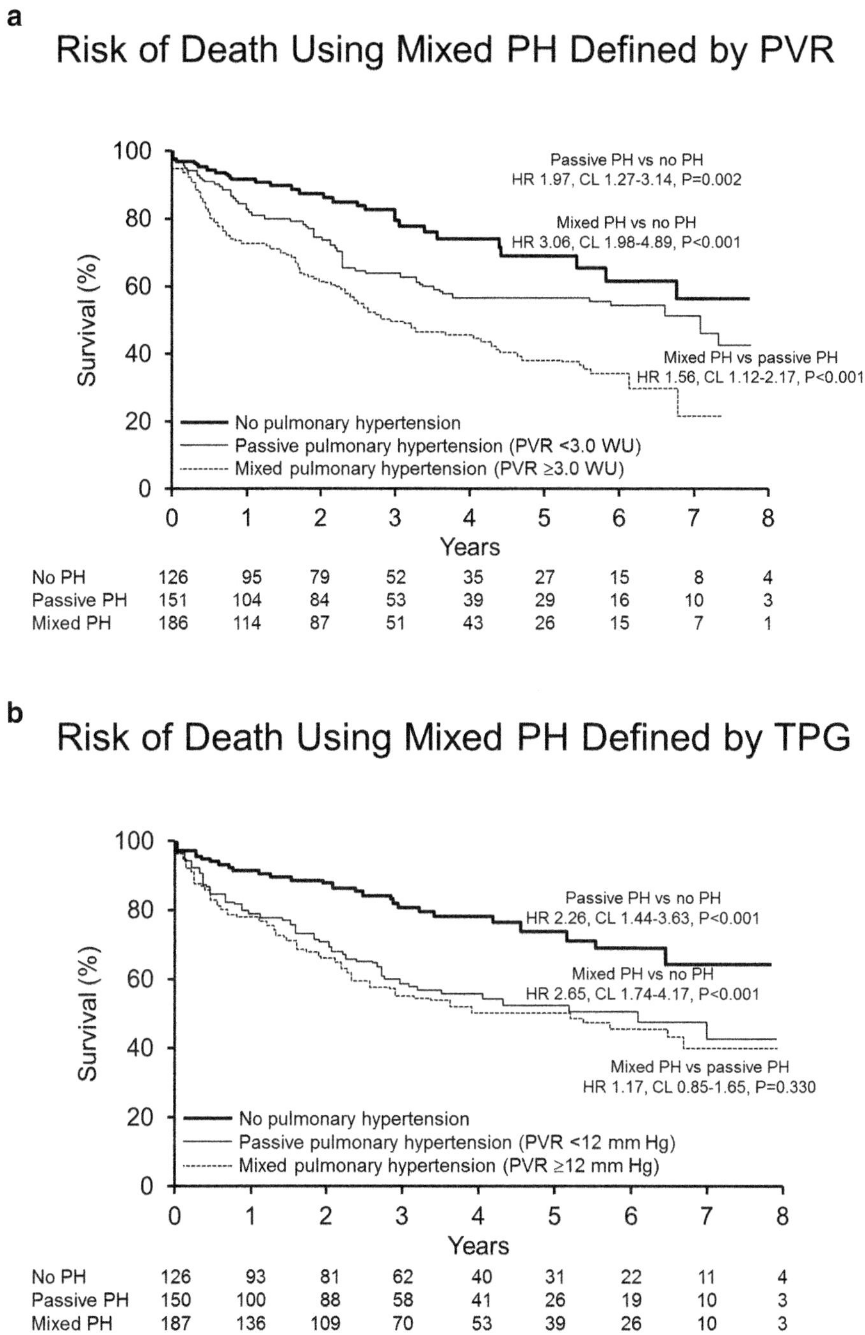

Fig. 5.3 Survival of HFREF patients with PH. (**a**) Kaplan–Meier estimates of survival in patients with heart failure of reduced left ventricular ejection fraction (HFREF) relative to passive pulmonary hypertension (PH) and mixed PH as defined by pulmonary vascular resistance (PVR) < or ≥3.0 Wood units (WU) and no PH. (**b**) Kaplan–Meier estimates of survival in patients with HFREF relative to passive PH and mixed PH as defined by transpulmonary gradient (TPG) < and ≥12 mmHg and no PH. Reproduced with permission [2]

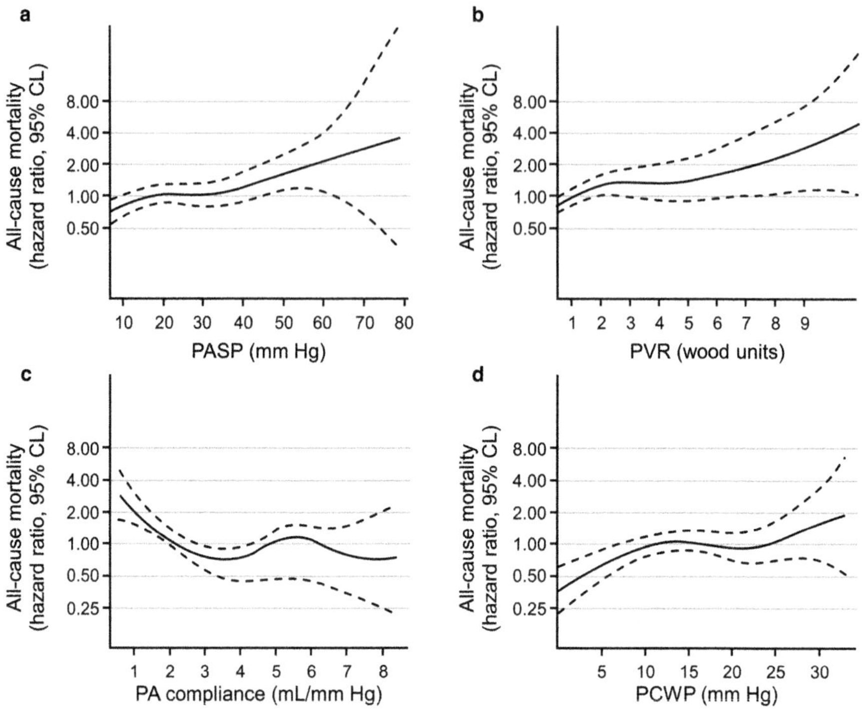

Fig. 5.4 All-cause mortality and hemodynamic parameters. (**a**) Unadjusted risk (hazard ratio [HR]: 95 % confidence limits [CL]) of all-cause mortality for sPAP analyzed as continuous variables. (**b**) Unadjusted risk (HR: 95 % CL) of all-cause mortality for PVR analyzed as continuous variables. (**c**) Unadjusted risk (HR: 95 % CL) of all-cause mortality for PAC analyzed as continuous variables. (**d**) Unadjusted risk (HR: 95 % CL) of all-cause mortality for PCWP analyzed as continuous variables. *PA* pulmonary artery, *PASP* pulmonary artery systolic pressure, *PCWP* pulmonary capillary wedge pressure, *PVR* pulmonary vascular resistance. Reproduced with permission [2]

Table 5.2 Acute hemodynamic effects of nitroprusside in a patient with LV systolic failure and mixed pulmonary hypertension

	Blood pressure	RA	PA	PCW	TPG	CO/CI	PVR
Baseline	120/74	21	88/35/57	26	31	5.7/2.8	5.5
NTP	100/37	13	47/20/31	16	15	7.0/3.5	2.1

RA right atrial pressure, *PA* pulmonary artery pressure (systolic, diastolic, mean), *PCW* pulmonary capillary wedge pressure, *TPG* transpulmonary gradient, *CO/CI* cardiac output, cardiac index, *PVR* pulmonary vascular resistance, *NTP* 1 μcg/kg/min sodium nitroprusside

study. Patients in the active monitoring group ended up on higher doses of angiotensin-converting enzyme inhibitors and beta-blockers, and were more likely to end up on nitrates, also suggesting that more active titration of a standard heart failure program is advantageous over a more passive approach [9]. *The take-home message*

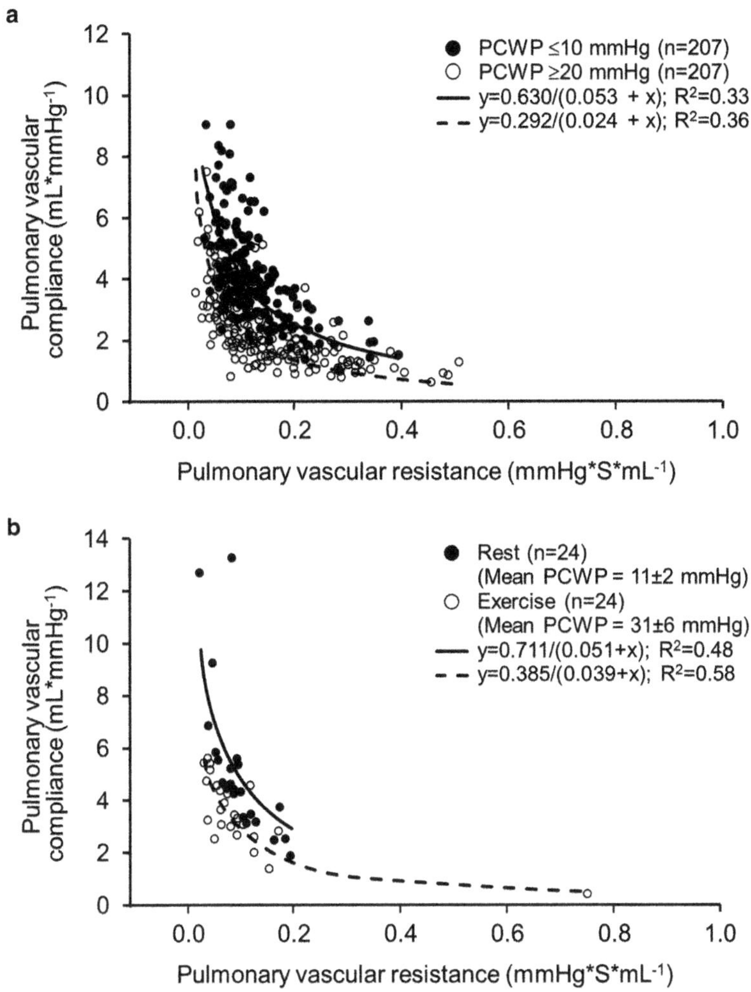

Fig. 5.5 Effect of pulmonary vascular resistance–compliance relationship (RPA–CPA) relationship by change in pulmonary capillary wedge pressure (PCWP) within an individual patient. (**a**) RPA–CPA for each patient is plotted at two different study times: at a low PCWP (PCWP ≤ 10 mmHg) and at a high PCWP (PCWP ≥ 20 mmHg). (**b**) Effect of increasing PCWP during supine exercise on RPA-CPA in 24 patients with early heart failure with preserved ejection fraction. Reproduced with permission [8]

here is that the most proven approach to pulmonary hypertension in the setting of LV systolic failure is to actively adjust standard heart failure therapies to optimal levels [8].

Other factors which may contribute to pulmonary hypertension in left heart failure include sleep disordered breathing, which may be central, obstructive, or mixed, and is quite common. Hypoxemia of any cause will aggravate pulmonary hypertension and right heart failure, and should be aggressively sought out and corrected. The possibility of concomitant pulmonary emboli must also be carefully considered.

Patients with HFrEF who have a more exaggerated rise in pulmonary artery pressures during exercise have worse exercise capacity and outcomes compared to patients without such a response [10]. In patients with PHHFrEF despite what is felt to be optimal medical therapy, case series and small randomized trials suggest the potential for phosphodiesterase-5 inhibition (PDE5i) to improve exercise tolerance and cardiac output response to exercise [11]. These encouraging preliminary data resulted in an NIH-funded multicenter study that was to have examined the impact of PDE5i with tadalafil in patients with PHHFrEF despite optimal medical therapy (Pitch-HF). Unfortunately this trial was not completed. It is hoped this concept will be studied further in the future. At the present time, use of PDE5i in PHHFrEF cannot be endorsed outside of research protocols.

Riociguat, the first in a new class of drugs which act via stimulation of soluble guanylate cyclase, was recently studied in a placebo-controlled, randomized trial of patients with PHHFrEF [12]. This trial did not reach its prespecified primary endpoint of a reduction in mean pulmonary artery pressure, but did result in a drop in pulmonary vascular resistance and systemic vascular resistance, with improvement in cardiac output and in Minnesota Living with Heart Failure scores [13]. Given the failure of the study to meet its primary endpoint, these additional analyses must be considered hypothesis generating, and suggest that additional studies of riociguat with more wisely chosen primary endpoints may be of value.

Heart Failure with Preserved Ejection Fraction

Approximately half of heart failure occurs in patients with preserved left ventricular ejection fraction (HFpEF). Most of these patients have accompanying pulmonary hypertension, and the severity of pulmonary hypertension is associated with prognosis [14]. Patients presenting with a syndrome compatible with HFpEF need careful scrutiny in an effort to identify specific diseases that may require very different management strategies. These include infiltrative cardiomyopathies such as amyloidosis, restrictive cardiomyopathy, and constrictive pericarditis. Traditional therapy for HFpEF includes optimal blood pressure control and use of diuretics. There are no proven treatments for HFpEF. A small randomized study of sildenafil in patients with HFpEF suggested improvement in hemodynamics, but the patient population was very unusual and very different from the usual HFpEF phenotype, having right atrial pressures on average over 20 mmHg, so the applicability of such results is highly questionable [15]. The robustly designed and executed, NIH-funded RELAX trial of PDE5i in HFpEF was recently completed [16, 17]. In this study, patients were randomized to receive sildenafil or placebo. The primary endpoint was peak oxygen consumption on cardiopulmonary exercise testing. Presence of pulmonary hypertension was not necessary for study inclusion, but many of the patients did have pulmonary hypertension. Sildenafil had no effect on peak oxygen consumption, 6 min walk, nor a composite hierarchical endpoint that included death, hospitalization for cardiovascular or renal causes, and quality of life. Furthermore, there were statistically significant adverse changes in creatinine, cystatin C, uric acid, N-terminal pro brain natriuretic peptide, and endothelin-1. Accordingly, PDE5i as a treatment strategy cannot currently be endorsed for use in patients with HFpEF. The search for differing therapeutic approaches to HFpEF must continue, but is complicated by the divergent phenotypic pictures of HFpEF, and the fact that such patients are at substantial risk of clinical events not directly related to their HFpEF.

The need to identify and treat other causes of pulmonary hypertension such as pulmonary emboli, hypoxemia, and sleep-disordered breathing in patients with HFpEF applies in a fashion similar to that discussed with regard to HFrEF. Key points regarding pulmonary hypertension in left heart disease are summarized in Table 5.3.

Pulmonary Hypertension Accompanying Chronic Lung Disease

Pulmonary hypertension accompanying chronic lung disease generally falls under World Health Organization (WHO) Group III (ventilatory disorders and hypoxic lung disease). This category of diseases represents a substantial challenge, and much is unknown regarding pathogenesis and management of pulmonary hypertension in this context. A systematic approach to evaluation of pulmonary hypertension is described in Table 5.4. A number of general principles should be considered.

1. Correct hypoxemia and hypoventilation as fully as possible. Hypoxemia is a potent pulmonary vasoconstrictor, aggravates right ventricular dysfunction, and increases risk of arrhythmia.
2. Aside from oxygen and correction of hypoventilation if present, along with use of diuretics in the setting of cor pulmonale, there are no approved treatments for this condition.
3. An effort should be made to determine if the patient is best described as having Group I pulmonary arterial hypertension (PAH) with a comorbidity of some intrinsic lung disease. This requires considering the context and severity of both the pulmonary hypertension and the lung disease. If there are risk factors for Group I PAH, this may assist with assessing the probability that the pulmonary hypertension appropriately falls within that purview. It is strengthened if the severity of the Group III disease process is mild or moderate.

Table 5.3 Key points regarding pulmonary hypertension in left heart disease

• Exclude superimposed thromboembolic disease. Ventilation/perfusion lung scanning is an excellent tool in this regard, avoiding risk of contrast nephropathy, and being highly sensitive for thromboembolism
• Actively seek and correct nocturnal and daytime hypoxemia. Sleep-disordered breathing is common in left heart disease, and will aggravate the biventricular failure
• Optimize left heart filling pressures by methodical titration of left heart therapies including vasodilators and diuretics
• Right heart catheterization with acute nitroprusside challenge can be helpful in understanding the extent to which optimization of vasodilator therapy may improve pulmonary hypertension and cardiac output. Additional correction of volume overload will further improve both LV filing pressures and pulmonary hypertension
• Regarding PH with Heart Failure with reduced Ejection Fraction:
– In advanced HFrEF, it may not be possible acutely to correct left heart filling pressures adequately to know whether the pulmonary hypertension would be reversible if this could be achieved. This is especially relevant in patients being considered for heart transplantation. Leaving a pulmonary artery catheter in place and using a combination of inotropes and intravenous diuretics for a few days may further clarify reversibility of the pulmonary hypertension. In some cases placement of a left ventricular assist device as a "bridge to decision" may be necessary to clarify reversibility of pulmonary hypertension with normalization of LV filling pressures
– If right atrial pressure is disproportionately high compared to the pulmonary artery occlusion pressure, then an LVAD may not be sufficient to correct the RV failure. Consideration of biventricular support or a total artificial heart as bridge to transplant would be a preferred approach
• Regarding PH with Heart Failure with preserved Ejection Fraction:
– HFpEF is not a free-standing diagnosis. Think carefully about the possibility of more specific diagnoses. Common pitfalls include failure to consider:
Constrictive pericarditis, which is potentially curable with pericardiectomy
Amyloidosis (AL, familial, or senile). Treatment options here can include chemotherapy or stem cell transplantation in AL amyloid, combined heart-liver transplant in familial amyloid, and cardiac transplantation in senile amyloid
Restrictive cardiomyopathy (familial or idiopathic)
Nonobstructive hypertrophic cardiomyopathy
– In advanced HFpEF of any cause, the extent of reversibility of pulmonary hypertension may be difficult to ascertain due to inability to correct LV filling pressures, with persistence of elevated PVR despite best efforts. Assessment of PA diastolic to wedge gradient may be useful in predicting probable hemodynamics at time of transplant. Placement of a total artificial heart as a bridge to transplant can be considered
– The RELAX trial showed no benefit of PDE5i in HFpEF, and there was evidence of worse renal function and higher endothelin and natriuretic peptide levels

4. Consider the possibility of superimposed thromboembolic disease.
5. Assess the extent to which the pulmonary hypertension is resulting in right ventricular failure. This includes assessment of resting parameters, and may also include assessing whether there is limitation to cardiac output upon exertion. The presence of right ventricular failure suggests a greater potential for pulmonary

Table 5.4 Comprehensive approach to pulmonary hypertension with chronic lung disease

Step 1: Phenotypic characterization of chronic lung disease	
Past medical history	Tobacco use: Pack years and date of cessation
	Exposure: Dust, mold, smoke, occupational exposures
	Query regarding signs and symptoms of sleep apnea, hypoventilation
	Query regarding anorexigen, illicit drug use including methamphetamines
	Family history of pulmonary hypertension, other lung disease
Pulmonary exam	Hyperresonance, AP diameter expiratory prolongation, wheeze, rhonchi
	Dry (Velcro) rales or wet rales
	Is there evidence of cyanosis? (Lips, ears, extremities)
CXR	Hyperinflation, bullae
	Interstitial infiltrates
	Pulmonary vascularity
	Cardiac size
Characterization of lung parenchyma	High resolution CT chest
Exclusion of concomitant thromboembolic disease	Ventilation/perfusion lung scan
	CT angiogram if V/Q equivocal
Lung function	Complete pulmonary function tests with DLCO
Hypoxia burden	(a) Overnight oximetry
	(b) 6-min walk
	(c) Rest and exercise arterial blood gases
	(d) Oxygen titration
	(e) Formal polysomnography
Step 2: Assessment for intrapulmonary shunt	
(a) Radioisotopic shunt study (selected cases)	
(b) CT angio if radioisotope shunt study positive (in selected cases)	
Step 3: Phenotypic characterization of cardiac status	
Past medical history	Hypertension (duration, therapy)
	Diabetes mellitus
	Coronary artery disease
	Valvular heart disease
	Prior congenital heart surgery, e.g., ASD or VSD closure
	Diuretic requirements including duration and dose
	Arrhythmia
Cardiac exam	Are features of possible RV failure present?
	(a) Jugular venous pressure elevation, V wave of tricuspid regurgitation
	(b) Hepatomegaly, pulsatile liver, ascites
	(c) Lower extremity edema

(continued)

Table 5.4 (continued)

Characterization of cardiac morphology and assessment for cardiac shunt	1. Transthoracic echocardiography with Doppler and bubble study
	(a) RA, RV, LA, LV chamber size
	(b) Septal displacement and paradoxical motion? "D"-shaped LV?
	(c) RV function (TAPSE, strain, visual appearance)
	(d) Tricuspid, other valve regurgitation or stenosis
	(e) LV function (systolic and diastolic)
	(f) IVC size and respiratory variation (estimate right atrial pressure)
	2. Transesophageal echocardiography (in selected cases)
	(a) Atrial septal defect, partial anomalous pulmonary venous return
Step 4: Hemodynamic characterization	
Right heart catheterization	1. Complete shunt run
	2. Oxygen challenge in event of hypoxemia to assess reversibility of hypoxemia and PH
	3. Vasodilator testing:
	(a) Consider nitric oxide if PCW normal
	(b) Consider nitroprusside if PCW high and adequate systemic blood pressure
	4. N-terminal pro-brain natriuretic peptide or brain natriuretic peptide levels

hypertension therapy. Phenotypic presentations and suggestions for evaluation and management principles are provided in Table 5.5.

Pulmonary Hypertension in the Context of Chronic Obstructive Pulmonary Disease

The mechanisms of development of pulmonary hypertension in the setting of chronic obstructive pulmonary disease (COPD) have been the subject of considerable recent interest. Pulmonary hypertension is usually mild in COPD, and is associated with hypoxemia and hypercapnia [18]. Recent analyses of explanted lungs from patients with COPD undergoing lung transplantation have demonstrated that the extent of pulmonary arterial lesions (rated using the Heath and Edwards classification scheme) correlates with the severity of pulmonary hypertension [19]. In that study, 38 % of patients had a mean PAP ≥ 25 mmHg, and only 4 % (10 of 247) had severe PH defined as a mean PAP ≥ 35 mmHg. Mechanisms of pulmonary hypertension in COPD have recently been reviewed in detail, and include direct

Table 5.5 Phenotypes and implications of pulmonary hypertension in chronic lung disease

Scenario	Severity of pulmonary hypertension	Additional steps	Pulmonary hypertension management
Stable COPD or ILD	*Mild* (echo RVSP<50, preserved RV function)	Assess LV systolic and diastolic function, Left atrial size, and risk factors for HFpEF	Correction of hypoxemia
			Control systemic BP
			Manage left heart disease
	Moderate to severe (echo RVSP>50, and/or evidence of RV enlargement/dysfunction, clinical features of cor pulmonale, elevated BNP)	Assess LV systolic and diastolic function, left atrial size, and risk factors for HFpEF	Correction of hypoxemia
		Exclude pulmonary emboli	Control systemic BP
		Consider risk factors for Group I PAH	Manage left heart disease
		Consider right heart catheterization	Hemodynamics consistent with moderate to severe PAH; normal LA size; parenchymal lung disease is mild to moderate: Consider possibility of Group I PAH with comorbidity of other lung disease; consider PAH therapy
Mixed restrictive/obstructive lung disease with severe hypoxemia	*Severe* (substantial RV failure)	Same as row above	Correction of hypoxemia
			Diuretics
			Hemodynamics demonstrate elevated right atrial pressure, reduced cardiac output and normal pulmonary capillary wedge: Consider possibility of pulmonary vasodilator therapy

vasoconstrictive effects of hypoxia, destruction of the pulmonary vascular bed and lung parenchyma, inflammatory and proliferative signaling resulting in vascular remodeling, toxic effects of factors such as tobacco, and genetic susceptibility (Fig. 5.6) [20, 21]. Oxygen therapy is the only therapy known to change the course of pulmonary hypertension in COPD [22, 23].

The very low prevalence of severe pulmonary hypertension has made it difficult to study the effect of vasodilators in such patients in a robust fashion. Studies of vasodilators in COPD to date have primarily examined acute or short-term hemodynamic effects, including impact on exercise hemodynamics. In a study of 15 patients with COPD, 9 of whom had PH, it was found that the patients with PH had lower stroke volumes than those without, but 3 months of sildenafil therapy had no impact

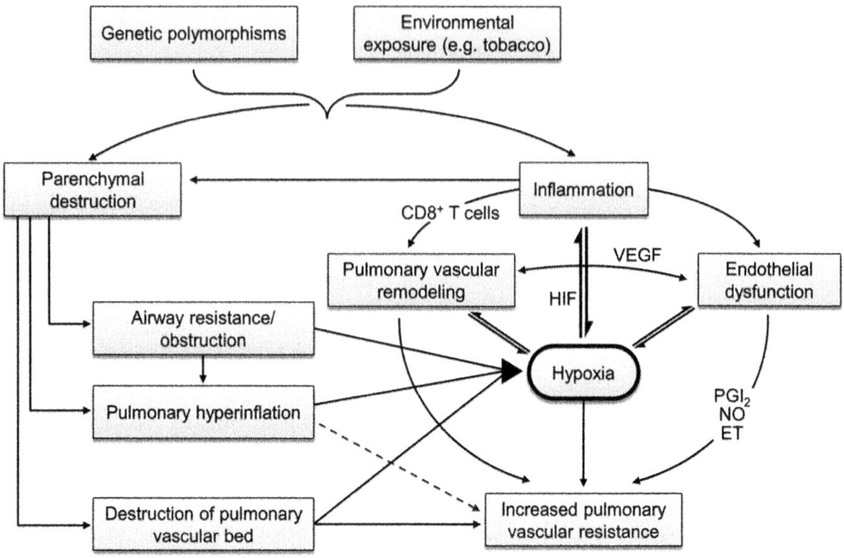

Fig. 5.6 Pathogenic mechanisms of pulmonary hypertension in COPD. The complex interactions between each of the pathogenic mechanisms which may lead to an increased pulmonary vascular resistance in subjects with COPD. In COPD, genetic and environmental exposures contribute to the development of parenchymal destruction and inflammation. Parenchymal destruction alters respiratory mechanics and causes destruction of the pulmonary vascular bed, which leads to hypoxia and contributes directly toward an increased pulmonary vascular resistance. Inflammation is likely to be intimately involved in pulmonary vascular remodeling and endothelial dysfunction, which also leads to hypoxia and increased pulmonary vascular resistance. The schema highlights the central role of hypoxia but also indicates that hypoxia is not essential to the development of an increased pulmonary vascular resistance in COPD. *VEGF* vascular endothelial growth factor, *HIF* hypoxia-inducible factors, *PGI2* prostacyclin, *NO* nitric oxide, *ET* endothelin. Reproduced with permission [20]

on stroke volume or exercise capacity [24]. A single-dose study of sildenafil in patients with COPD demonstrated an attenuation of rise in PA pressure with exercise, but no impact on cardiac output, stroke volume, or exercise capacity; only 5 of those patients had resting pulmonary hypertension [25]. A 1-month randomized cross-over study of sildenafil in COPD (without requirement for PH) showed no improvement in exercise capacity, with worsening of the alveolar-arterial oxygen gradient, symptoms, quality of life, and rate of adverse events [26]. A study of bosentan in COPD demonstrated no improvement in 6 min walk distance, and again with worsening of hypoxemia and quality of life [27]. Prostaglandin E1 has been shown to reduce pulmonary artery pressures and increase cardiac output in decompensated COPD, with little effect on oxygenation at the lower dose studied, but with slight worsening of oxygenation at the higher dose studied [28]. Short-term prostacyclin infusion has been shown to drop PVR in some patients with COPD [29].

Anecdotal reports and small case series have suggested the possibility of a role for prostanoid administration in the small subset of patients with severely impaired hemodynamics (low cardiac output, severe RV failure) in the setting of severe hypoxemic lung disease. Such therapy will not improve arterial oxygenation in most circumstances unless a patent foramen ovale is present and right to left shunting is lessened by reducing right atrial pressure. However, an increase in cardiac output can occur, which may improve peripheral tissue oxygen delivery and result in some symptomatic improvement. Such an approach must be considered anecdotal at this time, but worthy of additional study.

Pulmonary Hypertension in Interstitial Lung Disease

Pulmonary hypertension accompanies a variety of parenchymal lung diseases that exhibit interstitial patterns, including connective tissue diseases, sarcoidosis, and Langerhans cell histiocytosis, and is associated with worse exercise tolerance and outcome than in patients with these disorders in the absence of pulmonary hypertension [30–34]. The phenotypic spectrum of pulmonary hypertension in these disorders is wide, and, as with the case in COPD, there is the risk of aggravating ventilation/perfusion mismatching and hypoxemia with vasodilating agents. In general terms, the more severe the right heart failure (based upon noninvasive assessments such as physical signs of right heart failure, diuretic requirement, brain natriuretic peptide levels, and echocardiographic findings, plus invasive assessments of right atrial pressure, cardiac output, and confirmation of normal left heart filling pressures), the more likely it is that there may be a positive clinical response to pulmonary vasodilator therapy. Pulmonary hypertension and RV failure that seems disproportionate to the severity of the parenchymal lung disease may also be a clue to those rather unusual patients who seem to benefit from pulmonary vasodilator therapy. Much additional work is necessary to ultimately provide more clear guidance regarding which patients and which agents are most appropriate for treatment of these diverse patient groups.

Pulmonary Hypertension in Patients with Cystic Fibrosis

Pulmonary hypertension in patients with cystic fibrosis is usually mild, even in advanced disease, but occasionally can be severe [35]. Presence of pulmonary hypertension is likely a marker of more advanced disease; some studies have shown an association with survival, and others have not [36]. Some of these patients have elevated pulmonary capillary wedge pressures, so this possibility must be kept in mind when assessing pulmonary hypertension in cystic fibrosis. Pulmonary acceleration time measured by Doppler echocardiography has recently been shown to be a predictor of need for lung transplantation in cystic fibrosis [37]. Pulmonary acceleration time correlates inversely with pulmonary artery pressure, and is a useful measurement particularly in settings where there may not be sufficient tricuspid regurgitation to estimate right heart pressures by the Bernoulli technique. Pulmonary acceleration time less than 101 ms was associated with worse FEV1 and worse nocturnal oxygen saturation, and with shorter time to lung transplantation. In the latter regard, pulmonary acceleration time was a better marker than estimated pulmonary artery pressure. Additional studies of this parameter appear warranted.

Pulmonary Hypertension in Patients with Sleep-Disordered Breathing

Obstructive sleep apnea is common, particularly in the Western world, and increasing in prevalence, related to the epidemic of obesity. Many patients who have Group I PAH have obstructive sleep apnea as a comorbidity, and it should be evaluated and managed in usual fashion. Pulmonary hypertension in patients with isolated obstructive sleep apnea is usually mild [38]. When pulmonary hypertension is more severe, careful scrutiny for causes outside of sleep apnea is essential. A small randomized study has demonstrated that treatment with CPAP results in improvement in pulmonary hypertension in patients with obstructive sleep apnea [39]. In patients with obesity-hypoventilation syndrome, pulmonary hypertension and cor pulmonale can be severe, and connote a worrisome prognosis [40, 41]. This syndrome classically has been diagnosed on the basis of arterial blood gases demonstrating a $pCO_2 \geq 45$ mmHg, but a recent analysis has suggested that a $HCO_3 > 27$ mmol/L is a useful criterion [42, 43]. In such patients, correction of the hypoventilation is the principle strategy, along with use of diuretics for symptomatic management of right heart failure. There is no established role for pulmonary vasodilator therapy in such patients.

Conclusion

Pulmonary hypertension frequently accompanies a wide range of cardiac and pulmonary diseases, and nearly invariably is associated with a worse prognosis than those diseases in the absence of pulmonary hypertension. Careful thought must be given to understanding the root causes of the pulmonary hypertension, characterizing the hemodynamics, and appropriately treating the underlying condition. The role of pulmonary vasodilatory agents in such disorders is generally not well defined, in some situations can cause harm, and should only be considered when the underlying heart or lung disease is otherwise optimally managed with conventional agents. As a general principle, the more severe the right heart failure, the more likely that there could be a role for pulmonary vasodilator therapy. Much additional research is needed in order to better understand the optimal role of pulmonary vasodilator therapy in patients with these varied cardiac and pulmonary disorders.

References

1. Fang JC, DeMarco T, Givertz MM, Borlaug BA, Lewis GD, Rame JE, et al. World Health Organization Pulmonary Hypertension Group 2: Pulmonary hypertension due to left heart disease in the adult—a summary statement from the Pulmonary Hypertension Council of the International Society for Heart and Lung Transplantation. J Heart Lung Transplant. 2012;31(9): 913–33.
2. Miller WL, Grill DE, Borlaug BA. Clinical features, hemodynamics, and outcomes of pulmonary hypertension due to chronic heart failure with reduced ejection fraction pulmonary hypertension and heart failure. JACC Heart Fail. 2013;1(4):290–9.
3. Adamson PB, Gold MR, Bennett T, Bourge RC, Stevenson LW, Trupp R, et al. continuous hemodynamic monitoring in patients with mild to moderate heart failure: Results of the Reducing Decompensation Events Utilizing Intracardiac Pressures in Patients With Chronic Heart Failure (REDUCEhf) Trial. Congest Heart Fail. 2011;17(5):248–54.
4. Goland S, Czer LSC, Kass RM, De Robertis MA, Mirocha J, Coleman B, et al. Pre-existing pulmonary hypertension in patients with End-stage heart failure: impact on clinical outcome and hemodynamic follow-up after orthotopic heart transplantation. J Heart Lung Transplant. 2007;26(4):312–8.
5. Braunwald E, Braunwald NS, Ross J, Morrow AG. Effects of mitral-valve replacement on the pulmonary vascular dynamics of patients with pulmonary hypertension. N Engl J Med. 1965;273(10):509–14.
6. Vincens JJ, Temizer D, Post JR, Edmunds LH, Herrmann HC. Long-term outcome of cardiac surgery in patients with mitral stenosis and severe pulmonary hypertension. Circulation. 1995;92(9):137–42.
7. Nair PK, Kormos RL, Teuteberg JJ, Mathier MA, Bermudez CA, Toyoda Y, et al. Pulsatile left ventricular assist device support as a bridge to decision in patients with end-stage heart failure complicated by pulmonary hypertension. J Heart Lung Transplant. 2010;29(2):201–8.
8. Tedford RJ, Hassoun PM, Mathai SC, Girgis RE, Russell SD, Thiemann DR, et al. Pulmonary capillary wedge pressure augments right ventricular pulsatile loading. Circulation. 2012;125(2): 289–97.
9. Cheng J, Brockman R, Pina I, Gao Y, Wei S, Aguel F, et al. CardioMEMS Champion HF Monitoring system. FDA review of P100045. http://www.fdagov/downloads/Advisory Committees/CommitteesMeetingMaterials/MedicalDevices/MedicalDevices AdvisoryCommittee/CirculatorySystemDevicesPanel/UCM284020pdf. Accessed 8 Dec 2011.
10. Lewis GD, Murphy RM, Shah RV, Pappagianopoulos PP, Malhotra R, Bloch KD, et al. Pulmonary vascular response patterns during exercise in left ventricular systolic dysfunction predict exercise capacity and outcomes. Circ Heart Fail. 2011;4(3):276–85.
11. Lewis GD, Shah R, Shahzad K, Camuso JM, Pappagianopoulos PP, Hung J, et al. Sildenafil improves exercise capacity and quality of life in patients with systolic heart failure and secondary pulmonary hypertension. Circulation. 2007;116(14):1555–62.
12. Ghio S, Bonderman D, Felix SB, Ghofrani HA, Michelakis ED, Mitrovic V, et al. Left ventricular systolic dysfunction associated with pulmonary hypertension riociguat trial (LEPHT): rationale and design. Eur J Heart Fail. 2012;14(8):946–53.
13. Bonderman D, Ghio S, Felix SB, Ghofrani H-A, Michelakis E, Mitrovic V, et al. Riociguat for patients with pulmonary hypertension caused by systolic left ventricular dysfunction: a phase IIb double-blind, randomized, placebo-controlled, dose-ranging hemodynamic study. Circulation. 2013;128(5):502–11.
14. Lam CSP, Roger VL, Rodeheffer RJ, Borlaug BA, Enders FT, Redfield MM. Pulmonary hypertension in heart failure with preserved ejection fraction: a community-based study. J Am Coll Cardiol. 2009;53(13):1119–26.
15. Guazzi M, Vicenzi M, Arena R, Guazzi MD. Pulmonary hypertension in heart failure with preserved ejection fraction: a target of phosphodiesterase-5 inhibition in a 1-year study. Circulation. 2011;124(2):164–74.

16. Redfield MM, Borlaug BA, Lewis GD, Mohammed SF, Semigran MJ, LeWinter MM, et al. PhosphdiesteRasE-5 inhibition to improve CLinical Status and EXercise capacity in diastolic heart failure (RELAX) trial: rationale and design. Circ Heart Fail. 2012;5(5):653–9.
17. Redfield MM, Chen HH, Borlaug BA, et al. Effect of phosphodiesterase-5 inhibition on exercise capacity and clinical status in heart failure with preserved ejection fraction: A randomized clinical trial. JAMA. 2013;309(12):1268–77.
18. Andersen KH, Iversen M, Kjaergaard J, Mortensen J, Nielsen-Kudsk JE, Bendstrup E, et al. Prevalence, predictors, and survival in pulmonary hypertension related to end-stage chronic obstructive pulmonary disease. J Heart Lung Transplant. 2012;31(4):373–80.
19. Carlsen J, Hasseriis Andersen K, Boesgaard S, Iversen M, Steinbrüchel D, Bøgelund AC. Pulmonary arterial lesions in explanted lungs after transplantation correlate with severity of pulmonary hypertension in chronic obstructive pulmonary disease. J Heart Lung Transplant. 2013;32(3):347–54.
20. Wrobel JP, Thompson BR, Williams TJ. Mechanisms of pulmonary hypertension in chronic obstructive pulmonary disease: A pathophysiologic review. J Heart Lung Transplant. 2012; 31(6):557–64.
21. Barbera JA. Mechanisms of development of chronic obstructive pulmonary disease-associated pulmonary hypertensoin. Pulm Circ. 2013;3(1):160–4.
22. Weitzenblum E, Sautegeau A, Ehrhart M, Mammosser M, Pelletier A. Long-term oxygen therapy can reverse the progression of pulmonary hypertension in patients with chronic obstructive pulmonary disease. Am Rev Respir Dis. 1985;131(4):493–8.
23. Continuous or nocturnal oxygen therapy in hypoxemic chronic obstructive lung disease: a clinical trial. Ann Intern Med 1980;93(3):391–8.
24. Rietema H, Holverda S, Bogaard HJ, Marcus JT, Smit HJ, Westerhof N, et al. Sildenafil treatment in COPD does not affect stroke volume or exercise capacity. Eur Respir J. 2008;31(4): 759–64.
25. Holverda S, Rietema H, Bogaard HJ, Westerhof N, Postmus PE, Boonstra A, et al. Acute effects of sildenafil on exercise pulmonary hemodynamics and capacity in patients with COPD. Pulm Pharmacol Ther. 2008;21(3):558–64.
26. Lederer DJ, Bartels MN, Schluger NW, Brogan F, Jellen P, Thomashow BM, et al. Sildenafil for chronic obstructive pulmonary disease: a randomized crossover trial. COPD. 2012;9(3): 268–75.
27. Stolz D, Rasch H, Linka A, Di Valentino M, Meyer A, Brutsche M, et al. A randomised, controlled trial of bosentan in severe COPD. Eur Respir J. 2008;32(3):619–28.
28. Naeije R, Melot C, Mols P, Hallemans R. Reduction in pulmonary hypertension by prostaglandin E1 in decompensated chronic obstructive pulmonary disease. Am Rev Respir Dis. 1982; 125(1):1–5.
29. Jones K, Higenbottam T, Wallwork J. Pulmonary vasodilation with prostacyclin in primary and secondary pulmonary hypertension. Chest. 1989;96(4):784–9.
30. Behr J, Ryu JH. Pulmonary hypertension in interstitial lung disease. Eur Respir J. 2008;31(6): 1357–67.
31. Ryu JH, Krowka MJ, Swanson KL, Pellikka PA, McGoon MD. Pulmonary hypertension in patients with interstitial lung diseases. Mayo Clin Proc. 2007;82(3):342–50.
32. Nadrous HF, Pellikka PA, Krowka MJ, Swanson KL, Chaowalit N, Decker PA, et al. The impact of pulmonary hypertension on survival in patients with idiopathic pulmonary fibrosis. Chest. 2005;128(6 Suppl):616S–7.
33. Nadrous HF, Pellikka PA, Krowka MJ, Swanson KL, Chaowalit N, Decker PA, et al. Pulmonary hypertension in patients with idiopathic pulmonary fibrosis. Chest. 2005;128(4):2393–9.
34. Chaowalit N, Pellikka PA, Decker PA, Aubry M-C, Krowka MJ, Ryu JH, et al. Echocardiographic and clinical characteristics of pulmonary hypertension complicating pulmonary langerhans cell histiocytosis. Mayo Clin Proc. 2004;79(10):1269–75.

35. Belle-van Meerkerk G, Cramer MJ, Kwakkel-van Erp JM, Nugroho MA, Tahri S, de Valk HW, et al. Pulmonary hypertension is a mild comorbidity in end-stage cystic fibrosis patients. J Heart Lung Transplant. 2013;32(6):609–14.
36. Venuta F, Tonelli AR, Anile M, Diso D, De Giacomo T, Ruberto F, et al. Pulmonary hypertension is associated with higher mortality in cystic fibrosis patients awaiting lung transplantation. J Cardiovasc Surg (Torino). 2012;53(6):810–7.
37. Damy T, Burgel PR, Pepin JL, Boelle PY, Cracowski C, Murris-Espin M, et al. Pulmonary acceleration time to optimize the timing of lung transplant in cystic fibrosis. Pulm Circ. 2012;2(1):75–83.
38. Golbin JM, Somers VK, Caples SM. Obstructive sleep apnea, cardiovascular disease, and pulmonary hypertension. Proc Am Thorac Soc. 2008;5(2):200–6.
39. Arias MA, García-Río F, Alonso-Fernández A, Martínez I, Villamor J. Pulmonary hypertension in obstructive sleep apnoea: effects of continuous positive airway pressure: a randomized, controlled cross-over study. Eur Heart J. 2006;27(9):1106–13.
40. Marik PE. The malignant obesity hypoventilation syndrome (MOHS). Obes Rev. 2012;13(10):902–9.
41. Marik PE, Desai H. The emergent malignant obesity hypoventilation syndrome: a New critical care syndrome. J Intensive Care Med. 2013;28(3):200.
42. Macavei VM, Spurling KJ, Loft J, Makker HK. Diagnostic predictors of obesity-hypoventilation syndrome in patients suspected of having sleep disordered breathing. J Clin Sleep Med. 2013;9(9):879–84.
43. Basoglu OK, Tasbakan MS. Comparison of clinical characteristics in patients with obesity hypoventilation syndrome and obese obstructive sleep apnea syndrome: a case-control study. Clin Respir J. 2014;8(2):167–74.

Chapter 6
Chronic Thromboembolic Pulmonary Hypertension

William R. Auger and Peter F. Fedullo

Abstract Chronic thromboembolic pulmonary hypertension (CTEPH) is a potential outcome in approximately 1–4 % of patients having experienced one or more acute pulmonary embolic events. Despite this recognized complication of acute thromboembolic disease, this clinical entity remains underdiagnosed. The importance of diagnosing CTEPH in any pulmonary hypertensive patient centers on the realization that, with surgical thromboendarterectomy, a potential cure for this form of pulmonary hypertension is currently available. For those patients with inoperable chronic thromboembolic pulmonary hypertension, recent advances in the development of pulmonary hypertensive specific medical therapy now offer hope for an improvement in pulmonary hemodynamics and functional status. This chapter presents an updated review of the epidemiology, pathophysiology, clinical presentation, assessment, and treatment options for those patients with chronic thromboembolic pulmonary hypertension.

Keywords Exertional dyspnea • Pulmonary embolism • Chronic thromboembolic disease • Pulmonary hypertension • Pulmonary thromboendarterectomy

Introduction

In 1990, Dr. Kenneth Moser and coworkers, pioneers in the evaluation and management of chronic thromboembolic pulmonary hypertension (CTEPH), noted in a review of the topic that the list of investigative opportunities presented by this disease entity was substantial [1]. Over the past quarter century, many of these challenges have been satisfactorily met, others remain, while new ones have arisen. While recognition of CTEPH as one of the most curable forms of pulmonary hypertension has grown throughout this period of time, identification of patients who are at risk and the pathophysiologic mechanisms underlying the transition from acute to

W.R. Auger, M.D. (✉) • P.F. Fedullo, M.D.
Division of Pulmonary and Critical Care Medicine, University of California, San Diego, 9300 Campus Point Drive, La Jolla, CA 92037, USA
e-mail: bauger@UCSD.edu

J.R. Klinger, R.P. Frantz (eds.), *Diagnosis and Management of Pulmonary Hypertension*, Respiratory Medicine 12, DOI 10.1007/978-1-4939-2636-7_6

organized thromboembolic disease remain elusive. With advancement of the imaging technologies of computerized tomography and magnetic resonance, the opportunity to detect chronic thromboembolic disease has been advanced, though the criteria for diagnosis, and particularly the description of *operable* chronic thromboembolic disease, remain incomplete. The global expansion of specialized centers for the evaluation and treatment of patients with chronic thromboembolic disease has resulted in the ability to care for a greater number of patients afflicted with this previously fatal disorder. However, the selection criterion for patients who might be considered candidates for thromboendarterectomy, the therapy which offers the greatest chance for a cure, varies considerably. Although the availability of pulmonary hypertensive medical therapy has expanded over the past decade, the patients with CTEPH who would be best treated with these medications remain incompletely defined. This chapter provides an overview of the most recent information addressing issues in the evaluation and management of patients with chronic thromboembolic disease.

Epidemiology

The incidence of chronic thromboembolic pulmonary hypertension (CTEPH) following an initial or recurrent episode of pulmonary embolism remains a matter of considerable debate. Widely disparate estimates of the incidence of the disease have been reported over the past decade, ranging from 0.57 to 8.8 % in patients with an initial episode of pulmonary embolism and from 13.4 to 37.5 % in those with recurrent events [2–7]. A similar divergence in estimated disease incidence is associated with acute pulmonary embolism (ranging from as few as 80,000 incidence cases to as many as 600,000 annually in the United States), highlighting the difficulty encountered clinically in accurately detecting and evaluating disorders of the right ventricle and pulmonary vascular bed [8–11].

In the largest of the studies assessing the incidence of CTEPH, a cohort screening study involving 866 survivors of acute pulmonary embolism, four patients were ultimately diagnosed with CTEPH (confirmed by right heart catheterization) for a cumulative incidence of 0.57 % in the overall population and 0.80 % in patients in whom CTEPH was objectively confirmed or excluded [5]. It is estimated that the number of pulmonary thromboendarterectomy (PTE) procedures performed in the United States approximates 300–500 annually, with 150 of these being done at the University of California, San Diego, and the remainder at other national referral sites. Assuming that 100,000–200,000 cases of acute pulmonary embolism occur annually in the United States with a 2-year survival rate of 60 %, an incidence of CTEPH requiring surgical intervention of approximately 1 % would seem a reasonable estimate [12].

Factors contributing to uncertainty regarding the incidence of CTEPH include the limited number of long-term studies which have been undertaken in patients with acute embolism and, in those that have, differences in the populations studied (unselected versus consecutive versus referral), the echocardiographic criteria utilized to define pulmonary hypertension (pulmonary artery systolic pressure >30 mmHg versus >35 mmHg versus >40 mmHg), the inconsistent use of cardiac catheterization to confirm the presence of pulmonary hypertension and to exclude other potential etiologies, and the criteria utilized to determine surgical eligibility [2–7].

It is now generally accepted that CTEPH is a consequence of acute pulmonary embolism. Despite the prevalence of the disease, acute embolism remains incompletely defined in terms of its long-term hemodynamic and ventilatory outcomes. Substantial anatomic resolution occurs in the majority of patients experiencing an embolic event. Recent data, however, would suggest that this resolution is often incomplete and may be associated with both physiologic and functional impairment [13–17].

Stevinson and coworkers evaluated 109 previously healthy patients 6 months after experiencing symptomatic, hemodynamically submassive pulmonary embolism. At the time of presentation, 50 % of patients had echocardiographic evidence of RV dysfunction, a figure consistent with that found in other series [16]. Six months later, 25 % of the patients continued to demonstrate echocardiographic evidence of RV dysfunction and 25 % had evidence of functional limitation as determined by a 6-min walk test <330 m or subjective functional limitation with a NYHA class > II. Similar evidence of right ventricular dysfunction and functional limitation following hemodynamically submassive pulmonary embolism, albeit with a lower incidence, has been reported by Kline and coworkers [15]. Wartski and coworkers in a follow-up study of 157 patients enrolled in the THESEE (Tinzaparine ou Heparine Standard: Evaluations dans l'Embolie Pulmonaire) trial reported that residual pulmonary vascular obstruction >5 % was documented in 66 % of patients, including 13 (8.3 %) with a residual obstruction of at least 50 % 3 months following the event [14]. Functional limitation in the absence of overt pulmonary hypertension following acute embolism would appear to result from two physiologic abnormalities related to the residual pulmonary vascular obstruction and its effect on right ventricular function, that is, an increase in dead space ventilation and an inability to optimally augment cardiac output to sufficiently meet exercise oxygen demands [18–20].

Based on current data, an expansion in the utilization of thrombolytic therapy in patients with hemodynamically submassive embolism does not appear to reduce the subsequent incidence of CTEPH. Outcome studies of thrombolytic therapy in pulmonary embolism have predominantly utilized mortality and short-term imaging and hemodynamic resolution as endpoints, not long-term hemodynamic outcome or functional status. The limited data available, however, suggest that the overall extent of embolic resolution is equivalent in patients treated with heparin or thrombolytic agents [21, 22]. Recently published data from the PEITHO (Pulmonary Embolism Thrombolysis Trial) trial, evaluating the role of tenecteplase in patients with intermediate-risk embolism and RV dysfunction, demonstrated a reduction in the rate of hemodynamic compromise within a week of diagnosis, compared to those patients receiving heparin anticoagulation alone. However, the long-term benefit of early thrombolysis in this patient group as it relates to the prevention of right heart compromise over time was not a study endpoint [23].

A central confounding factor in defining the true incidence of CTEPH has been a failure to more precisely characterize the entire disease spectrum. Initial clinical interests centered on those with advanced pulmonary hypertension potentially requiring PTE surgery. Because of the high perioperative mortality associated with a thromboendarterectomy, its utilization was limited in those with less severe disease [24]. The major focus of clinical and investigative effort, therefore, centered on the preoperative evaluation, surgical management, and postoperative care of patients with advanced pulmonary hypertension. However, recent insight into the natural history of acute embolism coupled with the introduction of pulmonary hypertension-specific medical therapy and a decline in the PTE mortality rate below 1 % in those with less severe disease should result in an expansion of that focus [25, 26]. The syndrome of chronic thromboembolic disease should be recognized as a continuum encompassing not only overt thromboembolic pulmonary hypertension but also postembolic right ventricular dysfunction that can occur during exercise and respiratory compromise from dead space ventilation, clinical entities which can be referred to as thromboembolic-related respiratory insufficiency (TERRI). If the entire spectrum of disease is included, therefore, it is probable that the incidence of chronic cardiopulmonary disease associated with pulmonary embolism is several-fold higher than the 1 % estimate of those who ultimately go on to require thromboendarterectomy.

The importance of establishing the diagnosis of CTEPH is further underscored by the observation that long-term survivorship in the absence of appropriate treatment is poor. And as is the case in other forms of pulmonary hypertension, prognosis correlates to the degree of pulmonary hypertension and right heart dysfunction at the time of diagnosis. In a study conducted during a period when therapeutic options were limited, 5-year survival rate in patients with CTEPH was 30 % when the mean pulmonary artery pressure at the time of presentation was between 40 and 50 mmHg; when the mean pulmonary artery pressure was greater than 50 mmHg, survivorship at 5 years declined to approximately 10 % [27]. In a more recent report, CTEPH patients with mean pulmonary artery pressures above 30 mmHg experienced a poorer prognosis [28].

Predisposing Factors and Pathophysiology

CTEPH results from a prior episode of pulmonary embolism regardless of whether that episode was symptomatic or not. It is not at all surprising that approximately 25 % of patients with CTEPH do not provide a history of prior venous thromboembolism given the known frequency of asymptomatic embolism, the frequency with which the diagnosis of acute embolism is overlooked in favor of other alternatives, and the known incidence of asymptomatic pulmonary embolism associated with proximal venous thrombosis [29–31].

Despite extensive investigation, only two identifiable thrombophilic tendencies have been associated with CTEPH. Antiphospholipid antibodies have been encountered in approximately 10–20 % of patients [32, 33]. An elevated level of Factor VIII was identified as a risk factor in a study of 122 patients with CTEPH compared to 88 patients with nonthrombotic pulmonary arterial hypertension and 82 healthy controls [34]. The prevalence of antithrombin III, protein C, protein S deficiency, and the prothrombin G20210A appears to be no higher than that in the general population. Preliminary evidence suggested that activated protein C resistance is no more common in patients with CTEPH than in the general population. However, a more recent, retrospective trial did demonstrate that factor V Leiden mutation was more frequent in CTEPH than in other forms of pulmonary hypertension (29 % versus 7.8 %) [35]. Although no consistent defect in fibrinolytic activity has been identified, fibrinogen variants resulting in fibrin resistant to lysis have been identified in certain patients with CTEPH [36, 37].

In terms of clinical risk factors, the presence of prior embolism is obviously the most common. The larger the embolic event, the more severe the hemodynamic impairment at the time of presentation, and the presence of residual pulmonary hypertension following the event appears to contribute to the eventual development of CTEPH [38, 39]. A history of recurrent embolic events resulting in progressive occlusion of the pulmonary vascular bed is also strongly associated with disease development [2–7].

A number of associated conditions have been linked to the development of the disease including prior major surgery, obesity, cancer, congestive heart failure, and the presence of ventriculo-atrial shunts [29, 40]. All, however, are also associated with the development of acute embolism. The one disease process associated with CTEPH which does not have a strong association with acute embolism is a history of splenectomy which in one series was reported to occur in 22 of 57 (38.6 %) patients referred to a single clinical center [41]. In the recently published European Registry, splenectomy was present in 3.4 % of patients, 1.9 % in those considered operable and 5.7 % in those inoperable [29]. No mention was made whether these patients had an associated hemoglobinopathy. The basis for the association between splenectomy and CTEPH is uncertain. In part, it may be related to the reactive thrombocytosis that occurs post-splenectomy. In patients with thalassemia, a procoagulant status of thalassemic red cells has been recognized. Abnormal expression of phosphatidylserine on the surface of erythrocytes may trigger the coagulation cascade [40, 42].

Although insufficiently studied, it is possible that genetic risk factors contribute to the development and therefore incidence of CTEPH. Clinical experience with this disease process has amply demonstrated that equivalent degrees of pulmonary vascular obstruction can result in wide differences among individuals in the long-term pulmonary hemodynamic response and that progression of pulmonary hypertension occurs in the absence of additional large vessel obstruction. Studies of microvascular changes in CTEPH have shown indistinguishable vascular lesions from those seen in idiopathic pulmonary arterial hypertension as well as dysfunctional pulmonary arterial cell function [43–47]. It is currently hypothesized that acute embolism in predisposed patients is simply the initiating event in a process that ultimately results in pathologic alterations at the small vessel level, the physiologic perturbations responsible for these anatomic alterations under investigation [48–50].

Clinical Presentation

Early in the course of the disease, the clinical presentation of CTEPH can be subtle. This contributes to the delay in diagnosis, making it necessary to maintain a high index of suspicion in those patients presenting with exertional dyspnea without apparent cause or without a prior history of venous thromboembolism. Atypical chest pain, episodic hemoptysis [51], a nonproductive cough, and palpitations are rarely presenting complaints. Evidence of right heart dysfunction such as peripheral edema, severe exercise limitation and associated chest discomfort, exertional dizziness, or syncopal episodes can be manifest late in the disease.

Physical exam findings can be equally deceptive early in the natural history of CTEPH. With advancing pulmonary hypertension though, clinical presentation and exam findings are similar to that seen in other forms of pulmonary hypertension including a right ventricular impulse, a split second heart sound with accentuation of the pulmonic component, a murmur of tricuspid regurgitation, and a right ventricular S_4 gallop. As right ventricular failure develops, jugular venous distension, peripheral edema, hepatomegaly, ascites, and a right-sided S_3 may be evident. An exam finding that can be useful in distinguishing small vessel from large vessel variants of pulmonary hypertension is the presence of pulmonary flow murmurs or bruits [52]. An auscultatory finding in approximately 30 % of patients with CTEPH, the bruit results from turbulent flow across partially obstructed, medium- to large-sized pulmonary vessels. They have not been described in small vessel pulmonary hypertensive disorders. However, they are not unique to patients with chronic thromboembolic disease, having been described in other disease states which involve large pulmonary arteries, such as congenital branch stenoses or large vessel pulmonary arteritis. Additional exam findings in the CTEPH patient might include peripheral cyanosis, alerting the clinician to the possibility of a right-to-left shunt through a patent foramen ovale. Examination of the lower extremities may disclose superficial varicosities and venous stasis skin discoloration in those individuals who have experienced prior venous thrombosis.

Evaluation for Chronic Thromboembolic Disease

Following an episode of pulmonary embolism, routine cardiopulmonary screening has a low yield in the detection of CTEPH [53]. Standard pulmonary function testing is most useful in evaluating for coexisting parenchymal lung disease or airflow obstruction, providing nonspecific information as it relates to the presence or absence of chronic thromboembolic disease. In approximately 20 % of CTEPH patients with parenchymal scarring from prior lung infarction, a mild to moderate restrictive defect may be detected [54]. Similarly, a modest reduction in single breath diffusing capacity for carbon monoxide (DLco) may be present in some CTEPH patients, though a normal value does not exclude the diagnosis [55].

A severe reduction in DLco should raise concerns that the distal pulmonary vascular bed is significantly compromised, making it imperative that an alternative diagnosis other than CTEPH be considered. Furthermore, some CTEPH patients will exhibit some degree of hypoxemia, and if measured, elevated dead space ventilation [20], both worsening with exercise. These findings reflect a moderate ventilation-perfusion mismatch and an inadequate cardiac output response to exercise with a reduction in mixed venous oxygen saturation [56]. Marked hypoxemia at rest implies severe right heart dysfunction or the presence of a considerable right-to-left shunt, such as through a patent foramen ovale.

Early in the course of chronic thromboembolic disease, the chest radiograph may be unremarkable. With disease progression and the development of pulmonary hypertension, enlargement of the proximal pulmonary vascular bed typically occurs, and with chronic thromboembolic involvement of the main or lobar pulmonary arteries, this central PA enlargement can be asymmetric. This is not a radiographic finding in those patients with small vessel disease pulmonary hypertension [57]. As the right ventricle adapts to the rise in pulmonary vascular resistance, radiographic signs of chamber enlargement, such as obliteration of the retrosternal space and prominence of the right heart border, can be observed [58]. Without coexisting parenchymal lung disease, interstitial-alveolar markings within the lung fields are atypical. However, relatively avascular lung regions can be appreciated if an organized thrombus has compromised blood flow to that area (Fig. 6.1). In these poorly perfused lung regions, consequences of lung injury such as peripheral alveolar opacities, linear scar-like lesions, and pleural thickening may be found.

Transthoracic echocardiography is often the first objective indication as to the presence of elevated pulmonary pressures or right ventricular compromise. Current technology allows for estimates of pulmonary artery systolic pressure (using Doppler

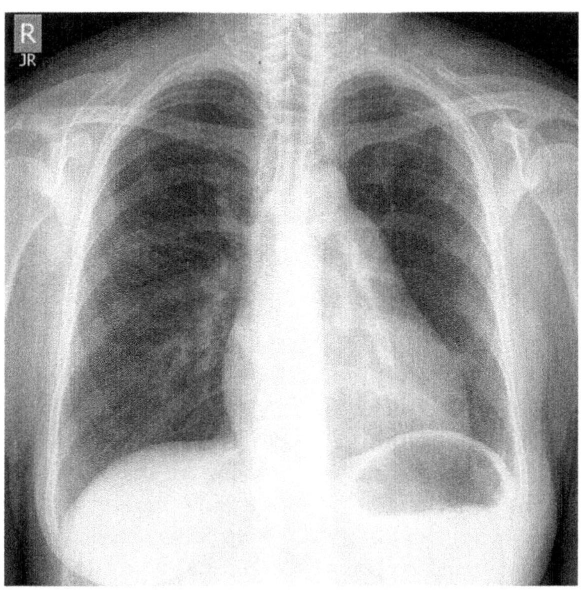

Fig. 6.1 Chest X-ray showing reduced vascular markings throughout left lung caused by large pulmonary embolism

analysis of the degree of tricuspid regurgitation), along with cardiac output and RV performance [59]. Enlargement of the right heart chambers, tricuspid regurgitation as a result of this chamber enlargement, flattening or paradoxical motion of the interventricular septum, encroachment of an enlarged right ventricle on the left ventricular cavity, and impaired left ventricular diastolic dysfunction that it is not the result of primary left ventricular or valvular heart disease are findings in patients with significant pulmonary hypertension [60, 61]. Contrast echocardiography using intravenous agitated saline can detect the presence of an intracardiac shunt, such as a patent foramen ovale or a previously undetected septal defect. In a patient with symptomatic chronic thromboembolic disease who has an echocardiogram that shows only minimal elevation of pulmonary artery pressures or modest right ventricular compromise at rest, an exercise stress echocardiogram may demonstrate a substantial rise in pulmonary artery pressures or dilatation of the right ventricle.

To a large extent, computed tomographic (CT) angiography of the pulmonary vessels has replaced ventilation-perfusion (V/Q) scintigraphy in the evaluation of patients with suspected acute pulmonary embolic disease. However, the V/Q scan continues to provide essential information in the pulmonary hypertensive patient, and can often be the first indication that chronic thromboembolic disease should be considered. This study serves as a valuable screening test for this disease [62]. In a single center, retrospective survey comparing V/Q scanning with CT angiography in 227 pulmonary hypertensive patients, there was a sensitivity of 97.4 % for V/Q scanning compared to 51 % for CT angiography in the detection of chronic thromboembolic disease [63]. In a more recent study of 12 CTEPH patients, Soler and colleagues demonstrated that SPECT perfusion scintigraphy was more sensitive in detecting obstructed vascular segments when compared to CT pulmonary angiography, with a sensitivity of 62 ± 4.1 % versus 47.8 ± 2.9 %, respectively [64]. Further, the interpretation of an abnormal perfusion pattern can assist in the differentiation between disorders involving the central or proximal vascular bed from those primarily affecting the peripheral pulmonary circulation. In chronic thromboembolic disease, at least one and more commonly several segmental or larger mismatched perfusion defects are present. For those patients with small vessel pulmonary vascular disease, perfusion scans either are normal or exhibit a "mottled" appearance characterized by nonsegmental defects [65, 66]. Exceptions include cases of pulmonary veno-occlusive disease or pulmonary capillary hemangiomatosis in which multiple, larger mismatched defects have been reported [67, 68]. As important has been the observation that a relatively normal perfusion pattern on V/Q scan excludes the diagnosis of surgically accessible chronic thromboembolic disease (Fig. 6.2).

It has also been established that the magnitude of perfusion defects exhibited by CTEPH patients with operable disease may understate the degree of pulmonary vascular obstruction determined by angiography [69]. The plausible explanation for this finding is that during the process of thrombus organization, proximal vessel thromboemboli may recanalize or narrow the vessel in such a manner that radiolabeled macroaggregated albumin may traverse the area of partial obstruction, creating gray zones or regions of relative hypoperfusion. Therefore, chronic thromboembolic disease should be considered and further evaluation for operable disease should

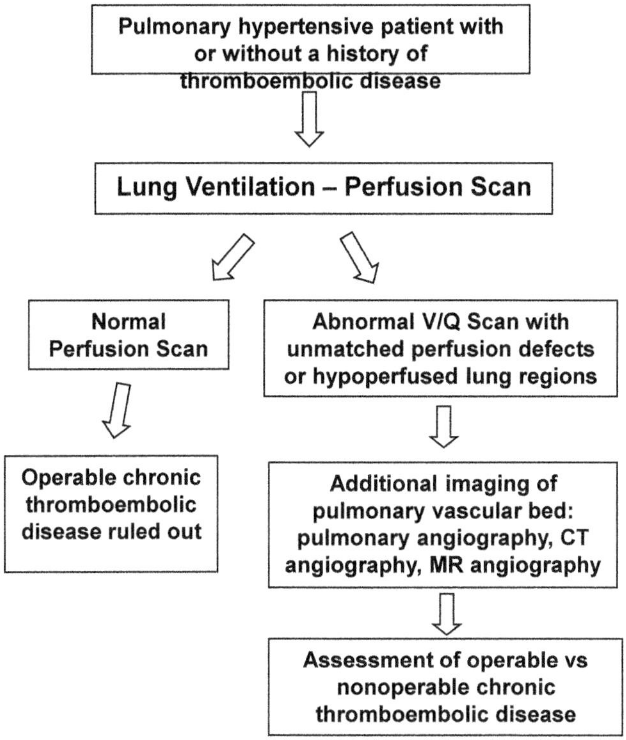

Fig. 6.2 Diagnostic approach to the evaluation of CTEPH. *CT* computed tomography, *MR* magnetic resonance. Adapted from Hoeper et al. [62]

proceed even if the V/Q scan demonstrates a limited number of mismatched perfusion defects, or lung regions which are relatively "hypoperfused."

The next step in the evaluation of patients with suspected chronic thromboembolic disease is to more clearly image the pulmonary vascular bed, to not only establish the diagnosis but also define the extent and location of lesions. Prior to the availability of computed tomographic angiography and magnetic resonance imaging of the chest, conventional pulmonary angiography was the principal means of achieving these goals in the evaluation of patients for pulmonary thromboendarterectomy surgery. It can be considered the gold standard in providing a "map" for surgery, against which other modalities are to be measured. Under essentially all circumstances, a properly performed bi-plane angiogram will provide sufficient information on which to base a decision regarding chronic thrombus location, and as a result, surgical accessibility. The angiographic appearance of chronic thromboembolic disease bears little resemblance to that of the well-defined, intraluminal filling defects of acute pulmonary embolism. Instead, the angiographic patterns encountered in chronic thromboembolic disease reflect the complex patterns of organization and recanalization that occur following an acute thromboembolic event.

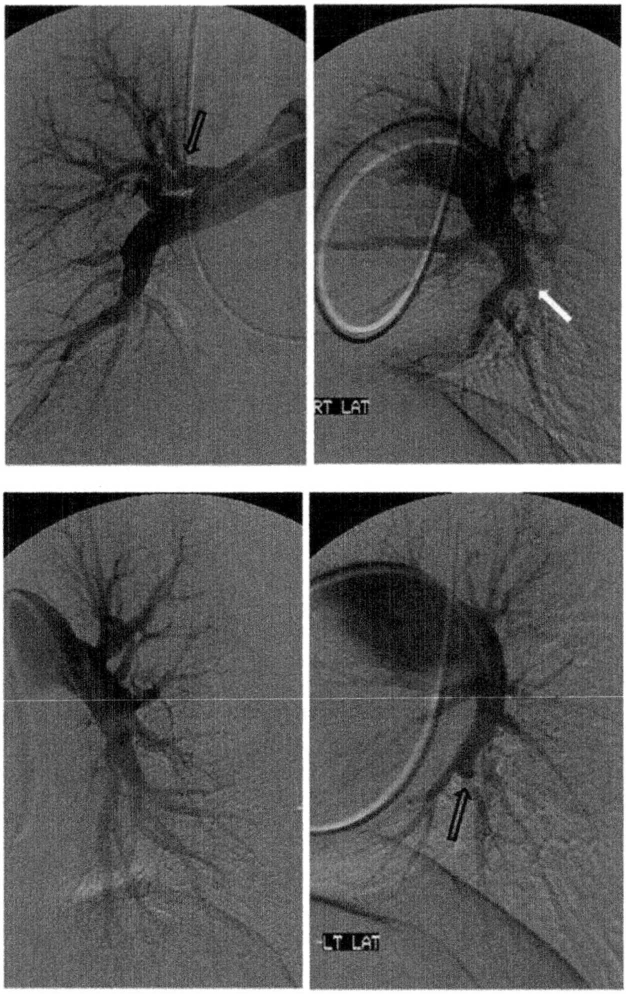

Fig. 6.3 Conventional pulmonary angiogram in a CTEPH patient. *Open arrows*: "web" narrowing of the proximal segmental arteries. *Closed arrow*: "pouch" defect occluding the posterior branch to the right lower lobe. *Lateral views* providing better definition of the pulmonary vascular anatomy that is less apparent on anteroposterior views

Several angiographic patterns have been described in chronic thromboembolic disease that correlate with material removed at the time of surgery [70]. These include "pouch defects," pulmonary artery webs or bands, intimal irregularities, abrupt, frequently angular narrowing of the major pulmonary arteries, and complete obstruction of main, lobar, or segmental vessels at their point of origin (Figs. 6.3 and 6.4). In the majority of CTEPH patients, two or more of these angiographic findings are present, typically involving both lungs.

With the advances in computed tomographic (CT) angiography of the chest, and greater availability and use of this technology in assessing the pulmonary vascular

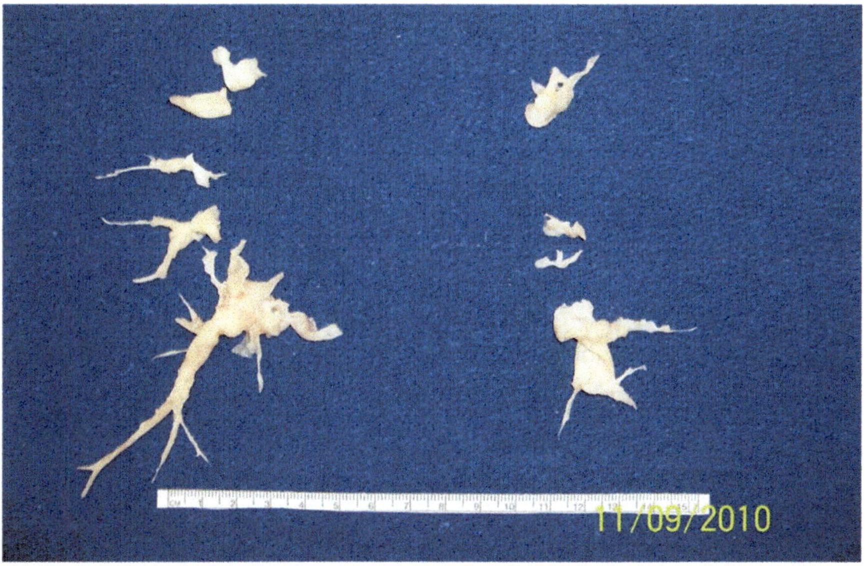

Fig. 6.4 Chronic thromboembolic material endarterectomized from the pulmonary vessels depicted in the pulmonary angiogram in Fig. 6.2. Ruler is 15 cm in length

bed, CT is playing an expanded role in the evaluation of the pulmonary hypertensive patient for chronic thromboembolic disease. There are a number of CT findings which have been described in patients with chronic thromboembolic disease. These include mosaic perfusion of the lung parenchyma; enlargement of the central pulmonary arteries and right heart chambers; variability in the size of lobar and segmental-level vessels with a reduction in vessel caliber of those involved with chronic thrombi; and peripheral, scar-like lesions in poorly perfused lung regions. With contrast enhancement of the pulmonary vasculature during CT imaging, organized thrombus can be seen to line the pulmonary vessels, often in an eccentric manner. Associated narrowing of pulmonary arteries, web strictures, "pouch defects," and other irregularities of the intima may also be appreciated [71, 72] (Figs. 6.5 and 6.6). These CT findings are distinct from the intraluminal filling defects of acute thromboemboli and primary pulmonary vascular tumors [73]. With appropriate timing of the intravenous contrast bolus for CTA, opacification of the pulmonary and systemic circulations is possible. In addition to the pulmonary vascular bed, this allows examination of a number of cardiac features including cardiac chamber size, position and shape of the interventricular septum, the presence of congenital cardiac abnormalities, anomalous pulmonary venous drainage, and the size and distribution of collateral vessels arising from the systemic arterial circulation (bronchial arteries off the aorta, coronary vessels) [72, 74]. What remains incompletely validated is the utility of CT angiography in determining operability in certain subgroups of CTEPH patients. This is particularly important as operative techniques allow for resection of chronic thromboembolic material at the segmental vessel level.

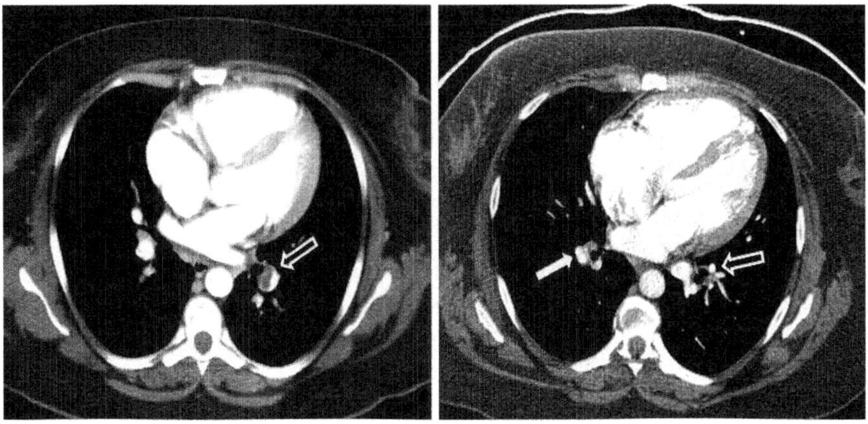

Fig. 6.5 Transition from acute to organized, chronic thromboembolic lesions (*open arrows*) occurring over 4 months on antithrombotic therapy. Vessel narrowing in the absence of intraluminal defects has occurred. Intimal thickening, a small web and vessel narrowing can be seen at the level of the distal right descending pulmonary artery (*closed arrow*). The chronic thromboembolic material removed at surgery is pictured in Fig. 6.3

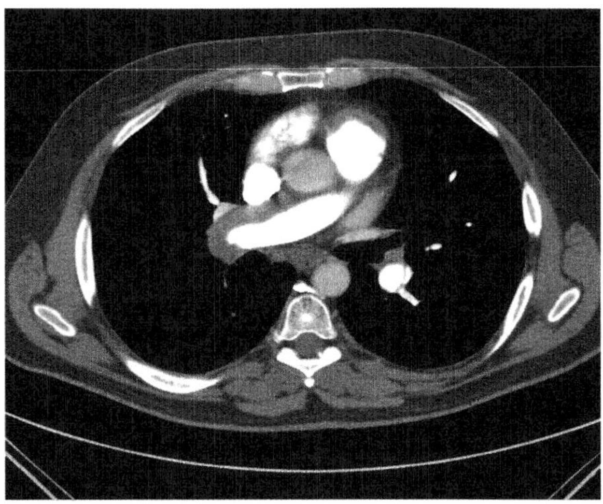

Fig. 6.6 CT angiogram in a CTEPH patient, demonstrating lining thrombus right main and interlobar arteries, with an intravascular web … a remnant of an acute pulmonary embolus … in the left descending pulmonary artery

Clinical experience has demonstrated that the absence of lining thrombus or thickened intima of the *central* vessels on CT does not exclude the diagnosis of chronic thromboembolic disease or the possibility of surgical intervention. Studies directly comparing CT with pulmonary angiography are limited. In one such study, CT and digital angiography were nearly equivalent in terms of identifying complete vessel occlusion at the segmental level. However, for nonocclusive changes, CT was significantly inferior to angiography [75]. Accuracy of CT has improved with technological advances in scanners. In a recent study of 44 patients with suspected CTEPH,

Sugiura and colleagues compared pulmonary digital subtraction angiography with enhanced, electrocardiogram gated 320-slice CT in the detection of thrombi within the pulmonary vascular bed. The sensitivity and specificity of CT to detect chronic thromboembolic lesions were 97.0 % and 97.1 % at the main and lobar vessel level; at the segmental level, the corresponding numbers were 85.8 % and 94.6 %, respectively [76].

In addition, there is considerable value for CT in detecting disorders of the pulmonary parenchyma and mediastinum. For CTEPH patients with coexisting interstitial lung disease or emphysema, CT will be able to define the extent and location of the parenchymal lung process. Reperfusion of severely diseased lung parenchyma following an endarterectomy is likely to result in an undesirable outcome, and thereby should exclude a patient from surgical consideration. For those patients whose V/Q scan demonstrates absence or near-complete absence of perfusion to an entire lung, CT is an essential study to rule out extrinsic pulmonary vascular compression from mediastinal adenopathy, fibrosis, or neoplasm [77].

Expanding experience using magnetic resonance (MR) imaging and magnetic resonance angiography (MRA) to visualize the pulmonary vascular bed in patients with chronic thromboembolic pulmonary hypertension has established this imaging modality as a reliable means to determine surgical candidacy for CTEPH patients [78]. Kreitner and colleagues have shown that contrast-enhanced MRA is able to demonstrate the vascular changes typical for CTE disease. In a study of 34 CTEPH patients, wall-adherent thromboembolic material involving the central pulmonary arteries down to the segmental level could be demonstrated; intraluminal webs and bands as well as abnormal vessel tapering and "cutoffs" were also detected. Further they showed that MRA was superior to digital subtraction angiography in determining the proximal location of resectable chronic thromboembolic material [79]. An additional study comparing magnetic resonance techniques with conventional contrast angiography involved 29 patients with either CTEPH or idiopathic pulmonary arterial hypertension (IPAH). Nikolaou and colleagues showed that the combined interpretation of MR perfusion imaging and MR angiography led to a correct diagnosis of IPAH or CTEPH in 26 (90 %) of 29 patients when compared to the reference diagnosis based on V/Q scintigraphy, digital subtraction angiography, or CT angiography. The interpretation of MR angiography alone had a sensitivity of 71 % for wall-adherent thrombi, 50 % for webs and bands, and between 83 and 86 % for detection of complete vessel obstruction and free-floating thrombi when compared to DSA or CT angiography [80]. More recently, Rajaram and colleagues retrospectively evaluated the accuracy of contrast-enhanced MR angiography compared to CT pulmonary angiography in a group of 53 CTEPH patients. The sensitivity and specificity of MRA in detecting proximal and distal vessel chronic thromboembolic disease were 98 and 94 %, the sensitivity of MR diagnosis of central vessel disease considerably improved when images were analyzed with unenhanced proton MRA (50–88 %). Overall, MRA identified more stenosis, poststenotic dilatation, and occlusive lesions when compared with CT angiography in this particular study [81]. However, in a small study of 24 CTEPH patients in whom all three diagnostic modalities were performed within a 3-day period, Ley and colleagues compared digital subtraction angiography, ECG-gated multidetector CT angiography, and contrast-enhanced MR angiography in the detection of vascular changes associated with chronic thromboembolic disease. Based on comparison with reference standards, it was concluded that multidetector CT provided the best image quality and highest level of sensitivity and specificity for detection of vascular abnormalities at the main, lobar, and segmental levels [82].

Additional features of magnetic resonance imaging that can be useful in the evaluation of CTEPH patients include cine imaging which allows an assessment of RV and LV function, providing data on end-systolic and end-diastolic volumes, ejection fraction, and muscle mass [83, 84]. Furthermore, phase contrast imaging may be used to measure cardiac output, along with pulmonary and systemic arterial flow. In CTEPH patients undergoing PEA, this technique has been used to measure changes in aortic and pulmonary arterial blood flow before and after surgery [79].

Surgical Approach to Chronic Thromboembolic Disease

The goals in the evaluation of patients with suspected CTEPH are to first establish the diagnosis, and then to determine whether or not pulmonary thromboendarterectomy is feasible. The appropriate interpretation of the angiographic studies reviewed in the previous section determines the proximal extent, and as a result, the surgical accessibility of the organized thrombi present. Equally essential in the determination of whether any particular CTEPH patient is a surgical candidate, particularly as it relates to an assessment of perioperative risks, is defining the severity of pulmonary hypertension and the degree of cardiac dysfunction at rest with right heart catheterization. Early surgical experience supported the observation that patients with severe pulmonary hypertension (pulmonary vascular resistance >1,000 dyn/s/cm^{-5}) bear a greater perioperative mortality risk. Hartz et al. reported that a preoperative PVR over 1,100 dyn/s/cm^{-5} was associated with 41 % mortality—compared to less than 6 % if PVR was less than 1,100 dyn/s/cm^{-5} [85]. Dartevelle and colleagues reported an increased postoperative mortality of 20 % for patients with preoperative PVR over 1,200 dyn/s/cm^{-5} compared to 4 % mortality if the preoperative PVR was less than 900 dyn/s/cm^{-5} [86]. Although the San Diego group has reported a declining overall operative mortality risk following thromboendarterectomy surgery over the past several years, the most recent report reveals that in 500 patients operated between 2006 and 2010, those patients with a preoperative PVR > 1,000 dyn/s/cm^{-5} experienced a mortality rate of 4.1 % compared to 1.6 % in those patients with a PVR less than 1,000 dyn/s/cm^{-5} [25].

For symptomatic CTEPH patients with minimal pulmonary hypertension at rest, exercise hemodynamic measurements should be undertaken. In these cases it is likely the normal compensatory mechanisms of recruitment and dilation of the pulmonary vasculature have been overcome, and with exercise, an elevation in pulmonary artery pressure as cardiac output increases can be observed. This hemodynamic information provides objective evidence to explain an individual's symptoms, and may reflect a reduction in pulmonary vascular reserve from chronic thrombotic obstruction of a limited amount of the pulmonary vasculature, or equally plausible, an indication of a clinically relevant stage in the development of severe CTEPH in which there is coexisting small vessel hypertensive changes.

There are a number of considerations in the determination of whether an individual patient with CTEPH might be a candidate for thromboendarterectomy surgery (Table 6.1). Despite advancements in diagnostics and an expanding surgical experience, there remains considerable subjectivity in this assessment. The most critical factor determining operative candidacy is the presence of surgically accessible chronic thromboembolic lesions, as established by angiographic (conventional, CT, MR) studies. However, interpretative experience and knowledge of surgical capabilities at any specialized clinical center will dictate what lesions can be endarterectomized. As surgical experience is gained, not only is it possible to resect main pulmonary artery and lobar level disease, but also more distal, segmental chronic thromboembolic lesions [25]. Although early experience with PTE surgery focused on the treatment of patients with pulmonary hypertension and right heart dysfunction, indications for surgical intervention have expanded to include those patients with chronic thromboembolic disease who experience exertion-related pulmonary hypertension, as well as those who are primarily symptomatic from elevated dead space ventilation [20].

As important is the recognition when surgical intervention might be ill-advised. Patients exhibiting significant comorbidities (e.g., severe emphysema, end-stage malignancies) that not only place them at extraordinary perioperative risk, but would prevent the hemodynamic and functional status benefit following PTE surgery from being realized should not be considered operative candidates. Furthermore, when the degree of pulmonary hypertension appears out of proportion to the extent of accessible chronic thromboembolic disease apparent by angiography, and surgical resection is not expected to result in a substantive improvement in pulmonary hemodynamics, surgery should be avoided. With appropriate waveform analysis, data obtained with right heart catheterization has the potential to objectively assess the degree of concurrent small vessel disease in CTEPH, essentially "partitioning" the different elements (proximal versus distal) of pulmonary vascular resistance.

Table 6.1 Selection of patients for pulmonary thromboendarterectomy

• Surgically accessible CTE[a] disease (main, lobar, segmental) with:
1. Pulmonary hypertension and right heart dysfunction, or
2. Exertion associated pulmonary hypertension, or
3. Elevated dead space ventilation
• Relative contraindications:
1. Pulmonary hypertension out of proportion to the extent of CTE present
2. Endarterectomy of CTE lesions not expected to improve pulmonary hemodynamics
3. Comorbidities to a degree post-PTE hemodynamic and functional benefits would not be realized

[a]Chronic thromboembolic

Though specialized equipment is required and obtaining adequate occlusion waveforms may be difficult in this patient population, the available data from this technique underscores the heterogeneity of pulmonary vascular lesions present in CTEPH. Patients with operable disease usually exhibit a greater degree of upstream resistance (Rup) [87]. This information may further predict outcomes following endarterectomy. In a small series of 26 CTEPH patients, Kim and colleagues, utilizing pulmonary artery occlusion waveform analysis, demonstrated an inverse correlation between the percent upstream resistance and postoperative mean pulmonary artery pressure and pulmonary vascular resistance. In addition, all 4 deaths in this series occurred in patients in whom the Rup was less than 60 % [88]. This finding, however, was not observed in Toshner's study, where both CTEPH patients who died following endarterectomy exhibited an upstream resistance of 68 and 73 % [87].

Pulmonary thromboendarterectomy is the unique surgical intervention to remove obstructive, adherent chronic thromboembolic lesions from within the pulmonary vascular bed. During the three decades since the first attempts in the early 1960s to surgically treat CTEPH, there were a number of essential technical modifications which have led to the current success of this procedure [89–91]. Performance of a median sternotomy provides access to the central pulmonary vessels of both lungs, while avoiding disruption of the extensive bronchial artery collateral circulation and pleural adhesions that may develop following longstanding pulmonary arterial obstruction. Furthermore, if additional cardiac procedures are necessary, such as coronary artery bypass or valve surgery, there is access to the heart via the sternotomy [92]. The use of cardiopulmonary bypass with periods of hypothermic circulatory arrest is a mainstay of the surgical procedure. Deep hypothermia provides for tissue protection, while intermittent circulatory arrest periods avoids back-bleeding from bronchial artery to pulmonary artery anastomoses and provides the necessary bloodless field to perform the meticulous and optimal dissection of chronic thromboembolic material from the pulmonary vessels. The importance of this phase of the operation has grown as dissection from the segmental arteries has become technically feasible, making adequate visualization of these more distal vessels imperative [25]. Modifications of this technique have been employed with the intent of minimizing neurologic risks of deep hypothermia and circulatory arrest periods. Those described include the use of moderate hypothermia (23–32 °C), aortic bronchial artery occlusion with a balloon catheter, shortening circulatory arrest periods (20 min periods to 7 min) with more frequent reperfusion periods, antegrade cerebral artery perfusion with and without total circulatory arrest, and application of negative pressure in the left ventricle [93–97]. Whether any of these technical modifications result in substantive benefits in postoperative outcomes has not been convincingly established. However, within the experience of a single practice over a prolonged period, utilizing moderate hypothermia and shorter circulatory arrest periods, Morsolini and colleagues demonstrated an improvement in postoperative respiratory function with a reduction in ventilator days and postoperative infections, along with a trend toward fewer neurologic events despite an increase in total circulatory arrest times [97].

Published results have shown that the majority of patients undergoing PTE surgery experience both short- and long-term pulmonary hemodynamic improvement as a result of this operation. A reduction in mean pulmonary artery pressure with augmentation in cardiac outcome is a consistent observation, though results vary between experienced centers [25, 29, 98–101]. In a recent report of the surgical outcomes in a series of 500 patients undergoing PTE between 2006 and 2010, Madani and colleagues showed a reduction in PVR from a preoperative mean value of 719.0 ± 383.2 to 253.4 ± 148.6 dyn/s/cm^{-5} postoperatively. Mean preoperative pulmonary artery pressure was 45.5 ± 11.6 mmHg, declining to 26.0 ± 8.4 mmHg after surgery. The preoperative cardiac output in this group of patients was 4.3 ± 1.4 L/min, improving to 5.6 ± 1.4 L/min postoperatively [25]. As longer term data have become available, the hemodynamic and resultant functional status improvements are sustained in most patients. A favorable impact on long-term survivorship is also noted [102–106].

Though the definition of residual pulmonary hypertension varies between reporting centers, there are patients who do not achieve normal pulmonary pressures and right heart function following PTE surgery. Occurrence estimates vary between 5 and 35 % of operated patients, though long-term information as to what level of residual pulmonary hypertension negatively impacts functional status and survivorship is lacking [102, 105, 107–109]. Possible explanations for this postoperative outcome include residual chronic thromboembolic disease that could not be surgically resected, or a significant amount of coexisting distal vasculopathy.

Mortality rates reported from centers performing PTE surgery have declined over the years, currently in the range of 2.2–11.4 % [25, 98–101], the lower perioperative mortality figures at centers with more extensive experience. For "low risk" patients based on a preoperative PVR < 1,000 dyn/s/cm^{-5}, postoperative mortality rates have been reported to be as low as 1.3 % [110]. However, the presence of residual pulmonary hypertension post-endarterectomy represented a considerable risk factor for doing poorly in the postoperative period; this same study noting a mortality rate of 30.6 % for those individuals left with a PVR > 500 dyn/s/cm^{-5} following surgery. However, as has been the experience for CTEPH centers worldwide, the overall decline in mortality rates reflects expanding surgical capabilities, better understanding of the natural history of the disease leading to earlier and more selective surgical referral, improved diagnostic techniques, and better coordinated postoperative care.

Medical Therapy for Chronic Thromboembolic Disease

Over the past couple decades, a number of novel pulmonary arterial hypertension (PAH) specific medical therapies, including prostacyclin analogs, endothelin receptor antagonists (ERA), phosphodiesterase-5 (PDE-5) inhibitors, and most recently, stimulators of soluble guanylate cyclase (sGC), have been developed and proven to be effective in the treatment of various types of small vessel pulmonary arterial disease. With the heterogeneity in pulmonary vascular lesions known to exist in CTEPH [43, 111], and especially given the similarities in small vessel pathology shared with idiopathic PAH, efficacy studies have understandably been pursued in subgroups of patients with chronic thromboembolic disease [26]. Acknowledging that the optimal treatment option for patients with CTEPH is a thromboendarterectomy, the most targeted subgroup where medical therapy has been tested includes those patients deemed to have *inoperable* CTEPH. Other patient groups where PAH specific medical therapy might prove to be of benefit are in post-thromboendarterectomy patients exhibiting residual pulmonary hypertension and as a "therapeutic bridge" in those patients with operable chronic thromboembolic disease who exhibit severe pulmonary hypertension and right heart dysfunction. Only a limited amount of information is available examining disease modifying therapies for each of these indications.

The majority of data addressing medical therapy for inoperable CTEPH come from trials with the dual endothelin receptor antagonist, bosentan. In a meta-analysis involving 11 studies comprising 269 patients (39 patients with persistent pulmonary hypertension following endarterectomy), treatment with bosentan was associated with an improvement in 6-min walk distance (6MWD) of 35.9 m after 3–6 months of therapy, with further modest gain of 21 m at 1 year for patients receiving drug for a more extended period. Approximately 25 % of patients experienced an improvement in NYHA functional class at 3–6 months. Hemodynamic data available from 7 studies (185 patients) revealed a weighted improvement in cardiac index (0.23 L/min/m^2) and weighted reductions in mean pulmonary artery pressure (2.62 mmHg); 5 studies (164 patients) reported a weighted mean reduction of PVR -159.7 dyn/s/cm^{-5} (20 % of baseline) [112]. The only randomized controlled trial examining the efficacy of bosentan in inoperable CTEPH was reported in 2008. Jais and colleagues enrolled 157 patients (bosentan use in 77 patients), with approximately 28 % having previously undergone PTE surgery. Compared to baseline, 16-week treatment with bosentan resulted in an improvement in pulmonary hemodynamic parameters: a 24.1 % reduction in PVR, a decline in total pulmonary resistance (treatment effect: −193 dyn/s/cm^{-5}) with a rise in cardiac index (treatment effect: 0.3 L/min/m^2). There was also a decrease in NT-proBNP levels (−622 ng/L) in the bosentan-treated patients relative to those receiving placebo. However, at 16 weeks, there was no definable improvement in exercise capacity (6MWD) and no statistically significant treatment effect of bosentan on WHO functional class [113].

Available studies examining the efficacy of other classes of PAH specific medical therapy for patients with inoperable CTEPH are even more limited. In a double-blind, placebo-controlled, 12-week pilot study, Suntharalingham and colleagues enrolled 19 patients with inoperable CTEPH, assessing the benefit of sildenafil (9 patients receiving drug) in this group. Although there was no significant difference detected in 6MWD (primary end point), an improvement in WHO functional class and PVR was noted. Control subjects were then transferred to open-label sildenafil use and reassessed at 12 months. Significant improvement in 6-min walk distance, activity and symptom scores (CAMPHOR), cardiac index, PVR, and NT-proBNP values (1,000 to 811 pg/mL) was noted [114]. In a larger patient group, Reichenberger and colleagues conducted an open-label study of sildenafil (50 mg three times a day) in 104 patients with inoperable CTEPH. After 3 months of therapy, there was a modest decrease in pulmonary vascular resistance (863 ± 38 to 759 ± 62 dyn/s/cm^{-5}), with an increase in 6MWD from 310 ± 11 to 361 ± 15 m; this distance further improved to 366 ± 18 m after 12 months of sildenafil [115]. In a single center uncontrolled observational study, 28 patients with severe inoperable CTEPH were treated with subcutaneous treprostinil. Right heart catheterization was repeated in 19 patients after 19 ± 6.3 months of treatment. Treprostinil therapy was associated with not only a significant reduction in PVR but also an improvement in 6MWD, WHO functional class, BNP levels, and cardiac output. Five-year survival rate was 53 % compared with 16 % in untreated historical controls [116]. The use of intravenous epoprostenol in patients with inoperable CTEPH has also been examined. Cabrol and colleagues retrospectively analyzed 27 patients with inoperable CTEPH who were treated with epoprostenol. After 3 months of therapy, there was a decrease in mean pulmonary artery pressure (56 ± 9 to 51 ± 8 mmHg), total pulmonary resistance (29.3 ± 7.0 to 23.0 ± 5.0 U/m^2), and an increase in 6MWD of 66 m. NYHA functional class improved by one class in 11 of 23 patients [117]. Riociguat, a soluble guanylate cyclase stimulator and the first such agent in this unique class of PAH modifying therapies, has been trialed in patients with pulmonary hypertension and inoperable CTEPH. In a multicenter, open-label, uncontrolled phase II trial, 41 patients with inoperable CTEPH (four patients also receiving bosentan) were treated with riociguat for 12 weeks. An overall improvement in 6MWD of 55 m (17.0–105.0) from a baseline of 390.0 m (330.0–441.0) was noted. In a subgroup of 30 patients undergoing follow-up right heart catheterization, there was a significant decline in mean PA pressure (median improvement of -4.5 mmHg from a baseline of 42.5 mmHg), accompanied by a significant decrease in PVR and SVR, along with a rise in cardiac index [118]. A double-blind, placebo-controlled study of 261 patients examining the efficacy of riociguat in the treatment of inoperable, residual, or recurrent CTEPH demonstrated a placebo corrected difference in 6-min walk distance of 46 m at 16 weeks [119]. Positive secondary endpoints included a 246 dyn/s/cm^{-5} placebo corrected change in pulmonary vascular resistance, and improvement in functional class and NT-proBNP levels. This important study has resulted in specific regulatory approval of riociguat to treat inoperable or residual thromboembolic pulmonary hypertension.

Additional information regarding the use of PAH specific medical therapy in patients with residual pulmonary hypertension following PTE surgery is limited to data extracted from studies involving patients with inoperable disease. Condliffe and colleagues performed a retrospective observational study analyzing patients with inoperable CTEPH as well as those with persistent post-PTE pulmonary hypertension. Seventy of the 198 patients who survived PTE surgery (35 %) exhibited persistent pulmonary hypertension which was defined as a mean PA pressure ≥25 mmHg and PVR of 240 mmHg dyn/s/cm^{-5} or greater. Using treatment criteria of a mean PA pressure of 30 mmHg or greater and/or WHO functional class III or worse, 8 % of survivors were receiving disease modifying therapy at 3 months, with an increase to 18 % at 2 years following surgery. An intention-to-treat analysis of patients with a baseline 6MW test demonstrated the average improvement in distance walked was 97.0 ± 14.6 m at 3 months and 103.1 ± 22.7 m at 12 months. One- and three-year survival for those with post-PTE pulmonary hypertension was 99 % and 94 %, which was nearly identical for those patients without residual pulmonary hypertension [102]. In the BENEFiT study, as noted above, bosentan had a significantly positive effect on pulmonary hemodynamics but not on exercise capacity, both in patients with inoperable CTEPH and those with persistent pulmonary hypertension after PTE [113].

Medical therapy has also been used as a "therapeutic bridge" prior to thromboendarterectomy, the presumption being that if pulmonary hypertension and right heart function can be improved in high-risk patients, a reduction in postoperative mortality might be realized. Nagaya and colleagues administered intravenous prostacyclin at a mean dose of 6 ± 1 ng/kg/min for a duration of 46 ± 12 days prior to PTE surgery in 12 patients with operable CTEPH, each with a PVR > 1,200 dyn/s/cm^{-5}. This resulted in a significant preoperative reduction in PVR, 1,510 ± 53–1,088 ± 58 dyn/s/cm^{-5} and a decline in plasma BNP levels. Postoperatively, one patient in the treatment group died (8.3 %) during the first 30 days, none in the group of 21 patients with a preoperative PVR < 1,200 dyn/s/cm^{-5}. Most notable in study was the observation that the pulmonary hemodynamic outcome in both patient groups was comparable [120]. More recently, Reesink and colleagues conducted a randomized, controlled single-blind study using bosentan as a bridge to pulmonary endarterectomy surgery. Twenty-five patients with operable CTEPH were enrolled, 13 receiving bosentan for 16 weeks. Comparative differences from baseline between the groups, with therapeutic benefit achieved in those patients receiving bosentan, showed a change in total pulmonary resistance of 299 dyn/s/cm^{-5}, mean PA pressure 11 mmHg, cardiac index of 0.3 L/min/m^2, and 6MWD of 33 m. However, postoperative pulmonary hemodynamic outcomes were similar between the patient groups (though postoperative mean PA pressure and TPR were lower in the bosentan group, this did not achieve statistical significance). Three patients died in the no-bosentan group postoperatively, compared to no deaths in the bosentan-treated patients. Otherwise, for those who survived surgery, the short-term postoperative clinical course between groups was comparable (ICU days, ventilator days, occurrence of lung injury) [121].

Additional investigation is necessary as to the indications and optimal use of PAH specific medical therapies in patients with chronic thromboembolic pulmonary hypertension. Presented data suggest modest improvements in functional status and pulmonary hemodynamics in patients with inoperable CTEPH at short-term follow-up. However, a recent longer term observational study (32 patients over a mean follow-up of 3.4 years) revealed that even with advancement of medical therapies, the 1- and 3-year rates of freedom from clinical worsening were 74 % and 60 %, respectively. Mortality during this time period was 34 % (11 of 32 patients) [122]. These findings further underscore the importance of ensuring that the chronic thromboembolic lesions in any individual are inoperable given the superior hemodynamic outcomes achieved with thromboendarterectomy surgery.

Disease modifying therapy also appears to have benefit for those patients with residual pulmonary hypertension following surgery. The level of pulmonary hypertension that is clinically important and the appropriate time to initiate therapy following surgery are issues that require clarification. Existing data have not justified the routine use of PAH specific medical therapy in patients with *operable* CTEPH, though there may be clinical benefit achieved in a subgroup of these patients with severe pulmonary hypertension and right heart dysfunction. Jensen and colleagues, in a retrospective analysis of patients referred for PTE surgery between 2005 and 2007, suggested that use of PAH specific medical therapy in patients with surgical CTEPH (19.9 % of patients in 2005, 37.0 % in 2007) was associated with a significant delay in time to referral, without having a discernible benefit on postoperative hemodynamic outcomes [123].

Percutaneous Transluminal Pulmonary Angioplasty

Recently, percutaneous transluminal pulmonary angioplasty (PTPA) has been recognized as an alternative approach to PTE especially in patients who exhibit lesions in segmental, subsegmental, and more distal pulmonary arteries. This approach, first described for treatment of CTEPH in 2001 [124], utilizes balloon angioplasty to open pulmonary arterial vessels that are partially occluded by thrombotic lesions. A wire is passed distal to the partially occluding lesion and balloon expansion is used to compress the lesion and dilate the vessel. Pulmonary vascular lesions in segmental or more distal arteries that indicate intravascular bands or webs, intimal irregularities, or abrupt narrowing are most appropriate for this approach. Lesions than exhibit pouch defects and complete vascular occlusion are usually not amenable to PTPA. Patients with large proximal clot burden are more likely to derive greater benefit from PTE but may be considered for this approach if they have other comorbidities that make their operative risk unacceptable or if the patient is unwilling to undergo surgery. Although experience with this technique is still limited, a recent, retrospective analysis at a single center found that the 2-year outcome in patients selected for PTPA was similar to that of those undergoing PTE [125]. This study examined the outcome of 136 results with CTEPH. Twenty-nine patients received medical therapy only, 39 underwent PEA, and 68 underwent PTPA.

Patients were treated with PTPA if they rejected PEA or if they had increased perioperative risk of PEA due to advanced age, poor physical condition, right heart failure, or comorbidities. Mean pulmonary arterial pressure (mPAP) and PVR decreased 46 and 49 %, respectively, in the PTE group and 40 and 49 % in the PTPA group. The 2-year survival rate was 97 % in the PTE group and 98.5 % in those treated with PTPA. The occurrence of right heart failure and revascularization was 2.6 and 2.8 % for those treated with PTE and 2.9 and 2.9 % for those undergoing PTPA. Complications of PTPA included reperfusion pulmonary edema, 7.0 %; hemosputum or hemoptysis, 5.6 %; vessel dissection, 2.3 %; pulmonary artery perforation by guidewire, 0.9 %. Patients reviewed in this study were highly selected and treated by a team of physicians with extensive experience in this technique. Randomized prospective studies are needed to determine true differences in safety and efficacy between PTE and PTPA, but at the present time, PTPA may provide a reasonable alternative to PTE in properly selected patients who are unwilling to undergo surgery or who have a high risk of perioperative complications.

References

1. Moser KM, Auger WR, Fedullo PF. Chronic major-vessel thromboembolic pulmonary hypertension. Circulation. 1990;81:1735–43.
2. Pengo V, Lensing ASA, Prins MH, Marchiori A, Davidson BL, Tiozzo F, et al. Incidence of chronic thromboembolic pulmonary hypertension after pulmonary embolism. N Engl J Med. 2004;350:2257–64.
3. Miniati M, Monti S, Bottai M, Scoscia E, Bauleo C, Tonelli L, et al. Survival and restoration of pulmonary perfusion in a long-term follow-up of patients after acute pulmonary embolism. Medicine. 2006;85:253–62.
4. Becattini C, Agnelli G, Pesavento R, Silingardi M, Poggio R, Taliani MR, et al. Incidence of chronic thromboembolic pulmonary hypertension after a first episode of pulmonary embolism. Chest. 2006;130:172–5.
5. Klok FA, van Kralingen KW, van Dijk APJ, Heyning FH, Vliegen HW. Prospective cardiopulmonary screening program to detect chronic thromboembolic pulmonary hypertension in patients after acute pulmonary embolism. Haematologica. 2010;95:970–5.
6. Korkmaz A, Ozlu T, Ozsu S, Kazaz Z, Bulbul Y. Long-term outcomes in acute pulmonary thromboembolism: the incidence of chronic thromboembolic pulmonary hypertension and associated risk factors. Clin Appl Thromb Hemost. 2012;18:281–8.
7. Dentali F, Donadini M, Gianni M, Bertolini A, Squizzato A, Venco A, et al. Incidence of chronic pulmonary hypertension in patients with previous pulmonary embolism. Thromb Res. 2009;124:256–8.
8. Dalen JE, Alpert JS. Natural history of pulmonary embolism. Prog Cardiovasc Dis. 1975;17:259–70.
9. Anderson FA, Wheeler HB, Goldberg RJ, Hosmer DW, Patwardhan NA, Jovanovic B, et al. A population-based perspective of the hospital incidence and case-fatality rates of deep vein thrombosis and pulmonary embolism. The Worcester DVT study. Arch Intern Med. 1991;151:933–8.
10. Silverstein MD, Heit JA, Mohr DN, Petterson TM, O'Fallon WM, Melton 3rd LJ. Trends in the incidence of deep vein thrombosis and pulmonary embolism. A 25-year population-based study. Arch Intern Med. 1998;158:585–93.
11. Tapson VT. Acute pulmonary embolism. N Engl J Med. 2008;358:1037–52.
12. Klok FA, Zondag W, van Kralingen KW, van Dijk AP, Tamsma JT, Heyning FH, et al. Patient outcomes after acute pulmonary embolism. A pooled survival analysis of different adverse events. Am J Respir Crit Care Med. 2010;181:501–6.
13. Nijkeuter M, Hovens MMC, Davidson BL, Huisman MV. Resolution of thromboemboli in patients with acute pulmonary embolism. Chest. 2006;129:192–7.
14. Wartski M, Collignon M-A, for the THESEE Study Group. Incomplete recovery of lung perfusion after 3 months in patients with acute pulmonary embolism treated with antithrombotic agents. J Nucl Med. 2000;41:1043–8.
15. Kline JA, Steuerwald MT, Marchik MR, Hernandez-Nino J, Rose GA. Prospective evaluation of right ventricular function and functional status 6 months after acute submassive pulmonary embolism: frequency of persistent or subsequent elevation in estimated pulmonary artery pressure. Chest. 2009;136:1202–10.

16. Stevinson BG, Hernandez-Nino J, Rose G, Kline JA. Echocardiographic and functional cardiopulmonary problems 6 months after first-time pulmonary embolism in previously healthy patients. Eur Heart J. 2007;28:251702524.
17. Grifoni S, Olivotto I, Cecchini P, Pieralli F, Camaiti A, Santoro G, et al. Short-term clinical outcome of patients with acute pulmonary embolism, normal blood pressure, and echocardiographic right ventricular dysfunction. Circulation. 2000;101:2817–22.
18. Sun X-G, Hansen JE, Oudiz RJ, Wasserman K. Exercise pathophysiology in patients with primary pulmonary hypertension. Circulation. 2001;104:429–35.
19. Zhai Z, Murphy K, Tighe H, Wang C, Wilkins MR, Gibbs JS, et al. Differences in ventilatory inefficiency between pulmonary arterial hypertension and chronic thromboembolic pulmonary hypertension. Chest. 2011;140:1284–91.
20. van der Plas MN, Reesink HJ, Roos CM, van Steenwijk RP, Kloek JJ, Bresser P. Pulmonary endarterectomy improves dyspnea by the relief of dead space ventilation. Ann Thorac Surg. 2010;89:347–52.
21. Konstantinides S, Tiede N, Geibel A, Olschewski M, Just H, Kasper W. Comparison of alteplase versus heparin for resolution of major pulmonary embolism. Am J Cardiol. 1998;82:966–70.
22. Daley MJ, Lat I. Clinical controversies in thrombolytic therapy for the management of acute pulmonary embolism. Pharmacotherapy. 2012;32:158–72.
23. Meyer G, Vicaut E, Danays T, Agnelli G, Becattini C, Beyer-Westendorf J, Bluhmki E, Bouvaist H, Brenner B, Couturaud F, Dellas C, Empen K, Franca A, Galiè N, Geibel A, Goldhaber SZ, Jimenez D, Kozak M, Kupatt C, Kucher N, Lang IM, Lankeit M, Meneveau N, Pacouret G, Palazzini M, Petris A, Pruszczyk P, Rugolotto M, Salvi A, Schellong S, Sebbane M, Sobkowicz B, Stefanovic BS, Thiele H, Torbicki A, Verschuren F, Konstantinides SV, PEITHO Investigators. Fibrinolysis for patients with intermediate-risk pulmonary embolism. N Engl J Med. 2014;370(15):1402–11.
24. Fedullo PF, Auger WR, Kerr KM, Kim NH. Chronic thromboembolic pulmonary hypertension. Semin Respir Crit Care Med. 2003;24(3):273–86.
25. Madani MM, Auger WR, Pretorius V, Sakakibara N, Kerr KM, Kim NK, et al. Pulmonary endarterectomy: recent changes in a single institution's experience of more than 2,700 patients. Ann Thorac Surg. 2012;94:97–103.
26. Bresser P, Pepke-Zaba J, Jaïs X, Humbert M, Hoeper MM. Medical therapies for chronic thromboembolic pulmonary hypertension. An evolving treatment paradigm. Proc Am Thorac Soc. 2006;3:594–600.
27. Riedel M, Stanek V, Widimsky J, Prerovsky I. Longterm follow-up of patients with pulmonary thromboembolism. Late prognosis and evolution of hemodynamics and respiratory data. Chest. 1982;81:151–8.
28. Lewczuk J, Piszko P, Jagas J, Porada A, Wojciak S, Sobkowicz B, et al. Prognostic factors in medically treated patients with chronic pulmonary embolism. Chest. 2001;119:818–23.
29. Pepke-Zaba J, Delcroix M, Lang I, et al. Chronic thromboembolic pulmonary hypertension. Results from an international prospective registry. Circulation. 2011;124:1973–81.
30. Stein PD, Matta F, Mussani MH. Silent pulmonary embolism in patients with deep venous thrombosis. A systematic review. Am J Med. 2010;123:426–31.
31. Pineda LA, Hathwar VS, Grant BJ. Clinical suspicion of fatal pulmonary embolism. Chest. 2001;120:791–5.
32. Wolf M, Boyer-Neumann C, Parent F, Eschwege V, Jaillet H, Meyer D, et al. Thrombotic risk factors in pulmonary hypertension. Eur Respir J. 2000;15(2):395–9.
33. Lang IM, Pesavento R, Bonderman D, Yuan JX-J. Risk factors and basic mechanisms of CTEPH—a current understanding. Eur Resp J. 2013;41(2):462–8 [Epub ahead of print].
34. Bonderman D, Turecek PL, Jakowitsch J, Weltermann A, Adlbrecht C, Schneider B, et al. High prevalence of elevated clotting factor VIII in chronic thromboembolic pulmonary hypertension. Thromb Haemost. 2003;90(3):3726.
35. Wong CL, Szydio R, Gibbs S, Laffan M. Hereditary and acquired thrombotic risk factors for chronic thromboembolic pulmonary hypertension. Blood Coagul Fibrinolysis. 2010;21:201–6.

36. Morris TA, Marsh JJ, Chiles PG, Magana MM, Liang NC, Soler X, et al. High prevalence of dysfibrinogenemia among patients with chronic thromboembolic pulmonary hypertension. Blood. 2009;114:1929–36.
37. Suntharalingam J, Goldsmith K, van Marion V, Long L, Treacy CM, Dudbridge F, et al. Fibrinogen Aa Thr312Ala polymorphism is associated with chronic thromboembolic pulmonary hypertension. Eur Respir J. 2008;31:736–41.
38. Ribeiro A, Lindmarker P, Johnsson H, Juhlin-Dannfelt A, Jorfeldt L. Pulmonary embolism: one-year follow-up with echocardiography doppler and five-year survival analysis. Circulation. 1999;99:1325–30.
39. de Perrot M, Fadel E, McRae K, Tan K, Slinger P, Paul N, et al. Evaluation of persistent pulmonary hypertension after acute pulmonary embolism. Chest. 2007;132:780–5.
40. Kim NH, Lang IM. Risk factors for chronic thromboembolic pulmonary hypertension. Eur Respir Rev. 2012;12:27–31.
41. Jais X, Ioos V, Jardim C, Sitbon O, Parent F, Hamid A, et al. Splenectomy and chronic thromboembolic pulmonary hypertension. Thorax. 2005;60:1031–4.
42. Cappellini MD, Grespi E, Cassinerio GE, Bignamini D, Fiorelli G. Coagulation and splenectomy: an overview. Ann N Y Acad Sci. 2005;1054:317–24.
43. Moser KM, Bloor CM. Pulmonary vascular lesions occurring in patients with chronic major vessel thromboembolic pulmonary hypertension. Chest. 1993;103:685–92.
44. Yao W, Firth AL, Sacks RS, Ogawa A, Auger WR, Fedullo PF, et al. Identification of putative endothelial cells ($CD34^+CD133^+Flk\text{-}1^+$) in endarterectomized tissue of patients with chronic thromboembolic pulmonary hypertension. Am J Physiol Lung Cell Mol Physiol. 2009; 296:L870–8.
45. Firth AL, Yao W, Ogawa A, Madani MM, Lin GY, Yuan JX. Multipotent mesenchymal progenitor cells are present in endarterectomized tissues from patients with chronic thromboembolic pulmonary hypertension. Am J Physiol Cell Physiol. 2010;298:C1217–25.
46. Sakao S, Hao H, Tanabe N, Kasahara Y, Kurosu K, Tatsumi K. Endothelial-like cells in chronic thromboembolic pulmonary hypertension: crosstalk with myofibroblast-like cells. Respir Res. 2011;12:109.
47. Maruoka M, Sakao S, Kantake M, Tanabe N, Kasahara Y, Kurosu K, et al. Characterization of myofibroblasts in chronic thromboembolic pulmonary hypertension. Int J Cardiol. 2012; 159(2):119–27.
48. Firth AL, Yau J, White A, Chiles PG, Marsh JJ, Morris TA, et al. Chronic exposure to fibrin and fibrinogen differentially regulates intracellular Ca^{2+} in human pulmonary arterial smooth muscle and endothelial cells. Am J Physiol Lung Cell Mol Physiol. 2009;296:L979–86.
49. Ogawa A, Firth AL, Yao W, Madani MM, Kerr KM, Auger WR, et al. Inhibition of mTOR attenuates store-operated Ca^{2+} entry in cells from endarterectomized tissues of patients with chronic thromboembolic pulmonary hypertension. Am J Physiol Lung Cell Mol Physiol. 2009;297:L666–76.
50. Zabini D, Nagaraj C, Stacher E, Lang IM, Nierlich P, Klepetko W, et al. Angiostatic factors in the pulmonary endarterectomy material from chronic thromboembolic pulmonary hypertension patients cause endothelial dysfunction. PLoS One. 2012;7(8):e43793.
51. Reesink HJ, van Delden OM, Kloek JJ, Jansen HM, Reekers JA. Embolization for hemoptysis in chronic thromboembolic pulmonary hypertension: report of two cases and review of the literature. Cardiovasc Intervent Radiol. 2007;30:136–9.
52. Auger WR, Moser KM. Pulmonary flow murmurs: a distinctive physical sign found in chronic pulmonary thromboembolic disease. Clin Res. 1989;37:145A.
53. Surie S, Gibson NS, Gerdes VE, Bouma BJ, van Eck-Smit BL, Buller HR, et al. Active search for chronic thromboembolic pulmonary hypertension does not appear indicated after acute pulmonary embolism. Thromb Res. 2010;125:e202–5.
54. Morris TA, Auger WR, Ysrael MZ, Olson LK, Channick RN, Fedullo PF, et al. Parenchymal scarring is associated with restrictive spirometric defects in patients with chronic thromboembolic pulmonary hypertension. Chest. 1996;110:399–403.

55. Steenhuis LH, Groen HJM, Koeter GH, van der Mark TW. Diffusion capacity and haemodynamics in primary and chronic thromboembolic pulmonary hypertension. Eur Respir J. 2000;16:276–81.
56. Kapitan KS, Buchbinder M, Wagner PD, Moser KM. Mechanisms of hypoxemia in chronic thromboembolic pulmonary hypertension. Am Rev Respir Dis. 1989;139:1149–54.
57. Woodruff III WW, Hoeck BE, Chitwood Jr WR, Lyerly HK, Sabiston Jr DC, Chen JTT. Radiographic findings in pulmonary hypertension from unresolved embolism. Am J Roentgenol. 1985;144:681–6.
58. Satoh T, Kyotani S, Okano Y, Nakanishi N, Kunieda T. Descriptive patterns of severe chronic pulmonary hypertension by chest radiography. Respir Med. 2005;99:329–36.
59. Blanchard DG, Malouf PJ, Gurudevan SV, Auger WR, Madani MM, Thistlethwaite P, et al. Utility of right ventricular Tei index in the noninvasive evaluation of chronic thromboembolic pulmonary hypertension before and after pulmonary thromboendarterectomy. J Am Coll Cardiol Img. 2009;2:143–9.
60. Raisinghani A, Ben-Yehuda O. Echocardiography in chronic thromboembolic pulmonary hypertension. Semin Thorac Cardiovasc Surg. 2006;18:230–5.
61. Mahmud E, Sadehgi HM, Raisinghani A, Hassankhani A, Strachan GM, Auger WR, et al. Correlation of left ventricular diastolic filling characteristics with right ventricular overload and pulmonary artery pressure in chronic thromboembolic pulmonary hypertension. J Am Coll Cardiol. 2002;40:318–24.
62. Hoeper MM, Barbera JA, Channick RN, Hassoun PM, Lang IM, Manes A, et al. Diagnosis, assessment, and treatment of non-pulmonary arterial hypertension pulmonary hypertension. J Am Coll Cardiol. 2009;54:S85–96.
63. Tunariu N, Gibbs SJ, Win Z, Gin-Sing W, Graham A, Gishen P, et al. Ventilation-perfusion scintigraphy is more sensitive than multidetector CTPA in detecting chronic thromboembolic disease as a treatable cause of pulmonary hypertension. J Nucl Med. 2007;48:680–4.
64. Soler X, Kerr KM, Marsh JJ, Renner JW, Hoh CK, Test VJ, et al. Pilot study comparing SPECT perfusion scintigraphy with CT pulmonary angiography in chronic thromboembolic pulmonary hypertension. Respirology. 2012;17:180–4.
65. Lisbona R, Kreisman H, Novales-Diaz J, Derbekyan V. Perfusion lung scanning: differentiation of primary from thromboembolic pulmonary hypertension. Am J Roentgenol. 1985;144: 27–30.
66. Powe JE, Palevsky HI, McCarthy KE, Alavi A. Pulmonary arterial hypertension: value of perfusion scintigraphy. Radiology. 1987;164:727–30.
67. Bailey CL, Channick RN, Auger WR, Fedullo PF, Kerr KM, Yung GL, et al. "High probability" perfusion lung scans in pulmonary venoocclusive disease. Am J Respir Crit Care Med. 2000;162:1974–8.
68. Rush C, Langleben D, Schlesinger RD, Stern J, Wang NS, Lamoureux E. Lung scintigraphy in pulmonary capillary hemangiomatosis: a rare disorder causing primary pulmonary hypertension. Clin Nucl Med. 1991;16:913–7.
69. Ryan KL, Fedullo PF, Davis GB, Vasquez TE, Moser KM. Perfusion scan findings understate the severity of angiographic and hemodynamic compromise in chronic thromboembolic pulmonary hypertension. Chest. 1988;93:1180–5.
70. Auger WR, Fedullo PF, Moser KM, Buchbinder M, Peterson KL. Chronic major- vessel chronic thromboembolic pulmonary artery obstruction: Appearance at angiography. Radiology. 1992;183:393–8.
71. Castaner E, Gallardo X, Ballasteros E, Andreu M, Pallardo Y, Mata JM, et al. CT diagnosis of chronic pulmonary thromboembolism. Radiographics. 2009;29:31–50.
72. Willemink MJ, van Es HW, Koobs L, Morshuis WJ, Snijder RJ, van Hesewijk JPM. CT evaluation of chronic thromboembolic pulmonary hypertension. Clin Radiol. 2012;67: 277–85.
73. Kerr KM. Pulmonary artery sarcoma masquerading as chronic thromboembolic pulmonary hypertension. Nat Clin Pract Cardiovasc Med. 2005;2:108–12.

74. McKie SJ, Hardwick DJ, Reid JH, Murchison JT. Features of cardiac disease demonstrated on CT angiography. Clin Radiol. 2005;60:31–8.
75. Pitton MB, Kemmerich G, Herber S, Schweden F, Mayer E, Thelen M. [Chronic thromboembolic pulmonary hypertension: diagnostic impact of multislice CT and selective pulmonary DSA]. Rofo. 2002;174:474–9.
76. Sugiura T, Tanabe N, Matsuura Y, Shigeta A, Kawata N, Jujo T, et al. Role of 320-slice computed tomography in the diagnostic workup of patients with chronic thromboembolic pulmonary hypertension. Chest. 2012;143:1070–7 [Epub ahead of print].
77. McMann C, Gopalan D, Sheares K, Screaton N. Imaging in pulmonary hypertension, part 2: large vessel disease. Postgrad Med J. 2012;88:317–25.
78. Kreitner K-F, Kunz RP, Ley S, Oberholzer K, Neeb D, Gast KK, et al. Chronic thromboembolic pulmonary hypertension—assessment by magnetic resonance imaging. Eur Radiol. 2007;17:11–21.
79. Krietner K-F, Ley S, Kauczor H-U, Mayer E, Kramm T, Pitton MB, et al. Chronic thromboembolic pulmonary hypertension: pre- and postoperative assessment with breath-hold magnetic resonance techniques. Radiology. 2004;32:535–43.
80. Nikolaou K, Schoenberg SO, Attenberger U, Scheidler J, Dietrich O, Kuehn B, et al. Pulmonary arterial hypertension: diagnosis with fast perfusion imaging and high-spatial-resolution MR angiography—preliminary experience. Radiology. 2005;236:694–703.
81. Rajaram S, Swift AJ, Capener D, Telfer A, Davies C, Hill C, et al. Diagnostic accuracy of contrast-enhanced MR angiography and unenhanced proton MR imaging compared with CT angiography in chronic thromboembolic pulmonary hypertension. Eur Radiol. 2012;22: 310–7.
82. Ley S, Ley-Zaporozhan J, Pitton MB, Schneider J, Wirth GM, Mayer E, et al. Diagnostic performance of state-of-the-art imaging techniques for morphological assessment of vascular abnormalities in patients with chronic thromboembolic pulmonary hypertension (CTEPH). Eur Radiol. 2012;22:607–16.
83. Alfakih K, Reid S, Jones T, et al. Assessment of ventricular function and mass by cardiac magnetic resonance imaging. Eur Radiol. 2004;14:1813–22.
84. Beygui F, Furber A, Delepine S, et al. Routine breath-hold gradient echo MRI-derived right ventricular mass, volumes and function: accuracy, reproducibility and coherence study. Int J Cardiovasc Imaging. 2004;20:509–16.
85. Hartz RS, Byme JG, Levitsky S, Park J, Rich S. Predictors of mortality in pulmonary thromboendarterectomy. Ann Thorac Surg. 1996;62:1255–60.
86. Darteville P, Fadel E, Mussot S, et al. Chronic thromboembolic pulmonary hypertension. Eur Respir J. 2004;23:637–48.
87. Toshner M, Suntharalingam J, Fesler P, Soon E, Sheares KK, Jenkins D, et al. Occlusion pressure analysis role in partitioning of pulmonary vascular resistance in CTEPH. Eur Respir J. 2012;40:612–7.
88. Kim HS, Fesler P, Channick RN, Knowlton KU, Ben-Yehuda O, Lee SH, et al. Preoperative partitioning of pulmonary vascular resistance correlates with early outcome after thromboendarterectomy for chronic thromboembolic pulmonary hypertension. Circulation. 2004;109: 18–22.
89. Daily PO, Auger WR. Historical perspective: surgery for chronic thromboembolic disease. Semin Thorac Cardiovasc Surg. 1999;11:143–51.
90. Winkler MH, Rohrer CH, Ratty SC, Jamieson S, Dembitsky W, Moser K, et al. Perfusion techniques of profound hypothermia and circulatory arrest for pulmonary thromboendarterectomy. J Extra-Corp Tech. 1990;22:57–60.
91. Madani MM, Jamieson SW. Technical advances of pulmonary endarterectomy for chronic thromboembolic pulmonary hypertension. Semin Thorac Cardiovasc Surg. 2006;18:243–9.
92. Thistlethwaite PA, Auger WR, Madani MM, Pradhan S, Kapelanski DP, Jamieson SW. Pulmonary thromboendarterectomy combined with other cardiac operations: indications, surgical approach, and outcome. Ann Thorac Surg. 2001;72:13–9.

93. Hagl C, Khaladj N, Peters T, Hoeper MM, Logemann F, Haverich A, et al. Technical advances of pulmonary thromboendarterectomy for chronic thromboembolic pulmonary hypertension. Eur J Cardiothorac Surg. 2003;23:776–81.
94. Thompson B, Tsui SSL, Dunning J, Goodwin A, Vuylsteke A, Latimer R, et al. Pulmonary endarterectomy is possible and effective without the use of complete circulatory arrest—the UK experience in over 150 patients. Eur J Cardiothorac Surg. 2008;33:157–63.
95. Mikus PM, Mikus E, Martin-Suarez S, Galie N, Manes A, Pastore S, et al. Pulmonary endarterectomy: an alternative to circulatory arrest and deep hypothermia: mid-term results. Eur J Cardiothorac Surg. 2008;34:159–63.
96. Lafci G, Tasoglu I, Ulas MM, Yalcinkaya A, Cagli K. Pulmonary endarterectomy with use of moderate hypothermia and antegrade cerebral perfusion without circulatory arrest. Tex Heart Inst J. 2012;39:65–7.
97. Morsolini M, Nicolardi S, Milanesi E, Sarchi E, Mattiucci G, Klersy C, et al. Evolving surgical techniques for pulmonary endarterectomy according to the changing features of chronic thromboembolic pulmonary hypertension patients during 17-year single-center experience. J Thorac Cardiovasc Surg. 2012;144:100–7.
98. Mayer E, Jenkins D, Lindner J, D'Armini A, Kloek J, Meyns B, et al. Surgical management and outcome of patients with chronic thromboembolic pulmonary hypertension: results from an international prospective registry. J Thorac Cardiovasc Surg. 2011;141:702–10.
99. Ogino H, Ando M, Matsuda H, Minatoya K, Sasaki H, Nakanishi N, et al. Japanese single-center experience of surgery for chronic thromboembolic pulmonary hypertension. Ann Thorac Surg. 2006;82:630–6.
100. de Perrot M, McRae K, Shargall Y, Pletsch L, Tan K, Slinger P, et al. Pulmonary thromboendarterectomy for chronic thromboembolic pulmonary hypertension: the Toronto experience. Can J Cardiol. 2011;27:692–7.
101. Maliyasena VA, Hopkins PMA, Thomson BM, Dunning J, Wall DA, et al. An Australian tertiary referral center experience of the management of chronic thromboembolic pulmonary hypertension. Pulm Circ. 2012;2:359–64.
102. Condliffe R, Kiely DG, Gibbs JS, Corris PA, Peacock AJ, Jenkins DP, et al. Improved outcomes in medically and surgically treated chronic thromboembolic pulmonary hypertension. Am J Respir Crit Care Med. 2008;177:1122–7.
103. Saouti N, Morshuis WJ, Heijmen RH, Snijder RJ. Long-term outcome after pulmonary endarterectomy for chronic thromboembolic pulmonary hypertension: a single institution experience. Eur J Cardiothorac Surg. 2009;35:947–52.
104. Freed DH, Thomson BM, Tsui SSL, Dunning JJ, Sheares KK, Pepke-Zaba J, et al. Functional and haemodynamic outcome 1 year after pulmonary thromboendarterectomy. Eur J Cardiothorac Surg. 2008;34:525–30.
105. Corsico AG, D'Armini AM, Cerveri I, Klersy C, Ansaldo E, Niniano R, et al. Long term outcome after pulmonary thromboendarterectomy. Am J Respir Crit Care Med. 2008;178:419–24.
106. Ishida K, Masuda M, Tanabe N, Matsumiya G, Tatsumi K, Nakajima N. Long-term outcome after pulmonary endarterectomy for chronic thromboembolic pulmonary hypertension. J Thorac Cardiovasc Surg. 2012;144:321–6.
107. Bonderman D, Skoro-Sajer N, Jakowitsch J, Adlbrecht C, Dunkler D, Taghavi S, et al. Predictors of outcome in chronic thromboembolic pulmonary hypertension. Circulation. 2007;115:2153–8.
108. Thistlethwaite PA, Kemp A, Du L, Madani MM, Jamieson SW. Outcomes of pulmonary thromboendarterectomy for treatment of extreme thromboembolic pulmonary hypertension. J Thorac Cardiovasc Surg. 2006;131:307–13.
109. Freed DH, Thomson BM, Berman M, Tsui SSL, Dunning J, Sheares KK, et al. Survival after pulmonary thromboendarterectomy: effect of residual pulmonary hypertension. J Thorac Cardiovasc Surg. 2011;141:383–7.
110. Jamieson SW, Kapelanski DP, Sakakibara N, Manecke GR, Thistlethwaite PA, Kerr KM, et al. Pulmonary endarterectomy: experience and lessons learned in 1,500 cases. Ann Thorac Surg. 2003;76:1457–64.

111. Yi ES, Kim H, Ahn H, Strother J, Morris T, Masliah E, et al. Distribution of obstructive intimal lesions and their cellular phenotypes in chronic pulmonary hypertension. A morphometric and immunohistochemical study. Am J Respir Crit Care Med. 2000;162:1577–86.
112. Becattini C, Manina G, Busti C, Gennarini S, Agnelli G. Bosentan for chronic thromboembolic pulmonary hypertension: findings from a systemic review and a meta-analysis. Thromb Res. 2010;126:e51–6.
113. Jais X, D'Armini A, Jansa P, Torbicki A, Delcroix M, Ghofrani HA, et al. Bosentan for treatment of inoperable chronic thromboembolic pulmonary hypertension: BENEFiT (Bosentan effects in iNopErable Forms of chronIc Thromboembolic pulmonary hypertension), a randomized, placebo-controlled trial. J Am Coll Cardiol. 2008;52:2127–34.
114. Suntharalingham J, Treacy CM, Doughty NJ, Goldsmith K, Soon E, Toshner MR, et al. Long-term use of sildenafil in inoperable chronic thromboembolic pulmonary hypertension. Chest. 2008;134:229–36.
115. Reichenberger F, Voswinckel R, Enke B, Rutsch M, El Fechtail E, Schmehl T, et al. Long-term treatment with sildenafil in chronic thromboembolic pulmonary hypertension. Eur Respir J. 2007;30:922–7.
116. Skoro-Sajer N, Bonderman D, Wiesbauer F, Harja E, Jakowitsch J, Klepetko W, et al. Treprostinil for severe inoperable chronic thromboembolic pulmonary hypertension. J Thromb Haemost. 2007;5:483–9.
117. Cabrol S, Souza R, Jais X, Fadel E, Ali RH, Humbert M, et al. Intravenous epoprostenol in inoperable chronic thromboembolic pulmonary hypertension. J Heart Lung Transplant. 2007;26:357–62.
118. Ghofrani HA, Hoeper MM, Halank M, Meyer FJ, Staehler G, Behr J, et al. Riociguat for chronic thromboembolic pulmonary hypertension and pulmonary arterial hypertension: a phase II study. Eur Respir J. 2010;36:792–9.
119. Ghofrani HA, D'Armini AM, Grimminger F, et al. Riociguat for the treatment of chronic thromboembolic pulmonary hypertension. N Engl J Med. 2013;369:319–29.
120. Nagaya N, Sasaki N, Ando M, Ogino H, Sakamaki F, Kyotani S, et al. Prostacyclin therapy before pulmonary thromboendarterectomy in patients with chronic thromboembolic pulmonary hypertension. Chest. 2003;123:338–43.
121. Reesink HJ, Surie S, Kloek JJ, Tan HL, Tepaske R, Fedullo PF, et al. Bosentan as a bridge to pulmonary endarterectomy for chronic thromboembolic pulmonary hypertension. J Thorac Cardiovasc Surg. 2010;139:85–91.
122. Scholzel B, Post MC, Thijs Plokker HW, Snijder RJ. Clinical worsening during long-term follow-up in inoperable chronic thromboembolic pulmonary hypertension. Lung. 2012;190: 161–7.
123. Jensen KW, Kerr KM, Fedullo PF, Kim NH, Test VJ, Ben-Yehuda O, et al. Pulmonary hypertensive medical therapy in chronic thromboembolic pulmonary hypertension before pulmonary thromboendarterectomy. Circulation. 2009;120:1248–54.
124. Feinstein JA, Goldhaber SZ, Lock JE, Ferndandes SM, Landzberg MJ. Balloon pulmonary angioplasty for treatment of chronic thromboembolic pulmonary hypertension. Circulation. 2001;103(1):10–3.
125. Inami T, Kataoka M, Ando M, Fukuda K, Yoshino H, Satoh T. A new era of therapeutic strategies for chronic thromboembolic pulmonary hypertension by two different interventional therapies; pulmonary endarterectomy and percutaneous-transluminal pulmonary angioplasty. PLoS One. 2014;9(4):e94587.

Chapter 7
Schistosomiasis-Associated Pulmonary Arterial Hypertension

Rita de Cassia dos Santos Ferreira, Angela Pontes Bandeira, and Ana Lúcia Coutinho Domingues

Abstract Schistosomiasis is the third most common endemic disease and has been considered the most common cause of pulmonary arterial hypertension (PAH) in the world. Around 6 % of people with chronic schistosomiasis in endemic areas are affected. Schistosomiasis-associated pulmonary arterial hypertension (Sch-PAH) is classified by the World Health Organization as group 1 pulmonary arterial hypertension because it has clinical, pathological, and hemodynamic characteristic that are similar to idiopathic pulmonary arterial hypertension. Sch-PAH is a severe disease that affects mainly middle-aged women. Symptoms and signs of right-heart insufficiency may be present, such as dyspnea, syncope, and peripheral edema. It has been demonstrated that Sch-PAH has a more benign clinical course and a better survival than idiopathic pulmonary hypertension. There are few reports of any beneficial effect from specific therapy directed toward group 1 PAH in this population of patients. The mechanisms responsible for the development of pulmonary hypertension in patients with schistosomiasis are unknown. There is growing evidence that vessel obstruction and granulomatous reaction to pulmonary embolization of eggs is not the sole mechanism that causes the disease. Further studies are needed to better elucidate the pathogenesis of Sch-PAH and to develop targeted therapies for this devastating disease.

Keywords Pulmonary hypertension • Pulmonary arterial hypertension • Schistosomiasis • Parasitic disease • *Schistosoma mansoni*

R.C.S. Ferreira, Ph.D. (✉)
Department of Pneumology, Hospital das Clínicas - Universidade Federal de Pernambuco, Av Prof Moraes Rego 1235, Cidade Universitária, Recife, PE 50670-901, Brazil
e-mail: rita.pneumo@gmail.com

A.P. Bandeira, M.D.
University of Pernambuco, Recife, Brazil

A.L.C. Domingues, Ph.D.
Health Sciences Centre, Federal University of Pernambuco, Recife, Brazil

J.R. Klinger, R.P. Frantz (eds.), *Diagnosis and Management of Pulmonary Hypertension*, Respiratory Medicine 12, DOI 10.1007/978-1-4939-2636-7_7

Abbreviations

6MWT	6-min walk test
CT	Computed tomography
HIV	Human immunodeficiency virus
IL	Interleukin
INF γ	Interferon γ
mPAP	Mean pulmonary artery pressure
PAH	Pulmonary arterial hypertension
PAP	Pulmonary artery pressure
PAOP	Pulmonary artery occlusion pressure
PASP	Pulmonary artery systolic pressure
PH	Pulmonary hypertension
PVR	Pulmonary vascular resistance
PWP	Pulmonary wedge pressure
Sch-PAH	Schistosomiasis-associated pulmonary arterial hypertension
TGF β	Transforming growth factor β
Th cells	T helper cells
TNF α	Tumuor necrosis factor α

Introduction

Schistosomiasis is a parasitic disease that is acquired from infected freshwater snails. It is considered to be the third most important endemic disease in the world and it is estimated that 240 million people are infected with the *Schistosoma* species worldwide. The most common organisms reported are *Schistosoma japonicum*, *S. haematobium*, and *S. mansoni* [1], the latter being responsible for almost all cases of pulmonary hypertension [2]. The disease is endemic in 74 countries, including those of Eastern South America, the Caribbean Islands, East Asia, some parts of China, and the Middle East. However, more than 80 % of infected people are found in sub-Saharan Africa. Approximately 6 % of those afflicted develop pulmonary hypertension making schistosomiasis the leading cause of pulmonary arterial hypertension (PAH) in the world [3].

Schistosomiasis

People become infected with *Schistosoma* through contact with contaminated water due to agricultural, domestic, and recreational activities (Fig. 7.1). The parasite's life cycle (Figs. 7.2 and 7.3) involves a freshwater snail host that is penetrated by miracidia, the larvae released from the eggs deposited in the urine (*S. haematobium*)

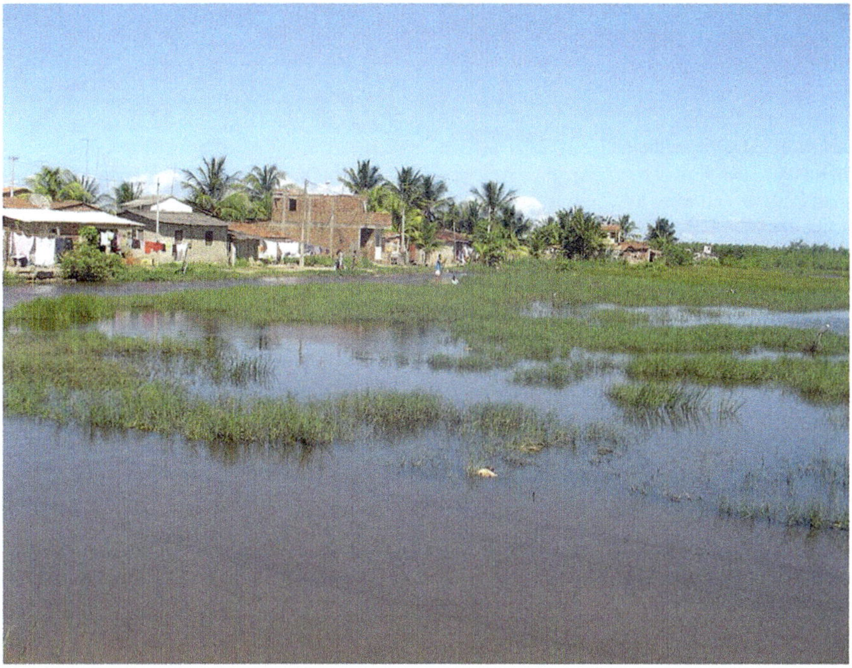

Fig. 7.1 An endemic area of schistosomiasis in Northeast of Brazil, where conditions of poor sanitation favor the dissemination of the disease

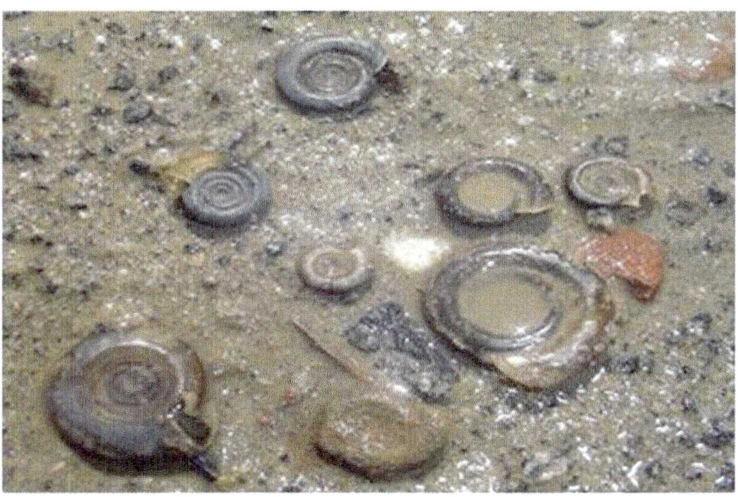

Fig. 7.2 *Biomphalaria glabrata*, a snail host of *Schistosoma mansoni*, found in Brazil

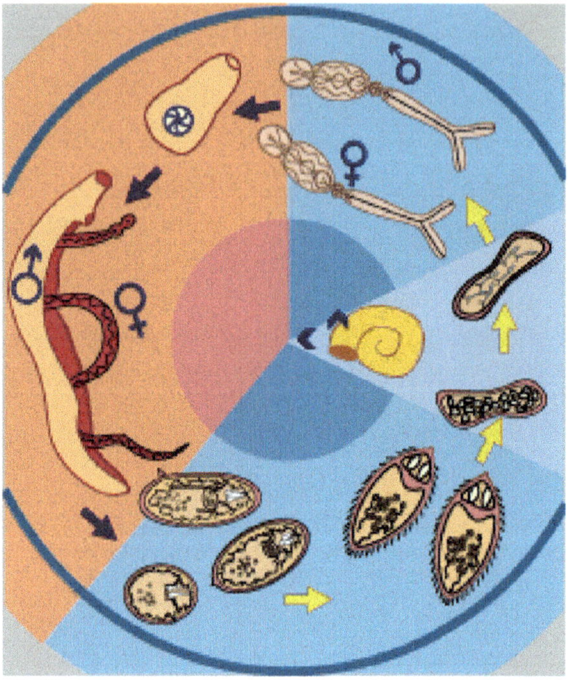

Fig. 7.3 Life cycle of schistosomiasis (WHO 2012): *Blue*: Eggs from the parasite are released in the water and hatch into miracidia. The miracidia infects the snail host. The snail releases cercariae into water. *Orange*: Cercariae penetrate the human skin exposed to water and the worms go to target organ where they mate and release eggs. Most of these are excreted in the feces (*S. mansoni* and *S. japonicum*) and urine (*S. haematobium*)

or feces (*S. mansoni* and *S. japonicum*) of infected people. These miracidia multiply asexually within the snail where they become sporocysts before being released as cercariae. After 4–6 weeks, hundreds of motile, forked-tail cercariae go into the water and penetrate the normal skin of a human host and transform into schistosomula. After 2–3 days, the schistosomula reach the lungs by venous circulation. Around the ninth day of infection, they go through the systemic circulation into the liver where they remain while maturing into adult worms and mating. Eventually, adult worms make their way to the mesenteric vein (*S mansoni* and *S. japonicum*) or to the vesical plexus and veins draining the ureters (*S. haematobium*) where they reside and lay their eggs. *S. mansoni* enter the systemic circulation on the fourth week. The adult worms mate and migrate to the superior hemorrhoidal plexus and inferior mesenteric vein, where the females lay their eggs. The adult worms can live for up to 30 years, with an average of 5–10 years, producing up to 300 ova per day [2, 4]. A great proportion of these (60 %) are eliminated with feces that will hatch with water contact, releasing the miracidium and initiating a new cycle.

Many eggs that are not eliminated from the body via feces are transported via the hepatic portal vein to the liver where they become lodged and cause granuloma formation. The inflammatory reaction within the granulomas is a stimulus to the production of fibrosis. After many years of infections and reinfections, large sheets of fibrosis can be formed in the liver, depending on the parasite burden and the patient's immune response leading to a condition known as Symmer's fibrosis. The hepatocytes are not destroyed, but the fibrosis around the portal vein causes a blockage of hepatic blood flow and secondary portal hypertension. This leads to the opening of portal systemic anastomoses to decompress the portal system [5, 6]. These collaterals may permit the passage of worms and eggs into the pulmonary circulation and induce an immune response and granulomatous reaction in the pulmonary arterial bed leading to pulmonary arterial vascular remodeling and development of PAH in some individuals [7].

Schistosomiasis has a very large spectrum of clinical manifestations [5]. In the acute phase, a macula-papular rash can occur at the site of penetration of cercariae into the skin. This skin reaction occurs some hours after the exposure, can last for several days, and usually disappears spontaneously. It is named cercarial dermatitis and occurs more commonly in people who have not been exposed to the parasite, previously. The lungs can be affected in the acute and chronic phase of the disease. The acute phase, known as Katayama syndrome, occurs predominantly in people that come from non-endemic areas or nonimmune hosts. It is a systemic hypersensitivity reaction that appears a few weeks (16–90 days) after infection and is caused by the passage of migrating schistosomula and egg antigens through the lungs and other parts of the body.

Clinical symptoms include fever, chills, weight loss, headache, anorexia, nausea, vomiting, dry cough, dyspnea, wheezing, and diarrhea. Physical exam may reveal hepatomegaly, splenomegaly, and skin lesions. Liver abscess, brain pseudo-tumors, and myeloradiculopathy are also described in a small number of cases. The symptoms last for 2–12 weeks. Hypereosinophilia is a hallmark of this phase. Eggs of the parasites can be found in the feces about 40 days after infection. A chest X-ray can reveal micronodules, pulmonary condensations, and pleural effusion [2]. On chest computed tomography (CT) nodular lesions can be seen, sometimes with a halo signal and ground glass pattern [8] (Fig. 7.4). This syndrome is believed to be the result of an immunologic process that occurs in nonimmune patients as a reaction to circulating parasite antigens [9, 10].

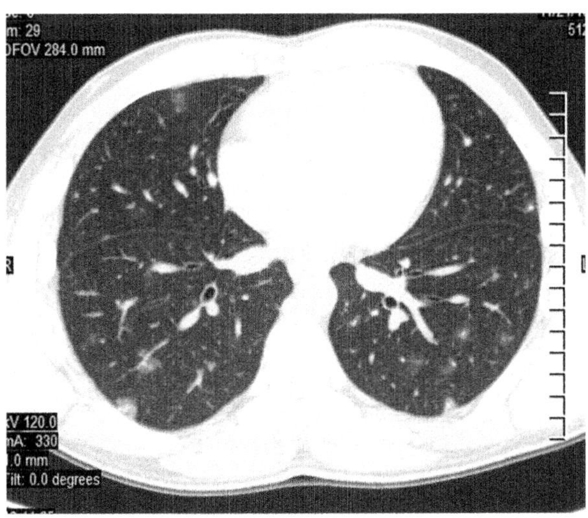

Fig. 7.4 Computed tomography of the thorax of a 29-year-old male patient with Katayama syndrome showing subpleural and peribronchovascular nodules, some with halo sign, and focal ground glass opacities

Chronic schistosomiasis appears several months or years after infection and patients can be asymptomatic or present variable manifestations. The hepatointestinal form can present with abdominal pain and intestinal transit alterations, with or without mild periportal fibrosis and without portal hypertension. This can result in iron-deficiency anemia and constitutional symptoms such as weight loss, malnutrition, and chronic fatigue. The associated hepatomegaly, particularly enlargement of the left lobe with periportal fibrosis, defines the hepatic form. The hepatoesplenic form is associated with splenomegaly in addition to the intestinal symptoms. It is one of the most severe manifestations of the disease, due to portal hypertension that leads to the formation of esophageal and hemorrhoidal variceals that can rupture, leading to severe bleeding that is often the main cause of death in these patients [5, 6].

Patients with chronic *S. haematobium* infection have chronic inflammation of the venous plexus around the bladder, resulting in hematuria, fibrosis with ureteral obstruction, and nephrolithiasis. Squamous cell carcinoma of the bladder can also develop. Other manifestations of the disease include pseudo-tumor formation, glomerulonephritis, infertility in women, neurologic manifestations, and ectopic disease in the eyes, skin, and urogenital tract [2, 4].

Hepatopulmonary syndrome and pulmonary arterial hypertension (PAH) are the two main types of chronic pulmonary manifestations. Hepatopulmonary syndrome is characterized by the presence of portal hypertension, arterial hypoxemia, and intrapulmonary vascular dilatation [11]. It can be found in 10 % of patients with the hepatosplenic form of schistosomiasis [12]. This form was previously defined as the cyanotic form of schistosomiasis, a more severe phase of hepatopulmonary syndrome, described by Faria et al. [13]. Schistosomiasis-associated pulmonary arterial hypertension (PAH) (Sch-PAH) is defined as an increase in mean pulmonary arterial pressure (mPAP) $\geq$25 mmHg at rest and pulmonary wedge pressure (PWP) $\leq$15 mmHg in the setting of schistosomotic disease [13].

Epidemiology

As described earlier, nearly 240 million people are infected with the *Schistosoma* species in the world and about 10 % have severe disease [1, 14]. The true prevalence of Sch-PAH in these individuals is unknown, because the majority of the studies are hospital based with small samples and without a uniform definition of the schistosomal disease and accurate assessment of pulmonary arterial pressure (PAP). A recent systematic review noted that more than 50 % of the studies reporting prevalence of Sch-PAH were from Brazil and less than 20 % from Africa, which accounts for the major burden of schistosomiasis disease [15]. In a rare study that used a random community-based sample, investigators found that the prevalence of Sch-PAH in infected people with schistosomiasis ranged from 0 to 28.3 % (4 ± 8 %). When only people with hepatosplenic disease were considered, the prevalence ranged from 0 to 60 % (18.1 ± 15.9 %) and when the proportion of pulmonary hypertension (PH) was estimated in areas endemic for *S. mansoni*, it was 6.3–46.5 %. The study concluded that the prevalence of PH is 6.1 % in those infected with schistosomiasis, and 15.1 % in patients with hepatosplenic schistosomiasis, and that Sch-PAH represents 30.8 % of all causes of PH in areas where schistosomiasis is endemic [15]. In these studies, there was no homogeneity in the definition of PH. Some studies defined PH on clinical grounds or histologically. Others assess PH by echocardiogram using different limits of systolic pressures, and others assessed PH by cardiac catheterization. Moreover, several studies did not use exclusion criteria for other causes of PH or other liver diseases in these prevalence studies.

Schistosoma mansoni is the only species present in Brazil where 2.5–6 million people are infected. It continues to cause severe forms of the disease, being responsible for at least 700 hospital admissions and 492 deaths a year. The disease is endemic in nine states and has focal transmission areas in ten states [16]. Two important hemodynamic series found mPAP > 20 mmHg in 23 % of 137 patients [17] and 13 % of 141 patients [18] with portal hypertension. De Cleva et al. [19] found a median mPAP of 20–25 mmHg in 8 (22 %) and mPAP > 25 mmHg in 2 (6 %) of 36 patients with hepatosplenic disease, before they underwent surgery for esophagogastric devascularization and splenectomy or distal splenorenal shunt in order to avoid digestive hemorrhage from esophageal varices. Lapa et al. [20] reported a prevalence of 18.5 % (IC 95 %: 10.8–29.5 %) in patients with a hepatosplenic form of the disease from a PH referral center in Sao Paulo, Brazil. In that study, PH was defined as pulmonary systolic arterial pressure (PSAP) > 40 mmHg as assessed by transthoracic echocardiogram. However, only 7.8 % (IC 95 %: 3.3–16.7 %) had mPAP ≥ 25 mmHg on the right-heart catheterization and only 4.7 % (IC 95 %: 1.5–12.7 %) of all cases had precapillary PH with pulmonary artery occlusion pressure (PAOP) < 15 mmHg. At the same time, PWP has been reported to represent up to 30 % of the PH patients followed up at referral centers in Brazil [21–23].

One limitation of prevalence studies in Sch-PAH is that it is believed that PH occurs almost exclusively in people with the hepatosplenic form of schistosomiasis, which limits the populations studied. These patients represent only 5 % of infected people and this strategy can underestimate the true prevalence [15]. Few studies have included patients without this severe form of schistosomiasis. Lambertucci et al. [24] conducted a study in an endemic area, where 66.3 % of the population had schistosomiasis. Abdominal ultrasound revealed liver fibrosis in 54 % of examined subjects (246) and 25 (11.7 %) of 213 subjects were submitted to echocardiogram showed evidence of PH. However, PASP was estimated by pulmonary arterial acceleration time and the median value found was 31 ± 8.8 mmHg. In another hospital-based study in Brazil, Ferreira et al. [25] found a prevalence of 10.7 % (CI 95 %: 5–19.4 %) using echocardiographic assessment of pulmonary arterial pressure (PAP) in 84 consecutive patients attending an outpatient schistosomiasis clinic who were found to have periportal fibrosis on abdominal ultrasound. The authors included patients with the hepatointestinal and hepatosplenic form of schistosomiasis and defined PH as PASP > 35 mmHg; however, all patients with PH had PASP ≥ 40 mmHg.

Considerably less information is available regarding the prevalence of Sch-PAH in Africa. Studies carried out in the Sudan, Zimbabwe, and Ethiopia found very low levels of Sch-PAH, but these studies were not recent and were not specifically aimed at this problem [15]. In sub-Saharan Africa, where most people infected with schistosoma live, studies of prevalence of PH are lacking.

In general, if we consider that around 200 million people have schistosomiasis in the world, and that of these 120 million have symptomatic disease and 5 % have hepatosplenic disease, approximately 270,000 patients may have Sch-PAH, making it the main cause of PAH in the world [3].

Pathology

Pulmonary vascular remodeling in PAH is characterized by intimal thickening, medial smooth muscle cell hypertrophy, and fibrosis and obstructive lesions of distal precapillary vessels known as plexiform lesions. Inflammatory infiltrate is often demonstrated around the adventitia of the affected vessels. Plexiform lesions consist of a network of vascular channels lined by endothelial cells and a core of myofibroblastic or less well-differentiated cells. These changes are nearly always seen in cases of severe idiopathic PAH (IPAH) and PAH associated with HIV infection, liver cirrhosis, CREST syndrome, and congenital left to right cardiac shunts [26]. These histologic features have also been described in Sch-PAH [27], and, in addition to the similar degree of increase in PAP and pulmonary vascular resistance (PVR), justified the classification of Sch-PAH as group 1 PAH [28].

In the initial pathologic description of Shaw and Ghareeb [29], focal and widespread pulmonary arterial lesions in patients who died of Sch-PAH were attributed to the direct action of the eggs attacking the arterioles. The eggs were demonstrated in the arteriolar lumen producing necrosis of the inner layers of the vessels, with posterior obliteration of the lumen by endarteritis. Intimal thickening, hypertrophy of the media, and collagenous thickening of the adventitia were described along with recanalization by new tortuous vessels called angiomatoid structures. Granulomas were described around extravascular eggs. In 1954, Faria described similar pathologic alterations encountered in specimens of lungs obtained in necropsies: endarteritis in small pulmonary arterial branches, necrotizing arteritis, thrombosis, and intimal fibrous thickenings. However, granulomatous reaction around the vessels was rarely seen and the pulmonary vascular changes found were not directly related to the presence of eggs. The author suggested that the anatomical changes caused by the *Schistosoma*'s eggs had a secondary role in the pathogenesis of PAH. Interestingly, patients with schistosomiasis without cor pulmonale exhibited eggs retained in smaller branches of the vessels, probably because there was less endarteritis in these cases, permitting the passage of eggs more distally. The most important changes seen were in the intima and media layers of pulmonary arteries and arterioles. The lumen of the vessels could have been filled by concentric or eccentric mass of fibrous tissue associated with medial hypertrophy [30]. Plexiform lesions were demonstrated in more than 80 % of lungs obtained in necropsy studies. These structures continued distally with dilated angiomatoid thin-walled channels [31, 32]. Other authors believed that the embolization of eggs was necessary for the occurrence of arteritis and that PAH would be the result of a peripheral vascular blockage caused by the disseminated granulomata [33, 34].

Recently, a study of 18 lung specimens from individuals who had died from Sch-PAH demonstrated plexiform lesions in all samples and 89 % showed evidence of arterial medial thickening. Only 4 (22 %) of the 18 samples had granuloma, contrasting with prior studies, and *S. mansoni* eggs in pulmonary samples were not found. A dark pigment was found adjacent to vascular lesions. Its origin is not known, but it had an identical appearance to anthracotic pigment [35].

Pathogenesis

In schistosomiasis, most of the pathology is caused by the T-cell-dependent immune response of the host directed against the eggs of the parasite, which results in chronic granulomatous inflammation and ultimately in fibrosis [36]. The main organ affected is the liver where the eggs of the parasites are trapped along the periportal tissues, which leads to inflammation, tissue eosinophilia, collagen deposition, and fibrosis of the periportal spaces with secondary portal-vein obstruction and subsequent portal hypertension and development of collateral vessels [6]. The granuloma formation is a process which is predominantly CD4+ T helper (Th) cell dependent. The CD4+ Th cell response evolves from a Th1- to a Th2-dominated response following egg production. The type 1 T-cell response occurs with the liberation of several cytokines: IL-1, IL-12, interferon-y (INF-γ), transforming growth factor-β (TGF-β), and TNF-α. They modulate the release of several chemokines. After the liberation of eggs and egg-derived antigens, a Th2 cell response is elicited to limit the primary response, which occurs around 8 weeks from infection. In this phase the liberation of IL-4, IL-5, IL-10, and IL-13 predominates. The formation of granulomas seems to limit the infectious process, in spite of the fact that it provokes the main pathology of the disease [36–38]. The Th1- and Th2-associated cytokines have different roles in the regulation of fibrogenesis. For example, IL-13 has an important role in fibrogenesis whereas TNF-α, INF-γ, and IL-12 seem to have an anti-fibrotic activity and IL-10 has an important regulatory effect in the balance of Th1 and Th2 responses, clearly regulating liver pathology. It is produced from Treg cells and/or Th2 cells. There is some agreement that chronically infected patients with intestinal, hepatointestinal, and hepatosplenic forms of the disease have a dominant Th2 cytokine profile [39, 40], whereas a predominance of the Th1 cytokines is observed in acutely infected patients [36, 37, 39].

Much less is known about the immune mechanisms in Sch-PAH. Today it is recognized that inflammation is an important aspect of most types of PAH and that T-cells, and other immunomodulatory cells are part of this process [41]. In PAH, there appears to be an initial insult to the endothelium, such as hypoxia, mechanical stress, or an infectious process. Secondarily, an inflammatory process occurs which leads to the activation of an immune response and cytokine and chemokine production that propagates this inflammation and leads to the production of growth factors, culminating in vascular remodeling [41]. Genetic determinants may also be important in the development of PAH [42]. In familial PAH, 80 % of patients have a mutation in the gene encoding the bone morphogenetic protein receptor type 2 (BMPR II), a member of the TGF-β superfamily. This mutation is also found in 25 % of patients with IPAH. This mutation is the most important known risk factor to PAH and may interact with environmental agents including chronic infection to initiate the development of PAH. It is not yet known if this type of mutation enhances the development of PAH in patients infected with schistosomiasis.

Perivascular infiltration of inflammatory cells around remodeled vessels has consistently been demonstrated in animal models of PAH, including the mouse model of Sch-PAH and in patients with IPAH [43]. The cells involved are T-cells, macrophages, B cells, mast cells, and dendritic cells in the adventitia and media of muscular pulmonary arteries. With the activation of the immune response, cytokines and chemokines are produced, propagating further inflammation and associated production of growth factors which drive vascular remodeling. In IPAH there is an elevation of serum levels of cytokines, including IL-1-β, IL-6, and IL-8 and chemokines such as chemokine ligand 2/monocyte chemotactic protein-1, CCL5, and CXC3CL1/fractalkine [44]. IL-6 and TGF-β induce differentiation of TH17 cells that are highly proinflammatory. Treg cells also participate in the process balancing Th1 and Th2 responses [41].

In schistosomiasis, the passage of eggs into pulmonary capillaries through portosystemic anastomoses is the main mechanism historically proposed for the development of PAH. PH was felt to occur due to mechanical obstruction of distal pulmonary vessels due to egg impaction, focal arteritis, and inflammation related to the formation of granulomas around the eggs. Crosby et al. [45] showed that infected mice with eggs in the lungs had significant pulmonary hypertension, vascular remodeling, and right ventricular hypertrophy, whereas infected mice without lung egg deposition did not exhibit these changes. Pulmonary vascular remodeling was more severe in arterioles near granulomas, suggesting that the presence of eggs and granulomas drove the process of vascular remodeling in this model of Sch-PAH [45]. However, this model is not entirely applicable to human disease, because Sch-PAH can occur without portal hypertension. Furthermore, in animal models, mice are infected with cercariae and then rechallenged with intravenous administration of eggs that can go directly to the lungs in an attempt to mimic what is supposed to occur in humans via the development of collateral shunts. In this model, infected mice develop a widespread arterial vasculopathy, often with a perivascular inflammatory cellular infiltrate, with pulmonary vascular remodeling affecting media and intimal layers of pulmonary arteries, but without plexiform lesions [35, 43]. These alterations were reduced in mice lacking IL-13RαR1, with loss of the IL-13 function, in a nonstatistically significant manner, while in mice lacking IL-13Rα2, with gain of the IL-13 function, there was an increase in intimal thickness. These infected animals had an increase in right ventricle maximum pressure, mainly if they had a gain of the IL-13 function. Enhanced IL-13 signaling caused PAH in this model. The authors suggested that the enhanced lung inflammatory response triggered by the challenge with eggs correlates with the development of experimental Sch-PAH. The granulomas formed are composed of macrophages, eosinophils, and cells containing smooth muscle actin, which could represent myofibroblasts and/or differentiated smooth muscle cells [43]. Crosby et al. [45] demonstrated that IL-13 but not IL-4 stimulated the migration of pulmonary artery smooth muscle cells in transwell assays. Altered TGF-β signaling was investigated through the expression of Smad2/3 in lungs of schistosomiasis-infected mice and their expression was increased in granulomas and pulmonary arteries. Nevertheless, the absolute levels of TGF-β were not altered in infected mice [45]. In specimens of human lungs obtained at autopsy, there was an intense p-Smad2/3 activity in the smooth muscle cells with thickened media and in vascular channels within the plexiform lesions [35]. Smads are proteins that can be phosphorylated after the attachment of TGF-β in cell receptors and which can move to the nucleus of cells, altering essential cell functions. There is evidence that the TGF-β system stimulates the proliferation of pulmonary arterioles in PAH, and leads to vasculogenesis, including intimal hyperplasia and growth of the medial layer [42, 46]. More recently, Graham et al. [47] demonstrated that a mouse model of Sch-PAH submitted to pharmacological blockage of the TGF-β ligand and receptor and that mice lacking Smad3 were significantly protected from pulmonary vascular remodeling and PAH. This blockage also led to a decrease in IL-4 and IL-13 concentrations [47]. Accordingly, Ferreira et al. [48] demonstrated significantly increased serum levels of TGF-β1 in patients with Sch-PAH compared with patients with schistosomiasis without PAH, suggesting that this growth factor may contribute to vascular remodeling in this disease. Studies using animal models demonstrated a correlation between cytokines and pulmonary remodeling and between the numbers of muscularized small peripheral vessels and the lung egg burden. In these models pulmonary vascular remodeling is characterized by a marked perivascular inflammatory infiltrate, heterogeneous severe thickening of the media of small pulmonary arteries, and the occurrence of plexiform-like lesions in the absence of PAH [45].

It is interesting to note that in the animal model of Sch-PAH, the development of disease requires mice sensitization with cercariae prior to intravenous egg administration, suggesting that a potent pulmonary inflammatory response and inflammatory cell infiltrate are needed rather than the hepatic disease with shunting of eggs and parasites to lungs. The injection of eggs alone was not sufficient to cause right ventricular hypertension, so the embolic disease alone does not seem to cause experimental PAH [43]. Studies with lung samples collected at autopsies of individuals with Sch-PH demonstrated pulmonary vascular remodeling with plexiform lesions and arterial medial thickening in all 18 samples examined, but failed to find eggs of the parasite. Antibodies against *S. mansoni*-soluble egg antigens (SEA) did not detect significant amounts of egg antigens in the human lung species, although they were identified in lungs of experimentally infected mouse and human intestine specimens. Rare fragments of *S. mansoni* eggs in human lung specimens were only identified using anti-SEA antibodies within granulomas and not adjacent to the pulmonary vascular lesions. In spite of the presence of vascular remodeling in patients who died of Sch-PAH, significant immunohistochemically antigenic material was not found, suggesting that after an initial acute inflammatory response, vascular lesions are established and can progress or persist independently of the presence of the antigens. These findings corroborate with the persistence of vascular remodeling in patients treated against the parasite [35]. On the other hand, a total or partial regression of liver lesions occurs with parasite treatment [49].

Clinical Presentation of Sch-PAH

In endemic areas, chronic pulmonary disease is common and PH is the most severe complication of the disease. It is almost exclusively found in *Schistosomiasis mansoni* [7] and is more commonly encountered in patients with hepatosplenic disease. In one study from Brazil, 48.9 % of patients with Sch-PAH had the hepatosplenic form of schistosomiasis, 27.6 % had hepatointestinal disease, and 23.4 % were splenectomized [50]. In Brazil, the splenectomy has been used as a treatment for upper digestive hemorrhage secondary to rupture of esophageal varices [51, 52]. The fact that almost 30 % of patients with Sch-PAH had the hepatointestinal form of the disease suggests that pulmonary embolism of worms or eggs through portosystemic anastomoses is not a prerequisite for the development of PH in schistosomiasis [50].

There are no clinical symptoms that are characteristic of Sch-PAH as compared to other types of PAH. Patients generally have symptoms that are the result of progressive right heart failure such as dyspnea on exertion, weakness, fatigue, cough, giddiness and syncope, palpitation, and chest pain that are the main symptoms [25]. Hemoptysis can also occur. Chest pain is usually caused by right ventricular angina and syncope results from depressed cardiac output and low systemic blood pressure. On physical exam, the lungs are usually clear. Peripheral edema, ascites, anasarca, or jugular vein distension can be seen. A prominent pulmonic component of the second heart sound may be present along with right ventricular heave and murmurs of tricuspid or pulmonic valve insufficiency. Less commonly, patients exhibit cyanosis and rarely digital clubbing is seen. Hepatomegaly secondary to schistosomal disease (left lobe enlargement) or congestion and splenomegaly can be seen in patients with the hepatosplenic form [7, 53].

Patients with Sch-PAH are usually middle aged and are more often women. In a study by Japiassu et al. [54], the mean age was 46.9 ± 12.6 years and 70.6 % were women. About half of the patients are in NYHA functional class III or IV at the time of presentation [54, 55].

Diagnosis Workup

In patients suspected of Sch-PAH, the aim of the diagnostic workup is to confirm or exclude the diagnosis of both PAH and schistosomiasis. At the same time, other causes of PH and liver disease need to be evaluated. Finally, the severity of the disease and the patient's prognosis should be assessed.

Diagnosis of Schistosomiasis

The diagnosis of schistosomiasis is based on a suggestive epidemiological history with the identification of parasite eggs in stool examination or rectal biopsy. Some patients may refer a history of treatment of the disease. Nevertheless the great majority of patients with chronic disease present no viable eggs on stools and the diagnosis is made by abdominal ultrasound findings of left liver enlargement or periportal fibrosis with or without splenomegaly (hepatosplenic and hepatointestinal forms, respectively) [5–7]. Periportal fibrosis is often classified in accordance with Niamey methods as pattern C (peripheral periportal thickening), pattern D (central periportal thickening), pattern E (central periportal thickening with echogenic patches expanding into parenchyma), or pattern F (very advanced central and peripheral periportal thickening) [56]. Serologic testing is not a viable tool in endemic areas, because a great proportion of individuals will have prior exposure to infection and present antibodies to *Schistosoma* without developing chronic schistosomal disease [57].

PAH Diagnosis

Echocardiogram with Doppler ultrasound is the main tool used to evaluate PAP in patients suspected of Sch-PAH. Abnormalities seen on echocardiogram are the same as those demonstrated in patients with other causes of PAH, including right ventricular and atrial chamber enlargement, bowing of the interventricular septum toward the left ventricle during diastole, and an increased pressure gradient across the tricuspid valve [58]. Although there is a good correlation between measurements of PAP pressure obtained by echocardiogram and right heart catheterization, echocardiogram is less accurate and can underestimate or overestimate PAP pressure in a significant number of individuals [59]. It is helpful to exclude other causes of PAH, such as congenital left to right cardiac shunts, left ventricular dysfunction, or valvular heart disease. As in other causes of PAH, some echocardiographic signs are associated with a poorer prognosis, including the presence of a pericardial effusion and a tricuspid annular plane systolic excursion (TAPSE) <1.5 [60].

Electrocardiography can demonstrate right ventricular hypertrophy or strain, signs of right atrial enlargement and right bundle branch block, and the presence of arrhythmias [53], but it lacks sensitivity for diagnoses of PH.

Right heart catheterization is a mandatory step to confirm the diagnosis of PAH and estimate the severity of the disease. It is important to confirm the presence of precapillary pulmonary hypertension by demonstrating an elevated PAP and a normal pulmonary capillary wedge pressure (PWP) ($\leq$15 mmHg) and to measure the cardiac index, pulmonary arterial saturation of oxygen, and pulmonary vascular resistance (PVR). Right heart catheterization also allows acute pulmonary vasodilator testing to determine if the patient may respond to treatment using calcium channel blockers [60, 61]. In the study of Japiassu et al. [54], most cases were considered to be severe. In this study, pulmonary vasoreactivity testing with inhaled nitric oxide was positive in only 3 patients (3.5 %). Increased PVR was associated with worse functional class and shorter 6-min walking distance (6-min walk test, 6MWT). There were also significant correlations between pulmonary artery oxygen saturation and functional class and 6MWT. This study found that PVR was a more reliable parameter of disease severity than mPAP or cardiac index [54]. Other studies suggest that Sch-PAH patients have less severe hemodynamic derangements at diagnosis than patients with IPAH. In one study [55], mPAP and PVR were lower in Sch-PAH and cardiac output was higher, but no differences were seen in right atrial or pulmonary capillary wedge pressure. In this study no schistosomotic patient had an acute response to vasodilator challenge, compared to 16.2 % of patients who responded in the idiopathic group [55].

Chest radiography can be helpful in the initial evaluation of the Sch-PAH patients. A PA and lateral chest film can reveal reticulations, cardiomegaly secondary to dilatation of the right ventricle and atrium, enlarged main pulmonary arteries with tapering of the distal vasculature, prominent hila, and straightening or camber of the pulmonary arch in more than 50 % of the patients with pulmonary hypertension (Fig. 7.5) [25]. Aneurismal dilatation of the pulmonary trunk has also been reported [62].

Similar to other forms of PAH, pulmonary function tests are usually normal or demonstrate mild restrictive or obstructive defects [25]. When present, it is important to further evaluate significant obstructive or restrictive patterns to ensure that other pulmonary diseases that can be responsible for PH are not present [60, 61, 63]. Computed tomography (CT) pulmonary angiogram and vantilation-perfusion scintigraphy to assess interstitial lung disease and thromboembolic disease that could account for PH should be considered in these cases [60, 64]. Chest CT findings commonly seen in other forms of PAH such as increased ratio of pulmonary trunk to ascending aorta, dilatation of right cardiac chambers, bulging or straightening of the interventricular septum, tapering of intrapulmonary arteries, dilatation of peripheral vessels, increased segmental artery-to-bronchus ratio, and mosaic pattern of attenuation are also seen in Sch-PAH (Fig. 7.6) [65]. In one study of 44 patients with Sch-PAH, multidetector chest CT revealed a pulmonary trunk diameter of 4.31 ± 1.16 cm (range: 2.2–7.8 cm), right pulmonary artery diameter of 3.21 ± 0.79 cm (range 1.90–4.2 cm), and left pulmonary artery diameter of 2.97 ± 0.73 cm (range

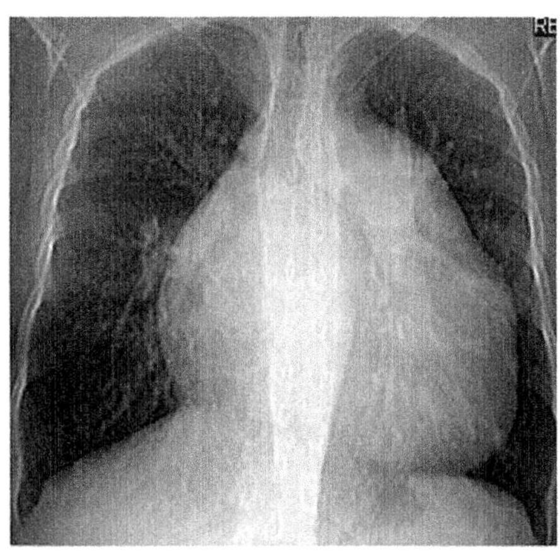

Fig. 7.5 X-ray of a patient with schistosomiasis-associated pulmonary hypertension showing cardiomegaly due to increased right ventricle and atria and bulging of the pulmonary artery trunk

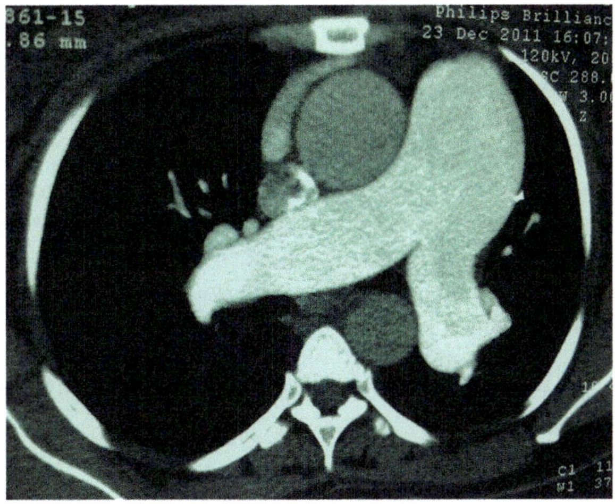

Fig. 7.6 Computed tomography of the thorax of a 42-year-old female patient with schistosomiasis-associated pulmonary hypertension, showing enlarged diameter of pulmonary artery trunk compared with the diameter of aorta

1.60–5.4 cm). 29.5 % of the patients had calcified nodules, 15.9 % had undetermined nodules, and 13.6 % both types of nodules [66].

The 6 minute walk test (6MWT) is a simple, inexpensive, and standardized test that can be helpful in assessing prognosis and response to treatment [60, 67]. In the series of Sch-PAH reported by Japiassu et al., the mean 6MWT was 360.1 ± 75.3 m in patients with NYHA class I/II and 158.8 ± 95.5 m in patients with NYHA class III/IV [54].

Blood Tests and Immunology

Serological tests to detect HIV infection, connective tissue disease, and hepatitis are routinely performed in the evaluation of PAH [60, 61] and should be done in patients suspected of Sch-PAH as well. In Sch-PAH, serum levels of AST, ALT, and bilirubin are usually normal, but the levels of alkaline phosphatase and γ-GT tend to be higher [32]. Eosinophilia may be present in patients having continuous exposure to the parasite and active infection. The serum brain natriuretic peptide level, as in other forms of PAH, can be used as a prognostic marker and to follow the response to therapy [60, 68, 69].

Treatment

Treatment of Sch-PAH should first be directed toward control of schistosomal infection. The administration of praziquantel in patients with Sch-PAH is recommended because it is targeted at killing the adult worms, thereby preventing further dissemination of eggs, and because it halts the progression of disease. Prednisone at a dose of 1 mg/kg/day, starting one day prior with a slow taper over 4 weeks, is also recommended, because praziquantel can elicit acute cor pulmonale. Contrary to the reversion or reduction of liver lesions and fibrosis that can be seen following treatment of schistosomiasis [49, 72], parasite treatment seems to have little or no effect on cardiac manifestations including PH [7]. Perhaps a better response to treatment could be expected if the treatment was administered in the initial phase of the development of the pulmonary vascular remodeling. Crosby et al. demonstrated that treatment with praziquantel reversed pulmonary vascular remodeling and prevented pulmonary hypertension in a mouse model of Sch-PAH [71]. On the other hand, only one case has reported improvement in pulmonary hemodynamics after treatment of schistosomiasis alone in a human patient with Sch-PAH [72].

Diuretics, supplemental oxygen, and angiotensin receptor antagonist are commonly used to reduce right ventricular overload and improve symptoms in patients with Sch-PAH. Beta blockers have been used to help prevent variceal bleeding in patients with hepatic and hepatosplenic schistosomiasis, but their effects are uncertain in patients with Sch-PAH [73]. Benefits of anticoagulants in these patients have not been studied and caution must be observed in those with portal hypertension and esophageal varices or other bleeding risks.

There are few studies regarding the use of specific PAH treatments for patients with Sch-PAH patients and those that exist consist of case reports or small case series [62, 74–76]. Bandeira et al. reported a favorable response to sildenafil in 13 functional class III/IV patients with Sch-PAH [74]. Significant improvement in functional class and 6MWT was observed, as well as a reduction in PASP, without significant adverse effects [74]. Loureiro et al. found significant improvement in pulmonary hemodynamics as assessed by cardiovascular magnetic resonance in seven patients with Sch-PAH who were treated with sildenafil for 3 months [75]. In a retrospective study of 12 functional class III/IV Sch-PAH patients treated for 34.9 ± 15.5 months, seven patients received phosphodiesterase-5 inhibitors, four received endothelin receptor antagonists, and one was given both as initial therapy [76]. The drugs were well tolerated and the majority of patients (9 of 12) improved at least one functional class. Cardiac index, 6MWT distance, and PVR also improved significantly, but no significant difference was seen in mPAP. Based on these limited findings and the similarities between Sch-PAH and other forms of PAH, the use of specific PAH therapy in patients with Sch-PAH is recommended following presently available guidelines for the treatment of WHO group 1 PAH [77]. Caution and careful monitoring of liver function should be used when treating hepatosplenic schistosomiasis patients with endothelin receptor antagonists. Considering the very low percentage of Sch-PAH patients with a positive pulmonary vasodilator response [54, 55], it is unlikely that calcium channel blockers will be effective in Sch-PAH patients and may be quite dangerous in those with right heart failure or limited cardiac output.

Prognosis

A survival study carried out in Sao Paulo, Brazil, enrolled 54 Sch-PAH patients and 95 IPAH patients. The schistosomotic patients were treatment naïve, whereas 94 % of IPAH patients were treated with specific IPAH drugs. Survival rates at 1, 2, and 3 years were 95.1 %, 95.1 %, and 85.9 % for Sch-PAH and 95 %, 86 %, and 82 %, for IPAH patients, respectively ($p=0.49$). The presence of high mPAP or PVR, NYHA class IV, or low 6MWT distance were associated with poorer prognosis. The survival rates presented in both groups were higher when compared to the survival estimated by the National Institute of Health equation for IPAH patients, suggesting that Sch-PAH patients have a more favorable hemodynamic profile at diagnosis and a more benign clinical course, even without treatment compared with IPAH patients [55]. A recent survival study with PAH patients in the USA found that the 7-year survival rate was significantly better than the median survival of 3 years reported in the NIH registry, probably reflecting the new therapies for PAH. In this analysis, the subgroup of portopulmonary hypertension had a worse 2-year survival than patients with IPAH [78]. In conclusion, Sch-PAH patients have better prognosis in general when compared to other forms of PAH including PAH associated with portopulmonary hypertension.

Conclusions

Chronic schistosomal infection is likely the leading cause of PAH in the world. Although there are many questions regarding the mechanisms by which schistosomal infection induces pulmonary vascular remodeling that is similar to that seen in other forms of PAH, it appears that Sch-PAH is not due to mechanical obstruction of pulmonary vessels by parasite ova, alone. It is not known if there is a genetic susceptibility that increases the risk of PAH in schistosomiasis as occurs in heritable or IPAH. Shunting of portal blood into the systemic veins and inflammatory responses to parasite ova likely contribute to pulmonary vascular disease in Sch-PAH. Proper diagnosis entails establishing a diagnosis of schistosomiasis and excluding other causes of PAH. Treatment of Sch-PAH is aimed at eradication or control of schistosomal infection, treatment of right heart failure, and implementation of PAH-specific therapies mindful of the limited data on their efficacy and their potential adverse effects on cardiac output and liver function. Presently, the understanding of the pathological features, treatment response, and overall prognosis of Sch-PAH lags behind what is known about other forms of PAH. In order to advance the treatment of this serious disease, further studies of the pathogenesis and clinical management of Sch-PAH are needed along with the development of strategies that retard the spread of schistosomal infection and lead to the earlier diagnosis of schistosomal disease.

References

1. WHO. Schistosomiasis. A major public health problem. [Internet]. http://www.who.int/schistosomiasis/en/. Accessed 6 Nov 2012.
2. Ross AG, Bartley PB, Sleigh AC, Olds GR, Li Y, et al. Schistosomiasis. N Engl J Med. 2002;346:1212–20.
3. Graham BB, Bandeira AP, Morrell NW, Butrous G, Tuder RM. Schistosomiasis-associated pulmonary hypertension. Pulmonary vascular disease: the global perspective. Chest. 2010; 137(6 Suppl):20S–9.
4. Gryseels B, Polman K, Clerinx J, Kestens L. Human schistosomiasis. Lancet. 2006;368: 1106–18.
5. Domingues ALC, Ferraz AAB. Doença Hepática Esquistossomótica. In: Coelho J, editor. Aparelho Digestivo: Clínica e Cirurgia. São Paulo: Editora Atheneu; 2012. p. 1559–75.
6. Strauss E. Hepatosplenic schistosomiasis: a model for the study of portal hypertension. Ann Hepatol. 2002;1(1):6–11.
7. Morris W, Knauer CM. Cardiopulmonary Manifestations of Schistosomiasis. Semin Respir Infect. 1997;12(2):159–70.
8. Waldman ADB, Day JH, Shaw P, Bryceson ADM. Subacute pulmonary granulomatous schistosomiasis: high resolution CT appearances—another cause of the halo sign. Br J Radiol. 2001;74:1052–5.
9. Lambertucci JR. Acute schistosomiasis mansoni: revisited and reconsidered. Mem Inst Oswaldo Cruz. 2010;105(4):422–35.
10. Ross AG, Vicker D, Olds GR, Snah S, McManus DP. Katayama syndrome. Lancet Infect Dis. 2007;7:218–24.
11. Porres-Aguillar M, Altamirano JT, Torr-Delgadillo A, Charlton MR, Duarte-Rojo A. Portopulmonary hypertension and hepatopulmonary syndrome: a clinician-oriented overview. Eur Respir Rev. 2012;21(125):223–33.
12. Ferreira RCS, Domingues ALC, Markman Filho B, Veras FHAP, Batista LJB. Albuquerque Filho, ES Hepatopulmonary syndrome in patients with Schistosoma mansoni periportal fibrosis. Acta Trop. 2009;111:119–24.
13. Faria JL, Barbas JV, Fujioka T, Lion M.F, Andradre e Silva U, Décourt LV. Pulmonary schistosomotic arteriovenous fistulas producing a new cyanotic syndrome in Manson's schistosomiasis. Am Heart J. 1959;58:556–7.
14. WHO. Schistosomiasis. Weekly epidemiological record. 2011;86:73–80.
15. Ward TJC, Fenwick A, Butrous G. The prevalence of pulmonary hypertension in schistosomiasis: a systematic review. PVRI Rev. 2011;3(1):12–21.
16. Sistema de Vigilância em Saúde. Esquistossomose. [Internet]. http://portal.saude.gov.br/portal/saude/profissional/area.cfm?id_area=1551. Accessed 6 Nov 2012
17. Guimaraes AC, Alves Jr AR, Santos-Filho A, Esteves JP, Vinhaes LS, Abreu WN, Souza JÁ, Bina JC, Prata AR. Blood gas changes and pulmonary hemodynamics in portal hypertension due to *schistosomiasis mansoni*. Rev Inst Med Trop Sao Paulo. 1977;19:80–93.
18. Vinhaes LSA, Guimarães AC, Santos A, Abreu WN, Esteves JP, Bina JC, Prata AR. A circulação pulmonar na síndrome de hipertensão portal esquistossomótica. Interrelacões radiológico-hemodinâmicas. Arq Bras Cardiol. 1977;30:13–8.
19. De Cleva R, Herman P, D'Albuquerque LA, Pugliese V, Santarem OL, Saad WA. Pre- and postoperative systemic hemodynamic evaluation in patients subjected to esophagogastric devascularization plus splenectomy and distal splenorenal shunt: a comparative study in schistosomal portal hypertension. World J Gastroenterol. 2007;13:5471–5.
20. Lapa M, Dias B, Jardim C, Fernandes CJ, Dourado PM, Figueiredo M, Farias A, Tsutsui J, Terra-Filho M, Humbert M, Souza R. Cardiopulmonary manifestations of hepatosplenic schistosomiasis. Circulation. 2009;119:1518–23.
21. Bandeira AP, Mattos SS, Armstrong A, Marques FFS, Ferraz NCM. Clinical characteristics of pulmonary arterial hypertension in patients from northeast. Arq Bras Cardiol. 2007; 89(Suppl):94.

22. Lapa MS, Ferreira EVM, Jardim C, Martins BCS, Arakaki JSO, Souza R. Clinical characteristics of pulmonary hypertension patients in two reference centers in the city of São Paulo. Rev Assoc Med Bras. 2006;52(3):139–43.
23. Machado C, Brito I, Souza D, Correia LC. Etiological frequency of pulmonary hypertension in a reference outpatient clinic in Bahia. Brazil Arq Bras Cardiol. 2009;93:629–36.
24. Lambertucci JR, Gerspacher-Lara R, Pinto-Silva RA, Barbosa MM, Teixeira R, Barbosa HF, Serufo JC, Rezende DF, Drummond SC, Rayes AA. O projeto Queixadinha: a morbidade e o controle da esquistossomose em área endêmica no nordeste de Minas Gerais, Brasil. Rev Soc Bras Med Trop. 1996;29(2):127–35.
25. Ferreira RC, Domingues AL, Bandeira AP, Markman-Filho B, Albuquerque-Filho ES, Correia de Araújo AC, Batista LJB, Markman M, Campelo ARL. Prevalence of pulmonary hypertension in patients with schistosomal liver fibrosis. Ann Trop Med Parasitol. 2009;103:129–43.
26. Tuder RM, Marecki JC, Richter A, Fijalkowska SF. Pathology of pulmonary hypertension. Clin Chest Med. 2007;28:23–42.
27. Tuder RM. Pathology of pulmonary arterial hypertension. Semin Respir Crit Care Med. 2009;30:376–85.
28. Simonneau G, Robbins IM, Beghetti M, Channick RN, Delcroix M, Denton CP, Elliott CG, Gaine SP, Gladwin MT, Jing Z, Krowka MJ, Langleben D, Nakanishi N, Souza R. Updated Clinical Classification of Pulmonary Hypertension. J Am Coll Cardiol. 2009;54:S43–54.
29. Shaw AFB, Ghareeb AA. Pathogenesis of pulmonary schistosomiasis in Egypt with special reference to Ayerza's disease. J Pathol Bacteriol. 1938;46:401–24.
30. Faria JL. CorPulmonale in Manson's Schistosomiasis I. Frequency in Necropsy Material: Pulmonary Vascular changes caused by Schistosome Ova. Am J Pathol. 1954;30:167–93.
31. Chaves E. The Pathology of the Arterial Pulmonary Vasculature in Manson's Schistosomiasis. Dis Chest. 1966;50(1):72–7.
32. Sadigursky M, Andrade ZA. Pulmonary changes in schistosomal cor pulmonale. Am J Trop Med Hyg. 1982;31(4):779–84.
33. Andrade ZA, Andrade SG. Pathogenesis of schistosomal pulmonary arteritis. Am J Trop Med Hyg. 1970;19(2):305–10.
34. Andrade ZA. Pathology of human schistosomiasis. Mem Inst Oswaldo Cruz. 1987;82 Suppl 4:17–23.
35. Graham BB, Chabon J, Bandeira A, Espinheira L, Butrous G, Tuder RM. Significant intrapulmonary Schistosoma egg antigens are not present in schistosomiasis-associated pulmonary hypertension. Pulm Circ. 2011;1(4):456–61.
36. Abath FGC, Morais CNL, Montenegro CEL, Wynn TH, Montenegro SML. Immunopathogenic mechanisms in schistosomiasis: what can be learnt from human studies? Trends Parasitol. 2006;22(2):85–91.
37. Morais CNL, Souza JR, Melo WG, Aroucha ML, Miranda P, Domingues ALC, Abath FGC, Montenegro SML. Cytokine profile associated with chronic and acute human schistosomiasis mansoni. Mem Inst Oswaldo Cruz. 2008;103(6):561–8.
38. Wilson MS, Mentink-Kane MM, Pesce JT, Ramalingam TR, Thompson R, Wynn TA. Immunopathology of schistosomiasis. Immunol Cell Biol. 2007;85(2):148–54.
39. Caldas RC, Campi-Azevedo AC, Oliveira LFA, Silveira AMS, Oliveira RC, Gazzinelli G. Human schistosomiasis mansoni: Immune responses during acute and chronic phases of the infection. Acta Trop. 2008;108(2–3):109–17.
40. Yu L, Sun X, Yang F, Yang J, Shen J, Wu Z. Inflammatory cytokines IFN-ϒ, IL-4, IL-13 and TNF-α alterations in schistosomiasis: a meta-analysis. Parasitol Res. 2012;110(4):1547–52.
41. Price LC, Wort SJ, Perros F, Dormüller P, Huertas A, Montani D, Cohen-Kaminsky S, Humbert M. Inflammation in Pulmonary Arterial Hypertension. Chest. 2012;141(1):210–21.
42. Newman JH, Phillips JA. Narrative review: the enigma of pulmonary arterial hypertension: new Insights from genetic studies. Ann Intern Med. 2008;148(4):278–83.
43. Graham BB, Mentink-Kane MM, El-Haddad H, Purnell S, Zhang L, Zaiman A, Redente EF, Riches DWH, Hassoun PM, Bandeira AP, Champion HC, Butrous G, Wynn TA, Tuder RM. Schistosomiasis-Induced Experimental Pulmonary Hypertension. Role of Interleukin-13 Signaling. Amer. J Pathol. 2010;177(3):1549–61.

44. Souza PRS, Souza ALS, Negrão-Correa D, Teixeira AL, Teixeira MM. The role of chemokines in controlling granulomatous inflammation in Schistosoma mansoni infection. Acta Trop. 2008;108:135–8.
45. Crosby A, Jones FM, Southwood M, Stewart S, Schermuly R, Butrous G, Dunne DW, Morrel NW. Pulmonary Vascular Remodeling Correlates with Lung Eggs and Cytokines in Murine Schistosomiasis. Am J Respir Crit Care Med. 2010;181:279–88.
46. Goumans M, Liu Z, Dijke P. TGF-β signaling in vascular biology and dysfunction. Cell Res. 2009;19:116–27.
47. Graham BB, Chabon J, Gebreab L, Poole J, Debella E, Davis L, Tanaka T, Sanders L, Dropcho N, Bandeira A, Vandivier RW, Champion HC, Butrous G, Wang X, Wynn TA, Tuder RM. Transforming growth factor-β signaling promotes pulmonary hypertension caused by *Schistosoma mansoni*. Circulation. 2013;128:1354–64.
48. Ferreira RCS, Montenegro SML, Domingues ALC, Bandeira AP, Silveira CAM, Leite LAC, Pereira CA, Fernandes IM, Mertens AB, Almeida MO. TGF beta and IL 13 in schistosomiasis mansoni associated pulmonary arterial hypertension; a descriptive study with comparative groups. BMC Infect Dis. 2014;14:282.
49. Ruiz-Guevara R, Noya BA, Valero SK, Lecuna P, Garassini M, Noya O. Achados clínicos e no ultra-som pré e pós tratamento com praziquantel em pacientes venezuelanos com esquistossomose. Rev Soc Bras Med Trop. 2007;40(5):505–11.
50. Bandeira AP, Ferreira RCS, Japiassu FAA, Silveira CAM, Oliveira M, Mertens AB, Domingues ALC. Clinical and hemodynamic characteristics of patients with schistosomal pulmonary arterial hypertension attended in PROCAPE—Recife, Brazil. International Symposium on Schistosomiasis; 16–19 Sept 2012, Belo Horizonte, Brazil; 2012, p. 192.
51. Conceição MJ, Argento CA, Vieira OM, Takiya CM, Chagas VL. Surgical indication in Schistosomiasis mansoni portal hypertension—follow-up from 1985 to 2001. Mem Inst Oswaldo Cruz. 2002;97 Suppl 1:165–6.
52. Ferraz AAB, Araújo JRJGC, Ferraz EM. Tratamento cirúrgico da esquistossomose mansônica. In: Moraes IN, editor. Tratado de Clínica Cirúrgica. 1st ed. São Paulo: Editora Roca; 2005. p. 1331–43.
53. Barbosa MM, Lamounier JA, Oliveira EC, Souza MV, Marques DS, Silva AA, Lambertucci JR. Pulmonary hypertension in Schistosomiasis mansoni. Trans R Soc Trop Med Hyg. 1996;90(6):663–5.
54. Japyassú FAA, Mendes AA, Bandeira AP, Oliveira FRA, Sobral Filho DS. Hemodynamic Profile of Severity at Pulmonary Vasoreactivity Test in Schistosomiasis Patients. Arq Bras Cardiol. 2012;99(3):789–96.
55. dos Santos Fernandes CJ, Jardim CV, Hovnanian A, Hoette S, Dias BA, Souza S, Humbert M, Souza R. Survival in Schistosomiasis-Associated Pulmonary Arterial Hypertension. J Am Coll Cardiol. 2010;56(9):715–20.
56. Richter J, Domingues ALC, Barata CH, Prata AR, Lambertucci JR. Report of the second satellite symposium on ultrasound in schistosomiasis. Mem Inst Oswaldo Cruz. 2001;96(Suppl):151–6.
57. Schwartz E. Pulmonary schistosomiasis. Clin Chest Med. 2002;23(2):443.
58. Roberts JD, Forfia PR. Diagnosis and assessment of pulmonary vascular disease by Doppler echocardiography. Pulm Circ. 2011;1(2):160–81.
59. Fisher MR, Forfia PR, Chamera E, Housten-Harris T, Champion HC, Girgis RE, Corretti MC, Hassoun PM. Accuracy of Doppler echocardiography in the hemodynamic assessment of pulmonary hypertension. Am Respir Crit Care Med. 2009;179(7):615–21.
60. Galiè N, Hoeper MM, Humbert M, Torbicki A, Vachiery J, Barbera JA, Beghetti M, Corris P, Gaine S, Gibbs JS, Gomez-Sanchez MA, Jondeau G, Klepetko W, Opitz C, Peacock A, Rubin L, Zellweger M, Simonneau G. Guidelines for diagnosis and treatment of pulmonary hypertension. The Task Force for the diagnosis and treatment of pulmonary hypertension of the European Society of Cardiology (ESC) and the European Respiratory Society (ERS) endorsed by the International Society of Heart and Lung Transplantation (ISHLT). Eur Respir J. 2009;34:1219–63.

61. Barst RJ, McGoon M, Torbicki A, Sitbon O, Krowka MJ, Olschewski H, Gaine S. Diagnosis and differential assessment of pulmonary arterial hypertension. J Am Coll Cardiol. 2004; 43(12 Suppl S):S40–7.
62. Correa RA, Moreira MVSC, Saraiva JMS, Mancuzo EV, Silva LCS, Lambertucci JR. Treatment of schistosomiasis-associated pulmonary hypertension. J Bras Pneumol. 2011;37(2):272–6.
63. McGoon M, Gutterman D, Steen V, Barst R, McCrory DC, Fortin TA, Loyd JE. Screening, Early Detection, and Diagnosis of Pulmonary Arterial Hypertension: ACCP Evidence-Based Clinical Practice Guidelines. Chest. 2004;126:14–34.
64. Tunariu N, Gibbs SJR, Win Z, Gin-Sing W, Graham A, Gishen P, Al-Nahhas A. Ventilation-perfusion scintigraphy is more sensitive than multidetector CTPA in detecting chronic thromboembolic pulmonary disease as a treatable cause of pulmonary hypertension. J Nucl Med. 2007;48(5):680–4.
65. Grosse C, Grosse A. CT Findings in Diseases Associated with Pulmonary Hypertension: A Current Review. RadioGraphics. 2010;30:1753–77.
66. Ferreira RCS, Mertens AB, Oliveira M, Silveira CAM, Bandeira AP, Domingues ALC, Buril R. Computed tomography in pulmonary hypertension caused by schistosomiasis. international symposium on schistosomiasis; 16–19 Sept 2012; Belo Horizonte, Brazil, p. 191.
67. Miyamoto S, Nagaya N, Satoh T, Kyotani S, Sakamaki S, Fujita M, Nakanishi N, Miyatake K. Clinical correlates and prognostic significance of six-minute walk test in patients with primary pulmonary hypertension: comparison with cardiopulmonary exercise testing. Am J Respir Crit Care Med. 2000;161(2 Pt 1):487–592.
68. McLaughlin VV, Presberg KW, Doyle RL, Abman SH, McCrory DC, Fortin T, Ahearn G. Prognosis of Pulmonary Arterial Hypertension: ACCP Evidence-Based Clinical Practice Guidelines. Chest. 2004;126:78–92.
69. Yap LB, Murkerjee D, Timms PM, Ashrafian H, Coghlan JG. Natriuretic Peptides, Respiratory Disease, and the Right Heart. Chest. 2004;126:1330–6.
70. Homeida MA, el Tom I, Nash T, Bennet JL. Association of therapeutic activity of praziquantel with reversal of Symmer's fibrosis induced by Schistosoma mansoni. Am J Trop Med Hyg. 1991;45(3):360–5.
71. Crosby A, Jones FM, Kolosionek E, Southwood M, Purvis I, Soon E, Butrous G, Dunne DE, Morrell NW. Praziquantel reverses pulmonary hypertension and vascular remodeling in murine schistosomiasis. Am J Respir Crit Care Med. 2011;184(4):467–73.
72. Bourée P, Piveteau J, Gerbal JL, Halpen G. Pulmonary arterial hypertension due to bilharziasis. Apropos of case due to Schistosoma haematobium having been cured by praziquantel. Bull Soc Pathol Exot. 1999;83(1):66–71.
73. So PP, Davies RA, Chandy G, Stewart D, Beanlands RS. Usefulness of beta-blocker therapy and outcomes in patients with pulmonary hypertension. Am J Cardiol. 2012;109(10):1504–9.
74. Bandeira AP, Mendes AA, Santos-Filho P, Sa DT, Loureiro R. Clinical efficacy of oral sildenafil in severe pulmonary hypertension in patients with chronic pulmonary schistosomiasis. Circulation. 2004;110(17 Supplement III):296.
75. Loureiro R, Mendes A, Bandeira A, Cartaxo H, Sá D. Oral Sildenafil improves functional status and cardiopulmonary hemodynamic in patients with severe pulmonary hypertension secondary to chronic pulmonary schistosomiasis: a cardiac magnetic resonance study (abstr). Circulation. 2004;110(Suppl III):572.
76. Fernandes CJCS, Dias BA, Jardim CVP, Hovnannian A, Hoette S, Morinaga LK, Souza S, Suesada M, Breda AP, Souza R. The Role of Target Therapies in Schistosomiasis-Associated Pulmonary Arterial Hypertension. Chest. 2012;141(4):923–8.
77. Galiè N, Corris PA, Frost A, Girgis RE, Granton J, Jing ZC, Klepetko W, McGoon MD, McLaughlin VV, Preston IR, Rubin LJ, Sandoval J, Seeger W, Keogh A. Updated treatment algorithm of pulmonary arterial hypertension. J Am Coll Cardiol. 2013;62(25 Suppl):D60–72.
78. McGoon MD, Miller DP. REVEAL: a contemporary US pulmonary arterial hypertension registry. Eur Respir Rev. 2012;21(123):8–18.

Chapter 8
Approach to the Patient with Elevated Pulmonary Arterial Pressure

Jason S. Fritz and Harold I. Palevsky

Abstract Pulmonary hypertension (PH) refers to a mean pulmonary arterial pressure ≥25 mmHg and may be related to elevations in left atrial pressure, pulmonary vascular resistance, cardiac output, or combinations thereof. When the mechanism of PH is related to an elevation in vascular resistance, the term pulmonary *arterial* hypertension is used, and may occur in the presence or absence of certain associated conditions. Identification of this subset is important as these patients are at an elevated risk of morbidity and mortality related to progressive right heart failure. Symptoms are nonspecific, and the clinician must maintain a high index of suspicion in order to minimize diagnostic delay, particularly when the history and results of ancillary testing do not suggest an alternative explanation for cardiopulmonary symptoms. Echocardiography provides valuable information that can aid the clinician in estimating the degree of PH, as well as gauge the likelihood that any observed elevations in pulmonary pressures are related to left atrial hypertension. In addition, relatively simple metrics of right ventricular size and function can be obtained. When such abnormalities exist in isolation, the clinician should have a high suspicion for pulmonary vascular disease. Right heart catheterization remains the gold standard for confirming the presence of PH, determining its hemodynamic basis, and guiding therapeutic decisions. Assessing hemodynamics with exercise may be informative in patients with predominantly exertional symptoms who display normal or equivocal values at rest.

Keywords Pulmonary hypertension • Diagnosis • Right heart failure • Diastolic dysfunction • Echocardiography

J.S. Fritz, M.D. • H.I. Palevsky, M.D. (✉)
Pulmonary Vascular Disease Program, Pulmonary, Allergy, and Critical Care Division, Department of Medicine, Penn Presbyterian Medical Center, Perelman School of Medicine at the University of Pennsylvania, 51 N. 39th St., PHI Building, Suite 120, Philadelphia, PA 19104, USA
e-mail: Harold.Palevsky@uphs.upenn.edu

J.R. Klinger, R.P. Frantz (eds.), *Diagnosis and Management of Pulmonary Hypertension*, Respiratory Medicine 12, DOI 10.1007/978-1-4939-2636-7_8

Abbreviations

2DE	2-Dimensional echocardiography
6MWT	6-min Walk test
ABG	Arterial blood gas
AcT	Acceleration time
ANA	Antinuclear antibody
ANCA	Antineutrophil cytoplasmic antibody
APAH	Associated pulmonary arterial hypertension
APVD	Anomalous pulmonary venous drainage
ASD	Atrial septal defect
AV	Aortic valve
BMPR2	Bone morphogenetic protein receptor type 2
BNP	Brain natriuretic peptide
CO	Cardiac output
CPET	Cardiopulmonary exercise test
CT	Computed tomography
CTA	Computed tomographic angiography
CTD	Connective tissue disease
CTEPH	Chronic thromboembolic pulmonary hypertension
CXR	Chest X-ray
DLco	Diffusing capacity of the lung for carbon monoxide
ECG	Electrocardiogram
FVC	Forced vital capacity
FVE	Flow velocity envelope
HFpEF	Heart failure with preserved ejection fraction
HIV	Human immunodeficiency virus
HPAH	Heritable pulmonary arterial hypertension
IPAH	Idiopathic pulmonary arterial hypertension
IVC	Inferior vena cava
JVD	Jugular venous distention
LA	Left atrium
LV	Left ventricle
LVEF	Left ventricular ejection fraction
LVH	Left ventricular hypertrophy
mPAP	Mean pulmonary artery pressure
MV	Mitral valve
NIH	National Institutes of Health
NYHA	New York Heart Association
PAH	Pulmonary arterial hypertension
PASP	Pulmonary artery systolic pressure
PCWP	Pulmonary capillary wedge pressure
PDA	Patent ductus arteriosus
PE	Pulmonary embolism

PFT	Pulmonary function test
PH	Pulmonary hypertension
PIOPED	Prospective Investigation of Pulmonary Embolism Diagnosis
PoPH	Portopulmonary hypertension
PSG	Polysomnogram
PVOD	Pulmonary veno-occlusive disease
PVR	Pulmonary vascular resistance
Q_p	Pulmonary blood flow
Q_s	Systemic blood flow
RA	Right atrium
RAP	Right atrial pressure
RHC	Right heart catheterization
RNP	Ribonucleoprotein
ROC	Receiver operating characteristic
RV	Right ventricle
RVOT	Right ventricular outflow tract
RVSP	Right ventricular systolic pressure
SLE	Systemic lupus erythematosus
SVR	Systemic vascular resistance
TAPSE	Tricuspid annular plane systolic excursion
TGG-β	Transforming growth factor beta
TR	Tricuspid regurgitation
TR_{vel}	Velocity of the tricuspid regurgitation jet
V/Q	Ventilation/perfusion
VSD	Ventricular septal defect
WHO	World Health Organization

Introduction

The evaluation of the patient with elevated pulmonary pressures requires a consistent and methodical approach aimed at identifying the correct etiology of the pulmonary hypertension (PH), assessing its physiologic impact, and choosing appropriate therapy. A recent population-based echocardiographic study from Olmsted County, Minnesota, suggests that up to 20 % of the general population exhibits an estimated right ventricular systolic pressure (RVSP) >35 mmHg (although this threshold may include individuals who do not have PH as determined by invasive testing) [1]. This fraction is likely to be significantly higher among patients referred for subspecialty evaluation [2, 3]. The identification of PH may be the result of a deliberate search in a dyspneic patient known to be at risk for PH (e.g., screening a patient with systemic sclerosis), or alternatively, may be found incidentally when diagnostic testing (i.e., an echocardiogram) is performed for another reason. The clinical classification of PH is divided into five groups, most recently updated at the 2013 Fifth World Symposium on PH held in Nice, France [4], and takes into account both hemodynamics and underlying pathophysiology (Table 8.1). The list of conditions associated with PH is long, however, and establishing a precise etiologic diagnosis is crucial to inform both prognosis and therapeutic strategy. Due to its grave implications for long-term survival if left untreated, early diagnosis of pulmonary *arterial* hypertension (PAH) is essential to allow institution of appropriate disease-modifying therapies. However, symptoms are often nonspecific and the presence of common comorbidities can create diagnostic confusion and delay accurate diagnosis [5], underscoring the importance of a methodical evaluation. Despite increasing awareness and scientific study of pulmonary vascular diseases over recent decades, certain tests recommended by current diagnostic algorithms [6–8] for the evaluation of PH remain underutilized [9]. Contemporary registries confirm the unfortunate reality that 70–80 % of PAH patients are in New York Heart Association (NYHA) functional classes III or IV at time of diagnosis [10–12], a statistic that has changed little over the preceding 25 years [13]. This chapter will present a practical overview of the approach to a patient with documented or suspected pulmonary hypertension.

Hemodynamic Basis of PH: An Introduction with Clinical Correlation

While a more detailed overview of pulmonary hemodynamics is presented in Chap. 10, a working knowledge of the hemodynamic basis of PH is extremely helpful in directing the clinical approach to the patient and so will be reviewed here in brief.

Current guidelines define PH as mean pulmonary artery pressure (mPAP) ≥25 mmHg with the patient at rest [6–8]. The definition of abnormal PAP response to exercise was considered as part of the 2013 WHO Nice deliberations, but no consensus was reached due to the lack of available data. Changes in pulmonary vascular and left ventricular compliance with aging make it difficult to determine normal and abnormal rises in PAP during exercise leading to the recommendation that exercise-induced PAP not be included in the definition of pulmonary hypertension [14]. It is crucial to note that while the pressure cutoff of 25 mmHg defines the presence or absence of disease by convention, it provides no information regarding its etiology. Application of Ohm's law is used to describe the relationship between pressure and flow in the pulmonary circulation, but this assumes nonpulsatile, laminar flow within uniform, nondistensible vessels—all of which do not apply to the pulmonary vascular bed. With this limitation in mind, Ohm's law dictates that mPAP is the product of pulmonary blood flow (Q_p) and resistance across the pulmonary bed (pulmonary vascular resistance [PVR]), added to pulmonary venous pressure. In the absence of an anatomic shunt, Q_p is approximately equal to systemic blood flow (Q_s or cardiac output [CO]). Pulmonary venous pressure is difficult to measure directly in routine practice, so pulmonary capillary wedge pressure (PCWP) is used as a more readily obtained surrogate. Thus, an increase in mPAP may occur as a result of increases in Q_p, PVR, or PCWP (Fig. 8.1). Each will be discussed in turn below.

Table 8.1 Clinical classification of pulmonary hypertension [4]

Group	Subgroup
1. Pulmonary arterial hypertension (PAH)	1.1. Idiopathic PAH
	1.2. Heritable
	1.2.1. BMPR2
	1.2.2. ALK1, endoglin, SMAD9, CAV1, KCNK3
	1.2.3. Unknown
	1.3. Drug- and toxin-induced
	1.4. Associated with
	1.4.1. Connective tissue disease
	1.4.2. HIV infection
	1.4.3. Portal hypertension
	1.4.4. Congenital heart diseases
	1.4.5. Schistosomiasis
	1′. Pulmonary veno-occlusive disease (PVOD) and/or pulmonary capillary hemangiomatosis (PCH)
	1″. Persistent pulmonary hypertension of the newborn (PPHN)
2. Pulmonary hypertension owing to left heart disease	2.1. Left ventricular systolic dysfunction
	2.2. Left ventricular diastolic dysfunction
	2.3. Valvular disease
	2.4. Congenital/acquired left heart inflow/outflow obstruction and congenital cardiomyopathies
3. Pulmonary hypertension owing to lung diseases and/or hypoxia	3.1. Chronic obstructive pulmonary disease
	3.2. Interstitial lung disease
	3.3. Other pulmonary diseases with mixed restrictive and obstructive pattern
	3.4. Sleep-disordered breathing
	3.5. Alveolar hypoventilation disorders
	3.6. Chronic exposure to high altitude
	3.7. Developmental lung disease
4. Chronic thromboembolic pulmonary hypertension (CTEPH)	
5. Pulmonary hypertension with unclear multifactorial mechanisms	5.1. Hematologic disorders: myeloproliferative disorders, splenectomy, chronic hemolytic anemia
	5.2. Systemic disorders: sarcoidosis, pulmonary Langerhans cell histiocytosis, lymphangioleiomyomatosis, neurofibromatosis, vasculitis
	5.3. Metabolic disorders: glycogen storage disease, Gaucher disease, thyroid disorders
	5.4. Others: tumoral obstruction, fibrosing mediastinitis, chronic renal failure segmental PH

Reproduced with permission from reference [4]

ALK1 activin receptor-like kinase type 1, *BMPR2* bone morphogenetic protein receptor type 2, *HIV* human immunodeficiency virus

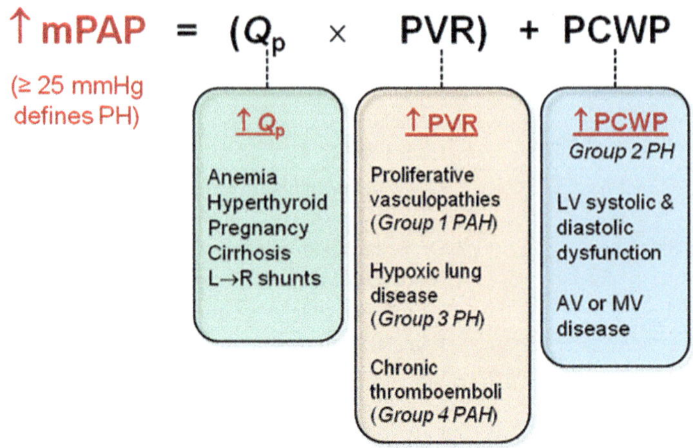

Fig. 8.1 Schematic representation of hemodynamic etiologies of increased pulmonary artery pressure. *mPAP* mean pulmonary arterial pressure, Q_p pulmonary blood flow, *PVR* pulmonary vascular resistance, *PCWP* pulmonary capillary wedge pressure, *LV* left ventricle, *PH* pulmonary hypertension, *PAH* pulmonary arterial hypertension, *AV* aortic valve, *MV* mitral valve

Elevated Q_p

Disorders associated with isolated elevations in pulmonary blood flow are relatively uncommon causes of pulmonary hypertension, since an otherwise healthy pulmonary vascular bed has the ability to recruit additional underperfused vasculature to accommodate increases in flow without a significant increase in pressure [15, 16]. In some circumstances, however, this reserve is impaired and elevations in Q_p may drive, at least in part, a rise in mPAP. Usually, diagnosis of the primary condition predates the discovery of pulmonary hypertension, and there are frequently other symptoms that tend to dominate the clinical picture rather than the pulmonary hypertension per se. For these reasons, disorders associated with isolated increases in CO are not explicitly represented as a separate etiologic category in the current PH classification scheme [4].

Systemic conditions classically associated with an elevated CO include chronic anemia, pregnancy, hyperthyroidism, liver disease, and left-to-right shunts on the basis of either congenital heart disease, arteriovenous fistulae, or certain other disorders (e.g., Paget's disease of bone, multiple myeloma). In anemia, elevated CO is a physiologic response aimed at maintaining adequate systemic oxygen delivery in the face of reduced oxygen carrying capacity. Modest levels of anemia commonly encountered in outpatient practice are not likely to cause significant elevations in CO, as a seminal hemodynamic study suggested a hemoglobin threshold of <7 g/dL is required to obligate a rise in CO in humans [17]. The increased metabolic demands of pregnancy imparted by the developing fetus also necessitate a rise in cardiac output, mediated by increases in both preload (due to plasma volume expansion) and heart rate and a reduction in systemic vascular resistance (SVR) [18]. Despite higher pulmonary blood flow, however, significant rises in PAP in healthy subjects typically do not occur presumably due to concomitant reductions in PVR [19]. Hyperthyroid states may be associated with elevated CO, wherein thyroid hormone can directly augment myocardial contractility as well as reduce SVR [20]. Interestingly, associations between abnormal thyroid function and PAH have been reported in up to half of such patients although hypothyroidism has been identified more commonly than hyperthyroidism [21, 22]. Thyroid disorders are particularly common in patients with APAH related to autoimmune disorders, potentially reflecting a common autoimmune basis in these patients. The potential pathogenic role of abnormal thyroid function in the development of PAH remains unclear; however, the association between thyroid dysfunction and pulmonary vascular disease is recognized by its inclusion in Group 5 (PH with unclear multifactorial mechanisms) of the current classification scheme [4].

Patients with end-stage renal failure who have an arteriovenous fistula for dialysis access are at risk for development of high cardiac output if the fistula flow becomes excessive. If such patients are undergoing hemodynamic catheterization, temporary occlusion of the fistula may enhance understanding of the contribution of the fistula to the high output state. Measurement of the fistula flow can be achieved by use of ultrasound or Fresenius clearance method [23]. If the fistula is resulting in excessive flow, banding of the fistula may be helpful. Arteriovenous malformations, particularly abdominal, also may result in high flow states.

Thus, while all these conditions can contribute to elevated cardiac output, they are rarely the sole cause of significant, symptomatic PH. However, they all may serve to unmask or exacerbate an underlying primary pulmonary vasculopathy (i.e., a process characterized by abnormal PVR) by superimposing an obligatorily increased Q_p on an already restricted pulmonary vascular bed. In such a scenario, the normal plasticity of the pulmonary circulation is impaired which results in higher mPAP at any given level of flow.

In the context of a discussion on elevated pulmonary blood flow and PH, two conditions deserve additional comment. The first relates to elevations in Q_p occurring in the context of a left-to-right anatomic shunt. Congenital defects in this category include ventricular septal defect (VSD), atrial septal defect (ASD), and patent ductus arteriosus (PDA), as well as more complex lesions such as truncus arteriosus, transposition of the great vessels, and syndromes characterized by single ventricle physiology. Anomalous pulmonary venous drainage (APVD) is another type of congenital defect associated with left-to-right shunting wherein one or more pulmonary veins return oxygenated blood to a systemic vein (most often the superior vena cava) or right atrium, and commonly co-exist with an ASD (usually sinus venosus type). In the case of VSD, ASD, or PDA, large defects typically present in infancy. However, smaller defects (in particular ASD) may go unnoticed for decades and not come to medical attention until well into adulthood [24, 25]. Initially, such anatomic defects cause PH by virtue of increased pulmonary blood flow mediated by the left-to-right shunt (elevated Q_p:Q_s), and PVR is normal. Over time, the increase in pulmonary blood flow can incite pathogenic changes within the pulmonary arterioles resulting in an obliterative pulmonary vasculopathy characterized by an elevated PVR. A higher pressure burden as seen in cases of VSD or PDA, combined with the detrimental effects of high flow and shear stress, may be an important factor in the more rapid development of pulmonary vascular disease in these subsets. As the process progresses, right-sided pressures increase, right ventricular insufficiency ensues, and the shunt may reverse (or become bidirectional) with resultant hypoxemia, known as Eisenmenger syndrome. Careful hemodynamic characterization with attention to the relative contributions of elevated Q_p and/or PVR to elevated PAP and utilization of pulmonary vasodilator challenge to assess reversibility are crucial to determine whether correction of the defect and/or institution of pulmonary vasoactive therapy is warranted.

Cirrhosis of the liver, particularly when advanced, is also associated with a hyperdynamic state characterized by elevated systemic and pulmonary blood flow, reduced SVR [26], and potentially increased cardiac filling pressures due to excessive salt and water retention. When abnormal pulmonary pressures are identified in this population, it is more frequently related to elevated cardiac output and/or PCWP [27, 28]. However, similar to the case of an anatomic shunt, it is critical to distinguish this scenario from that where the primary hemodynamic abnormality is an elevation in PVR. This latter condition is known as portopulmonary hypertension (PoPH) and occurs in ~5 % of patients with chronic liver disease being evaluated for liver transplant [28, 29]. The presence of portal hypertension is a prerequisite for the development of PoPH, although there is no clear association between the etiology or severity of portal hypertension and the presence or severity of PoPH [30, 31]. PoPH is classified within Group 1 of the current PH classification scheme, displays pathologic changes identical to those seen in idiopathic PAH [32], and harbors a worse prognosis compared to patients with chronic liver disease without PoPH [33, 34]. Significant, untreated PoPH is associated with increased mortality in the setting of liver transplantation [33, 35, 36] and may represent a contraindication to the procedure. Patients being evaluated for liver transplantation should be screened for pulmonary hypertension by echocardiography and if found should be further evaluated by right heart catheterization [37].

Elevated PCWP

Elevation in left atrial pressure and subsequent pulmonary venous hypertension, as reflected by elevated PCWP, is the final common pathway by which various forms of left heart disease can cause PH. Systolic, restrictive, or infiltrative cardiomyopathies as well as mitral or aortic valvular disease all can lead to a rise in left atrial pressure that is transmitted back to the pulmonary arteries via the pulmonary veins. Heart failure with preserved ejection fraction (HFpEF) is increasingly recognized as a cause of chronic dyspnea, congestive heart failure, and PH. A community-based study of subjects ≥65 years of age suggests an overall prevalence of CHF of ~9 %, over half of which are associated with normal EF on echocardiography [38].

Comorbidities that frequently associate with HFpEF include older age, female sex, hypertension, atrial fibrillation, and obesity [39–41]. PH may be exceedingly common in elderly patients with HFpEF; a community-based echocardiographic study (wherein an RVSP ≥35 mmHg defined the presence of PH) has indicated an overall prevalence of PH in this population of 83 %, compared with 8 % in elderly hypertensive patients without HFpEF [42].

Occasionally, pulmonary venous hypertension may exist in the absence of left atrial hypertension in the setting of pathologic processes that primarily affect the pulmonary veins. Rarely, bulky adenopathy (such as that seen in sarcoidosis [43], tuberculosis [44], histoplasmosis, or other chronic granulomatous diseases or metastatic malignancy) or fibrosing mediastinitis [45] may lead to pulmonary vein obstruction. More recently, catheter ablation with pulmonary vein isolation, used for the treatment of atrial fibrillation, has been associated with the development of pulmonary vein stenosis and subsequent PH [46, 47].

Elevated PVR

Abnormalities in PVR may result from a broad array of pathophysiologic mechanisms, and thus, this hemodynamic abnormality encompasses a heterogeneous group of disorders spanning Groups 1, 3, 4, and 5 of the PH classification scheme. This chapter uses the term *PAH* (pulmonary arterial hypertension) to refer to conditions in this category wherein the primary pathophysiologic determinant is an elevated PVR.

Group 1 PAH

This group includes idiopathic (IPAH; formerly "primary pulmonary hypertension"), heritable (HPAH), and drug/toxin-mediated forms of pulmonary arterial hypertension as well as those associated with certain underlying conditions (APAH), namely congenital heart disease with left-to-right shunts, connective tissue disease (CTD), HIV infection, portal hypertension, and schistosomiasis infection. Two other rare forms of PH include pulmonary veno-occlusive disease (PVOD), characterized by obliterative lesions in the septal and preseptal pulmonary veins, and pulmonary capillary hemangiomatosis (PCH), characterized by extensive proliferation of the pulmonary capillaries into alveolar septa, bronchial walls, and the pleura; these entities are subclassified as Group 1′. PVOD may represent up to 10 % of PAH cases otherwise thought to be idiopathic [48]. It presents with symptoms similar to IPAH, but is associated with more severe derangements in oxygenation and diffusion capacity. PVOD can cause unique chest imaging findings not found in other forms of PH that should raise suspicion for this diagnosis (see section "Chest Computed Tomography (CT)"). Occult alveolar hemorrhage on bronchoalveolar lavage is also suggestive [49]. Patients with PVOD treated with pulmonary vasoactive therapy can develop life-threatening pulmonary edema due to pulmonary arteriolar vasodilation in the setting of fixed venous outflow obstruction [50].

All of the above entities are associated with similar pathologic findings within the pulmonary vascular bed, including medial hypertrophy, intimal and adventitial fibrosis, in situ thrombosis, and the advanced plexiform lesion [51]. As the disease process progresses and PVR rises, the afterload imposed on the right ventricle increases and higher pressures are required to maintain a given level of cardiac output.

Group 3 PH

Group 3 includes primarily respiratory-related disorders characterized by hypoxemia and/or hypoventilation, including all forms of obstructive and restrictive lung disease, neuromuscular or chest wall/skeletal disorders, and sleep-disordered breathing (obstructive sleep apnea and obesity hypoventilation syndrome). Patients in this group have been uniformly excluded from all of the pivotal, randomized, controlled trials of targeted PAH therapies. Although hypoxic vasoconstriction and subsequent vascular remodeling may be a final common pathway for the development of PH in many of these disparate conditions [52, 53] (discussed in greater detail in Chap. 4), other unique pathobiologic mechanisms exist that can contribute to elevations in PAP and PVR in each particular disorder. COPD, for example, is uniquely associated with hyperinflation, which can contribute to an elevated PVR due to increased alveolar pressure and compression of intra-alveolar vessels [54]. In idiopathic pulmonary fibrosis, there may be "spillover" of the inflammation in the epithelial compartment into the adjacent endothelial compartment, contributing to vascular obliteration and a rise in PVR [55, 56].

Group 4 PAH

Pulmonary arterial hypertension in this category is thought to occur from vascular obstruction due to recurrent embolic and/or in situ thrombotic events with organization and incorporation of the thrombotic material into the vessel wall. The incidence of chronic thromboembolic pulmonary hypertension (CTEPH) may be as high as 3.8 % up to 2 years after an embolic event [57]. However, because not all patients with CTEPH can recollect a discrete embolic event, the true incidence of the disease may be higher. While pulmonary arterial obstruction by organized thrombi is the *sine qua non* of CTEPH, patients can exhibit histopathologic changes in the small pulmonary arterioles that are indistinguishable from those seen in IPAH, and these have been observed to occur in regions of the lung spared from large-vessel obstruction [58].

Pulmonary thromboendarterectomy is a technically demanding procedure in which proximal organized thrombi are surgically removed. Individuals with more proximal, surgically accessible disease appear to derive the greatest benefit from the procedure [59], underscoring the importance of a meticulous characterization of the burden of pulmonary vascular disease and its location based on information from RHC, CT angiogram, pulmonary angiography, and, at some centers, pulmonary angioscopy [60]. Chapter 6 of this text presents a more in-depth discussion of CTEPH.

Group 5 PH

Group 5 represents a collection of disorders that have been associated with pulmonary arterial hypertension due to unique and/or ill-defined mechanisms. The current classification scheme subdivides such entities into specific categories, including hematologic (myeloproliferative disorders, splenectomy, chronic hemolytic anemias), systemic (sarcoidosis, pulmonary Langerhans cell histiocytosis, neurofibromatosis, lymphangioleiomyomatosis, neurofibromatosis, vasculitis), metabolic (glycogen storage disease, Gaucher disease, thyroid disorders), and other (tumor obstruction, fibrosing mediastinitis, chronic renal failure on dialysis).

Although some forms of Group 5 PH such as those associated with sarcoidosis and metabolic disorders closely resemble Group 1 PAH, every randomized controlled trial of PAH therapy has excluded patients with Group 5 disease.

Clinical Approach: History

A detailed history provides a wealth of information in the evaluation of a patient with known or suspected PH. Relevant elements of the history can provide information regarding the likelihood of PH being present, its potential cause or causes, and inform the clinician as to its severity and response to treatment.

The most common symptom associated with most forms of PH is dyspnea, particularly dyspnea on exertion. It is reported in virtually all patients and is often of a progressive nature. Other common symptoms include fatigue, exertional near-syncope or syncope, chest pain, edema, and palpitations [13]. The degree of dyspnea should be quantitated, and an assessment of functional class performed according to WHO criteria [61], modeled on the New York Heart Association functional class schema for patients with CHF (Table 8.2). Patients with PH may have a progressive decline in their functional capacity resulting in gradual curtailment of activities to a level where dyspnea is minimized. This can result in an apparent overestimation of functional ability by some patients, which can be elucidated with an assessment of specific activities and asking the patient how easily he or she can perform such activities now as compared with a point in the past (e.g., "How easy is it for you to climb two flights of stairs now as compared with 6 months or a year ago?" or "Are there any activities you used to do that you have stopped recently?"). Soliciting the perspective of a close contact can be helpful in corroborating or refining the patient's assessment. Young patients, particularly those who are athletic or

Table 8.2 WHO functional class assessment for PH

Class I	Patients with PH but without resulting limitation of physical activity. Ordinary physical activity does not cause undue dyspnea or fatigue, chest pain, or near-syncope.
Class II	Patients with PH resulting in slight limitation of physical activity. They are comfortable at rest. Ordinary physical activity causes undue dyspnea or fatigue, chest pain, or near-syncope.
Class III	Patients with PH resulting in marked limitation of physical activity. They are comfortable at rest. Less than ordinary activity causes undue dyspnea or fatigue, chest pain, or near-syncope.
Class IV	Patients with PH with inability to carry out any physical activity without symptoms. These patients manifest sights of right heart failure. Dyspnea and/or fatigue may even be present at rest. Discomfort is increased by any physical activity.

Reproduced with permission from [61]

PH pulmonary hypertension

otherwise very fit, may report only a decrement in their ability to tolerate prolonged exercise which may be erroneously ascribed to deconditioning; this may in fact represent early pulmonary vascular disease with an impaired CO response to higher workloads.

The development of exertional chest discomfort or syncope is a potentially ominous sign of significant right ventricular (RV) ischemia and/or dysfunction and should impart an element of expediency to the diagnostic workup or modification of treatment in cases of known PAH. Anginal chest pain in PAH may arise due to increased oxygen demand from increased RV muscle mass, reduced oxygen supply due to reduced right coronary artery flow with impaired microcirculation due to right ventricular hypertrophy, and in some cases compression of the left main coronary artery by an enlarged pulmonary artery [62, 63]. In the seminal, prospective primary pulmonary hypertension registry, syncope eventually occurred in >1/3 of subjects [13] and is caused by the inability of the RV to increase CO in the face of increased demand and/or systemic vasodilation. Beyond the impairment to flow attributed to elevations in PVR, pathologic ventricular interaction results in reduced left ventricular diastolic compliance, which further limits the ability to maintain left ventricular stroke volume and adequate systemic perfusion pressure [64–67]. The abrupt onset of dyspnea in a patient with other clinical features to suggest PH should prompt consideration of acute pulmonary embolism (PE), either in isolation or superimposed on a background of chronic thromboembolic disease.

During the initial diagnostic phase, additional historical elements should be elicited to help formulate the differential diagnosis. A relatively short survey of comorbid conditions and possible associated symptoms will help the clinician quickly discern potential etiologic categories that may account for PH, and is summarized in Table 8.3. From a statistical perspective, given the relative rarity of idiopathic PAH, one should maintain a high index of suspicion of secondary pulmonary hypertension, keeping in mind that the most common cause of right heart failure is left heart failure. As such, consideration of various forms of left heart disease should be a priority in otherwise "undifferentiated" PH. Significant left ventricular systolic

Table 8.3 Historical elements and associated signs and symptoms pertinent to the evaluation of known or suspected pulmonary hypertension

Focused historical elements	Associated signs or symptoms	PH category
Family history of pulmonary hypertension, sudden death, or ill-defined heart failure		Group 1
Known congenital heart disease, protracted illness during infancy, "blue baby"	Cyanosis, polycythemia	
Use of prescription weight loss pills ("fen-phen" or congeners), methamphetamine use		
Known or suspected HIV/AIDS, IV drug use	Generalized wasting, "track marks"	
Liver disease or cirrhosis	Ascites, jaundice, encephalopathy, varices, or hemorrhoids	
Travel to or residence in areas with endemic Schistosomiasis	Malnutrition/wasting, hepatosplenomegaly	
Known or suspected connective tissue disease	Rash, telangiectasias, Raynaud's phenomenon, photosensitivity, sclerodactyly, esophageal problems, oral ulcers	
Valvular disease, coronary disease, cardiomyopathy, atrial fibrillation	Orthopnea, paroxysmal nocturnal dyspnea	Group 2
Smoking history, any "chronic lung problems," occupational exposures, sleep disturbances	Chronic cough or sputum production, snoring, witnessed apneas	Group 3
Prior history of deep venous thrombosis or pulmonary embolism, hypercoagulable state	Asymmetric edema	Group 4
Myoproliferative disorder, splenectomy, chronic dialysis		Group 5

PH pulmonary hypertension

dysfunction or aortic or mitral valvular disease is usually readily apparent on transthoracic 2DE. An increasingly common clinical problem is that of differentiating pulmonary venous hypertension related to HFpEF (PH-HFpEF) and PAH. As discussed previously, PH appears to be a common occurrence in HFpEF [42]. Echocardiographic clues to the presence of HFpEF include Doppler features of significant diastolic filling abnormality and presence of left atrial enlargement. Conversely, some patients with PAH, particularly when more advanced, may display echocardiographic evidence of impaired left ventricular filling due to pathologic ventricular interaction [68]. In a cross-sectional study comparing PH-HFpEF and PAH, historical features more frequently associated with PH-HFpEF included older age and the presence of systemic hypertension or coronary artery disease [69]. (It should be mentioned that in this study, those with PH-HFpEF had some element of pulmonary vascular disease as the authors required an elevation in PVR or transpulmonary gradient as part of the definition of PH-HFpEF.) However, it is important to recognize that the presence of PAH is not protective against the development of these more common comorbidities and thus can co-exist. Moreover, while the classic presentation of IPAH is that of a young woman with progressive dyspnea, PAH is being diagnosed with increased frequency in the elderly; contemporary registries suggest that ≥20 % of PAH subjects are >60 years of age [10, 11].

If suspicion of left heart disease as a primary cause of PH is relatively low, then a thorough search should be undertaken to identify other associated or secondary causes of PH. Connective tissue diseases are the most common underlying conditions predisposing to the development of PAH, and as such CTD features should be sought out. In a single-center cohort of elderly patients (>65 years of age) referred for evaluation of PH, the presence of CTD was found to be a strong predictor of PAH [70]. Scleroderma (both limited and diffuse forms) and mixed connective tissue disease are the two specific CTDs most commonly associated with PAH, followed by systemic lupus erythematosus (SLE), and less frequently rheumatoid arthritis, polymyositis/dermatomyositis, and Sjögren syndrome [11, 71, 72]. Occasionally, PAH may occur in the absence or precede the development of other symptoms or exam findings to suggest scleroderma ("scleroderma *sine* scleroderma") or another specific CTD. A directed history aimed at symptoms of esophageal dysfunction, Raynaud's phenomenon and autoantibody testing may help identify a "latent" CTD [73, 74]. A history of medical problems in the postnatal period or childhood heart murmur should be obtained as a clue to potential underlying congenital heart disease. The presence of chronic cough, sputum production, or wheezing may indicate underlying obstructive or restrictive lung disease. Snoring, witnessed apneas, morning headaches, or excessive daytime sleepiness suggests the presence of sleep-disordered breathing. A prior history of deep venous thrombosis or PE may raise the suspicion for CTEPH, although 25–50 % of CTEPH patients lack prior knowledge of any thrombotic event [75–77]. Large PE, unprovoked and/or multiple embolic events, younger age, or the presence of certain medical conditions, such as splenectomy, ventriculo-atrial shunts, inflammatory bowel disease, or positive antiphospholipid antibodies, may predispose to the development of CTEPH [57, 76, 78].

A social history should be performed, documenting any pertinent travel or occupational history, anorexigen (Aminorex or fenfluramine derivatives) or recreational (stimulants, including amphetamine compounds [79]) drug exposure, and risk factors for liver cirrhosis, HIV or viral hepatitis infection. While PAH associated with HIV infection remains relatively rare, the diagnosis should be considered in any patient with HIV with dyspnea of unknown origin, irrespective of the level of immune compromise [80]. A family history is necessary to assess for heritable PAH, which in a majority of cases is caused by mutations in the gene encoding the TGF-β receptor BMPR2 and displays an autosomal dominant pattern of inheritance [81–84]. However, due to incomplete penetrance, patients with heritable PAH may not always recollect a family member known to be afflicted with the disease. Alternatively, affected family members of previous generations may have been misdiagnosed as having another cardiopulmonary condition given a relative lack of awareness of PAH in preceding decades.

Clinical Approach: Physical Examination

In concert with a focused history, the physical examination can offer critical insights into the possible causes of PH and it severity. An anatomic-based approach is presented here.

Head and Neck

Underlying conditions that can predispose to PH often have manifestations in the head and neck. Sarcoidosis may be associated with cranial nerve deficits, parotid or lacrimal gland enlargement, ocular findings (uveitis, conjunctival nodules), or hypopigmentation around the hairline. Lymphadenopathy might suggest sarcoidosis or a lymphoproliferative disorder. Scleral icterus suggests hepatobiliary dysfunction. Proptosis in conjunction with an enlarged thyroid may be indicative of Graves' disease. An enlarged tongue, or periorbital purpura, may suggest systemic amyloidosis. Stigmata of connective tissue disease include malar rash, oral ulcers, loss of naso-labial folds, microstomia, and telangiectasias. A preponderance of telangiectasias involving mucous membranes should also raise suspicion of hereditary hemorrhagic telangiectasia (Osler-Weber-Rendu syndrome). A short, thick neck with low-riding soft palate or tonsillar crowding should raise the possibility of obstructive sleep apnea. Hypoxemic patients may display peri-oral cyanosis. Ulceration of the nasal septum may be seen in either sarcoidosis or ANCA-associated vasculitis. Aortic stenosis may result in a delayed carotid upstroke, whereas a bounding pulse may indicate aortic insufficiency or a hyperdynamic circulation, as seen in advanced cirrhosis, hyperthyroid states, or left-to-right shunting. An assessment of jugular venous pressure should be made in all patients as a surrogate for right atrial pressure; prominent *v* waves within the venous pulse contour indicate the presence of tricuspid regurgitation.

Cardiovascular

For obvious reasons, a careful cardiac examination is required in all patients with suspected PH. A prominent pulmonary component of the second heart sound (P_2) heard best over the left sternal border in the second to fourth intercostal space is present in most patients with idiopathic PAH, but requires practice to appreciate [13]. Regurgitant murmurs related to tricuspid, and less commonly pulmonic, insufficiency may be found. An RV lift and right-sided S_4 are clues to RV hypertrophy. A right-sided S_3 indicates compromised RV function and correlates with reduced cardiac output [13]. Right-sided gallops are best appreciated along the left sternal border. Fixed splitting of the second heart sound is observed in the setting of an ASD; a pansystolic murmur may indicate the presence of a VSD, whereas a constant, machine-like murmur is classically associated with a PDA. Murmurs associated with either aortic or mitral valve pathology and S_3 or S_4 gallops heard best towards the apex suggest underlying left-sided heart disease. Systemic hypotension with a narrow pulse pressure, tachycardia, and cool extremities are ominous signs of a low cardiac output state. Patients suspected of having left-to-right shunting should undergo a search for arteriovenous communications, including iatrogenic fistulae such as those created intentionally for hemodialysis or inadvertently during femoral vascular cannulation.

Pulmonary

Patients with idiopathic, heritable, or toxin-mediated PAH typically have an unremarkable pulmonary examination. In patients with PH due to left-sided heart disease and cardiogenic edema, rales may be appreciated along with dullness to percussion signifying the presence of pleural effusions; the latter finding may also be associated with liver disease. Fine, Velcro-type rales suggest fibrotic lung disease. Wheezing or rhonchi should prompt consideration of chronic obstructive pulmonary disease. Patients with chronic thromboembolic disease may exhibit a pulmonary artery bruit, caused by turbulent blood flow through narrowed proximal pulmonary arteries. The bruit is heard best by auscultation of the interscapular area during a breath hold.

Gastrointestinal

Hepatomegaly, pulsatility of the liver, and ascites may be seen in the setting of chronic elevations in right heart pressure due to PH of any cause. Concomitant splenomegaly or the presence of caput medusae suggests underlying portal hypertension, whereas isolated splenomegaly may be indicative of a lymphoproliferative disorder. Ascites can be a presenting manifestation of constrictive pericarditis. Occasionally, patients with PAH treated with epoprostenol may develop ascites in the absence of portal hypertension [85]. Epoprostenol therapy also has been associated with progressive splenomegaly when used for the treatment of patients with portopulmonary hypertension [86, 87].

Skin, Muscles, and Joints

A thorough musculoskeletal and skin examination should be performed with particular attention to findings that may implicate an underlying connective tissue disease, such as skin thickening, sclerodactyly, rash, telangiectasias (which could also indicate liver cirrhosis), synovitis, or ulcerative lesions. Clubbing of the digits may be seen with interstitial or chronic hypoxemic lung disease, cystic fibrosis, bronchiectasis, thoracic malignancy, congenital cyanotic heart disease, pulmonary veno-occlusive disease (PVOD), and chronic inflammatory states such as inflammatory bowel disease or endocarditis. Muscle wasting may reflect generalized malnutrition or neuromuscular disease. In patients receiving vasodilator therapy for PAH (in particular prostacyclin analogues), flushing of the skin may be noted.

Diagnostic Testing

Echocardiography

In contemporary practice, 2DE remains the most common modality leading to suspicion of PH and the most common screening tool used to assess patients suspected of having PH. It can readily estimate pulmonary arterial systolic pressure (assuming certain conditions are met) and also provides supplementary anatomic and physiologic information that can help elucidate the underlying pathophysiologic mechanisms responsible for PH as well as gauge its severity vis-à-vis right heart function. 2DE is best used as a screening tool when PH is suspected due to the presence of certain symptoms or examination findings. 2DE is discussed in more detail in Chap. 9, but a brief discussion will be presented here.

When faced with an echocardiogram reporting elevations in pulmonary arterial systolic pressure (PASP), the clinician must attempt to answer several questions:

1. *Is the reported PASP accurate?*
2. *If accurate, does the patient indeed have PH?*
3. *If PH is present, what is the etiology?*
4. *To what degree is the presence of PH impacting circulatory function?*

2DE is an imperfect diagnostic test with limitations in both sensitivity and specificity. Nevertheless, an understanding of its strengths and limitations will allow the clinician to risk-stratify a patient with cardiopulmonary symptoms and help direct the remainder of the diagnostic evaluation.

Echocardiography laboratories typically calculate and report PASP using the modified Bernoulli principle, according to the following equation:

$$\mathrm{PASP} \approx \mathrm{RVSP} \approx 4 \times \mathrm{TR}_{\mathrm{vel}}{}^{2} + \mathrm{RAP}$$

PASP will equal RV systolic pressure (RVSP) in the absence of pulmonic valve stenosis. $\mathrm{TR}_{\mathrm{vel}}$ and RAP denote Doppler-derived velocity of the tricuspid regurgitation (TR) jet and an estimate of right atrial pressure, respectively. While there is some debate as to the upper limit of normal of 2DE-derived PASP, a value of 40 mmHg is reasonable based on the available evidence, although older subjects may require a higher cutoff [1, 88]. In carefully studied populations, there is a strong correlation between 2DE- and RHC-derived values for PASP using traditional linear regression analysis when comparative measurements are obtained in close temporal proximity [89, 90]. However, suboptimal visualization or improper Doppler interrogation of the TR jet may lead to inaccurate estimates of TR_{vel}; the error associated with this inaccuracy is then magnified exponentially. Also, some patients will have insufficient TR to measure TRvel. Estimates of RAP based on an assessment of inferior cava collapsibility are also prone to error [91]. Contemporary studies of PH referral populations using Bland-Altman analysis suggest that ~50 % of 2DE-derived PASP estimates are inaccurate; both over- and underestimation occur, though the magnitude of underestimation appears to be greater [91, 92]. Thus, 2DE estimates of PASP should be viewed as simply one piece of information as part of a broader 2DE assessment of the right heart–pulmonary circulation–left heart axis.

Because the hemodynamic definition of PH requires knowledge of the *mean* PAP, PASP from 2DE cannot be used to define the presence or absence of PH. Although techniques exist to derive mPAP from acceleration time within the RV outflow tract (RVOT) [93], they are not commonly reported on most echocardiograms. Alternatively, mPAP may be estimated using formulas based on PASP [94, 95]; however, such methods are not recommended to replace invasive determination of mPAP by RHC, wherein other hemodynamic variables pertinent to the evaluation of patients with suspected pulmonary vascular disease can be obtained.

If the 2DE-derived PASP is consistent with PH, perhaps the most critical issue the clinician faces is determining the likelihood that the PH is arterial (i.e., PAH) vs. venous (related to left atrial hypertension) in origin, given the ramifications for prognosis and management. In such cases, RHC is required to confirm (or refute) the suspicion and guide therapy. While RHC has a relatively low risk of complications, performing RHC on all patients with elevated PASP on 2DE is neither practical nor desirable. At present, the ideal approach to noninvasively gauge the pretest probability of pulmonary vascular disease so as to optimize use of RHC is unknown. In practice, this decision is influenced by several factors, including the patient's risk of harboring PAH, results of other noninvasive testing (discussed below), and features on 2DE.

Beyond estimation of PASP, a thorough survey of parameters of right and left heart chamber size and function can be extremely helpful in assessing the likelihood that PAH is present. In general, the greater the extent of abnormalities related to right heart size and/or function, the higher the likelihood of PAH. When abnormalities in left heart size and/or function dominate the echocardiographic picture, there is a greater likelihood of pulmonary venous hypertension [96]. Simple indices of right heart pressure or volume overload easily seen on an apical four-chamber view include an RV:LV size ratio >1, flattening or leftward bowing of the interventricular septum, and encroachment of the RV into the apex. The presence of a mid- or late-systolic "notch" within the RVOT Doppler flow velocity envelope strongly predicts the presence of a PVR >3 Wood units [97]. A reduced tricuspid annular plane systolic excursion (TAPSE) is an easily obtainable surrogate of compromised RV longitudinal shortening and cardiac output, and has prognostic value in PAH [98–100]. When such findings are seen in the absence of significant left heart abnormalities, the clinician should increase his/her suspicion that PAH is present. In contrast, left ventricular systolic or diastolic dysfunction, left ventricular enlargement or hypertrophy, left atrial enlargement, or significant aortic or mitral valvular disease suggests a substrate for increased left atrial pressure and thus pulmonary venous hypertension. A 2DE-based prediction rule incorporating left atrial size, Doppler-based parameters from the RVOT (acceleration time, presence of notching), and lateral mitral E:e′ (a surrogate for left atrial filling pressure) was recently shown to have an area under the receiver operator characteristic (ROC) curve of 0.92 for the identification of PAH [101]. A pericardial effusion, while not specific for PAH, has been consistently associated with a poor prognosis in this group [102–105]. Lastly, 2DE (with or without agitated saline contrast) may disclose evidence of an intracardiac shunt, which could be the cause of PH (e.g., ASD, VSD, PDA), or, in the case of a PFO, may explain significant shunt-type hypoxemia in a patient with idiopathic or other types of PAH and elevated right heart pressures. If suspicion of an intracardiac shunt is high but transthoracic 2DE is nondiagnostic, transesophageal echocardiography [106] or cardiac magnetic resonance [107] should be performed. A comparison of various 2DE parameters which can help the clinician distinguish pulmonary arterial vs. venous hypertension is provided in Table 8.4.

The issue of diastolic dysfunction in the context of PH deserves additional comment. The clinician should recognize that diastolic dysfunction may worsen with exercise due to further impairment in filling time secondary to increased heart rate, and as such may be underappreciated as a cause of exertional dyspnea based on 2DE parameters obtained at rest. In such situations, assessment of diastolic function with exercise 2DE may be informative [108]. While diastolic dys-

Table 8.4 Echocardiographic parameters to distinguish pulmonary arterial from pulmonary venous hypertension

Pulmonary arterial hypertension	Pulmonary venous hypertension
2-D Imaging	
Normal LV ejection fraction	Reduced LV ejection fraction
Normal or size or small (underfilled) LV	Dilated LV
Dilated RA/Normal LA	Normal RA/Dilated LA
No LVH	LVH
RV:LV size ratio > 1	RV:LV size ratio < 1
RV apex-forming	RV not apex-forming
Reduced RV function/TAPSE	Normal RV function/TAPSE
Doppler imaging	
Grade I or no diastolic dysfunction	Grade II–III diastolic dysfunction
Minimal or no mitral/aortic valve disease	≥Moderate mitral/aortic valve disease
Systolic notching of FVE in RVOT	No systolic notching of FVE in RVOT
AcT of FVE in RVOT <70 ms	AcT of FVE in RVOT >95 ms

Adapted with permission from [96]

LV left ventricle, *RA* right atrium, *LA* left atrium, *RV* right ventricle, *LVH* left ventricular hypertrophy, *TAPSE* tricuspid annular plane systolic excursion, *FVE* flow velocity envelope, *RVOT* right ventricular outflow tract, *AcT* acceleration time

function appears to be very common, particularly in the elderly or those with other comorbidities as discussed previously, patients with PAH due to pulmonary vascular disease may also exhibit impaired left ventricular relaxation as a consequence of pathologic right → left ventricular interaction [66, 109]. A recent study of idiopathic/heritable PAH patients found an 88 % prevalence of Grade 1 diastolic dysfunction (impaired relaxation) [68]. Thus, the simple presence of mild diastolic dysfunction or impaired relaxation in the setting of an elevated PASP should not be considered synonymous with pulmonary venous hypertension. Rather, the clinician should attempt to integrate this finding with the overall clinical picture and echocardiographic assessment of left and right heart function to arrive at an assessment of the likely etiology of PH.

Using 2DE as a screening tool in populations considered at high risk for PAH has been recommended by various professional societies, although this is largely based on expert opinion [6–8]. Regular screening with 2DE seems reasonable for patients with a family history of PAH or with known BMPR2 mutations given that ~20 % of carriers will ultimately develop PAH [110, 111]. In dyspneic patients with scleroderma but without significant lung disease, ~8 % will have PAH by RHC [112]. Screening of patients with the scleroderma spectrum of diseases is recommended. The DETECT study provides useful guidance in this regard [113]. Screening methods in this setting can include a combination of PFTs with diffusion capacity for carbon monoxide (DLco), serum levels of brain natriuretic peptide (BNP) or its N-terminal pro-hormone (NT-proBNP), and echocardiography. As mentioned previously, given the elevated morbidity associated with uncontrolled portopulmonary hypertension in the setting of liver transplantation, 2DE should be performed in all patients being considered for this procedure [37].

Chest X-ray (CXR)

Given its relative low cost and ease, the CXR can provide useful information in the evaluation of patients with suspected PH; however, its suboptimal sensitivity precludes its use as a primary screening modality [114]. General CXR findings of PH include enlarged main pulmonary arteries and right-sided cardiac chamber enlargement; however, such changes may not be apparent in less advanced PH. In the NIH primary PH registry, 90 % of subjects displayed prominence of the main pulmonary artery [13]. An obliterated retrosternal air space as visualized on the lateral projection specifically suggests RV hypertrophy. When PAH is present and related to increased PVR, rapid tapering (or "pruning") of the pulmonary arteries may be seen. In contrast, when PH is related to increases in left atrial pressure or high pulmonary flow from an anatomic shunt, increased vascular markings and Kerley B lines may be observed; a similar pattern is associated with PVOD where the resistance to blood flow through the small pulmonary veins can result in areas of increased pulmonary capillary pressure. Focal areas of oligemia or an abrupt cutoff of a pulmonary artery should raise suspicion for CTEPH [115], particularly when pleural abnormalities are present which may represent sequelae of prior infarcts [116, 117]. Calcification of the pulmonary arteries has been described in congenital heart disease with reversed shunts (Eisenmenger syndrome) [118], and occasionally large pulmonary artery aneurysms may develop in cases of long-standing PAH. CXR may be particularly useful in assessing for associated conditions that may cause PH, such as hyperinflation (COPD), increased reticulation/cystic changes/honeycombing (interstitial lung disease/pulmonary fibrosis), or reduced lung volumes that may be associated with hypoventilation (obesity hypoventilation syndrome, neuromuscular, or skeletal conditions).

Electrocardiogram (ECG)

Like CXR, the ECG is a readily obtainable ancillary tool that may corroborate a suspicion for PH, but is of limited sensitivity, particularly in the detection of early disease [114]. While a majority of patients with significant PAH will display findings of right axis deviation, RV hypertrophy or RV strain, up to 13 % of patients will have a normal ECG [13, 119]. Recently, a QRS duration of ≥120 ms was found to be an independent predictor of mortality in a small cohort of IPAH subjects [120]. When evaluating a patient with known PH who is clinically deteriorating, the ECG can confirm suspicion of a tachy- or bradyarrhythmia as a contributing factor.

Pulmonary Function Tests (PFTs) and Arterial Blood Gas (ABG) Analysis

PFTs are commonly obtained in the evaluation of the dyspneic patient. In the context of suspected PH, they are extremely important in determining whether airway or parenchymal lung processes are present which may account for PH (i.e., Group 3 PH). A mild restrictive defect may be seen in IPAH [13, 121] and may be related to bronchial and vascular smooth muscle hypertrophy [122] or respiratory muscle weakness [123, 124]. Interestingly, IPAH has also been associated with peripheral airway obstruction [125, 126]. Thus, mild perturbations in pulmonary function indices should not immediately implicate the presence of intrinsic lung disease, but should trigger consideration of such potential etiologies; in such cases, chest CT can be very useful in refining the clinical assessment. The attribution of PH to intrinsic parenchymal or airway disease engenders uncertainty when spirometric or lung volume parameters fall within moderate grades of dysfunction, as studies have not typically proven a strong correlation between the severity of lung disease and the presence or severity of PH, although PH is typically associated with more advanced lung disease [43, 127–133]. Recently, PH has been identified as a significant complication of the combined pulmonary fibrosis and emphysema syndrome [134, 135]. These patients may display relatively preserved ("pseudonormalized") spirometry and lung volumes due to the counterbalancing effects of coexistent restriction and obstruction, but typically have significant reductions in DLco and abnormal CT imaging.

It appears that an assessment of DLco may be a more specific marker of pulmonary vascular disease, particularly when reduced "out of proportion" to reductions in lung volumes. A reduced DLco is common in IPAH (found in 75 % of patients [121]), and in the scleroderma population may signal the occult presence or future development of PH [136]. In a cohort of scleroderma patients suspected of having PH based on certain clinical characteristics, a percent-predicted FVC/DLco ratio of >2 displayed a negative and positive predictive value of ~70 % for the diagnosis of PAH [137]. Utilizing a lower cutoff (>1.6) [138] may improve the sensitivity of this parameter for the detection of PAH, though comparative data are lacking. In practice, the finding of an isolated reduction in DLco in the absence of significant anemia should heighten one's suspicion for the presence of pulmonary vascular disease.

ABG analysis should be performed to confirm a suspected hypoventilatory disorder, and may also quantify severity of hypoxemia. If shunt physiology is suspected, the ABG should be performed after inspiring 100 % oxygen for 20–30 min via a tight-fitting mask which can permit estimation of the right-to-left shunt fraction (Q_s/Q_t) [139].

Ventilation-Perfusion (V/Q) Scintigraphy

The V/Q study remains an integral component of the workup of patients with suspected PH, mainly to exclude the presence of chronic thromboembolic disease. In CTEPH, perfusion images will demonstrate at least one (or multiple) segmental or larger mismatched defects [140, 141]. V/Q has demonstrated superior sensitivity over CT angiography for the diagnosis of CTEPH. In one study where digital subtraction pulmonary angiography was used as the reference standard, V/Q scan displayed 97.4 % sensitivity and 98.5 % negative predictive value for the diagnosis of CTEPH (where a positive test was defined as an intermediate or high probability result), whereas CT angiography only displayed 51.3 % sensitivity and 79.7 % negative predictive value [142]. Thus, a normal V/Q scan essentially rules out chronic thromboembolism. A positive scan, however, cannot be used to make definitive statements regarding the anatomic extent of clot burden as the V/Q tends to underestimate the amount of disease observed at pulmonary angiogram or endarterectomy [143]. Patients with IPAH may also display an abnormal pattern on V/Q, described as a diffuse patchy abnormality or "mottled" appearance [13]. While it has been suggested that a high-probability scan due to PVOD may mimic CTEPH [144], a larger series has recently failed to confirm this association [145]. Rarely, tumor microemboli can lead to a clinical presentation very similar to CTEPH with mismatched defects seen on V/Q scanning [146, 147]. If right-to-left shunt is suspected, the clinician can request additional perfusion images be obtained over the brain and kidneys; detection of tracer in these regions implicates the presence of an anatomic shunt [148], but does not disclose the specific location (intracardiac, intrapulmonary, etc.).

Chest Computed Tomography (CT)

When performed for other reasons, findings on CT that may suggest the presence of pulmonary hypertension include an enlarged pulmonary artery (>29 mm in diameter [149] or pulmonary artery:aorta diameter ratio >1 [150]) and/or enlarged right-sided cardiac chambers with or without septal shift [151, 152], pericardial effusion [153], or reflux of contrast into the IVC and hepatic veins in the setting of elevated right atrial pressure [154]. In patients with chronic dyspnea and clinical concern for PH, nonenhanced CT scanning of the chest should be considered to exclude parenchymal lung disease, particularly when suggested by examination or PFT findings. This may be particularly important in patients with collagen vascular diseases who may be at risk for various types of interstitial disease (e.g., nonspecific, usual, or lymphocytic interstitial pneumonia or organizing pneumonia). PVOD is associated with several specific findings on chest CT that may aid in identifying the diagnosis and are related to the consequences of postcapillary venular obstruction to pulmonary blood flow, such as bilateral pleural effusions, mediastinal lymphadenopathy, and prominence of the interlobular septae and/or centrilobular opacities [155, 156]. This pattern may also be seen with pulmonary venous hypertension arising from left heart disease.

Contrast-enhanced CT angiography (CTA) can provide useful information regarding the anatomy of the pulmonary vasculature. Results from the Prospective Investigation of Pulmonary Embolism Diagnosis (PIOPED) II study indicate that CTA has an overall sensitivity of 83 % for the diagnosis of acute PE; its NPV is 96 % when clinical pretest probability is low, but falls to only 60 % when clinical suspicion is high [157]. CTA may prove useful for mapping proximal clot burden in CTEPH, but displays limited sensitivity for the detection of peripheral small vessel involvement as discussed previously [142]. Endoluminal CTA findings of CTEPH include eccentric or concentric luminal irregularities, abrupt cutoffs, webs, and pouches [158]. Additional findings that may implicate CTEPH include bronchial artery dilation [159, 160] and mosaic attenuation of the lung parenchyma [158, 161], because of either hypoperfusion of obstructed segments or regional air trapping secondary to vascular-mediated alterations in small airway tone. CTA can also identify other nonthrombotic lesions of the pulmonary vascular bed. Takayasu's arteritis is a large-vessel vasculitis which may affect the pulmonary circulation in a significant number of cases and may be misdiagnosed as CTEPH [162]. The presence of concomitant aortic disease should raise the suspicion for Takayasu's, although isolated pulmonary arteritis has been reported [163]. Other CTA findings that may differentiate this entity from CTEPH include circumferential pulmonary arterial wall thickening and delayed mural enhancement [164, 165]. Pulmonary artery aneurysms may be seen in Behçet's disease [165, 166].

Overnight Oximetry and Polysomnography (PSG)

Overnight pulse oximetry in the home is a relatively simple test to search for nocturnal hypoxemia. Nocturnal oxygen desaturation may occur in the IPAH population in the absence of sleep-disordered breathing [167]. Correction with supplemental oxygen is intuitive but it is not known whether such a strategy improves outcomes. Standard polysomnography is the gold standard for the diagnosis of obstructive sleep apnea.

Exercise Testing

The 6-min walk test (6MWT) is a submaximal test of exercise capacity that has been employed extensively in the evaluation and management of patients with PH. It is inexpensive, reproducible, and easy to perform by most patients, even those with more advanced disease. In the PAH population, results from the 6MWT have been shown to correlate with functional class, hemodynamics (CO and total pulmonary resistance), as well as peak oxygen consumption as determined by cardiopulmonary exercise testing [168]. Contemporary, prospective cohort studies indicate that the 6MWT has independent prognostic value in PAH in addition to parameters related to right heart function [102, 169]. Although a matter of some debate, it appears that it is the absolute value of 6MWT that is prognostically most relevant rather than the magnitude of change over time, as studies have failed to show a consistent association between improvements in walk distance on-therapy and outcomes [170–172]. Values below 300–380 m at baseline or after a period of time on-treatment have been associated with a worse prognosis in various studies [168, 173–175].

Cardiopulmonary exercise testing (CPET) is a maximal exercise study which is more labor-intensive, but provides the most comprehensive, integrative assessment of cardiac, pulmonary, and peripheral muscle function at progressively higher workloads. Abnormalities on CPET associated with pulmonary vascular disease include a reduced peak oxygen uptake, increased ventilatory inefficiency (as reflected by an elevated ratio of minute ventilation to CO_2 production [V_E/V_{CO2}] and reduced end-tidal CO_2), and reduced oxygen pulse [176]; however, these are not specific to pulmonary vascular disease and can be seen in obstructive and restrictive disorders as well as left heart failure. This combination of derangements is more likely to represent PAH when other ancillary tests (chest imaging, PFTs, 2DE, etc.) do not suggest an alternate diagnosis. One study of IPAH subjects found peak oxygen uptake to be an independent predictor of mortality [177], prompting some to advocate a treat-to-target (goal-oriented) strategy incorporating this parameter to help guide therapeutic decisions [178]. However, this approach has not been externally validated and therefore the use of CPET for this purpose remains center-dependent. Marked elevation of V_E/V_{CO2} in the absence of major ventilatory abnormality on PFTs can be a sign of right-to-left shunting or thromboembolic PH. CPET is discussed in more detail in Chap. 11.

Serologic Tests

Serologic tests can provide useful information in establishing potential etiologies of PH as well as help guide therapy. From a diagnostic perspective, serologies play a central role in confirming chronic viral hepatitis or HIV infection. The presence of certain autoantibodies may suggest the presence of an underlying connective tissue disease when considered in the context of appropriate clinical features. In the original NIH primary PH registry, 29 % of subjects had a positive antinuclear antibody (ANA) [13]. In scleroderma, anticentromere antibodies are usually associated with limited disease, and anti-Scl-70 antibodies with diffuse disease. The presence of antibodies against U3-RNP (fibrillarin) is associated specifically with PAH [179, 180].

In cases of CTEPH, the only consistent hypercoagulable abnormality identified has been the presence of antiphospholipid antibodies, found in up to 20 % of cases [181, 182]. Most patients, however, do not have any identifiable abnormality in coagulation, and therefore the lack of any laboratory-identified hypercoagulable state cannot be used to exclude the possibility of CTEPH.

BNP and NT-proBNP are proteins released from myocardial tissue in the setting of pressure or volume overload. Serum levels of BNP peptides may be elevated in patients with PAH and RV dysfunction, and lower levels have been associated with better outcomes [102, 175, 183, 184]. It is important to note that BNP is not specific to the RV and can be elevated in left-sided congestive heart failure and in renal dysfunction. In cases where PH is suspected to be related to HFpEF, BNP may be particularly unreliable, as a recent study demonstrated that 29 % of symptomatic outpatients with HFpEF and hemodynamically confirmed elevations in PCWP had a normal BNP level [41]. Studies in left-sided heart failure suggest that elevations in BNP or NT-proBNP may be attenuated by obesity, possibly related to either underproduction or increased peripheral clearance by adipose tissue [185–187]. A recent analysis of a PAH cohort has shown that, despite higher right-sided filling pressures, obese PAH patients have lower BNP levels than those who are not obese [188].

Other laboratory tests frequently obtained include complete blood count and general chemistries including indices of renal and hepatic function. Anemia should raise suspicion of a possible hemolytic disorder in the appropriate clinical context. Among patients with nonhemolytic PAH, iron deficiency and/or frank anemia occurs in ~25–60 % and has been shown to be a negative prognostic factor [189–191]. Anemia can also be seen as a side effect of treatment with endothelin receptor antagonists (ERAs). Thrombocytopenia should raise consideration of cirrhosis, HIV infection, or autoimmune disease. Prostacyclin therapy can also induce thrombocytopenia which in some cases may be related to splenomegaly [86]. Right-sided heart failure can lead to congestive hepatopathy; this pattern usually is characterized by a predominant rise in unconjugated bilirubin with minimal elevation in alkaline phosphatase and transaminases [192], though more dramatic rises in these latter parameters can be seen with severe RV failure and low cardiac output. Alternatively, a predominant liver injury pattern with elevated transaminases has been associated with ERA therapy [193, 194] which is dose-dependent and reversible upon discontinuation. Hyponatremia occurs in the setting of right heart failure and has been associated with worse prognosis [195].

Right Heart Catheterization (RHC)

For reasons discussed previously, RHC remains the gold standard for the diagnosis and characterization of elevated pulmonary artery pressures and is discussed in detail in Chap. 10. RHC serves to confirm the presence of PH, elucidate its hemodynamic origin, and, in cases of precapillary PAH, assess the extent of pulmonary vasoreactivity in response to a short-acting pulmonary vasodilator. Distinguishing between pre- and postcapillary causes of PH is critical, and thus requires an accurate assessment of left-sided filling pressures. Pressure measurements should always be made at end expiration. Failure to do so, or using the digital average reported by the pressure recorder, may result in an underestimation of PCWP and thus misclassification of left heart disease as pulmonary arterial hypertension, particularly in patients with concomitant hypoxic lung disease or morbid obesity [196]. When there is a high suspicion for pulmonary venous hypertension but measured PCWP is normal or borderline, a direct measurement of left ventricular end-diastolic pressure (LVEDP) may help avoid misclassification [197]. RHC by itself is very safe with an extremely low risk of mortality (≤0.2 %) [198, 199].

Assessment of PA Pressures with Exercise

Given that many patients only complain of symptoms with a certain amount of activity, assessing the hemodynamic response to exercise makes intuitive sense to better characterize changes in pressures, flow, and resistance in an attempt to define the predominant pathophysiology. While previous definitions of PH included an exercise criterion (mPAP >30 mmHg at peak exercise), current consensus statements have eliminated a definition of exercise-induced PH [6, 7]. This decision was largely based on growing uncertainty as to what constitutes a normal physiologic response of the pulmonary vascular bed to exercise. A recent literature synthesis on the topic concluded that ~20 % of healthy subjects aged <50 years will exceed an mPAP of 30 mmHg when exercised in the supine position, with an upper limit of normal (defined as 2 standard deviations above the mean) of 37 mmHg at maximal exercise. Older healthy subjects (≥50 years) may in fact have greater rises in pulmonary pressures; in this subgroup, the mean mPAP during "slight" exercise was 29.4 ± 8.4 mmHg, yielding an upper limit of normal of 46 mmHg. Older subjects display higher PCWP with exercise than do younger subjects (16.8 ± 6.5 vs. 10.9 ± 3.9 mmHg) [200].

With these concerns is mind, data exist to suggest that exercise-induced PH may be clinically relevant. Grunig et al. have demonstrated greater rises in PASP with exercise in both asymptomatic carriers of the BMPR2 mutation [201] and relatives of patients with idiopathic and heritable PAH [202]. Tolle and colleagues described CPET characteristics of patients with exercise-induced PAH (defined as a maximum mPAP ≥30 mmHg with PCWP <20 mmHg). This group displayed decrements in aerobic capacity and hemodynamic perturbations that were intermediate between normals and those with resting PAH [203]. Steen et al. performed exercise 2DE on patients with scleroderma who, based on certain clinical characteristics, were deemed to be at higher risk for PH. Exercised-induced PH by 2DE was defined as an increase in the PASP of ≥20 mmHg from baseline. They found that 44 % of patients displayed a positive exercise 2DE, which was confirmed to be PAH by RHC in 81 % of patients; in 12.5 % of cases the positive 2DE was due to pulmonary venous hypertension from diastolic dysfunction [204]. Mild elevations in PA pressure with moderate exercise have been associated with reduced exercise capacity in scleroderma [205]. In a large registry of CTD-associated PAH in the United Kingdom, 16 % of patients in the absence of significant lung disease had exercise-induced PAH as defined by invasive hemodynamic criteria of a mean PAP over 30 mmHg during exercise. Of these, 19 % displayed progression to resting PAH and four out of five reported deaths in this subgroup were attributed to PAH [206]. At present, however, it is unknown whether specific interventions aimed at reducing peak PA pressures in these populations will have a benefit on longer-term outcomes. Recently, a small, uncontrolled pilot study of ambrisentan in scleroderma-spectrum patients with exercise-induced PAH suggested a beneficial effect on hemodynamics and 6-min walk distance [207].

Assessing invasive hemodynamics may be particularly helpful in patients without clear risk factors for PAH and where occult HFpEF is suspected. In a study of 55 patients with exertional dyspnea with normal LVEF, BNP level, and resting hemodynamics, 58 % of subjects displayed abnormal increases in left-heart filling pressures (defined as PCWP ≥25 mmHg) with exercise [208]. In the series of patients undergoing CPET and exercise RHC for the evaluation of unexplained dyspnea reported by Tolle et al., 27 % of subjects were identified as having left ventricular diastolic dysfunction [203].

Concluding Remarks

Pulmonary hypertension can occur in many contexts. Echocardiographic diagnosis of PH has become increasingly common due to increased use of 2DE for the assessment of various cardiac and pulmonary complaints. Differentiation of pulmonary arterial from pulmonary venous hypertension is crucial to identify patients with an elevated risk of morbidity and mortality and allow institution of appropriate therapies. Ultimately, the diagnosis of PAH must be made at right heart catheterization. A thorough history, physical examination, laboratory investigation, and use of ancillary tests will aid the clinician in formulating a pretest probability of pulmonary vascular disease.

Table 8.5 summarizes various clinical features that should trigger suspicion for the presence of pulmonary arterial hypertension. In general, the greater number of such features, the higher the likelihood of PAH. In such patients, RHC should be pursued, and measurement of exercise hemodynamics should be considered if resting values are not informative.

Table 8.5 Summary of clinical features that should increase suspicion for the presence of PAH

Predisposing conditions	Symptoms and exam findings	Echocardiogram	PFTs	ECG
• BMPR2 mutation carrier • Anorexigen or stimulant use • CTD • Portal hypertension • Congenital heart disease • Prior PE • HIV	• Progressive dyspnea • Edema • Ascites • Lack of orthopnea • Prominent P_2 • JVD • Lack of rales • Hepatomegaly	• Relatively normal left heart • Dilated or dysfunctional RV • Rightward septal shift	• Relatively normal spirometry and lung volumes • Reduced DLco • FVC%/ DLco% > 1.6–2.0	• Rightward axis • RV strain

BMPR2 bone morphogenetic protein receptor type 2, *CTD* connective tissue disease, *PE* pulmonary embolism, *HIV* human immunodeficiency virus, *JVD* jugular venous distention, *RV* right ventricle, *DLco* diffusing capacity of the lung for carbon monoxide, *FVC* forced vital capacity

References

1. Lam CS, Borlaug BA, Kane GC, et al. Age-associated increases in pulmonary artery systolic pressure in the general population. Circulation. 2009;119:2663–70.
2. Leung CC, Moondra V, Catherwood E, et al. Prevalence and risk factors of pulmonary hypertension in patients with elevated pulmonary venous pressure and preserved ejection fraction. Am J Cardiol. 2010;106:284–6.
3. Bursi F, McNallan SM, Redfield MM, et al. Pulmonary pressures and death in heart failure: a community study. J Am Coll Cardiol. 2012;59:222–31.
4. Simonneau G, Gatzoulis MA, Adatia I, et al. Updated clinical classification of pulmonary hypertension. J Am Coll Cardiol. 2013;62:D34–41.
5. Brown LM, Chen H, Halpern S, et al. Delay in recognition of pulmonary arterial hypertension: factors identified from the REVEAL Registry. Chest. 2011;140:19–26.
6. McLaughlin VV, Archer SL, Badesch DB, et al. ACCF/AHA 2009 expert consensus document on pulmonary hypertension a report of the American College of Cardiology Foundation Task Force on Expert Consensus Documents and the American Heart Association developed in collaboration with the American College of Chest Physicians; American Thoracic Society, Inc.; and the Pulmonary Hypertension Association. J Am Coll Cardiol. 2009;53:1573–619.
7. Galie N, Hoeper MM, Humbert M, et al. Guidelines for the diagnosis and treatment of pulmonary hypertension. Eur Respir J. 2009;34:1219–63.
8. McGoon M, Gutterman D, Steen V, et al. Screening, early detection, and diagnosis of pulmonary arterial hypertension: ACCP evidence-based clinical practice guidelines. Chest. 2004; 126:14S–34.
9. McLaughlin VV, Langer A, Tan M, et al. Contemporary trends in the diagnosis and management of pulmonary arterial hypertension: an initiative to close the care gap. Chest. 2013;143:324–32.
10. Thenappan T, Shah SJ, Rich S, et al. A USA-based registry for pulmonary arterial hypertension: 1982–2006. Eur Respir J. 2007;30:1103–10.
11. Humbert M, Sitbon O, Chaouat A, et al. Pulmonary arterial hypertension in France: results from a national registry. Am J Respir Crit Care Med. 2006;173:1023–30.
12. Badesch DB, Raskob GE, Elliott CG, et al. Pulmonary arterial hypertension: baseline characteristics from the REVEAL Registry. Chest. 2010;137:376–87.

13. Rich S, Dantzker DR, Ayres SM, et al. Primary pulmonary hypertension: a national prospective study. Ann Intern Med. 1987;107:216–23.
14. Hoeper MM, Bogaard HJ, Condliffe R, et al. Definitions and diagnosis of pulmonary hypertension. J Am Coll Cardiol. 2013;62:D42–50.
15. Brofman BL, Charms BL, Kohn PM, et al. Unilateral pulmonary artery occlusion in man; control studies. J Thorac Surg. 1957;34:206–27.
16. Harris P, Segel N, Bishop JM. The relation between pressure and flow in the pulmonary circulation in normal subjects and in patients with chronic bronchitis and mitral stenosis. Cardiovasc Res. 1968;2:73–83.
17. Brannon ES, Merrill AJ, Warren JV, et al. The cardiac output in patients with chronic anemia as measured by the technique of right atrial catheterization. J Clin Invest. 1945;24:332–6.
18. Robson SC, Hunter S, Boys RJ, et al. Serial study of factors influencing changes in cardiac output during human pregnancy. Am J Physiol. 1989;256:H1060–5.
19. Robson SC, Hunter S, Boys RJ, et al. Serial changes in pulmonary haemodynamics during human pregnancy: a non-invasive study using Doppler echocardiography. Clin Sci (Lond). 1991;80:113–7.
20. Klein I, Ojamaa K. Thyroid hormone and the cardiovascular system. N Engl J Med. 2001;344:501–9.
21. Chu JW, Kao PN, Faul JL, et al. High prevalence of autoimmune thyroid disease in pulmonary arterial hypertension. Chest. 2002;122:1668–73.
22. Li JH, Safford RE, Aduen JF, et al. Pulmonary hypertension and thyroid disease. Chest. 2007;132:793–7.
23. Badr B, Bories P, Marais R, et al. Transonic, thermodilution, or ionic dialysance to manage vascular access: which method is best? Hemodial Int. 2014;18:127–35.
24. Horvath KA, Burke RP, Collins Jr JJ, et al. Surgical treatment of adult atrial septal defect: early and long-term results. J Am Coll Cardiol. 1992;20:1156–9.
25. Engelfriet P, Meijboom F, Boersma E, et al. Repaired and open atrial septal defects type II in adulthood: an epidemiological study of a large European cohort. Int J Cardiol. 2008;126: 379–85.
26. Kowalski HJ, Abelmann WH. The cardiac output at rest in Laennec's cirrhosis. J Clin Invest. 1953;32:1025–33.
27. Castro M, Krowka MJ, Schroeder DR, et al. Frequency and clinical implications of increased pulmonary artery pressures in liver transplantation. Mayo Clin Proc. 1996;71:543–51.
28. Krowka MJ, Swanson KL, Frantz RP, et al. Portopulmonary hypertension: results from a 10-year screening algorithm. Hepatology. 2006;44:1502–10.
29. Fritz JS, Fallon MB, Kawut SM. Pulmonary vascular complications of liver disease. Am J Respir Crit Care Med. 2013;187:133–43.
30. Colle IO, Moreau R, Godinho E, et al. Diagnosis of portopulmonary hypertension in candidates for liver transplantation: a prospective study. Hepatology. 2003;37:401–9.
31. Hadengue A, Benhayoun MK, Lebrec D, et al. Pulmonary hypertension complicating portal hypertension: prevalence and relation to splanchnic hemodynamics. Gastroenterology. 1991; 100:520–8.
32. Edwards BS, Weir EK, Edwards WD, et al. Coexistent pulmonary and portal hypertension: morphologic and clinical features. J Am Coll Cardiol. 1987;10:1233–8.
33. Swanson KL, Wiesner RH, Nyberg SL, et al. Survival in portopulmonary hypertension: Mayo Clinic experience categorized by treatment subgroups. Am J Transplant. 2008;8:2445–53.
34. Kawut SM, Taichman DB, Ahya VN, et al. Hemodynamics and survival of patients with portopulmonary hypertension. Liver Transpl. 2005;11:1107–11.
35. Krowka MJ, Mandell MS, Ramsay MA, et al. Hepatopulmonary syndrome and portopulmonary hypertension: a report of the multicenter liver transplant database. Liver Transpl. 2004;10:174–82.
36. Krowka MJ, Plevak DJ, Findlay JY, et al. Pulmonary hemodynamics and perioperative cardiopulmonary-related mortality in patients with portopulmonary hypertension undergoing liver transplantation. Liver Transpl. 2000;6:443–50.

37. Murray KF, Carithers Jr RL. AASLD practice guidelines: evaluation of the patient for liver transplantation. Hepatology. 2005;41:1407–32.
38. Kitzman DW, Gardin JM, Gottdiener JS, et al. Importance of heart failure with preserved systolic function in patients>or=65 years of age. Am J Cardiol. 2001;87:413–9.
39. Klapholz M, Maurer M, Lowe AM, et al. Hospitalization for heart failure in the presence of a normal left ventricular ejection fraction: results of the New York Heart Failure Registry. J Am Coll Cardiol. 2004;43:1432–8.
40. Lee DS, Gona P, Vasan RS, et al. Relation of disease pathogenesis and risk factors to heart failure with preserved or reduced ejection fraction: insights from the Framingham Heart Study of the National Heart, Lung, and Blood Institute. Circulation. 2009;119:3070–7.
41. Anjan VY, Loftus TM, Burke MA, et al. Prevalence, clinical phenotype, and outcomes associated with normal B-type natriuretic peptide levels in heart failure with preserved ejection fraction. Am J Cardiol. 2012;110:870–6.
42. Lam CS, Roger VL, Rodeheffer RJ, et al. Pulmonary hypertension in heart failure with preserved ejection fraction: a community-based study. J Am Coll Cardiol. 2009;53:1119–26.
43. Nunes H, Humbert M, Capron F, et al. Pulmonary hypertension associated with sarcoidosis: mechanisms, haemodynamics and prognosis. Thorax. 2006;61:68–74.
44. Palevsky HI, Cone L, Alavi A. A case of false-positive high probability ventilation-perfusion lung scan due to tuberculous mediastinal adenopathy with a discussion of other causes of false-positive high probability ventilation-perfusion lung scans. J Nucl Med. 1991;32:512–7.
45. Berry DF, Buccigrossi D, Peabody J, et al. Pulmonary vascular occlusion and fibrosing mediastinitis. Chest. 1986;89:296–301.
46. Robbins IM, Colvin EV, Doyle TP, et al. Pulmonary vein stenosis after catheter ablation of atrial fibrillation. Circulation. 1998;98:1769–75.
47. Saad EB, Marrouche NF, Saad CP, et al. Pulmonary vein stenosis after catheter ablation of atrial fibrillation: emergence of a new clinical syndrome. Ann Intern Med. 2003;138:634–8.
48. Mandel J, Mark EJ, Hales CA. Pulmonary veno-occlusive disease. Am J Respir Crit Care Med. 2000;162:1964–73.
49. Montani D, Price LC, Dorfmuller P, et al. Pulmonary veno-occlusive disease. Eur Respir J. 2009;33:189–200.
50. Palmer SM, Robinson LJ, Wang A, et al. Massive pulmonary edema and death after prostacyclin infusion in a patient with pulmonary veno-occlusive disease. Chest. 1998;113:237–40.
51. Pietra GG, Capron F, Stewart S, et al. Pathologic assessment of vasculopathies in pulmonary hypertension. J Am Coll Cardiol. 2004;43:25S–32.
52. Fishman AP. Hypoxia on the pulmonary circulation: how and where it acts. Circ Res. 1976;38:221–31.
53. Stenmark KR, Fagan KA, Frid MG. Hypoxia-induced pulmonary vascular remodeling: cellular and molecular mechanisms. Circ Res. 2006;99:675–91.
54. Harris P, Segel N, Green I, et al. The influence of the airways resistance and alveolar pressure on the pulmonary vascular resistance in chronic bronchitis. Cardiovasc Res. 1968;2:84–92.
55. Heath D, Gillund TD, Kay JM, et al. Pulmonary vascular disease in honeycomb lung. J Pathol Bacteriol. 1968;95:423–30.
56. Ebina M, Shimizukawa M, Shibata N, et al. Heterogeneous increase in CD34-positive alveolar capillaries in idiopathic pulmonary fibrosis. Am J Respir Crit Care Med. 2004;169:1203–8.
57. Pengo V, Lensing AW, Prins MH, et al. Incidence of chronic thromboembolic pulmonary hypertension after pulmonary embolism. N Engl J Med. 2004;350:2257–64.
58. Moser KM, Bloor CM. Pulmonary vascular lesions occurring in patients with chronic major vessel thromboembolic pulmonary hypertension. Chest. 1993;103:685–92.
59. Thistlethwaite PA, Kaneko K, Madani MM, et al. Technique and outcomes of pulmonary endarterectomy surgery. Ann Thorac Cardiovasc Surg. 2008;14:274–82.
60. Shure D, Gregoratos G, Moser KM. Fiberoptic angioscopy: role in the diagnosis of chronic pulmonary arterial obstruction. Ann Intern Med. 1985;103:844–50.
61. Rubin LJ. Diagnosis and management of pulmonary arterial hypertension: ACCP evidence-based clinical practice guidelines. Chest. 2004;126:7S–10.

62. van Wolferen SA, Marcus JT, Westerhof N, et al. Right coronary artery flow impairment in patients with pulmonary hypertension. Eur Heart J. 2008;29:120–7.
63. Kawut SM, Silvestry FE, Ferrari VA, et al. Extrinsic compression of the left main coronary artery by the pulmonary artery in patients with long-standing pulmonary hypertension. Am J Cardiol. 1999;83:984–6. A910.
64. Louie EK, Rich S, Brundage BH. Doppler echocardiographic assessment of impaired left ventricular filling in patients with right ventricular pressure overload due to primary pulmonary hypertension. J Am Coll Cardiol. 1986;8:1298–306.
65. Kasner M, Westermann D, Steendijk P, et al. Left ventricular dysfunction induced by nonsevere idiopathic pulmonary arterial hypertension: a pressure-volume relationship study. Am J Respir Crit Care Med. 2012;186:181–9.
66. Stojnic BB, Brecker SJ, Xiao HB, et al. Left ventricular filling characteristics in pulmonary hypertension: a new mode of ventricular interaction. Br Heart J. 1992;68:16–20.
67. Gan CT, Lankhaar JW, Marcus JT, et al. Impaired left ventricular filling due to right-to-left ventricular interaction in patients with pulmonary arterial hypertension. Am J Physiol Heart Circ Physiol. 2006;290:H1528–33.
68. Tonelli AR, Plana JC, Heresi GA, et al. Prevalence and prognostic value of left ventricular diastolic dysfunction in idiopathic and heritable pulmonary arterial hypertension. Chest. 2012;141:1457–65.
69. Thenappan T, Shah SJ, Gomberg-Maitland M, et al. Clinical characteristics of pulmonary hypertension in patients with heart failure and preserved ejection fraction. Circ Heart Fail. 2011;4:257–65.
70. Pugh ME, Sivarajan L, Wang L, et al. Causes of pulmonary hypertension in the elderly. Chest. 2014;146:159–66.
71. Chung L, Liu J, Parsons L, et al. Characterization of connective tissue disease-associated pulmonary arterial hypertension from REVEAL: identifying systemic sclerosis as a unique phenotype. Chest. 2010;138:1383–94.
72. Launay D, Hachulla E, Hatron PY, et al. Pulmonary arterial hypertension, a rare complication of primary Sjogren syndrome: report of 9 new cases and review of the literature. Medicine (Baltimore). 2007;86:299–315.
73. Poormoghim H, Lucas M, Fertig N, et al. Systemic sclerosis sine scleroderma: demographic, clinical, and serologic features and survival in forty-eight patients. Arthritis Rheum. 2000;43: 444–51.
74. Toya SP, Tzelepis GE. The many faces of scleroderma sine scleroderma: a literature review focusing on cardiopulmonary complications. Rheumatol Int. 2009;29:861–8.
75. Simonneau G, Azarian R, Brenot F, et al. Surgical management of unresolved pulmonary embolism: a personal series of 72 patients. Chest. 1995;107:52S–5.
76. Bonderman D, Wilkens H, Wakounig S, et al. Risk factors for chronic thromboembolic pulmonary hypertension. Eur Respir J. 2009;33:325–31.
77. Pepke-Zaba J, Delcroix M, Lang I, et al. Chronic thromboembolic pulmonary hypertension (CTEPH): results from an international prospective registry. Circulation. 2011;124: 1973–81.
78. Bonderman D, Skoro-Sajer N, Jakowitsch J, et al. Predictors of outcome in chronic thromboembolic pulmonary hypertension. Circulation. 2007;115:2153–8.
79. Chin KM, Channick RN, Rubin LJ. Is methamphetamine use associated with idiopathic pulmonary arterial hypertension? Chest. 2006;130:1657–63.
80. Mehta NJ, Khan IA, Mehta RN, et al. HIV-related pulmonary hypertension: analytic review of 131 cases. Chest. 2000;118:1133–41.
81. Deng Z, Morse JH, Slager SL, et al. Familial primary pulmonary hypertension (gene PPH1) is caused by mutations in the bone morphogenetic protein receptor-II gene. Am J Hum Genet. 2000;67:737–44.
82. Lane KB, Machado RD, Pauciulo MW, et al. Heterozygous germline mutations in BMPR2, encoding a TGF-beta receptor, cause familial primary pulmonary hypertension. Nat Genet. 2000;26:81–4.

83. Cogan JD, Pauciulo MW, Batchman AP, et al. High frequency of BMPR2 exonic deletions/duplications in familial pulmonary arterial hypertension. Am J Respir Crit Care Med. 2006;174:590–8.
84. Aldred MA, Vijayakrishnan J, James V, et al. BMPR2 gene rearrangements account for a significant proportion of mutations in familial and idiopathic pulmonary arterial hypertension. Hum Mutat. 2006;27:212–3.
85. Jones DK, Higenbottam TW, Wallwork J. Treatment of primary pulmonary hypertension intravenous epoprostenol (prostacyclin). Br Heart J. 1987;57:270–8.
86. Findlay JY, Plevak DJ, Krowka MJ, et al. Progressive splenomegaly after epoprostenol therapy in portopulmonary hypertension. Liver Transpl Surg. 1999;5:362–5.
87. Touma W, Nayak RP, Hussain Z, et al. Epoprostenol-induced hypersplenism in portopulmonary hypertension. Am J Med Sci. 2012;344:345–9.
88. McQuillan BM, Picard MH, Leavitt M, et al. Clinical correlates and reference intervals for pulmonary artery systolic pressure among echocardiographically normal subjects. Circulation. 2001;104:2797–802.
89. Currie PJ, Seward JB, Chan KL, et al. Continuous wave Doppler determination of right ventricular pressure: a simultaneous Doppler-catheterization study in 127 patients. J Am Coll Cardiol. 1985;6:750–6.
90. Chan KL, Currie PJ, Seward JB, et al. Comparison of three Doppler ultrasound methods in the prediction of pulmonary artery pressure. J Am Coll Cardiol. 1987;9:549–54.
91. Fisher MR, Forfia PR, Chamera E, et al. Accuracy of Doppler echocardiography in the hemodynamic assessment of pulmonary hypertension. Am J Respir Crit Care Med. 2009;179:615–21.
92. Rich JD, Shah SJ, Swamy RS, et al. Inaccuracy of Doppler echocardiographic estimates of pulmonary artery pressures in patients with pulmonary hypertension: implications for clinical practice. Chest. 2011;139:988–93.
93. Kitabatake A, Inoue M, Asao M, et al. Noninvasive evaluation of pulmonary hypertension by a pulsed Doppler technique. Circulation. 1983;68:302–9.
94. Chemla D, Castelain V, Provencher S, et al. Evaluation of various empirical formulas for estimating mean pulmonary artery pressure by using systolic pulmonary artery pressure in adults. Chest. 2009;135:760–8.
95. Chemla D, Castelain V, Humbert M, et al. New formula for predicting mean pulmonary artery pressure using systolic pulmonary artery pressure. Chest. 2004;126:1313–7.
96. Roberts JD, Forfia PR. Diagnosis and assessment of pulmonary vascular disease by Doppler echocardiography. Pulm Circ. 2011;1:160–81.
97. Arkles JS, Opotowsky AR, Ojeda J, et al. Shape of the right ventricular Doppler envelope predicts hemodynamics and right heart function in pulmonary hypertension. Am J Respir Crit Care Med. 2011;183:268–76.
98. Forfia PR, Fisher MR, Mathai SC, et al. Tricuspid annular displacement predicts survival in pulmonary hypertension. Am J Respir Crit Care Med. 2006;174:1034–41.
99. Rajagopalan N, Saxena N, Simon MA, et al. Correlation of tricuspid annular velocities with invasive hemodynamics in pulmonary hypertension. Congest Heart Fail. 2007;13:200–4.
100. Ghio S, Klersy C, Magrini G, et al. Prognostic relevance of the echocardiographic assessment of right ventricular function in patients with idiopathic pulmonary arterial hypertension. Int J Cardiol. 2010;140:272–8.
101. Opotowsky AR, Ojeda J, Rogers F, et al. A simple echocardiographic prediction rule for hemodynamics in pulmonary hypertension. Circ Cardiovasc Imaging. 2012;5:765–75.
102. Benza RL, Miller DP, Gomberg-Maitland M, et al. Predicting survival in pulmonary arterial hypertension: insights from the Registry to Evaluate Early and Long-Term Pulmonary Arterial Hypertension Disease Management (REVEAL). Circulation. 2010;122:164–72.
103. Raymond RJ, Hinderliter AL, Willis PW, et al. Echocardiographic predictors of adverse outcomes in primary pulmonary hypertension. J Am Coll Cardiol. 2002;39:1214–9.
104. Hinderliter AL, Willis PW, Long W, et al. Frequency and prognostic significance of pericardial effusion in primary pulmonary hypertension. Am J Cardiol. 1999;84:481–4. A410.

105. Eysmann SB, Palevsky HI, Reichek N, et al. Two-dimensional and Doppler-echocardiographic and cardiac catheterization correlates of survival in primary pulmonary hypertension. Circulation. 1989;80:353–60.
106. Gorcsan III J, Edwards TD, Ziady GM, et al. Transesophageal echocardiography to evaluate patients with severe pulmonary hypertension for lung transplantation. Ann Thorac Surg. 1995;59:717–22.
107. Diethelm L, Dery R, Lipton MJ, et al. Atrial-level shunts: sensitivity and specificity of MR in diagnosis. Radiology. 1987;162:181–6.
108. Burgess MI, Jenkins C, Sharman JE, et al. Diastolic stress echocardiography: hemodynamic validation and clinical significance of estimation of ventricular filling pressure with exercise. J Am Coll Cardiol. 2006;47:1891–900.
109. Marcus JT, Vonk Noordegraaf A, Roeleveld RJ, et al. Impaired left ventricular filling due to right ventricular pressure overload in primary pulmonary hypertension: noninvasive monitoring using MRI. Chest. 2001;119:1761–5.
110. Loyd JE, Primm RK, Newman JH. Familial primary pulmonary hypertension: clinical patterns. Am Rev Respir Dis. 1984;129:194–7.
111. Loyd JE, Butler MG, Foroud TM, et al. Genetic anticipation and abnormal gender ratio at birth in familial primary pulmonary hypertension. Am J Respir Crit Care Med. 1995; 152:93–7.
112. Hachulla E, Gressin V, Guillevin L, et al. Early detection of pulmonary arterial hypertension in systemic sclerosis: a French nationwide prospective multicenter study. Arthritis Rheum. 2005;52:3792–800.
113. Coghlan JG, Denton CP, Grunig E, et al. Evidence-based detection of pulmonary arterial hypertension in systemic sclerosis: the DETECT study. Ann Rheum Dis. 2014;73:1340–9.
114. Algeo S, Morrison D, Ovitt T, et al. Noninvasive detection of pulmonary hypertension. Clin Cardiol. 1984;7:148–56.
115. Chitwood Jr WR, Sabiston Jr DC, Wechsler AS. Surgical treatment of chronic unresolved pulmonary embolism. Clin Chest Med. 1984;5:507–36.
116. Woodruff III WW, Hoeck BE, Chitwood Jr WR, et al. Radiographic findings in pulmonary hypertension from unresolved embolism. AJR Am J Roentgenol. 1985;144:681–6.
117. Satoh T, Kyotani S, Okano Y, et al. Descriptive patterns of severe chronic pulmonary hypertension by chest radiography. Respir Med. 2005;99:329–36.
118. Timpanelli AE, Steinberg I. Calcification of the pulmonary artery in patent ductus arteriosus with reversal of blood flow: report of four cases. Am J Med. 1961;30:405–17.
119. Ahearn GS, Tapson VF, Rebeiz A, et al. Electrocardiography to define clinical status in primary pulmonary hypertension and pulmonary arterial hypertension secondary to collagen vascular disease. Chest. 2002;122:524–7.
120. Sun PY, Jiang X, Gomberg-Maitland M, et al. Prolonged QRS duration: a new predictor of adverse outcome in idiopathic pulmonary arterial hypertension. Chest. 2012;141:374–80.
121. Sun XG, Hansen JE, Oudiz RJ, et al. Pulmonary function in primary pulmonary hypertension. J Am Coll Cardiol. 2003;41:1028–35.
122. Schindler MB, Bohn DJ, Bryan AC, et al. Increased respiratory system resistance and bronchial smooth muscle hypertrophy in children with acute postoperative pulmonary hypertension. Am J Respir Crit Care Med. 1995;152:1347–52.
123. Meyer FJ, Lossnitzer D, Kristen AV, et al. Respiratory muscle dysfunction in idiopathic pulmonary arterial hypertension. Eur Respir J. 2005;25:125–30.
124. de Man FS, van Hees HW, Handoko ML, et al. Diaphragm muscle fiber weakness in pulmonary hypertension. Am J Respir Crit Care Med. 2011;183:1411–8.
125. Fernandez-Bonetti P, Lupi-Herrera E, Martinez-Guerra ML, et al. Peripheral airways obstruction in idiopathic pulmonary artery hypertension (primary). Chest. 1983;83:732–8.
126. Meyer FJ, Ewert R, Hoeper MM, et al. Peripheral airway obstruction in primary pulmonary hypertension. Thorax. 2002;57:473–6.
127. Chaouat A, Bugnet AS, Kadaoui N, et al. Severe pulmonary hypertension and chronic obstructive pulmonary disease. Am J Respir Crit Care Med. 2005;172:189–94.

128. Thabut G, Dauriat G, Stern JB, et al. Pulmonary hemodynamics in advanced COPD candidates for lung volume reduction surgery or lung transplantation. Chest. 2005;127:1531–6.
129. Scharf SM, Iqbal M, Keller C, et al. Hemodynamic characterization of patients with severe emphysema. Am J Respir Crit Care Med. 2002;166:314–22.
130. Lettieri CJ, Nathan SD, Barnett SD, et al. Prevalence and outcomes of pulmonary arterial hypertension in advanced idiopathic pulmonary fibrosis. Chest. 2006;129:746–52.
131. Hurdman J, Condliffe R, Elliot CA, et al. Pulmonary hypertension in COPD: results from the ASPIRE registry. Eur Respir J. 2013;41:1292–301.
132. Patel NM, Lederer DJ, Borczuk AC, et al. Pulmonary hypertension in idiopathic pulmonary fibrosis. Chest. 2007;132:998–1006.
133. Lederer DJ, Arcasoy SM, Wilt JS, et al. Six-minute-walk distance predicts waiting list survival in idiopathic pulmonary fibrosis. Am J Respir Crit Care Med. 2006;174:659–64.
134. Mejia M, Carrillo G, Rojas-Serrano J, et al. Idiopathic pulmonary fibrosis and emphysema: decreased survival associated with severe pulmonary arterial hypertension. Chest. 2009;136:10–5.
135. Cottin V, Le Pavec J, Prevot G, et al. Pulmonary hypertension in patients with combined pulmonary fibrosis and emphysema syndrome. Eur Respir J. 2010;35:105–11.
136. Steen V, Medsger Jr TA. Predictors of isolated pulmonary hypertension in patients with systemic sclerosis and limited cutaneous involvement. Arthritis Rheum. 2003;48:516–22.
137. Hsu VM, Moreyra AE, Wilson AC, et al. Assessment of pulmonary arterial hypertension in patients with systemic sclerosis: comparison of noninvasive tests with results of right-heart catheterization. J Rheumatol. 2008;35:458–65.
138. Fischer A, Bull TM, Steen VD. Practical approach to screening for scleroderma-associated pulmonary arterial hypertension. Arthritis Care Res (Hoboken). 2012;64:303–10.
139. Chiang ST. A nomogram for venous shunt (Qs/Qt) calculation. Thorax. 1968;23:563–5.
140. Powe JE, Palevsky HI, McCarthy KE, et al. Pulmonary arterial hypertension: value of perfusion scintigraphy. Radiology. 1987;164:727–30.
141. Fedullo P, Kerr KM, Kim NH, et al. Chronic thromboembolic pulmonary hypertension. Am J Respir Crit Care Med. 2011;183:1605–13.
142. Tunariu N, Gibbs SJ, Win Z, et al. Ventilation-perfusion scintigraphy is more sensitive than multidetector CTPA in detecting chronic thromboembolic pulmonary disease as a treatable cause of pulmonary hypertension. J Nucl Med. 2007;48:680–4.
143. Ryan KL, Fedullo PF, Davis GB, et al. Perfusion scan findings understate the severity of angiographic and hemodynamic compromise in chronic thromboembolic pulmonary hypertension. Chest. 1988;93:1180–5.
144. Bailey CL, Channick RN, Auger WR, et al. "High probability" perfusion lung scans in pulmonary venoocclusive disease. Am J Respir Crit Care Med. 2000;162:1974–8.
145. Seferian A, Helal B, Jais X, et al. Ventilation/perfusion lung scan in pulmonary venoocclusive disease. Eur Respir J. 2012;40:75–83.
146. Sostman HD, Brown M, Toole A, et al. Perfusion scan in pulmonary vascular/lymphangitic carcinomatosis: the segmental contour pattern. AJR Am J Roentgenol. 1981;137:1072–4.
147. Roberts KE, Hamele-Bena D, Saqi A, et al. Pulmonary tumor embolism: a review of the literature. Am J Med. 2003;115:228–32.
148. Genovesi MG, Tierney DF, Taplin GV, et al. An intravenous radionuclide method to evaluate hypoxemia caused by abnormal alveolar vessels: limitation of conventional techniques. Am Rev Respir Dis. 1976;114:59–65.
149. Kuriyama K, Gamsu G, Stern RG, et al. CT-determined pulmonary artery diameters in predicting pulmonary hypertension. Invest Radiol. 1984;19:16–22.
150. Ng CS, Wells AU, Padley SP. A CT sign of chronic pulmonary arterial hypertension: the ratio of main pulmonary artery to aortic diameter. J Thorac Imaging. 1999;14:270–8.
151. Oliver TB, Reid JH, Murchison JT. Interventricular septal shift due to massive pulmonary embolism shown by CT pulmonary angiography: an old sign revisited. Thorax. 1998;53:1092–4.

152. Reid JH, Murchison JT. Acute right ventricular dilatation: a new helical CT sign of massive pulmonary embolism. Clin Radiol. 1998;53:694–8.
153. Baque-Juston MC, Wells AU, Hansell DM. Pericardial thickening or effusion in patients with pulmonary artery hypertension: a CT study. AJR Am J Roentgenol. 1999;172:361–4.
154. Yeh BM, Kurzman P, Foster E, et al. Clinical relevance of retrograde inferior vena cava or hepatic vein opacification during contrast-enhanced CT. AJR Am J Roentgenol. 2004;183:1227–32.
155. Swensen SJ, Tashjian JH, Myers JL, et al. Pulmonary venoocclusive disease: CT findings in eight patients. AJR Am J Roentgenol. 1996;167:937–40.
156. Resten A, Maitre S, Humbert M, et al. Pulmonary hypertension: CT of the chest in pulmonary venoocclusive disease. AJR Am J Roentgenol. 2004;183:65–70.
157. Stein PD, Fowler SE, Goodman LR, et al. Multidetector computed tomography for acute pulmonary embolism. N Engl J Med. 2006;354:2317–27.
158. Schwickert HC, Schweden F, Schild HH, et al. Pulmonary arteries and lung parenchyma in chronic pulmonary embolism: preoperative and postoperative CT findings. Radiology. 1994;191:351–7.
159. Kauczor HU, Schwickert HC, Mayer E, et al. Spiral CT of bronchial arteries in chronic thromboembolism. J Comput Assist Tomogr. 1994;18:855–61.
160. Hasegawa I, Boiselle PM, Hatabu H. Bronchial artery dilatation on MDCT scans of patients with acute pulmonary embolism: comparison with chronic or recurrent pulmonary embolism. AJR Am J Roentgenol. 2004;182:67–72.
161. Sherrick AD, Swensen SJ, Hartman TE. Mosaic pattern of lung attenuation on CT scans: frequency among patients with pulmonary artery hypertension of different causes. AJR Am J Roentgenol. 1997;169:79–82.
162. Kerr KM, Auger WR, Fedullo PF, et al. Large vessel pulmonary arteritis mimicking chronic thromboembolic disease. Am J Respir Crit Care Med. 1995;152:367–73.
163. Lie JT. Isolated pulmonary Takayasu arteritis: clinicopathologic characteristics. Mod Pathol. 1996;9:469–74.
164. Park JH, Chung JW, Im JG, et al. Takayasu arteritis: evaluation of mural changes in the aorta and pulmonary artery with CT angiography. Radiology. 1995;196:89–93.
165. Marten K, Schnyder P, Schirg E, et al. Pattern-based differential diagnosis in pulmonary vasculitis using volumetric CT. AJR Am J Roentgenol. 2005;184:720–33.
166. Hamuryudan V, Yurdakul S, Moral F, et al. Pulmonary arterial aneurysms in Behcet's syndrome: a report of 24 cases. Br J Rheumatol. 1994;33:48–51.
167. Rafanan AL, Golish JA, Dinner DS, et al. Nocturnal hypoxemia is common in primary pulmonary hypertension. Chest. 2001;120:894–9.
168. Miyamoto S, Nagaya N, Satoh T, et al. Clinical correlates and prognostic significance of six-minute walk test in patients with primary pulmonary hypertension: comparison with cardiopulmonary exercise testing. Am J Respir Crit Care Med. 2000;161:487–92.
169. Humbert M, Sitbon O, Chaouat A, et al. Survival in patients with idiopathic, familial, and anorexigen-associated pulmonary arterial hypertension in the modern management era. Circulation. 2010;122:156–63.
170. Savarese G, Paolillo S, Costanzo P, et al. Do changes of 6-minute walk distance predict clinical events in patients with pulmonary arterial hypertension?: a meta-analysis of 22 randomized trials. J Am Coll Cardiol. 2012;60:1192–201.
171. Gabler NB, French B, Strom BL, et al. Validation of 6-minute walk distance as a surrogate end point in pulmonary arterial hypertension trials. Circulation. 2012;126:349–56.
172. Rich S. The 6-minute walk test as a primary endpoint in clinical trials for pulmonary hypertension. J Am Coll Cardiol. 2012;60:1202–3.
173. Barst RJ, Rubin LJ, Long WA, et al. A comparison of continuous intravenous epoprostenol (prostacyclin) with conventional therapy for primary pulmonary hypertension. N Engl J Med. 1996;334:296–301.
174. Sitbon O, Humbert M, Nunes H, et al. Long-term intravenous epoprostenol infusion in primary pulmonary hypertension: prognostic factors and survival. J Am Coll Cardiol. 2002;40:780–8.

175. Fritz JS, Blair C, Oudiz RJ, et al. Baseline and follow-up 6-min walk distance and brain natriuretic peptide predict 2-year mortality in pulmonary arterial hypertension. Chest. 2013;143:315–23.
176. Arena R, Lavie CJ, Milani RV, et al. Cardiopulmonary exercise testing in patients with pulmonary arterial hypertension: an evidence-based review. J Heart Lung Transplant. 2010;29: 159–73.
177. Wensel R, Opitz CF, Anker SD, et al. Assessment of survival in patients with primary pulmonary hypertension: importance of cardiopulmonary exercise testing. Circulation. 2002;106: 319–24.
178. Hoeper MM, Markevych I, Spiekerkoetter E, et al. Goal-oriented treatment and combination therapy for pulmonary arterial hypertension. Eur Respir J. 2005;26:858–63.
179. Sacks DG, Okano Y, Steen VD, et al. Isolated pulmonary hypertension in systemic sclerosis with diffuse cutaneous involvement: association with serum anti-U3RNP antibody. J Rheumatol. 1996;23:639–42.
180. Okano Y, Steen VD, Medsger Jr TA. Autoantibody to U3 nucleolar ribonucleoprotein (fibrillarin) in patients with systemic sclerosis. Arthritis Rheum. 1992;35:95–100.
181. Auger WR, Permpikul P, Moser KM. Lupus anticoagulant, heparin use, and thrombocytopenia in patients with chronic thromboembolic pulmonary hypertension: a preliminary report. Am J Med. 1995;99:392–6.
182. Wolf M, Boyer-Neumann C, Parent F, et al. Thrombotic risk factors in pulmonary hypertension. Eur Respir J. 2000;15:395–9.
183. Nagaya N, Nishikimi T, Uematsu M, et al. Plasma brain natriuretic peptide as a prognostic indicator in patients with primary pulmonary hypertension. Circulation. 2000;102:865–70.
184. Fijalkowska A, Kurzyna M, Torbicki A, et al. Serum N-terminal brain natriuretic peptide as a prognostic parameter in patients with pulmonary hypertension. Chest. 2006;129:1313–21.
185. Mehra MR, Uber PA, Park MH, et al. Obesity and suppressed B-type natriuretic peptide levels in heart failure. J Am Coll Cardiol. 2004;43:1590–5.
186. Wang TJ, Larson MG, Levy D, et al. Impact of obesity on plasma natriuretic peptide levels. Circulation. 2004;109:594–600.
187. Bayes-Genis A, Lloyd-Jones DM, van Kimmenade RR, et al. Effect of body mass index on diagnostic and prognostic usefulness of amino-terminal pro-brain natriuretic peptide in patients with acute dyspnea. Arch Intern Med. 2007;167:400–7.
188. Batal O, Faulx M, Krasuski RA, et al. Effect of obesity on B-type natriuretic peptide levels in patients with pulmonary arterial hypertension. Am J Cardiol. 2012;110:909–14.
189. Ruiter G, Lankhorst S, Boonstra A, et al. Iron deficiency is common in idiopathic pulmonary arterial hypertension. Eur Respir J. 2011;37:1386–91.
190. Rhodes CJ, Howard LS, Busbridge M, et al. Iron deficiency and raised hepcidin in idiopathic pulmonary arterial hypertension: clinical prevalence, outcomes, and mechanistic insights. J Am Coll Cardiol. 2011;58:300–9.
191. Krasuski RA, Hart SA, Smith B, et al. Association of anemia and long-term survival in patients with pulmonary hypertension. Int J Cardiol. 2011;150:291–5.
192. Dunn GD, Hayes P, Breen KJ, et al. The liver in congestive heart failure: a review. Am J Med Sci. 1973;265:174–89.
193. Rubin LJ, Badesch DB, Barst RJ, et al. Bosentan therapy for pulmonary arterial hypertension. N Engl J Med. 2002;346:896–903.
194. Galie N, Olschewski H, Oudiz RJ, et al. Ambrisentan for the treatment of pulmonary arterial hypertension: results of the ambrisentan in pulmonary arterial hypertension, randomized, double-blind, placebo-controlled, multicenter, efficacy (ARIES) study 1 and 2. Circulation. 2008;117:3010–9.
195. Forfia PR, Mathai SC, Fisher MR, et al. Hyponatremia predicts right heart failure and poor survival in pulmonary arterial hypertension. Am J Respir Crit Care Med. 2008;177:1364–9.
196. Ryan JJ, Rich JD, Thiruvoipati T, et al. Current practice for determining pulmonary capillary wedge pressure predisposes to serious errors in the classification of patients with pulmonary hypertension. Am Heart J. 2012;163:589–94.

197. Halpern SD, Taichman DB. Misclassification of pulmonary hypertension due to reliance on pulmonary capillary wedge pressure rather than left ventricular end-diastolic pressure. Chest. 2009;136:37–43.
198. Mills SR, Jackson DC, Older RA, et al. The incidence, etiologies, and avoidance of complications of pulmonary angiography in a large series. Radiology. 1980;136:295–9.
199. Nicod P, Peterson K, Levine M, et al. Pulmonary angiography in severe chronic pulmonary hypertension. Ann Intern Med. 1987;107:565–8.
200. Kovacs G, Berghold A, Scheidl S, et al. Pulmonary arterial pressure during rest and exercise in healthy subjects: a systematic review. Eur Respir J. 2009;34:888–94.
201. Grunig E, Janssen B, Mereles D, et al. Abnormal pulmonary artery pressure response in asymptomatic carriers of primary pulmonary hypertension gene. Circulation. 2000;102:1145–50.
202. Grunig E, Weissmann S, Ehlken N, et al. Stress Doppler echocardiography in relatives of patients with idiopathic and familial pulmonary arterial hypertension: results of a multicenter European analysis of pulmonary artery pressure response to exercise and hypoxia. Circulation. 2009;119:1747–57.
203. Tolle JJ, Waxman AB, Van Horn TL, et al. Exercise-induced pulmonary arterial hypertension. Circulation. 2008;118:2183–9.
204. Steen V, Chou M, Shanmugam V, et al. Exercise-induced pulmonary arterial hypertension in patients with systemic sclerosis. Chest. 2008;134:146–51.
205. Kovacs G, Maier R, Aberer E, et al. Borderline pulmonary arterial pressure is associated with decreased exercise capacity in scleroderma. Am J Respir Crit Care Med. 2009;180:881–6.
206. Condliffe R, Kiely DG, Peacock AJ, et al. Connective tissue disease-associated pulmonary arterial hypertension in the modern treatment era. Am J Respir Crit Care Med. 2009;179:151–7.
207. Saggar R, Khanna D, Shapiro S, et al. Effect of ambrisentan treatment on exercise-induced pulmonary hypertension in systemic sclerosis: a prospective single-center, open-label pilot study. Arthritis Rheum. 2012;64:4072–7.
208. Borlaug BA, Nishimura RA, Sorajja P, et al. Exercise hemodynamics enhance diagnosis of early heart failure with preserved ejection fraction. Circ Heart Fail. 2010;3:588–95.

Chapter 9
Echocardiography

Paul Forfia

Abstract In this chapter we aim to explore the role of the echocardiographic-Doppler examination in the evaluation and management of patients with pulmonary hypertension (PH). Too often, the echo-Doppler examination is primarily viewed as a method of "screening" for the presence of PH by Doppler estimation of increased pulmonary arterial pressure (PAP). While Doppler pressure estimation is important, an overemphasis on PAP estimation often occurs without recognition of the inherent imprecision of these methods and importantly, often neglects critically important two-dimensional (2D) and additional Doppler parameters that provide pivotal diagnostic, prognostic, and therapy-guiding information. It is the integration of relevant 2D and Doppler parameters that provide a comprehensive view of the underlying pathophysiology of PH. For example, several signature findings, well studied and validated, will help in differentiating the two major causes of PH, namely, PH that is caused by pulmonary venous hypertension (PH_{PVH}) from PH that is caused by pulmonary vascular disease (PH_{PVD}).

Keywords Pulmonary hypertension • Echocardiogram • Echocardiography • Doppler ultrasound

Normal Anatomy and Physiology of Right Ventricle-Pulmonary Circulation Unit

The right ventricle (RV) lies anterior to the left ventricle (LV). They are separated by the interventricular septum (IVS) that is curved anteriorly, giving the RV a crescent shape. The RV free wall is a thin structure (3–5 mm) which extends from the anterior and posterior aspects of the IVS. The cavity of the RV is comprised of inflow (sinus) and outflow (conus) regions, separated by a muscular ridge called the crista supraventricularis. The outflow region is a smooth funnel shaped structure

P. Forfia, M.D. (✉)
Section of Cardiology, Department of Medicine, Temple University,
3401 N. Broad St., 9th Floor Parkinson Pavilion, Philadelphia, PA 19140, USA
e-mail: paul.forfia@tuhs.temple.edu

J.R. Klinger, R.P. Frantz (eds.), *Diagnosis and Management of Pulmonary Hypertension*, Respiratory Medicine 12, DOI 10.1007/978-1-4939-2636-7_9

that ends with the pulmonic valve (PV). In contrast, the inflow region includes several structures including the tricuspid valve (TV) apparatus (leaflets, chordae and papillary muscles) as well as the body of the RV. The moderator band is a muscle band that connects the RV free wall to the septum and, in addition to more extensive trabeculations and higher insertion of the TV, is one of the distinguishing features of the RV cavity from that of the LV [1, 2].

The morphology of the RV is designed to couple to a low resistance circuit, namely the pulmonary circulation. The thin-walled RV is capable of generating the same amount of flow as the LV due to the low resistance of the pulmonary vasculature. Should pulmonary vascular resistance increase, i.e., in pulmonary vascular disease (PVD), uncoupling of the RV-pulmonary circulation can occur manifesting by the classic morphological triad of increased RV size and altered shape, RV systolic dysfunction, and variable degrees of bowing of the IVS during systole and diastole. The extent of the above changes is contingent upon the degree of uncoupling of the RV-pulmonary circulation unit, which is often proportional to the rise in pulmonary vascular resistance. This critical observation forms the cornerstone of the echocardiographic assessment of PVD [3–6].

Adaptation to chronic pulmonary hypertension usually manifests as hypertrophy rather than dilation of the RV. This hypertrophy helps, as in the case of Eisenmenger's syndrome, to maintain the coupling of the RV-pulmonary circulation unit for longer periods of time, hence preserving RV function and perhaps accounting for the better prognosis of such patients compared with other forms of pulmonary arterial hypertension (PAH) [7].

Echocardiographic Variables in the Assessment of RV Function and Morphology

The use of Doppler echocardiography (DE) in the evaluation of patients with known or suspected PVD is centered on the assessment of the morphology and function of the RV. Both direct and indirect components of this assessment exist and have prognostic significance.

Measures of RV Systolic Function

Unlike the LV, the morphology of the RV, as discussed above, does not allow for accurate estimation of RV volumes, and hence RV ejection fraction (RVEF) by conventional 2D echocardiography. 3D echocardiography, on the other hand, holds promise in this regard given its accuracy and feasibility.

Recognizing the limitations of volumetric based global RV functional assessment, an alternative method for quantitative global RV functional assessment uses RV area rather than volume [8–10]. Right ventricular fractional area change (RVFAC)

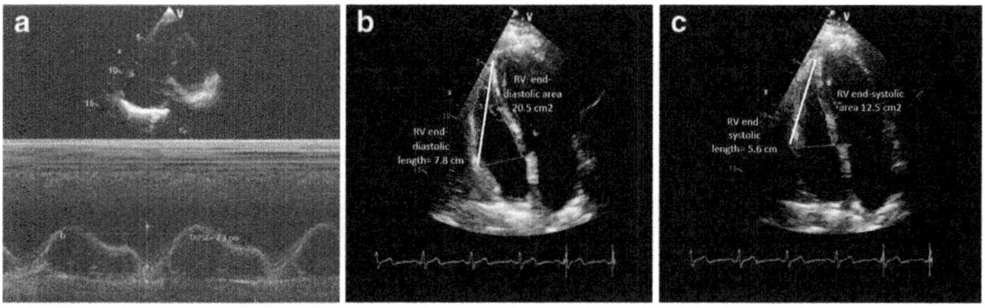

Fig. 9.1 (**a**) Tricuspid annular plane systolic excursion (TAPSE) in M-mode obtained in the apical four chamber view. The distance between the end-diastolic (*a*) and end-systolic points (*b*) is the TAPSE (2.3 cm). (**b**) Illustrates the RV end-diastolic length (7.8 cm) from the tricuspid valve plane to the RV apex. It also demonstrates the RV end-diastolic area (20.5 cm^2). (**c**) Represents the RV end-systolic length (5.6 cm). The difference between these two measurements is the 2D TAPSE (2.2 cm). It also demonstrates RV end-systolic area (12.5 cm^2). RVFAC is therefore [(20.5 − 12.5/20.5) × 100] = 40 %

is obtained from the apical four chamber view, using planimetry of the RV area at end-diastole and end-systole ([RVFAC = RV Area$_{ED}$ − RV Area$_{ES}$/RV Area$_{ED}$] × 100) [10]. However, limited visualization of the RV free wall, particularly when the RV is dilated, as well as suboptimal endocardial definition does limit the reproducibility and applicability of this measure in some instances (Fig. 9.1b, c) [8–10].

The orientation of muscle fibers of the RV dictates that the majority (77 %) of area change during systole occurs in the longitudinal direction [3, 11]. Systolic displacement of the RV base, referred to as tricuspid annular plane systolic excursion or (TAPSE) correlates strongly ($r = 0.79$–0.92) with RV ejection fraction derived from radionuclide angiography [4]. TAPSE can be derived from 2D echo or M-Mode and is highly reproducible due to its freedom from geometric assumptions and lack of reliance on endocardial definition (Fig. 9.1). A normal TAPSE ranges from 2.4 to 2.7 cm [11–14]. A TAPSE < 1.8 cm predicts a stroke volume index <29 ml/m^2 with 87 % accuracy, and is associated with increased hospitalization rates for right heart failure and decreased survival in patients with PAH [10, 12]. Ghio et al. recently showed in a PAH cohort that a TAPSE ≤ 1.5 cm was associated with a nearly three-fold higher event rate (death or emergent lung transplant) versus subjects with a TAPSE > 1.5 cm [15]. Of note, Raina et al. have demonstrated that compared to normal subjects, patients who undergo cardiac surgery demonstrate a change in the pattern of their RV contraction, such that their average TAPSE was 1.6 cm while maintaining normal global RV function. In the post-operative subjects, there was a loss of longitudinal RV contraction relative to transverse shortening. This is likely related to geometric changes in the RV that occur following pericardiotomy. Therefore, a global measure of RV function such as RVFAC is preferred in patients with prior cardiac surgery and pericardiotomy [16].

Another method of longitudinal RV function assessment utilizes the velocity of RV longitudinal shortening via tissue Doppler imaging TDI (denoted S'). S' correlates strongly with TAPSE and is similarly a reproducible method of RV function

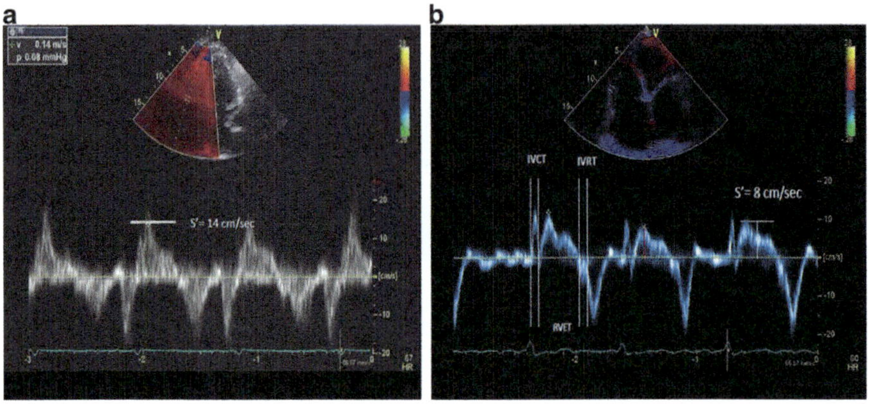

Fig. 9.2 Right ventricular Tissue Doppler imaging obtained along the basal one-third of the RV free wall in the longitudinal plane. The peak longitudinal shortening velocity is denoted as *S′* and is measured at 14 cm/s in panel (**a**), and 8 cm/s in panel (**b**). Right ventricular myocardial performance index (in panel **b**) can be obtained from the isovolumic contraction time (IVCT), relaxation time (IVRT), and ejection time (RVET)

assessment [17]. An *S′* <10 cm/s predicts a cardiac index <2.0 l/min/m^2 with 89 % sensitivity and 87 % specificity [18]. Additionally, the RV TDI signal can be integrated to measure the longitudinal tissue displacement, which is numerically identical to TAPSE. Using ROC curve analysis, an RV tissue displacement >1.5 cm predicted an RV stroke volume index ≥30 ml/m^2 (AUC 0.79); changes in RV tissue displacement strongly correlated to changes in RV stroke volume index in response to intravenous epoprostenol infusion (Fig. 9.2) [19].

The myocardial performance index (MPI) integrates systolic and diastolic parameters in a single measure. Using tissue Doppler signals the time intervals of isovolemic contraction (IVCT), isovolemic relaxation (IVRT), and RV ejection time (RVET) are measured to derive the MPI (IVRT + IVCT/RVET) (Fig. 9.2). A higher MPI value is associated with worse RV function and survival in PAH [20].

An additional method of assessing RV function is the averaged longitudinal RV free wall strain as assessed by speckle tracking [21]. In this study, persistence of or progression to a severe reduction in free wall systolic strain (<−12.5 %) at 6 months was associated with greater disease severity and diuretic use. higher mean pulmonary artery pressure, and poorer survival (4-year mortality 43 % vs. 23 %, $p = 0.002$). After adjusting for age, functional class, and RV strain at baseline, patients with ≥5 % improvement in RV free wall systolic strain had a greater than sevenfold lower mortality risk at 4 years (hazard ratio 0.13, 95 % confidence interval 0.03–0.50, $p = 0.003$).

All echocardiographic measures of RV function assessment are load (especially afterload) dependent. Although this can be viewed as a limitation, the fact that RV dysfunction in PAH is largely afterload dependent allows changes in RV function to inform the clinician on responses (or lack thereof) to PH specific medical therapy.

Right Ventricular Size, Shape, Septal Position

The first response of the RV to a rise in pulmonary arterial load is RV dilatation, which serves as a compensatory response which may assist in the maintenance of RV stroke volume (heterometric autoregulation). The normal RV measures approximately 2.5–3.5 cm at end-diastole, with a planimetered area of 15–18 cm^2. Of note, the presence of RV dilatation does not always signify RV systolic dysfunction. A dilated RV with normal or dynamic function often signifies excess preload only, with the rise in RV function occurring in response to volume loading and increased sarcomere length. This is often the case in primary tricuspid valve and pulmonic valve regurgitation as well as in the presence of systemic to pulmonary shunt conditions. A practical rule is that in the absence of moderate or greater tricuspid or pulmonic regurgitation, a dilated and hyperdynamic RV should alert the clinician to the presence of a systemic to pulmonary shunt.

A practical way to estimate RV size is to compare RV dimensions to LV dimensions (or area) in the apical four chamber view. RV dimensions are obtained at the RV base, approximately 1 cm apical of the tricuspid annulus. A diastolic RV/LV diameter ratio of 0.5–0.7 is considered normal, with increasing RV:LV ratios in patients with mild (0.8–1.0), moderate (1.1–1.4), and severe (≥1.5) RV dilatation. A useful rule of thumb is that the RV:LV ratio should be <1.0, and any value >1.0 is strongly suggestive of RV dilatation, often coinciding with RV dysfunction (Fig. 9.3) [22].

The apex of the heart is normally formed by the LV. In cases of RV enlargement related to increased RV afterload, the RV will occupy or share the apex of the heart (apex-forming RV). This is associated with widening (opening) of the angle of the RV apex which is normally acute in the apical four chamber view. Lopéz-Candeles

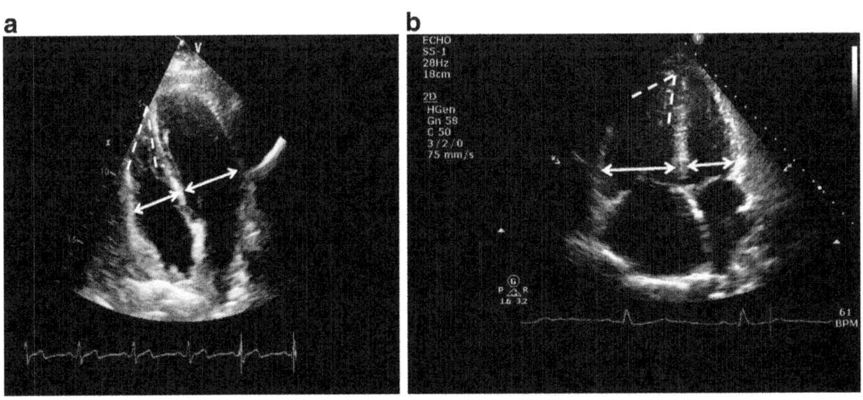

Fig. 9.3 (**a** and **b**) Apical four chamber view. Panel (**a**) demonstrates a normal RV:LV dimension ratio (<1.0) and normal RV shape, given the relative tapering of the RV dimension from base to apex. Note the relatively acute RV apex angle in this patient with a normal PVR. Panel (**b**) represents a patient with PAH, whom has a markedly increased RV:LV ratio (1.5). Note the relative lack of tapering of RV dimensions from base to apex and the open RV apex angle. The RV is apex-sharing with the LV. These findings is panel **b** are highly consistent with PH related to a high PVR

showed that a relatively large or "open" RV apical angle was a common finding in the setting of chronic pulmonary hypertension, relating inversely to decreases in TAPSE and RV fractional area change [23]. In our experience, a dilated and open RV apex angle is quite specific for PH related to high afterload conditions such as PAH and CTEPH. In PVH and other PH conditions where the PVR is normal, the RV apex angle will remain rather acute or "closed," imparting an inverted triangle shape to the RV, where the dimension tapers quickly from base to RV apex (Figure 9.3).

As the RV dilates, the potential space in the pericardium is obliterated leading to pericardial constraint. With increasing constraint of the heart, further dilatation of the RV leads to shifting of the IVS from right to left (an example of diastolic ventricular interdependence), leading to a fall in LV cavity size and impaired LV diastolic filling [24]. As a result, the transmitral Doppler filling pattern will demonstrate reversal of early (E) versus late (A) diastolic waveforms on pulsed wave Doppler mitral inflow (so-called E to A reversal) in patients with PAH or CTEPH [25]. Confusion can sometimes arise if the clinician wrongly assumes that reversal of E/A ratio (often reported as "Grade I diastolic dysfunction") equates to elevated LA pressure and hence attributes the PH to left sided diastolic dysfunction. In the presence of RV dilation and significant right to left septal shifting, the presence of a reversed E/A ratio is a strong indicator of normal left atrial pressure. Moreover, when septal IVS shift is due to PAH or CTEPH and alleviated by treatment, LV diastolic filling returns to normal [26, 27].

Additionally, RV dysfunction is associated with a delay in the time to peak RV contraction, which leads to mechanical RV/LV dyssynchrony [28]. This RV/LV dyssynchrony leads to systolic septal flattening which is characteristic of high RV afterload states. Magnetic resonance imaging studies have shown relatively strong correlations between the degree of RV systolic septal bowing and pulmonary vascular resistance [26, 28]. Systolic septal flattening is nearly always present in PAH and CTEPH, and thus functions as a reliable and practical indicator of increased pulmonary arterial afterload (Fig. 9.4).

Mild to moderate pericardial effusion is a common finding, occurring in about 50 % of patients with PAH [29]. It has long been recognized as poor prognostic sign in PAH, often signifying relative RV decompensation (Fig. 9.4b). The accumulation of pericardial fluid in PAH likely occurs due to chronically elevated RA pressure, which in turn impairs coronary venous return and results in transudation of fluid into the pericardial space [30]. Importantly, attempts at pericardial drainage (surgical or catheter based) should be avoided unless there is compelling evidence of tamponade, as the effusion is typically the result and not the cause of RV failure in this setting and mechanical drainage of the effusion in some series was associated with unacceptably high mortality rates [31]. Others have achieved success in draining pericardial effusions in PAH with low procedural mortality [32]. In our experience, in the absence of frank tamponade, pericardial effusions may resolve over weeks or months if the PAH and RV failure respond to diuresis and PH specific medical therapy.

RA enlargement is another indirect measure of RV dysfunction. An increased RA area index is predictive of increased mortality in PAH. While RA dilatation

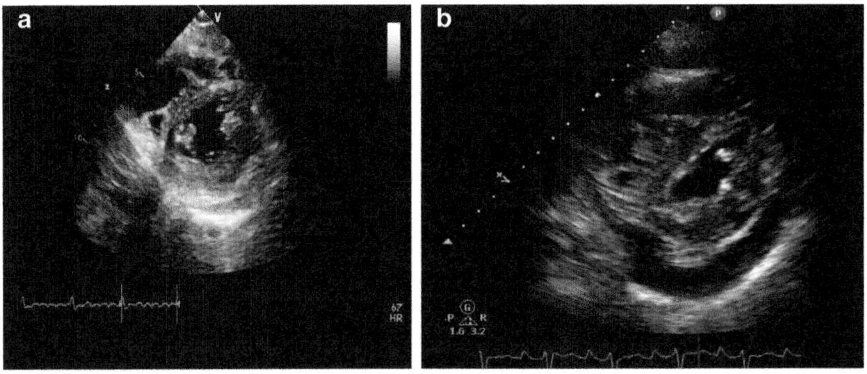

Fig. 9.4 (**a** and **b**) Short axis images at the midventricular level demonstrating mild (**a**), and more marked (**b**) systolic septal flattening in patients with mild, and more advanced pulmonary vascular disease. The presence of systolic septal flattening is present in PH associated with a high PVR, however, is typically absent in PH in the setting of a normal PVR (i.e., PVH). Also note the presence of a small to moderate size pericardial effusion (panel **b**), which is indicative of a high right atrial pressure, poor RV function and worse prognosis in PAH

might be seen as simply a marker of progressive RV failure and worsening TR, more recent work suggests that RA systolic function may account for upwards of 50 % of total longitudinal RV shortening in patients with PAH [33–35]. Therefore, the RA may play a larger role in maintaining total right heart function than previously appreciated.

Doppler Examination

Pulmonary arterial load (the afterload of the RV) and pulmonary artery pressure should not be viewed as synonymous. Afterload is the force that opposes flow, whereas pressure results from the interaction between flow and afterload. Since pressure does not oppose flow, it cannot be considered afterload. This fundamental physiologic distinction is supported by the fact that PA pressure correlates poorly with RV function and prognosis in patients with PAH [35]. Moreover, there are conditions where pressure is low and afterload is high (i.e., acute PE) and where pressure is high and afterload is low (i.e., systemic to pulmonary shunt with PH from high pulmonary blood flow). RV afterload is better represented by pulmonary vascular resistance rather than pressure. Thus, practically speaking when a clinician notes PH+RV dysfunction a high PVR should be suspected, whereas when PH is present without RV dysfunction, low PVR PH conditions are far more likely, such as left-sided diastolic HF.

Despite its shortcomings as a measure of RV afterload, PA pressure remains an important component in the evaluation of established or suspected pulmonary hypertension since some elevation is nearly always present in varying degrees in patients with PVD. A pulmonary artery systolic pressure (PASP) of 40 mmHg has been traditionally accepted as the upper limit of normal in most subjects, although the upper limit of PASP may be slightly higher in advancing age. The echocardiographic discovery of an elevated PA pressure is usually, although not ideally, what triggers further workup for PH, and therefore, it is important to review the echocardiographic assessment of PA pressure [36–38].

The PASP is most commonly estimated through continuous wave Doppler interrogation of the tricuspid regurgitant jet velocity, which provides an estimate of the pressure gradient between the RV and the RA [39]. This gradient, when added to RA pressure, should equal the systolic RV pressure, which in turn should equal PASP in the absence of pulmonic valve stenosis. In the latter case, the PASP can still be estimated by subtracting the gradient across the pulmonic valve from peak RV systolic pressure. This approach utilizes the modified Bernoulli equation: $\text{PASP} \approx 4v^2 +$ estimated RA. The v represents the velocity of the tricuspid regurgitant jet. The use of a high quality TR jet signal with a clearly defined peak velocity ensures the highest chance of an accurate and reproducible PASP estimate (Fig. 9.5).

The most common method of RA pressure assessment utilizes inferior vena cava (IVC) size and collapsibility with inspiration [40, 41]. Unfortunately, this method has not proved very reliable, likely because the size of the IVC is governed not only by the RA pressure, but also by the compliance of the IVC and the degree to which the negative pleural pressure is transmitted to it [42–44]. Another way of estimating RA pressure was recently described. Using the ratio of tricuspid inflow *E* velocity

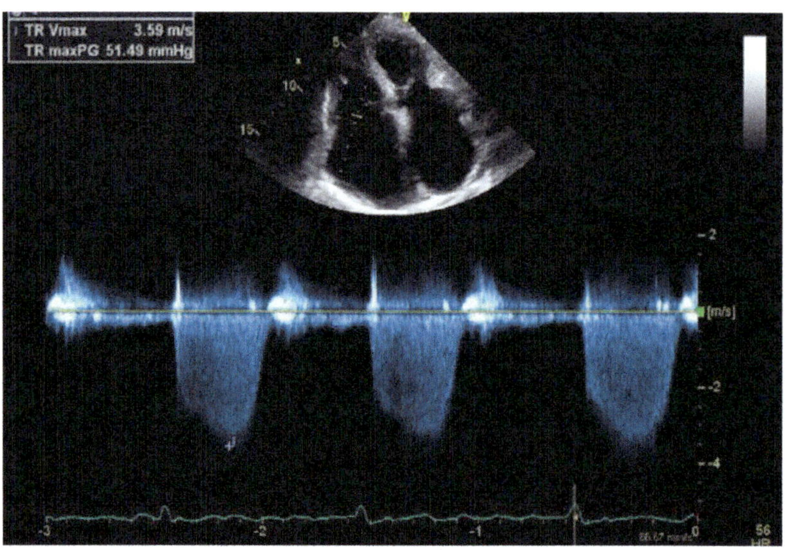

Fig. 9.5 Apical four chamber view with continuous wave Doppler interrogation across the tricuspid valve. The peak velocity is 3.6 m/s, thus estimating a pressure gradient between the right ventricle and right atrium of 51 mmHg. This added to an RA pressure estimate will estimate PA systolic pressure. The high quality Doppler signal with a clearly defined peak lends to more reproducible and reliable pressure estimation

to tricuspid annular tissue Doppler E_a wave velocity (E/E_a) yielded values that correlated well ($r=0.8$) with invasively measured pressures [45]. However, given the significant variation in these techniques, we prefer to use the clinically estimated RA pressure, when possible.

Data on the accuracy of Doppler echo assessment of PA pressure have been disappointing [42, 46]. This is largely due to the fact that in many patients the ideal conditions of a high quality TR jet signal, proper Doppler alignment, and accurate RA pressure estimation do not exist. Fisher et al. examined the correlation between Doppler estimated and invasively measured PA systolic pressure in a cohort of 65 patients with more severe pulmonary hypertension (62 % with pulmonary arterial hypertension) [42]. Using Bland-Altman analysis, 48 % of the patients had an estimated PA systolic pressure that was 10 mmHg or more different from invasively obtained measurements. Pressure overestimations were due to either overestimation of the peak velocity signal, or an overestimation of the RA pressure by IVC size and collapsibility assessment (Fig. 9.6). Underestimations were also common, and more pronounced (–30 mmHg) than overestimations (+19). Suboptimal TR jet signal quality was the most common reason for PASP underestimation (Fig. 9.6). Nonetheless, in the study by Fisher et al., the absence of TR did not necessarily equate to the absence of pulmonary hypertension, as four of the six subjects with no TR had severe pulmonary hypertension by catheterization. In addition, 12 of the 16 patients in whom PA pressure was underestimated by Doppler had evidence of RV enlargement and/or dysfunction on their Doppler echo exam. Thus, if the PASP estimate is <40 mmHg in the presence of significant RV dilation, dysfunction or

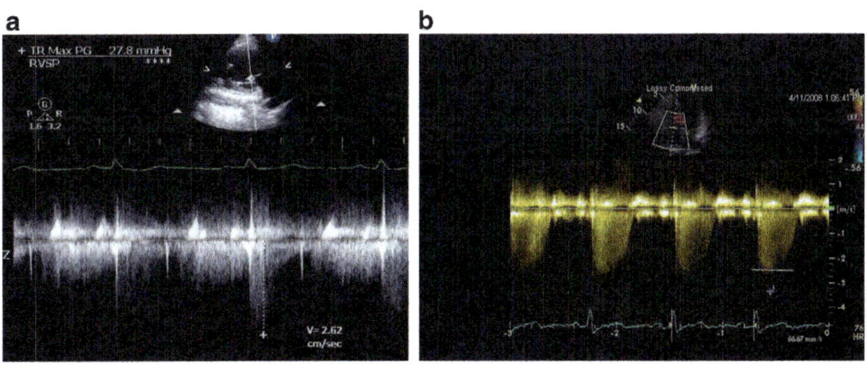

Fig. 9.6 (**a**) Example of pulmonary artery systolic pressure underestimation by continuous wave Doppler method. Note the Doppler signal dropout and a poorly defined peak TR velocity. The peak velocity is estimated at 2.62 m/s, estimating an RV to RA gradient of about 28 mmHg and PA systolic pressure of 40 mmHg. A right heart catheterization within 24 h of the echo examination revealed a pulmonary artery systolic pressure of 75 mmHg. (**b**) Example of pulmonary artery systolic pressure overestimation by the continuous-wave Doppler method. The reported peak velocity is 3.4 m/s, estimating a gradient between the RV and the RA of 46 mmHg. However, the true peak velocity is 2.3 m/s (denoted by horizontal line), estimating a RV-RA gradient of only 21 mmHg. This figure highlights the importance of measuring the peak velocity carefully, as the peak velocity is squared, thus amplifying the error

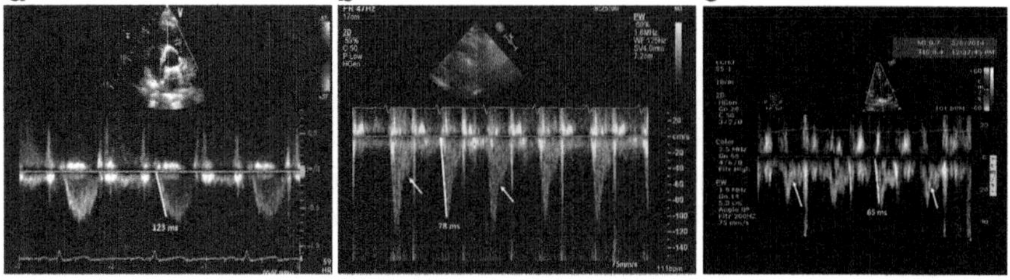

Fig. 9.7 Pulsed wave Doppler signals from the RV outflow tract. Panel (**a**) demonstrates a non-notched flow velocity envelope. Panel (**b**) is more triangular with a late-systolic notching pattern. Panel (**c**) has a pronounced mid-systolic notching pattern. The difference in the shape of the Doppler patterns is largely determined by differences in pulmonary vascular resistance, not PA pressure. Also shown are times to peak velocity or acceleration times (AcT) from the same pulse wave Doppler interrogation of the right ventricular outflow tract. Panel (**a**) an AcT=123 ms, consistent with normal mean pulmonary artery pressure and resistance. Panel (**b**) illustrates an AcT=78 ms, in a patient with a pulmonary vascular resistance (PVR) of 6 WU. Panel **c** demonstrates marked mid systolic notch and shorter AcT, in this case associated with a PVR of 11 WU

septal flattening, the clinician should remain highly suspicious for the presence of significant PH and the patient should be referred for right heart catheterization.

An alternative or complementary method of pulmonary artery pressure assessment utilizes the acceleration time (AcT) (Fig. 9.7) of the pulsed wave Doppler flow velocity envelope in the right ventricular outflow tract (RVOT Doppler) [mean PAP=79−0.45 (RVOT AcT)] [47]. This measure is simple, reproducible, and inversely correlates with mean PA pressure (mPAP). Moreover, AcT may be a better marker of pulmonary artery impedance/right ventricular afterload than pressure; thus, in two patients with equal mPAPs, the patient with a high AcT (i.e., >100 ms) will have a relatively normal PVR, whereas a patient with an AcT less than 100 ms is more likely to have an increased PVR and right ventricular afterload.

In addition to systolic and mean PA pressures, the diastolic PA pressure (PADP) can be derived from the end-diastolic point of the pulmonary regurgitation signal, again added to an estimate of right atrial pressure [48]. Alternatively, PADP can be estimated from the velocity obtained from the TR jet at the time of pulmonic valve opening [49, 50]. In either case, the accuracy of the method is contingent on the presence of PR or TR and the quality of the respective Doppler envelopes.

The most important thing to remember about Doppler derived PA pressure assessment is that it should be taken in the context of the clinical condition and, importantly, in the context of other echocardiographic features such as RV size, RV apex morphology, RV systolic function and septal position. Using this more integrated approach provides a far more comprehensive PH assessment and greatly offsets the potential for PH misdiagnosis by PASP Doppler estimation alone.

As discussed earlier, an elevated PVR is the hallmark of PH_{PVD}. Doppler echocardiography can also be used to estimate PVR. Abbas et al. showed that the ratio of trans-tricuspid flow velocity (surrogate of pressure) to the velocity-time interval obtained from the RV outflow tract (RVOT VTI) (surrogate of flow) closely correlates to PVR [51]. This approach estimates PVR well when PVR is low (<2 WU), but does not correlate well in the setting of elevated PVR (>8 WU) [52]. Additionally, as this ratio correlates with total pulmonary resistance (mPAP/cardiac output) rather than PVR alone, this measure could lead one to believe that an elevated ratio is related to elevated PVR (i.e., PVD), when the total pulmonary resistance is actually elevated secondary to left atrial hypertension. Another formula, proposed recently, derives PVR from the ratio of PASP to RVOT VTI, with a corrective constant (+3) in the setting of mid-systolic notching of the RVOT Doppler signal (*vide infra*). This method (PVR = [(PASP/RVOT VTI) + 3]) demonstrated an area under the curve (AUC) of 0.95 and 0.92 for PVR more than 3 and 5 WU, respectively, and was 98 % sensitive and 61 % specific for predicting PVR more than 3 WU [53].

A simpler approach to estimating PVR relies on the visual inspection of the pulsed wave Doppler profile in the RVOT (RVOT Doppler). In the setting of normal RV afterload (normal PVR), the RVOT Doppler signal is rounded and parabolic in shape, with no evidence of systolic deceleration or "notching" of the Doppler profile (Fig. 9.7a). In the setting of an increased PVR and decreased pulmonary artery compliance, the RVOT Doppler signal will demonstrate evidence of "notching," that can occur in late systole (Fig. 9.7b) or mid-systole (Fig. 9.7c). RVOT Doppler notching arises from alteration of the flow pattern exiting the RV due to early arrival of reflected pressures waves from a constricted and noncompliant pulmonary circulation [54–56]. Mid-systolic notching is 96 % specific for a PVR > 5 WU, a mean PVR of 9 WU, and is associated with a greater degree of right heart dysfunction than the late notch pattern, which is typically associated with a PVR of 3–6 WU and less severe right heart dysfunction [57]. In this study, a notched RVOT Doppler profile was strongly associated with a PVR > 3 WU (odds ratio 29:1), and was present in 100 % of patients with incident PAH. On the other hand, subjects with PH in the absence of Doppler notching are far more likely to have pulmonary venous congestion and left heart disease as the source of their PH (odds ratio 33:1). Visual inspection of the RVOT Doppler profile for the presence of absence of "notching" is a very simple, powerful, and practical way to detect PH_{PVD} and should be incorporated into the routine echo-Doppler examination of every patient with known or suspected PH.

Role of Echo-Doppler Beyond Initial Screening for PH

Pulmonary Arterial Hypertension (PAH)

As discussed previously, pulmonary vascular disease alters the normal structure of the right heart and Doppler flow profile in a consistent and reproducible manner, such that the presence of certain findings provides powerful diagnostic information irrespective of the Doppler PASP estimate. The echocardiographic features of idiopathic pulmonary arterial hypertension (IPAH) were described in the early 1970s by Goodman et al. [58]. They showed that the vast majority of patients with PAH had evidence of RV dilatation and systolic septal flattening. In a subsequent series, RV dilatation (98 %) and systolic septal flattening (90 %), were common, with a high prevalence of RV systolic dysfunction (76 %). In this same study, the investigators demonstrated a relatively low correlation between PAP estimated by Doppler and measured invasively ($r=0.31$) [59]. They also showed that the RVOT AcT was abnormal in the majority of the patients (AcT < 100 ms), which parallels the observation that the RVOT Doppler profile is consistently and reproducibly altered in PH_{PVD} (Doppler notching pattern), as shown by Arkles et al. [57] Bossone et al. also showed that moderate to severe TR was common as was the reversal of E/A ratio on mitral inflow Doppler. In fact, 70 % of the PAH patients demonstrated E to A reversal (grade 1 diastolic dysfunction) while none of the subjects had an elevated LA pressure on invasive measurement. As discussed above, transmitral Doppler E to A reversal in the setting of echo-Doppler features of PAH is a very strong indicator for the presence of normal LA pressure.

A notched RVOT Doppler profile has been observed in 100 % of patients with incident PAH. In contrast, the absence of RVOT notching in a patient with pulmonary hypertension strongly correlated with a PVR < 3 WU and a wedge pressure of >15 mmHg [57].

From a prognostic standpoint, it seems that either indirect or direct measure of impaired right heart performance can be associated with adverse outcome in PAH. The presence of a pericardial effusion is seen in about 15 % of patients with PAH and is associated with an adverse prognosis, likely related to chronically elevated right atrial pressure. Impaired LV diastolic filling (related to the degree of septal flattening and LV compression) and a high RA area index are also associated with worse outcome [35].

Similarly, an RV MPI ≥ 0.83 is associated with a lower event free survival at 5 years as opposed to those with RV MPI < 0.83 [20]. Others have demonstrated that in patients with PAH a TAPSE of <1.8 cm corresponded to higher catheter derived right atrial pressure, lower stroke volume index, greater RV dilatation and septal bowing, and a higher incidence of pericardial effusion. Two-year survival estimate for those patients was 50 % as opposed to 80 % for those with a TAPSE ≥ 1.8 cm [10].

Chronic Thromboembolic Pulmonary Hypertension (CTEPH)

In about 4 % of patients with prior pulmonary embolism (PE), incomplete clot resolution leads to residual obstruction in the pulmonary circulation, resulting in CTEPH. Unlike PAH, which is largely a disease of the small pulmonary vessels, the circulatory impedance in CTEPH arises from obstruction and remodeling of both large and small arteries [60, 61]. The small vessel disease component of CTEPH leads to similar 2D echocardiographic findings as PAH, with the triad of RV dilatation, RV systolic dysfunction and septal flattening being highly prevalent. Thus, any patient with these 2D echocardiographic findings should undergo ventilation perfusion scanning to exclude CTEPH. The presence of proximal, large vessel obstruction in CTEPH leads to relatively greater pulsatility in the pulmonary circulation, which can be appreciated by echo-Doppler examination or right heart catheterization in the form of a high PA pulse pressure relative to mean PA pressure (referred to as the fractional pulse pressure (FPP); PA pulse pressure/mean PA pressure). A FPP > 1.4 is very suggestive of CTEPH as opposed to PAH in which the FPP is usually around 0.8 [62, 63]. Doppler estimated FPP of 1.35 differentiates CTEPH from IPAH with a sensitivity of 95 % and a specificity of 100 % in one series [64].

In addition, it has long been observed that a notched RVOT Doppler profile is present in the setting of acute and chronic PE, owed to early arrival of reflected pressure and flow waves arising from proximal PA obstruction. Hence, RVOT Doppler notching is also seen in acute and chronic PE. Moreover, early or mid-systolic notching of the RVOT Doppler profile predicts the greatest benefit from pulmonary thromboendarterectomy (PTE) in CTEPH patients [55].

Acute Pulmonary Embolism

Pulmonary embolism (PE) is a very common cause of morbidity and mortality in the USA. Fortunately, most PE's are small and have little to no hemodynamic consequence, and are thus not appreciated by echocardiography [65]. However, in the setting of larger and more centrally located PE, the RV is exposed to a sudden and dramatic rise in afterload to which it is not well designed to overcome [66, 67]. This leads to a rapid uncoupling of the RV–PA circuit, abrupt RV dilatation, RV dysfunction and varying degrees of pulmonary hypertension [68, 69]. Due to the sudden rise in afterload and relative inability to generate normal or large stroke volumes, the degree of PH is typically less severe in acute PE with the PASP usually <60 mmHg (mean <40 mmHg) [65]. As a result, the degree of RV dilatation and dysfunction is more informative to clot burden in the PA circuit than the degree of PH [69]. Moreover, in the setting of acute PE, a McConnell's sign is frequently observed, referring to the relative sparing of transverse shortening of the distal one-third of the RV near the apex, while the remainder of the RV is hypokinetic (Fig. 9.8). This phenomenon likely results from tethering of the RV apex by a normal or hypercontractile LV through forces transmitted across the IVS and shared fibers between the LV and RV [70].

Longitudinal RV function is impaired in acute PE, and thus, a depressed TAPSE or RV TDI S′ is frequently observed [71]. Another signature finding of acute PE is the "60/60" sign, referring to an RVOT Doppler AcT < 60 ms combined with a PASP of <60 mmHg [72].

Occasionally in acute PE, embolus in transit can be appreciated on TTE, with mobile clot visualized in the RA, RV, or even in the RA partially traversing a patent foramen ovale. Embolus in transit represents a relative medical emergency that is associated with a high in hospital mortality and necessitates immediate consideration of aggressive therapies such as thrombolysis or embolectomy (catheter based or surgical) [73, 74].

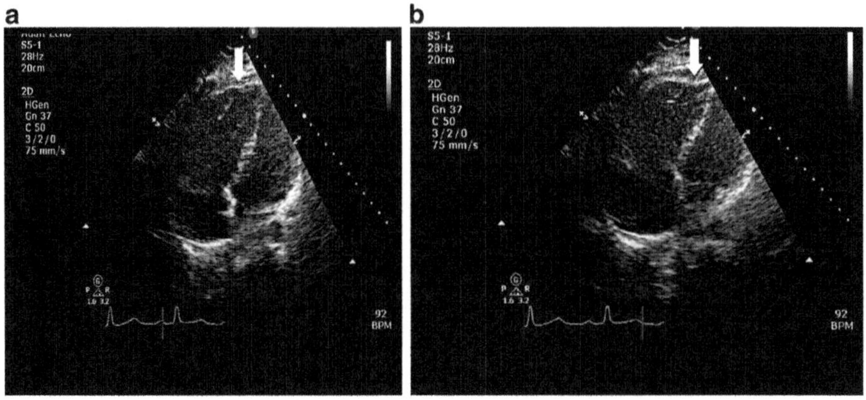

Fig. 9.8 McConnell's sign in a patient with a large pulmonary embolus. Note the systolic "buckling" of the distal one-third of the RV near the RV apex (panel **b** *wide arrow*). This finding is typically observed when RV afterload rises suddenly, rendering the RV dysfunctional and allowing tethering of the RV near the apex due to normal or hypderdynamic LV function

Systemic to Pulmonary Shunt Conditions

Systemic to pulmonary shunts (SPS) can be caused by a myriad of conditions both congenital (atrial or ventricular septal defects, etc.) and acquired (e.g., hemodialysis AV fistula). The extent of hemodynamic perturbation in SPS may depend on the size, location, and chronicity of the shunt. However, there are some common rules that we can discuss here. In general, a SPS leads to an increase in pulmonary blood flow and volume loading of the right heart. The volume overload of a SPS is typically well tolerated and manifests typically as a dilated RV with normal or hyperdynamic RV function. In fact, a dilated and hypercontractile RV serves as an important clue to the presence of a SPS, and also informs the clinician to the notion that the SPS has not yet been complicated by pulmonary vascular remodeling and a rising PVR. In contrast, in the event that an SPS leads to pulmonary vascular injury and a high PVR, the echo-Doppler findings may be indistinguishable from PAH.

In patients with a large, chronic SPS, severe pulmonary vascular remodeling can develop, leading to Eisenmenger syndrome (ES), where marked increases in the PVR lead to partial or complete reversal of the direction of the shunt and cyanosis. In this setting, the slow, gradual increase in afterload characteristically results in marked hypertrophy of the RV free wall. As such, the RV of ES is typically normal in cavity size with extreme RVH, heavy RV trabeculation and a prominent moderator band. The RV in ES is capable of maintaining relatively preserved RV function despite massively elevated PVR, which is an important reason why these subjects survive longer than their PAH counterparts despite a greater degree of PH. RV dilatation and systolic dysfunction in ES usually only occurs at the a very late stage of the disease [7].

Pulmonary Venous Hypertension

Pulmonary venous hypertension (PVH) is by far the most common cause of pulmonary hypertension, and can result from left sided cardiac congestion from varying combinations of LV systolic dysfunction, valvular dysfunction, or diastolic left heart dysfunction [75, 76].

It should be emphasized that a normal LV ejection fraction should not be taken to indicate the presence of a normal left atrial pressure. Simple 2D and Doppler findings provide critical insight into the presence of left heart dysfunction and left heart congestion and allows for rapid differentiation between PVH and PH related to pulmonary vascular disease [77, 78].

One of the most important clues to the presence of PVH is the presence of LA enlargement (LAE). Another important clue to the presence of PVH is the presence of LV hypertrophy (LVH). The combined presence of LAE and LVH provides the most important clue to a diagnosis of left sided heart failure in the presence of a normal LV ejection fraction [79].

The transmitral Doppler examination provides key evidence to the presence or absence of an elevated left atrial pressure [80]. Normal LV filling occurs in two phases; passive early filling represented by the E wave and late, active filling due to atrial contraction represented by the A wave. The A wave is absent in atrial fibrillation. Normally, the majority of diastolic filling occurs early and therefore the normal E/A ratio is >1.0 with an E wave deceleration time of 160–240 ms. Mild impairment of diastolic dysfunction (Grade I diastolic dysfunction) leads to a redistribution of the diastolic flow to the later part of diastole and hence a larger reliance on atrial contraction to empty the LA. In this case, the E/A ratio is E/A< 1.0. As discussed above, in the setting of a dilated and dysfunctional RV, Grade I diastolic dysfunction favors a normal LA pressure and thus a diagnosis of PAH. Grade II and III diastolic filling patterns indicate moderate and severe elevations of left atrial pressure, respectively. Moderate or greater degrees of aortic or mitral valve disease provide compelling evidence of PVH and serve as relatively simple ways to differentiate pure PVH from PAH. In addition, the relative absence of RV dilation, dysfunction and septal flattening in the setting of PH provide key insight to the presence of PVH.

Approach to Differentiating PH_{PVD} from PVH

While right heart catheterization is still considered the gold standard for differentiating PVH from PH_{PVD}, a simple echocardiographic scoring system allows rapid reliable differentiation of these two conditions.

Opotowsky et al. employed a scoring system using LA size, Doppler estimated LA pressure, and the RVOT Doppler profile. Using this approach, the echo score was able to differentiate PH_{PVD} from PVH with an AUC of 0.92 and differentiate Group I and II PH with an AUC of 0.97. No patient with an echo score <0 had PH_{PVD} (Fig. 9.9) [81].

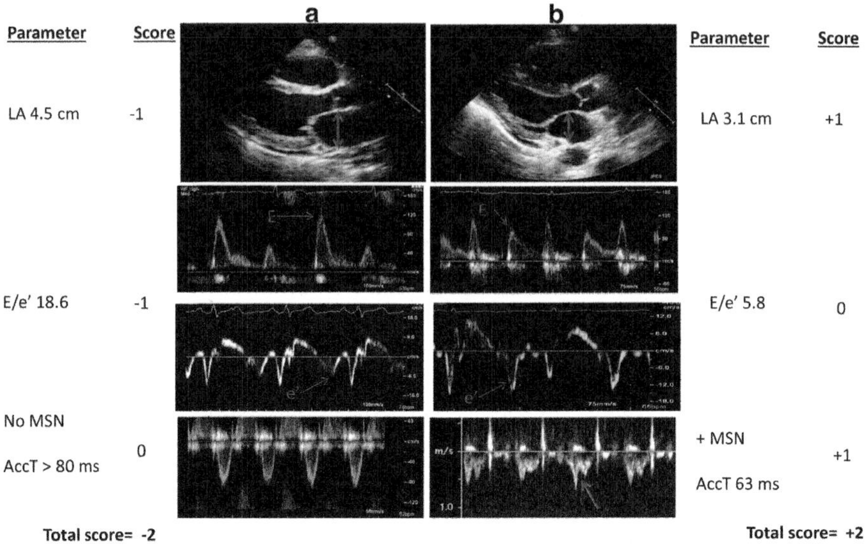

Fig. 9.9 Representative 2D and Doppler echocardiographic images , showing how echo score is derived from the routine images of left atrial size, ratio of transmitral E wave maximal velocity/ tissue Doppler early diastolic velocity (*E*/*e*′), and the shape of the pulsed wave Doppler tracing from the right ventricular outflow tract. Column **a** contains (top to bottom) 2D and Doppler images from a patient with left atrial enlargement, an increased *E*/*e*′, no evidence of "notching" of the pulsed wave Doppler profile in the RV outflow tract and a normal Doppler acceleration time (corresponding echo score = −2). Invasive hemodynamics: mean pulmonary artery pressure of 40 mmHg, pulmonary arterial wedge pressure 29 mmHg, and pulmonary vascular resistance of 2.0 mmHg/l/min. Column **b** contains (top to bottom) 2D and Doppler images from a patient with normal left atrial size, a normal *E*/*e*′, mid-systolic notching of the pulsed wave Doppler profile in the RV outflow tract and a shortened Doppler acceleration time (corresponding echo score = +2). Invasive hemodynamics: mean pulmonary artery pressure of 45 mmHg, pulmonary arterial wedge pressure 10 mmHg, and pulmonary vascular resistance of 8.8 mmHg/l/min. From [81]. Reprinted with permission from Wolters Kluwer Health

Assessment of Response to Therapy in PH_{PVD}

PAH

Galie et al. showed that many of the echocardiographic signature abnormalities in patients with IPAH and PAH associated with CTD improved with bosentan therapy [82]. Namely, improved RV MPI, reduced RV end systolic area, RV:LV diastolic area ratio, and pericardial effusion. Importantly, peak TR velocity did not change significantly, casting further doubt on the value of following this parameter in patients being treated for PAH. Brown et al. demonstrated that TAPSE increases in response to PH specific therapy in PAH; thus, serial TAPSE assessment may be an important and simple method for assessing the RV functional response to therapy in PAH. In this study, the rise in TAPSE positively correlated with a rise in cardiac stroke volume in response to PH therapy [83].

CTEPH

In patients who undergo successful PTE there is a demonstrable improvement in RV size, systolic function and septal flattening. LV diastolic filling also improves [84, 85].

Exercise Echocardiography

Assessment of PAP in response to exercise is an attractive approach to evaluating known or suspected pulmonary hypertension, based on three basic concepts: first, that a rise in PA pressure in response to exercise is always abnormal. Second, that a rise in PA pressure with exercise equates to the cause of a patient's dyspnea, and lastly, that the PASP can be accurately measured with exercise. Unfortunately, the literature on exercise physiology does not support the notion that PA pressure elevation with exercise is necessarily an abnormal response. Several studies, including both invasive and noninvasive assessment of PA pressure with exercise, have demonstrated that especially at higher exercise workloads, healthy subjects can have significant increases in PA pressure with exercise [86–88]. In these subjects, the rise in PA pressure was physiologic, with normal preservation of the pulmonary artery pressure–flow relationship. There is no consensus on what the normal PASP response is to exercise in a healthy aging population nor is there an adjustment for the rise in systemic BP with exercise. Furthermore, a rise in the PASP with exercise does not account for the degree to which left heart congestion is contributing to exercise related PH [89]. As a result, a rise in PASP with exercise may simply indicate exercise induced left heart congestion. Lastly, in our experience, Doppler pressure estimates are often inaccurate in the setting of exercise. Taken together, recent guidelines on the diagnosis and management of pulmonary hypertension state that no treatment decisions should be made on the bases of exercise echocardiography [37].

In our view, a more reliable and robust approach to exercise echocardiography should focus on evaluating the RV functional response to exercise. The finding of a small, hypercontractile RV at peak exercise has much different implications than an RV that becomes increasingly dilated and dysfunction with exercise.

Future Directions

Proper use of the echocardiographic-Doppler examination of patients with known or suspected pulmonary hypertension extends well beyond Doppler assessment of pulmonary arterial systolic pressure. The examination should incorporate measures of RV size, septal position, systolic function and Doppler physiology reflective of pulmonary vascular function in order to provide accurate and relevant information to the clinician. This more integrated echo-Doppler assessment is far more powerful in its approach and provides key differentiating features to the pathophysiology of PH on baseline assessment. Moreover, serial assessment of the right heart is essential to monitoring the response to therapy in PH related to pulmonary vascular disease.

References

1. Dell'italia LJ. Anatomy and physiology of the right ventricle. Cardiol Clin. 2012;30:167–87.
2. James TN. Anatomy of the crista supraventricularis: its importance for understanding right ventricular function, right ventricular infarction and related conditions. J Am Coll Cardiol. 1985;6:1083–95.
3. Rushmer RF, Crystal DK, Wagner C. The functional anatomy of ventricular contraction. Circ Res. 1953;1:162–70.
4. Kaul S, Tei C, Hopkins JM, Shah PM. Assessment of right ventricular function using two-dimensional echocardiography. Am Heart J. 1984;107:526–31.
5. Kerbaul F, Brimioulle S, Rondelet B, Dewachter C, Hubloue I, Naeije R. How prostacyclin improves cardiac output in right heart failure in conjunction with pulmonary hypertension. Am J Respir Crit Care Med. 2007;175:846–50.
6. Kuehne T, Yilmaz S, Steendijk P, Moore P, Groenink M, Saaed M, et al. Magnetic resonance imaging analysis of right ventricular pressure volume loops: In vivo validation and clinical application in patients with pulmonary hypertension. Circulation. 2004;110:2010–6.
7. Hopkins WE. The remarkable right ventricle of patients with Eisenmenger syndrome. Coron Artery Dis. 2005;16:19–25.
8. Schenk P, Globits S, Koller J, Brunner C, Artemiou O, Klepetko W, et al. Accuracy of echocardiographic right ventricular parameters in patients with different end-stage lung diseases prior to lung transplantation. J Heart Lung Transplant. 2000;19:145–54.
9. Ghio S, Recusani F, Klersy C, Sebastiani R, Laudisa ML, Campana C, et al. Prognostic usefulness of the tricuspid annular plane systolic excursion in patients with congestive heart failure secondary to idiopathic or ischemic dilated cardiomyopathy. Am J Cardiol. 2000;85:837–42.
10. Forfia PR, Fisher MR, Mathai SC, Housten-Harris T, Hemnes AR, Borlaug BA, et al. Tricuspid annular displacement predicts survival in pulmonary hypertension. Am J Respir Crit Care Med. 2006;174:1034–41.
11. Brown SB, Rania A, Katz D, Szerlip M, Wiegers SE, Forfia PR. Longitudinal shortening accounts for the majority of right ventricular contraction in normal subjects and in pulmonary arterial hypertension and improves after pulmonary vasodilator therapy. Chest. 2011;140(1): 27–33.
12. Lee CY, Chang SM, Hsiao SH, Tseng JC, Lin SK, Liu CP. Right heart function and scleroderma: Insights from tricuspid annular plane systolic excursion. Echocardiography. 2007;24:118–25.
13. Hammarström E, Wranne B, Pinto FJ, Puryear Y, Popp RL. Tricuspid annular motion. J Am Soc Echocardiogr. 1991;4:131–9.
14. López-Candales A, Dohi K, Rajagopalan N, Edelman K, Gulyasy B, Bazaz R. Defining normal variables of right ventricular size and function in pulmonary hypertension: an echocardiographic study. Postgrad Med J. 2008;84:40–5.
15. Ghio S, Klersy C, Magrini G, D'Armini AM, Scelsi L, Raineri C, et al. Prognostic relevance of the echocardiographic assessment of right ventricular function in patients with idiopathic pulmonary arterial hypertension. Int J Cardiol. 2010;140:272–8.
16. Raina A, Vaidya A, Gertz ZM, Chambers S, Forfia PR. J Heart Lung Transplant. 2013;32(8): 777–83.
17. Saxena N, Rajagopalan N, Edelman K, López-Candales A. Tricuspid annular systolic velocity: a useful measurement in determining right ventricular systolic function regardless of pulmonary artery pressures. Echocardiography. 2006;23:750–5.

18. Rajagopalan N, Saxena N, Simon MA, Edelman K, Mathier MA, López-Candales A. Correlation of tricuspid annular velocities with invasive hemodynamics in pulmonary hypertension. Congest Heart Fail. 2007;13:200–4.
19. Urheim S, Cauduro S, Frantz R, McGoon M, Belohlavek M, Green T, et al. Relation of tissue displacement and strain to invasively determined right ventricular stroke volume. Am J Cardiol. 2005;96:1173–8.
20. Yeo TC, Dujardin KS, Tei C, Mahoney DW, McGoon MD, Seward JB. Value of a Doppler-derived index combining systolic and diastolic time intervals in predicting outcome in primary pulmonary hypertension. Am J Cardiol. 1998;81:1157–61.
21. Hardegree EL, Sachdev A, Villarraga HR, Frantz RP, et al. Role of serial quantitative assessment of right ventricular function by strain in pulmonary arterial hypertension. Am J Cardiol. 2013;111(1):143–8.
22. Bommer W, Weinert L, Neumann A, Neef J, Mason DT, DeMaria A. Determination of right atrial and right ventricular size by two-dimensional echocardiography. Circulation. 1979;60:91–100.
23. López-Candales A, Dohi K, Iliescu A, Peterson RC, Edelman K, Bazaz R. An abnormal right ventricular apical angle is indicative of global right ventricular impairment. Echocardiography. 2006;23:361–8.
24. Bove AA, Santamore WP. Ventricular interdependence. Prog Cardiovasc Dis. 1981;23: 365–88.
25. Marcus JT, Gan CT, Zwanenburg JJ, Boonstra A, Allaart CP, Götte MJ, et al. Interventricular mechanical asynchrony in pulmonary arterial hypertension: Left-to-right delay in peak shortening is related to right ventricular overload and left ventricular underfilling. J Am Coll Cardiol. 2008;51:750–7.
26. Benza R, Biederman R, Murali S, Gupta H. Role of cardiac magnetic resonance imaging in the management of patients with pulmonary arterial hypertension. J Am Coll Cardiol. 2008;52: 1683–92.
27. Gan CT, Lankhaar JW, Marcus JT, Westerhof N, Marques KM, Bronzwaer JG, et al. Impaired left ventricular filling due to right-to-left ventricular interaction in patients with pulmonary arterial hypertension. Am J Physiol Heart Circ Physiol. 2006;290:H1528–33.
28. Mauritz GJ, Marcus JT, Westerhof N, Postmus PE, Vonk-Noordegraaf A. Prolonged right ventricular post-systolic isovolumic period in pulmonary arterial hypertension is not a reflection of diastolic dysfunction. Heart. 2011;97:473–8.
29. Hinderliter AL, Willis IV PW, Long W, Clarke WR, Ralph D, Caldwell EJ, et al. Frequency and prognostic significance of pericardial effusion in primary pulmonary hypertension. PPH Study Group. Primary pulmonary hypertension. Am J Cardiol. 1999;84:481–4.
30. Miller AJ. Some observations concerning pericardial effusions and their relationship to the venous and lymphatic circulation of the heart. Lymphology. 1970;3:76–8.
31. Hemnes AR, Gaine SP, Wiener CM. Poor outcomes associated with drainage of pericardial effusions in patients with pulmonary arterial hypertension. South Med J. 2008;101:490–4.
32. Fenstad ER, Le RJ, Sinak LJ, Maradit-Kremers H, et al. Pericardial effusions in pulmonary arterial hypertension: characteristics, prognosis, and role of drainage. Chest. 2013;144(5): 1530–8.
33. Raymond RJ, Hinderliter AL, Willis PW, Ralph D, Caldwell EJ, Williams W, Ettinger NA, Hill NS, Summer WR, de Boisblanc B, et al. Echocardiographic predictors of adverse outcomes in primary pulmonary hypertension. J Am Coll Cardiol. 2002;39:1214–9.
34. Sivak J, Raina A, Forfia P. Assessing the physiologic contribution of right atrial function to total right ventricular function in patients with and without pulmonary arterial hypertension. Am J Respir Crit Care Med. 2011;183:4999. Abstract.
35. McLaughlin VV, Presberg KW, Doyle RL, Abman SH, McCrory DC, Fortin T, et al. Prognosis of pulmonary arterial hypertension: ACCP evidence based clinical practice guidelines. Chest. 2004;126 Suppl 1:78S–92.
36. McQuillan BM, Picard MH, Leavitt M, Weyman AE. Clinical correlates and subjects. Circulation. 2001;104:2797–802.

37. McLaughlin VV, Archer SL, Badesch DB, Barst RJ, Farber HW, Lindner JR, et al. ACCF/AHA 2009 expert consensus document on pulmonary hypertension a report of the American College of Cardiology Foundation Task Force on Expert Consensus Documents and the American Heart Association developed in collaboration with the American College of Chest Physicians; American Thoracic Society, Inc.; and the Pulmonary Hypertension Association. J Am Coll Cardiol. 2009;53:1573–619.
38. Berger M, Haimowitz A, Van Tosh A, Berdoff RL, Goldberg E. Quantitative assessment of pulmonary hypertension in patients with tricuspid regurgitation using continuous wave Doppler ultrasound. J Am Coll Cardiol. 1985;6:359–65.
39. Yock PG, Popp RL. Noninvasive estimation of right ventricular systolic pressure by Doppler ultrasound in patients with tricuspid regurgitation. Circulation. 1984;70:657–62.
40. Himelman RB, Stulbarg M, Kircher B, Lee E, Kee L, Dean NC, et al. Noninvasive evaluation of pulmonary artery pressure during exercise by saline-enhanced Doppler echocardiography in chronic pulmonary disease. Circulation. 1989;79:863–71.
41. Chan KL, Currie PJ, Seward JB, Hagler DJ, Mair DD, Tajik AJ. Comparison of three Doppler ultrasound methods in the prediction of pulmonary artery pressure. J Am Coll Cardiol. 1987;9:549–54.
42. Fisher MR, Forfia PR, Chamera E, Housten-Harris T, Champion HC, Girgis RE, et al. Accuracy of Doppler echocardiography in the hemodynamic assessment of pulmonary hypertension. Am J Respir Crit Care Med. 2009;179:615–21.
43. Brennan JM, Blair JE, Goonewardena S, Ronan A, Shah D, Vasaiwala S, et al. Reappraisal of the use of inferior vena cava for estimating right atrial pressure. J Am Soc Echocardiogr. 2007;20:857–61.
44. Kircher BJ, Himelman RB, Schiller NB. Noninvasive estimation of right atrial pressure from the inspiratory collapse of the inferior vena cava. Am J Cardiol. 1990;66:493–6.
45. Utsunomiya H, Nakatani S, Nishihira M, Kanzaki H, Kyotani S, Nakanishi N, et al. Value of estimated right ventricular filling pressure in predicting cardiac events in chronic pulmonary arterial hypertension. J Am Soc Echocardiogr. 2009;22:1368–74.
46. Rich JD, Shah SJ, Swamy RS, Kamp A, Rich S. Inaccuracy of Doppler echocardiographic estimates of pulmonary artery pressures in patients with pulmonary hypertension. Chest. 2011;139:988–93.
47. Kitabatake A, Inoue M, Asao M, Masuyama T, Tanouchi J, Morita T, et al. Noninvasive evaluation of pulmonary hypertension by a pulsed Doppler technique. Circulation. 1983;68:302–9.
48. Masuyama T, Kodama K, Kitabatake A, Sato H, Nanto S, Inoue M. Continuous wave Doppler echocardiographic detection of pulmonary regurgitation and its application to noninvasive estimation of pulmonary artery pressure. Circulation. 1986;74:484–92.
49. Lanzarini L, Fontana A, Lucca E, Campana C, Klersy C. Noninvasive estimation of both systolic and diastolic pulmonary artery pressure from Doppler analysis of tricuspid regurgitant velocity spectrum in patients with chronic heart failure. Am Heart J. 2002;144:1087–94.
50. Stephen B, Dalal P, Berger M, Schweitzer P, Hecht S. Noninvasive estimation of pulmonary artery diastolic pressure in patients with tricuspid regurgitation by Doppler echocardiography. Chest. 1999;116:73–7.
51. Abbas AE, Fortuin FD, Schiller NB, Appleton CP, Moreno CA, Lester SJ. A simple method for noninvasive estimation of pulmonary vascular resistance. J Am Coll Cardiol. 2003;41:1021–7.
52. Rajagopalan N, Simon MA, Suffoletto MS, Shah H, Edelman K, Mathier MA, et al. Noninvasive estimation of pulmonary vascular resistance in pulmonary hypertension. Echocardiography. 2009;26:489–94.
53. Opotowsky AR, Clair M, Afilalo J, et al. A simple echocardiographic method to estimate pulmonary vascular resistance. Am J Cardiol. 2013;112(6):873–82.
54. Furuno Y, Nagamoto Y, Fujita M, Kaku T, Sakurai S, Kuroiwa A. Reflection as a cause of mid-systolic deceleration of pulmonary flow wave in dogs with acute pulmonary hypertension: Comparison of pulmonary artery constriction with pulmonary embolisation. Cardiovasc Res. 1991;25:118–24.

55. Torbicki A, Kurzyna M, Ciurzynski M, Pruszczyk P, Pacho R, Kuch-Wocial A, et al. Proximal pulmonary emboli modify right ventricular ejection pattern. Eur Respir J. 1999;13:616–21.
56. Castelain V, Hervé P, Lecarpentier Y, Duroux P, Simonneau G, Chemla D. Pulmonary artery pulse pressure and wave reflection in chronicpulmonary thromboembolism and primary pulmonary hypertension. J Am Coll Cardiol. 2001;37:1085–92.
57. Arkles JS, Opotowsky AR, Ojeda J, Rogers F, Liu T, Prassana V, et al. Midsystolic 'notching' of the pulmonary artery Doppler flow profile identifies pulmonary vascular disease and RV dysfunction in a mixed PH cohort. Am J Respir Crit Care Med. 2009;179:A3399.
58. Goodman DJ, Harrison DC, Popp RL. Echocardiographic features of primary pulmonary hypertension. Am J Cardiol. 1974;33:438–43.
59. Bossone E, Duong-Wagner TH, Paciocco G, Oral H, Ricciardi M, Bach DS, et al. Echocardiographic features of primary pulmonary hypertension. J Am Soc Echocardiogr. 1999;12:655–62.
60. Dartevelle P, Fadel E, Mussot S, Chapelier A, Hervé P, de Perrot M, et al. Chronic thromboembolic pulmonary hypertension. Eur Respir J. 2004;23:637–48.
61. Fedullo PF, Auger WR, Kerr KM, Rubin LJ. Chronic thromboembolic pulmonary hypertension. N Engl J Med. 2001;345:1465–72.
62. Nakayama Y, Nakanishi N, Sugimachi M, Takaki H, Kyotani S, Satoh T, et al. Characteristics of pulmonary artery pressure waveform for differential diagnosis of chronic pulmonary thromboembolism and primary pulmonary hypertension. J Am Coll Cardiol. 1997;29: 1311–6.
63. Tanabe N, Okada O, Abe Y, Masuda M, Nakajima N, Kuriyama T. The influence of fractional pulse pressure on the outcome of pulmonary thromboendarterectomy. Eur Respir J. 2001;17: 653–9.
64. Nakayama Y, Sugimachi M, Nakanishi N, Takaki H, Okano Y, Satoh T, et al. Noninvasive differential diagnosis between chronic pulmonary thromboembolism and primary pulmonary hypertension by means of Doppler ultrasound measurement. J Am Coll Cardiol. 1998;31: 1367–71.
65. Miniati M, Monti S, Pratali L, Di Ricco G, Marini C, Formichi B, et al. Value of transthoracic echocardiography in the diagnosis of pulmonary embolism: results of a prospective study in unselected patients. Am J Med. 2001;110:528–35.
66. Guyton AC, Lindsey AW, Gilluly JJ. The limits of right ventricular compensation following acute increase in pulmonary circulatory resistance. Circ Res. 1954;2:326–32.
67. Kasper W, Geibel A, Tiede N, Bassenge D, Kauder E, Konstantinides S, et al. Distinguishing between acute and subacute massive pulmonary embolism by conventional and Doppler echocardiography. Br Heart J. 1993;70:352–6.
68. Jardin F, Dubourg O, Guéret P, Delorme G, Bourdarias JP. Quantitative two-dimensional echocardiography in massive pulmonary embolism: emphasis on ventricular interdependence and leftward septal displacement. J Am Coll Cardiol. 1987;10:1201–6.
69. Ribeiro A, Juhlin-Dannfelt A, Brodin LA, Holmgren A, Jorfeldt L. Pulmonary embolism: relation between the degree of right ventricle overload and the extent of perfusion defects. Am Heart J. 1998;135:868–74.
70. McConnell MV, Solomon SD, Rayan ME, Come PC, Goldhaber SZ, Lee RT. Regional right ventricular dysfunction detected by echocardiography in acute pulmonary embolism. Am J Cardiol. 1996;78:469–73.
71. Hsiao SH, Lee CY, Chang SM, Yang SH, Lin SK, Huang WC. Pulmonary embolism and right heart function: Insights from myocardial Doppler tissue imaging. J Am Soc Echocardiogr. 2006;19:822–8.
72. Kurzyna M, Torbicki A, Pruszczyk P, Burakowska B, Fijałkowska A, Kober J, et al. Disturbed right ventricular ejection pattern as a new Doppler echocardiographic sign of acute pulmonary embolism. Am J Cardiol. 2002;90:507–11.
73. Torbicki A, Galié N, Covezzoli A, Rossi E, De Rosa M, Goldhaber SZ, ICOPER Study Group. Right heart thrombi in pulmonary embolism: results from the International Cooperative Pulmonary Embolism Registry. J Am Coll Cardiol. 2003;41:2245–51.

74. Pierre-Justin G, Pierard LA. Management of mobile right heart thrombi: a prospective series. Int J Cardiol. 2005;99:381–8.
75. Delgado JF, Conde E, Sánchez V, López-Ríos F, Gómez-Sánchez MA, Escribano P, et al. Pulmonary vascular remodeling in pulmonary hypertension due to chronic heart failure. Eur J Heart Fail. 2005;7:1011–6.
76. Moraes DL, Colucci WS, Givertz MM. Secondary pulmonary hypertension in chronic heart failure: the role of the endothelium in pathophysiology and management. Circulation. 2000;102:1718–23.
77. Tribouilloy CM, Enriquez-Sarano M, Rossi A, Tajik AJ, Seward JB. Determinants of the pulmonary artery pressure rise in left ventricular dysfunction. Cardiologia. 1997;42:1051–8.
78. Forfia PR. Approach to patients with heart failure and pulmonary hypertension. Curr Treat Options Cardiovasc Med. 2007;9:302–9.
79. Melenovsky V, Borlaug BA, Rosen B, Hay I, Ferruci L, Morell CH, et al. Cardiovascular features of heart failure with preserved ejection fraction versus nonfailing hypertensive left ventricular hypertrophy in the urban Baltimore community: the role of atrial remodeling/dysfunction. J Am Coll Cardiol. 2007;49:198–207.
80. Nishimura RA, Tajik AJ. Evaluation of diastolic filling of left ventricle in health and disease: Doppler echocardiography is the clinician's Rosetta Stone. J Am Coll Cardiol. 1997;30:8–18.
81. Opotowsky AR, Ojeda J, Rogers F, et al. A simple echocardiographic prediction rule for hemodynamics in pulmonary hypertension. Circ Cardiovasc Imaging. 2012;5:765–75.
82. Galiè N, Hinderliter AL, Torbicki A, Fourme T, Simonneau G, Pulido T, et al. Effects of the oral endothelin-receptor antagonist bosentan on echocardiographic and Doppler measures in patients with pulmonary arterial hypertension. J Am Coll Cardiol. 2003;41:1380–6.
83. Brown BS, Raina A, Katz D, Szerlip M, Weigers SE, Forfia RP. Longitudinal shortening accounts for the majority of right ventricular contraction and improves after pulmonary vasodilator therapy in normal subjects and patients with pulmonary arterial hypertension. Chest. 2011;140(1):27–33.
84. Casaclang-Verzosa G, McCully RB, Oh JK, Miller Jr FA, McGregor CG. Effects of pulmonary thromboendarterectomy on right-sided echocardiographic parameters in patients with chronic thromboembolic pulmonary hypertension. Mayo Clin Proc. 2006;81:777–82.
85. Menzel T, Kramm T, Wagner S, Mohr-Kahaly S, Mayer E, Meyer J. Improvement of tricuspid regurgitation after pulmonary thromboendarterectomy. Ann Thorac Surg. 2002;73:756–61.
86. Damato AN, Galante JG, Smith WM. Hemodynamic response to treadmill exercise in normal subjects. J Appl Physiol. 1966;21:959–66.
87. Wagner PD, Gale GE, Moon RE, Torre-Bueno JR, Stolp BW, Saltzman HA. Pulmonary gas exchange in humans exercising at sea level and simulated altitude. J Appl Physiol. 1986;61:260–70.
88. Bossone E, Rubenfire M, Bach DS, Ricciardi M, Armstrong WF. Range of tricuspid regurgitation velocity at rest and during exercise in normal adult men: implications for the diagnosis of pulmonary hypertension. J Am Coll Cardiol. 1999;33:1662–6.
89. Kovacs G, Berghold A, Scheidl S, Olschewski H. Pulmonary arterial pressure during rest and exercise in healthy subjects. A systematic review. Eur Respir J. 2009;34:888–94.

Chapter 10
Pulmonary Hemodynamics and Right Heart Catheterization

Saurabh Rajpal, Yonatan Buber, and Michael J. Landzberg

Abstract Hemodynamic assessment of the patient with pulmonary hypertension begins with a careful physical exam and is followed by several noninvasive tests and ultimately right heart catheterization. Proper interpretation of the considerable data that is generated by this process requires a firm working knowledge of the pulmonary circulation and right ventricle along with major factors that can affect pulmonary vascular tone and cardiac output. This chapter reviews normal cardiopulmonary physiology and provides an in depth approach to assessing pulmonary hemodynamics in patients with pulmonary vascular disease. A detailed discussion of the physical exam and techniques used for transthoracic echocardiogram and right heart catheterization are provided along with a guide to interpreting their results. The skills and diagnostic approaches presented are necessary for the proper diagnosis of pulmonary vascular disease and should be used to distinguish patients with pulmonary arterial hypertension from patients with pulmonary hypertension associated with left heart failure or chronic thromboembolic pulmonary hypertension.

Keywords Pulmonary hypertension • Pulmonary arterial pressure • Cardiac output • Pulmonary vascular resistance • Right heart catheterization • Pulmonary artery catheter

---

S. Rajpal, M.D.
Louisiana State University School of Medicine, Shreveport, LA, USA

Boston Adult Congenital Heart (BACH) and Pulmonary Hypertension Group, Brigham and Women's Hospital and Children's Hospital, Harvard Medical School, Boston, MA, USA

Y. Buber, M.D.
Boston Adult Congenital Heart (BACH) and Pulmonary Hypertension Group, Brigham and Women's Hospital and Children's Hospital, Harvard Medical School, Boston, MA, USA

Sheba Medical Center, Sackler School of Medicine, Tel Aviv, Israel

M.J. Landzberg, M.D. (✉)
Boston Adult Congenital Heart (BACH) and Pulmonary Hypertension Group, Brigham and Women's Hospital and Children's Hospital, Harvard Medical School, Boston, MA, USA

Department of Cardiology, Boston Children's Hospital,
300 Longwood Avenue, Bader, 2nd Floor, Boston, MA 02115, USA
e-mail: Mike.Landzberg@CARDIO.CHBOSTON.ORG

J.R. Klinger, R.P. Frantz (eds.), *Diagnosis and Management of Pulmonary Hypertension*, Respiratory Medicine 12, DOI 10.1007/978-1-4939-2636-7_10

Abbreviations

AT	Acceleration time
CCB	Calcium channel blocker
CP	Constrictive pericarditis
CTEPH	Chronic thromboembolic pulmonary hypertension
CVP	Central venous pressure
dPAP	Diastolic pulmonary artery pressure
DPG	Diastolic pressure gradient
FAC	Fractional area change
ICU	Intensive care unit
IJ	Internal jugular
IVC	Inferior vena cava
JVP	Jugular venous pulse
LAP	Left atrial pressure
LV	Left ventricle
mLAP	Mean left atrial pressure
MPA	Main pulmonary artery
mPAP	Mean pulmonary artery pressure
NO	Nitric oxide
PAH	Pulmonary arterial hypertension
PAOP	Pulmonary artery occlusion pressure
PAP	Pulmonary artery pressure
PBF	Pulmonary blood flow
PCWP	Pulmonary capillary wedge pressure
PH	Pulmonary hypertension
PVR	Pulmonary vascular resistance
RAP	Right atrial pressure
RCM	Restrictive cardiomyopathy
RHC	Right heart catheterization
RV	Right ventricle
RVH	Right ventricle hypertrophy
RVOT	Right ventricle outflow tract
RVSP	Right ventricular systolic pressure
sPAP	Systolic pulmonary artery pressure
TAPSE	Tricuspid annulus plane systolic excursion
TPG	Transpulmonary gradient
TRV	Tricuspid regurgitation velocity
TTE	Transthoracic echocardiography
VTI	Velocity time integral

Definition of Pulmonary Hypertension Based on Hemodynamics

The conventional definition of pulmonary hypertension (PH) used in clinical studies includes a mean pulmonary artery pressure (mPAP) of greater than 25 mmHg at rest in the setting of a normal pulmonary arterial wedge pressure of 15 mmHg or less with a pulmonary vascular resistance (PVR) greater than 3 Wood units [1, 2]. Cardiac catheterization and hemodynamic assessment are essential for the diagnosis of PH. Of note, the current US and European PH care guidelines do not support the use of pulmonary artery hypertension (PAH) specific medications without a hemodynamic evaluation by right heart catheterization [2, 3]. Table 10.1 lists the hemodynamic definition of pulmonary hypertension [3].

The Pulmonary Vasculature

The lung has a dual blood supply from the bronchial and pulmonary circulations. While bronchial blood flow is a small part (2 %) of the left ventricular output; the pulmonary circulation carries the entire output of the right ventricle (RV) which in the absence of significant intravascular shunting equals left ventricular output and supplies the lung with the mixed venous blood draining all the tissues of the body [4]. It is the blood in the pulmonary circulation that participates in the gas exchange process.

Table 10.1 Hemodynamic definitions of pulmonary hypertension [3]

Definition	Characteristics	Clinical group(s)
Pulmonary hypertension (PH)	Mean PAP ≥25 mmHg	All
Pre-capillary PH	Mean PAP ≥25 mmHg	1. Pulmonary arterial hypertension
	PWP ≤15 mmHg	3. PH due to lung diseases
	CO normal or reduced	4. Chronic thromboembolic PH
		5. PH with unclear and/or multifactorial mechanisms
Post-capillary PH	Mean PAP ≥25 mmHg	2. PH due to left heart disease
	PCWP >15 mmHg	
	CO normal or reduced	
Passive	TPG ≤12 mmHg	
Reactive (out of proportion)	TPG >12 mmHg	

CO cardiac output, *PAP* pulmonary artery pressure, *PCWP* pulmonary capillary wedge pressure, *PH* pulmonary hypertension, *TPG* transpulmonary gradient

Despite typically similar blood flow, the pulmonary and systemic circulation have major differences. The pulmonary artery and its branches have thinner walls (comprised of less smooth muscle and elastin), and greater internal diameters when compared to the systemic arteries; as well, there are no smaller denominators of pulmonary artery that correspond to the highly muscular systemic arterioles [5]. As the result of these factors the pulmonary arteries have lower resistance and are both more distensible and compressible when compared to systemic arteries (Fig. 10.1). The location of pulmonary vessels in the thorax subjects them to alveolar and intrapleural and intrathoracic pressure changes that occur with respiration [4, 5]. These characteristics combine to underscore the importance of considering transmural pressure gradient (during both spontaneous as well as mechanical ventilation) as a determinant of PVR. It is important to know during which respiratory phase pulmonary vascular pressures are measured and a standard should be followed when reporting such.

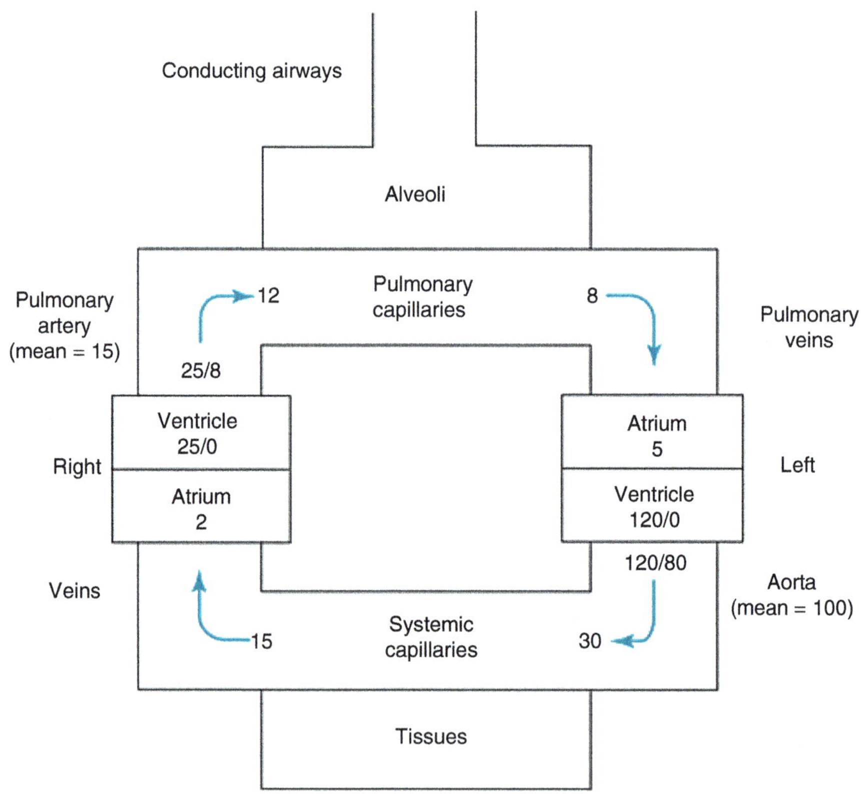

Fig. 10.1 Normal cardiac chamber pressures

Pulmonary Vascular Resistance (PVR)

PVR cannot be measured directly, but must be calculated. According to Hagen–Poiseuille's law that assumes laminar flow, non-compressible fluid and no flow acceleration, the pressure difference across a non-distensible tube is equal to flow multiplied by resistance represented by the equation $P1-P2=Q\times R$, where P1 is pressure at beginning of the tube, P2 is pressure at the end of the tube, Q is flow and R is resistance. Extrapolating this to pulmonary circulation, PVR = (mPAP − mLAP)/PBF, where PVR is pulmonary vascular resistance, mPAP is mean pulmonary artery pressure, mLAP is mean left atrial pressure and PBF is pulmonary blood flow which in the absence of significant intravascular shunting is equal to systemic cardiac output [4, 6].

As intravascular pressures, resistance, impedance, and afterload are lower in the pulmonary circulation as contrasted to the systemic arterial circulation, the left ventricle has greater metabolic demand and is thicker than the right ventricle. Under normal physiologic conditions, pulmonary arterial pressure (PAP) need not be as high as the systemic arterial pressure to overcome the effects of gravity, nor to distribute blood flow among several vascular beds. While in systemic circulation the majority of vascular resistance lies in the systemic arterioles, in the pulmonary circulation vascular resistance is evenly distributed among the pulmonary arteries, capillaries and veins. As the pulmonary circulation holds the same amount of blood with lower pressures, under normal circumstances PVR is one sixth to one ninth of the systemic vascular resistance. In addition to intrinsic vascular factors that regulate pulmonary vascular smooth muscle tone (Table 10.2), extravascular or mechanical factors (Table 10.3) are important in the regulation of PVR.

Gravitational Distribution of Pulmonary Blood Flow

Traditionally, gravity is considered to be an important factor affecting distribution of pulmonary blood flow (Fig. 10.2). In this classical model the lung is considered to have three zones: zone 1 has higher alveolar pressure than PAP and hence no blood flow occurs, in zone 3, PA and pulmonary vein pressure (PVP) are both greater than the alveolar pressure and hence blood flow occurs based on the pressure gradient between the PA and the PV, and in zone 2 PA pressure is higher than alveolar pressure and the driving force for pulmonary blood flow is the pressure difference between alveoli and pulmonary artery [7].

Although gravity has a measurable effect on pulmonary blood flow, recent studies have shown that gravity may not be the most important factor affecting distribution blood flow in lung as compared to anatomy and anatomic structure of the pulmonary arterial tree [8, 9]. While measuring PAP and PVR during catheterization this concept of zones of lungs is important to keep in mind especially if pressures are being measured in an upright patient.

Table 10.2 Factors affecting PVR specifically pulmonary vascular smooth muscle (modified from Levitzky MG. Chapter 4. Blood flow to the lung. In: Levitzky MG. eds. Pulmonary Physiology, 8e. New York, NY: McGraw-Hill; 2013)

Increase	Decrease
Stimulation of sympathetic innervation (may have greater effect by decreasing large vessel distensibility)	Stimulation of parasympathetic innervation (if vascular tone is already elevated)
Norepinephrine, epinephrine	Acetylcholine
Alpha adrenergic agonists	B-adrenergic agonists
PGF2A	PGE1
PGE2	PGI2
Thromboxane	Nitric oxide
Endothelin	Bradykinin
Angiotensin	
Histamine	
Alveolar hypoxia	
Alveolar hypercapnea	
Low pH	

Table 10.3 Factors affecting PVR—passive or mechanical factors (modified from Levitzky MG. Chapter 4. Blood flow to the lung. In: Levitzky MG. eds. Pulmonary physiology, 8e. New York, NY: McGraw-Hill; 2013)

Factor	Effect on PVR	Mechanism
Lung volume increase above functional residual capacity (FRC)	Increases	Lengthening and compression of alveolar vessels
Lung volume decrease above FRC	Increases	Compression of and less traction on extra-alveolar vessels
Increased pulmonary artery pressure; increased left atrial pressure; increased pulmonary blood volume; increased cardiac output	Decreases	Recruitment and distention *Long term effect of these factors could be elevation in PVR due to vascular remodeling*
Gravity; body position	Decreases in gravity-dependent regions of the lungs	Hydrostatic effects lead to recruitment and distention
Increased (more positive) interstitial pressure	Increases	Compression of vessels
Increased blood viscosity	Increases	Viscosity directly increases resistance
Positive-pressure ventilation		
Increased alveolar pressure	Increases	Compression and de-recruitment of alveolar vessels
Positive intrapleural pressure	Increases	Compression of extra-alveolar vessels; compression of vena cava decreases pulmonary blood flow and leads to derecruitment

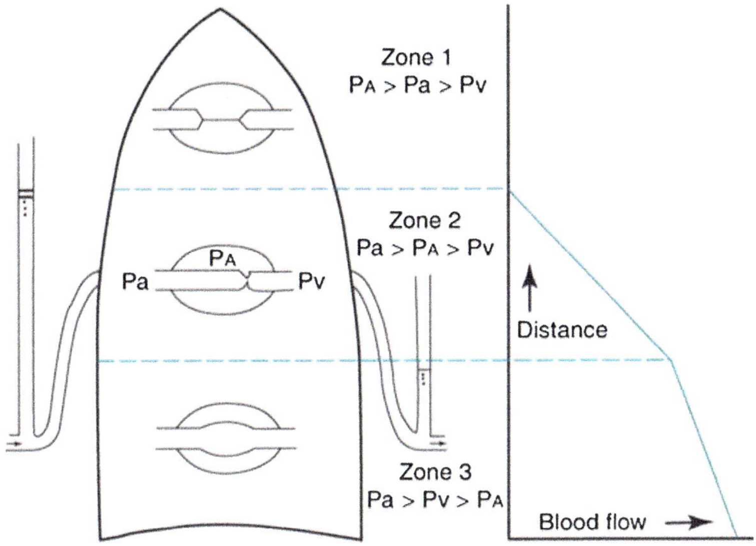

Fig. 10.2 Lung zones in gravitational distribution of pulmonary blood flow model

Hypoxic Pulmonary Vasoconstriction

Hypoxia has important physiologic effects on pulmonary vascular tone, typically balancing less ventilated and more poorly oxygenated alveoli with reduced blood flow under normal conditions. Arteriolar vasoconstriction (Fig. 10.3) in the less oxygenated alveoli, reduces the blood flow and hence decreases contamination of the pulmonary venous blood with poorly oxygenated blood [10].

Noninvasive Hemodynamic Assessment of Pulmonary Hypertension

Clinical Examination

The noninvasive evaluation of a patient starts with clinical examination. Patients who are using pulmonary vasodilator pharmacologic therapy have a distinct facial flushing which can mask effects of systemic arterial vasoconstriction due to low systemic cardiac output (and at times can simulate distributive physiology). Use of sphygmomanometric response of systemic blood pressure to valsalva maneuver is extremely useful in estimating pulmonary capillary wedge pressure (PCWP) [11]. Inflation of brachial cuff to blood pressure 15 points higher than systemic arterial systolic blood pressure, performance of valsalva maneuver for up to 10 s and observation of phase 2 response allows for reliable and reproducible estimation of PCWP.

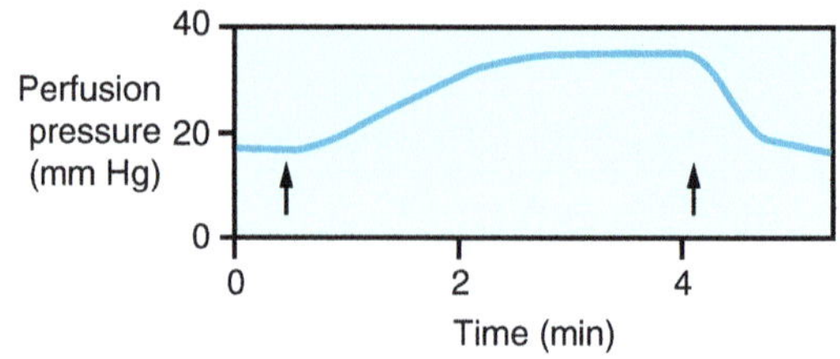

Fig. 10.3 Effect of hypoxia on vascular resistance of an isolated rat lung. The lung was perfused with blood at a constant flow. When the O_2 tension of the inspired air was reduced (between the *arrows*), the pulmonary resistance vessels constricted, as indicated by the substantial rise in perfusion pressure

Normally, Korotkoff sounds are heard during the initial phase of Valsalva then stop and return again at the end of Valsalva (phase 2). The persistence of Korotkoff sounds for either ≥4 beats but <10 s after the start of Valsalva, or for ≥10 s ("square root response") predicts elevated PCWP. Jugular venous pulsations (JVP) are elevated, at times with prominent "v" waves if significant tricuspid regurgitation is present. An elevated JVP signifies an elevated RV end diastolic pressure and hence RV failure and poor prognosis. Venous hypertension can also be examined by provoking the abdominojugular reflux sign, which indicates a volume-overloaded state and limited compliance of the systemic venous system. The abdominojugular reflux sign is provoked by applying consistent pressure over the right upper abdominal quadrant, for at least 10 s. A sustained rise of >3 cm in the venous pressure for at least 15 s is a positive response [12]. It is also important to note how quickly the JVP "falls" when the abdominal pressure is removed to assess the compliance of the systemic venous system.

Clubbing may be present and is a marker of chronic hypoxemia. The RV is anteriorly positioned, directly behind the sternum and chest wall; a palpable "right ventricular" heave is variably present when it is enlarged. Auscultation may include a loud pulmonary component of the second heart sound (P2), a holosystolic murmur of tricuspid regurgitation, a diastolic murmur of pulmonary insufficiency and a third sound of RV origin. Tricuspid regurgitation in the setting of markedly elevated RV systolic pressure and an enlarged RV may produce a high-pitched murmur. Lung sounds are usually normal; "wet" crackles suggest elevated left ventricular end diastolic pressure, disease, while "dry" inspiratory crackles may point towards interstitial lung disease [13]. Hepatomegaly, elevated JVP, peripheral edema, ascites, and cool extremities are consistent with low output right heart failure, indicating more advanced disease.

Chest X-Ray

A chest X-ray cannot be used for diagnosis of PH; however, certain findings can suggest important hemodynamics even though these findings are not sensitive or specific. An increased diameter of the right descending pulmonary artery may suggest significant elevated PAP. Increased hilar thoracic index (the horizontal distance between the outer borders of the right and left pulmonary arteries divided by the maximum transverse diameter of the thoracic cage. A ratio <0.35 is considered to be normal) is also suggestive of elevated PAP [14, 15]. In a prospective study of idiopathic pulmonary arterial hypertension (IPAH), the chest radiograph demonstrated prominence of the main pulmonary artery in 90 % of patients, enlarged hilar vessels in 80 %, and decreased peripheral vessels in 50 %. All three abnormalities were seen in just over 40 % of subjects, and the presence of all three abnormalities was associated with a higher mPAP and lower cardiac index [16]. The PCWP can be estimated by observing the vascular pattern and the presence of interstitial or alveolar edema on chest radiographs. It has been suggested that PCWP greater than 13 but less than 18 mmHg indicates the presence of vascular redistribution with relative hypervascularity of the upper lung fields. When PCWP is 18–25 mmHg, interstitial pulmonary edema is seen and when greater than 25 mmHg, alveolar edema and often pleural effusion is present [17, 18]. Such changes may be absent in the presence of remodeling changes within the pulmonary vascular bed.

CT Scan

CT scan and angiography are pivotal in diagnosing pulmonary embolism and chronic thromboembolic pulmonary hypertension (CTEPH), peripheral pulmonary arterial stenosis, and mechanical or other etiologies of obstruction within the pulmonary vasculature as causes of PH (as well as for ruling out significant primary parenchymal lung disease). However, for direct hemodynamic assessment of PH, CT has a limited role. Some CT findings that can predict hemodynamics include the main pulmonary artery (MPA) caliber, segmental artery to bronchus ratio [19, 20, 22], and presence of pericardial effusion [21]. MPA caliber greater than 29 mm measured 2 cm from the pulmonary valve has 84 % sensitivity, 75 % specificity, and 97 % positive predictive value for the presence of pulmonary arterial hypertension. Also, if the MPA has a maximum transverse diameter greater than that of the proximal ascending thoracic aorta, sensitivity is 70 %, specificity 92 %, and positive predictive value 96 % for the presence of pulmonary arterial hypertension. Segmental artery to bronchus ratio greater than 1.25 times the caliber of the adjacent bronchus suggests elevation of PAP [21] and pericardial thickening or effusion is suggestive of mPAP>35 mmHg.

MRI

The use of MRI in management of patients with PH is evolving. Phase contrast MRI calculated pulmonary vascular index, acceleration time (defined as time from onset of PA forward flow to maximum velocity), the ratio between acceleration time and RV ejection time are being evaluated to calculate PAP but results have been variable [23]. Kuehne and colleagues showed that PVR assessment using MRI-guided catheterization and MRI velocity mapping provided more reproducible results than the traditional thermodilution method. In addition, this technique seems to provide the ability to sample PVR more comprehensively (including both overall and branch-specific resistance) than can be achieved using Doppler guidewires [24].

Electrocardiogram

Electrocardiogram (ECG) lacks sensitivity and specificity in diagnosing PH. In patients with PH, sinus tachycardia may be the only abnormality present (EKG could be completely normal). RV strain, right ventricular hypertrophy (RVH), incomplete right bundle branch block and increased P wave amplitude are common findings [25]. On occasion, in patients in whom PAH attenuating treatment has been very effective, dramatic ECG changes from a pattern corresponding with RVH to a (near)-normal pattern have been reported [26]. P wave amplitude has been shown to predict prognosis in PAH [27].

Echocardiogram

The transthoracic echocardiogram (TTE) remains a core element of RV assessment with applications in the initial and longitudinal diagnosis and screening of pulmonary hypertension, discrimination between contributors to etiology, as well as in assessment of RV and valvular function. The European Society of Cardiology guidelines for the diagnosis and treatment of PH suggest the following: (1) PH is unlikely for tricuspid regurgitation velocity (TRV) ≤2.8 m/s, systolic PAP (sPAP) ≤ 36 mmHg (assuming RAP of 5 mmHg), and no additional echocardiographic signs of PH; (2) PH possible for TRV ≤ 2.8 m/s and sPAP ≤ 36 mmHg, but the presence of additional echocardiographic signs of PH or TRV of 2.9–3.4 m/s and SPAP of 37–50 mmHg with or without additional signs of PH; and (3) PH likely for TRV > 3.4 m/s and sPAP > 50 mmHg with or without additional signs of PH [3]. Combined with well-validated hemodynamic calculations, focused TTE can provide very close approximations of the pulmonary vascular and RV hemodynamics.

Systolic Pulmonary Artery Pressure (sPAP)

TTE-based estimation of sPAP most frequently relies upon determination of Doppler-based peak TVR and use of the modified Bernoulli equation (Δpressure = 4 × velocity [2]) to approximate differences between RV and right atrial (RA) pressure. Further addition of TTE-guided estimation of RA pressure (RAP) allows for calculation of RV systolic pressure (which in the absence of obstruction to RV outflow represents sPAP). As central venous pressure (CVP) and RAP are essentially equivalent in the absence of anatomic obstruction, the latter is commonly evaluated by measuring the size, flow patterns and the respiratory variation of the inferior vena cava (IVC). Generally, IVC diameter <2.1 cm and collapse greater than 50 % on inspiration would correspond to a normal RAP of 0–5 mmHg. The presence of either greater diameter or lesser collapse (but not both) correspond to RAP of 5–10 mmHg, and a diameter greater than 2.1 cm with less than 50 % collapse corresponds to a high RAP of 10–20 mmHg [28, 114]. These criteria are relatively poor indicators of RAP, however, and this should be acknowledged when estimating PAP [29]. Patients who cannot comply with taking a deep inspiration to demonstrate collapsibility of the IVC can be asked to perform a "sniff" maneuver, which causes a decrease in intrathoracic pressure.

Although widely accepted as a screening test, the precision of this echocardiographic estimate of PAP is modest. In studies that have compared echocardiographically estimated values and values measured by right heart catheterization (RHC), the mean difference ranged from 3 to 40 mmHg, and sPAP was underestimated with the echocardiographic method by >20 mmHg in 31 % of patients studied [30]. To minimize error in acquisition of the TR envelope by Doppler, it is recommended that TRV be measured in multiple views and the maximal velocity jet found should be used for the calculation. Inadequate regurgitant signals can be enhanced with the use of contrast. It should always be remembered that sPAP evaluation with Doppler methods, however, cannot definitively diagnose PH and has limited role in the decision to treat patients or to monitor therapy efficacy.

Mean Pulmonary Artery Pressure (mPAP)

The simplest method of calculating the mPAP may be by using sPAP as follows:

$$\text{mPAP} = 0.61 \times \text{sPAP} + 2\,\text{mmHg} \; [31].$$

As the only variable in the above equation is sPAP, this calculation carries the same pitfalls as measurement of sPAP mentioned above.

Doppler-based measure of diastolic pulmonary valve regurgitation may be difficult to obtain, and therefore may be absent on particular studies. When present and complete, use of the peak pulmonary valve regurgitation velocity (typically early in diastole) in the modified Bernoulli equation allows estimation of peak pressure difference between RV and PA in early diastole. The peak pulmonic regurgitation velocity represents the diastolic pressure gradient between the pulmonary artery and the RV. Adding the RAP to such calculation often provides acceptable estimation of mPAP (mPAP $= 4 \times$ (peak pulmonic valve regurgitation jet velocity)$^2 +$ RAP) [32].

RV–RA Mean Systolic Gradient

When TTE-based estimation of RAP is added to TR Doppler-velocity based approximation of peak systolic RA–RV systolic pressure difference, a value is obtained that has excellent correlation with mPAP measured during an invasive RHC [33]. Critical to use of this methodology is capture of complete and accurate tricuspid regurgitation Doppler envelope.

Diastolic Pulmonary Artery Pressure (dPAP)

Application of the modified Bernoulli equation to the end-diastolic pulmonary regurgitation velocity allows estimation of the end-diastolic gradient between the RV and PA, which, when added to the TTE-based estimation of RA pressure, estimates diastolic PA pressure, (dPAP), with a high correlation with invasive dPAP measurements [34]. Similar estimation can be obtained by Doppler-based assessment of the earliest systolic gradient at the time of pulmonary valve opening (closely approximating end-diastolic gradient between RV and PA) and adding TTE-based estimation of RA pressure, yielding estimate of dPAP [35, 36].

Pulmonary Vascular Resistance

Accurate assessment of PVR provides an understanding of the mechanism of elevated PAP and aids in selecting therapy for PH. As a result of its clinical importance, numerous TTE-based estimations of PVR have been developed. Noninvasively, one can relate trans-pulmonary gradient (TPG) to pulmonary blood flow by determining the ratio between the tricuspid regurgitation velocity and the velocity time integral of the pulmonary flow at the RV outflow tract. This equation simplifies to:

$$\begin{aligned}&10\times \text{tricuspid valve velocity}\\&/\text{velocity time integral at the RV outflow tract}\left(\text{RVOT}\right)\\&\approx \text{PVR}\left(\text{Wood units}\right)\end{aligned}$$

Individuals with ratios <0.2 have been demonstrated to likely have low PVR values (<2 WU), with 70 % sensitivity and 90 % specificity, even in the presence of increased Doppler sPAP [37].

Alternatively, relating sPAP by the heart rate-corrected velocity time integral (VTI) at the RVOT, namely sPAP/(HR × VTIRVOT), also estimates PVR but takes into account RAP and heart rate (cutoff value of 0.076 with >80 % sensitivity and specificity in a population with PVR > 15 Wood units) [38, 39].

Additional analysis of the pre-ejection systolic time (the period of the cardiac cycle between onset of tricuspid regurgitation and beginning of elevation of PAP) related to systolic acceleration time (period of time between the beginning of ejection and peak flow velocity), normalized for total systolic (ejection and non-ejection) time linearly correlates with invasively measured PVR between 0 and 9 Wood units [40].

An additional technique to estimate PVR is based on the fact that mid systolic notching of the RVOT envelope relates to pathologic wave reflection in the setting of elevated pulmonary artery impedance and PVR of at least 3 Woods units [41]. The ratio of sPAP Doppler to RVOT tract VTI with or without a constant value of 3 designates presence of RVOT VTI midsystolic notching. {PASP/RVOTVTI + 3 if midsystolic notching of RVOT envelope is present} provides superior agreement with catheterization estimates of PVR across a wide range of values.

Morphology of the Doppler Velocity Curves

The Doppler pulmonary flow velocity curve has a dome-like appearance in subjects with normal pulmonary pressures; this is transformed to a somewhat "triangular" shape in patients with PH. Acceleration time (AT) is decreased in the presence of elevated sPAP and mPAP, with peak velocity appearing earlier in systole. An AT <93 ms correlates well with invasive PAP elevation [42, 43]. At times of concomitant abnormality of PA compliance, capacitance or PVR, a second slower rise in velocity during mid-systolic flow deceleration can be observed, resulting in so-called "midsystolic notching" [44].

The combination of assessment of presence or absence of mid systolic notching of the RVOT envelope with estimate of Doppler acceleration time is one of the most utilized echocardiographic techniques to determine if PVR is elevated.

Estimates of RV Function

In response to pressure overload, the RF typically dilates and develops concentric hypertrophy. The TTE-based apical "4-chamber" view allows an expansive view of the heart. Transition of the RV from a triangular to a more globular or rounded shape can be demonstrated. Similarly as the RV expands in size, it may replace the LV in forming part or all of the cardiac apex. While quantification of the size of the RV remains a limitation of echocardiography, the ratio between the diastolic inflow diameters and the areas of the RV and the LV (0.6–1 mild, >1 severe) appear to correlate well with the degree of RV dilatation [45].

More complex methodology requires tracing of RV endocardium during systole and diastole to calculate the fractional are change (FAC) (RVFAC = (end-diastolic area − end-systolic area)/end-diastolic area × 100, normal being ≥35 %) as a correlate of RV systolic function [28, 46].

One of the most utilized indices of RV contractile function is perhaps one of the simplest to obtain. The longitudinal tricuspid annulus plane systolic excursion or TAPSE is calculated via M-mode echocardiography (though two-dimension estimates are often performed) of the right ventricular annulus. Normal values are >2.0 cm and are reduced in case of RV dysfunction [47]. Important limitations to this method include its dependency on proper image acquisition angle and RV load dependency, its focus on a small part of the RV myocardium, independent changes that occur after surgical or other penetration of the pericardium, and the fact that the tricuspid annulus motion may be very well affected by the overall heart motion [48]. TAPSE values of less than 1.8 cm correlate with worse 1 and 2 year prognosis in patients with groups 1 and 2 PH.

While the myocardial performance Tei index (sum of isovolumetric contraction time and isovolumetric relaxation time indexed to the total LV ejection time [(IVCT + IVRT)/(LVET)]) has been correlated with invasive hemodynamics and clinical outcomes, its use in care practice has been limited [49]. Additional complex hemodynamic assessments from TTE include tissue Doppler and strain assessment.

Current American Society of Echocardiography guidelines regarding right-heart assessment recommend that basal RV free wall $S' < 10$ cm/s should be considered a marker of RV dysfunction [28]. Mitral annular velocity should be checked to consider the presence of elevated left-sided filling pressures. Strain imaging can suggest RV dysfunction in the presence of decreased RV longitudinal strain and impairment of left ventricular segmental longitudinal and circumferential strain (when greater for the interventricular septum than for the LV free wall) [50].

The "reverse Bernheim effect" suggests RV and LV interaction such that poor RV function in the face of marked afterload can worsen LV filling and output [51]. The ratio of the long axis to short axis diameters of the left ventricle, both in diastole and in systole, otherwise known as the "eccentricity index" assesses LV compression, differentiates between volume and pressure overload, and is assessed on the two-dimensional short-axis view of the LV [52]. In addition, RV dilatation also causes abnormal left ventricular filling which may be assessed by evaluating the Doppler appearance of the mitral inflow. Abnormal relaxation pattern is often a surrogate to LV cavity compression in patients with more severe forms of PH.

The presence of pericardial effusion may be due in part to poor pericardial drainage in the setting of RA hypertension and lower cardiac output. While presence of effusion is a poor prognostic finding, tamponade is not a typically encountered clinical sequelae due to the high pressure in the RA and RV [53].

Right to left intravascular shunting (and resultant hypoxemia unresponsive to oxygen administration) through a patent foramen ovale can be demonstrated with agitated saline or echocardiographic contrast injection, and may be aggravated in the setting of elevation of RA pressure either at rest or with exercise,.

Right Heart Catheterization

Invasive hemodynamic assessment of PH is a dynamic process that often requires continuous recordings of multiple variables and thus, the need for RHC. For the assessment of PH, RHC typically includes vasoreactivity testing and may include exercise and fluid challenge as well as angiography. RHC remains essential for accurate diagnosis of most forms of PH including PAH. Standard of care practice guidelines strongly recommend that patients suspected of having PH after noninvasive evaluation undergo RHC prior to initiation of therapy.

Indications

In the evaluation of patients with PH, RHC is usually indicated for the following [2, 3]

(a) In all patients with PAH to confirm the diagnosis, to evaluate severity and to assist in selection of PAH specific therapy.
(b) For confirmation of efficacy of PAH-specific therapy.

Table 10.4 Essential components of invasive hemodynamic assessment [2]

Oxygen saturations (SVC, IVC, RA, RV, PA's, SA)
Right atrial pressure
Right ventricular pressure
Pulmonary artery pressure, systolic, diastolic, mean
Pulmonary arterial wedge pressure, left atrial pressure, or left ventricular end-diastolic pressure
Cardiac output/index
Pulmonary vascular resistance
Systemic blood pressure
Heart rate
Response to acute vasodilator

(c) For confirmation of hemodynamic effects of suspected clinical deterioration and as baseline for the evaluation of the effect of treatment escalation and/or combination therapy.

RHC may have limited benefit when an alternative diagnosis is obvious on non-invasive testing. Similarly, RHC may have specific but limited use when elevated PAP pressures on non-invasive testing can be explained by left heart disease, diastolic dysfunction, or chronic lung disease.

Table 10.4 lists the essential components of invasive hemodynamic assessment of PH. The addition of exercise testing, vasoreactivity testing or fluid challenge, and angiography to RHC is discussed in appropriate sections below.

Indications for Coronary Angiography with Right Heart Catheterization for Evaluation of Pulmonary Hypertension

It is not infrequent that assessment of coronary anatomy may carry import implications when performed as part of RHC to evaluate PH. The reasons for such include, but are not limited to, evaluation of the coronary anatomy as part of surgical planning, presence of coronary-fistula to the right-sided chambers as a possible source of left to right shunt, presence of atherosclerotic coronary artery disease as a possible reason for impaired LV function or elevated filling pressure, and evaluation of the anatomic relations between the coronary arteries and the pulmonary arteries for specific procedures (e.g., percutaneous prosthetic pulmonary valve implantation).

Safety

RHC, although technically demanding, is a safe procedure when performed by experienced operators [54]. Hoeper and colleagues reported on 5,727 RHC procedures retrospectively and 1,491 prospectively, for a total of 7,218 procedures. The overall number of serious adverse events was 76 (1.1 %, 95 % confidence interval 0.8–1.3 %). The most frequent complications were related to venous access (e.g., hematoma, pneumothorax), followed by arrhythmias and hypotensive episodes related to vagal reactions or pulmonary vasoreactivity testing. The vast majority of these complications were mild to moderate in intensity and resolved either spontaneously or after appropriate intervention. Four fatal events were recorded in association with any of the catheter procedures, resulting in an overall procedure-related mortality of 0.055 % (95 % confidence interval 0.01–0.099 %). Of the four fatal complications only two were related to the procedure itself (PA rupture and both electromechanical dissociation and intrapulmonary hemorrhage) [55]. Adequate patient preparation such as management of anticoagulation issues can help in reducing vascular access complications. It should be remembered that RHC as an elective, planned procedure is a very safe procedure and is very different from placement of a pulmonary artery catheter (PAC) in patients admitted to the intensive care unit (ICU) where the use of PAC has, in some studies, been associated with increased mortality. Also while a PAC placed in an ICU patient may stay in situ for several days, thus increasing vascular, infectious, and thromboembolic complications, diagnostic RHC is typically a short outpatient procedure lasting under an hour.

Patient Preparation

Policy regarding fasting status of patients, use of peripheral IV, and withholding of particular medications (such as hypoglycemics, vasodilators, diuretics, or anticoagulants) should be dependent upon individual laboratory preference, health status of the patient, and whether sedative use is planned. A clear plan for such though, should be constructed and documented. For example, the calculation of risk-benefit ratio of sustaining therapeutic INR up until catheterization for an individual patient in whom anticoagulation has been prescribed for mechanical mitral valve and atrial fibrillation may well be different than that of another patient in whom warfarin is prescribed for primary prevention of stroke with atrial fibrillation. Clear description of such logic should be available to personnel within the team assisting in catheterization (Table 10.5).

Sedation

While concern has been raised regarding safety and influence of sedatives used during catheterization on medical status and physiologic indices including loading conditions and inotropy, this is probably of minor concern unless liver and

Table 10.5 Anticoagulation management in case decision is made to withhold anticoagulation (modified from Massicotte A. A practice tool for the new oral anticoagulants. Can Pharm J (Ott). Jan 2014) [56]

Drug and creatinine clearance	Recommendation in preprocedure period	Recommendation in postprocedure period	Bridging with heparin needed
Warfarin	Stop 48 h prior until INR <1.7 (varies per institutional policy).	Resume therapy when hemostasis is adequate and clinical condition allows	Needed if moderate to high risk of thromboembolism
Dabigatran ≥80 ml/min	Stop 24 h before surgery.	Resume therapy when hemostasis is adequate and clinical condition allows	Needed only if patient cannot take oral medications and there is moderate to high risk of thromboembolism
Dabigatran 50 to <80 ml/min	Stop 1–2 days before surgery.	Resume therapy when hemostasis is adequate and clinical condition allows	Needed only if patient cannot take oral medications and there is moderate to high risk of thromboembolism
Dabigatran <30 ml/min	Stop at least 5 days before surgery.	Use alternative anticoagulation agent	NA
Rivaroxaban ≥30 ml/min	Stop at least 24 h before surgery.	Resume therapy when hemostasis is adequate and clinical condition allows	Needed only if patient cannot take oral medications and there is moderate to high risk of thromboembolism
Rivaroxaban <30 ml/min	Last dose on day −3.	Use alternative anticoagulation agent	NA
Apixaban >50 ml/min	Stop at least 24 h before surgery.	Resume therapy when hemostasis is adequate and clinical condition allows	Needed only if patient cannot take oral medications and there is moderate to high risk of thromboembolism

kidney functions are significantly impaired [57–59]. Nonetheless, it is becoming more common practice to avoid standard use of systemic sedation prior to or during RHC.

Right Heart Catheterization in a Mechanically Ventilated Patient

Complex influences by mechanical ventilation must be considered when assessing measured hemodynamics. Positive pressure ventilation, particularly in the setting of PEEP, variably increases RV afterload with resultant decline in RV contractility, and can contribute to elevated measure of PCWP particularly during inspiration [60, 61]. Additional influences may include baseline vascular and myocardial loading conditions and compliance of the chest wall and lungs. General practice is to discount meaningful influence of PEEP <10 cm H_2O on measured PCWP, with correction of PCWP when PEEP ≥10 cm H_2O by 2–3 cm for every 5 cm H_2O increment in PEEP [62, 63]. Another cause of falsely elevated PCWP in a mechanically ventilated patient is the monitoring catheter being located outside zone 3 (during positive pressure ventilation less of the lung is zone 3 due to elevated alveolar pressures). Care should be taken to demonstrate catheter tip placement within zone 3, gravitationally below the level of the left atrium [64].

Hemodynamic pressure measurements should reflect the time of most neutral intrathoracic pressure (in spontaneously respiring patients this occurs at end expiration, with converse in patients utilizing positive pressure ventilation), rather than sole recording of mean pressure. Esophageal manometry is rarely utilized to estimate the effects of high swings of intrathoracic pressure seen with labored breathing. When possible, the patient should be instructed to expire slowly to allow pressure recording that may assist in accuracy of hemodynamic measure [72].

Percutaneous Access Sites

Commonly used access sites include internal jugular (IJ) vein, femoral vein, brachial vein, and subclavian vein. Knowledge of prior procedures, venous and arterial obstructions, compressions, complex anatomical course and prior procedural complications is necessary to choose access site in an individual patient. The IJ vein is usually the preferred site because of its ease of access, lower complication rate and because it allows patients to be discharged early after procedure [54, 55, 65]. Proximal arm veins provide ready access to RHC, but catheter manipulation may be difficult and catheter size choice is limited. Some operators may prefer femoral vein if concomitant left heart catheterization is planned via femoral artery. Ultrasound guidance should be considered for both IJ and femoral access sites. Patients with kidney disease, congenital heart disease, pacemakers, or prior indwelling venous access for other reasons (e.g., TPN) are more likely to have had multiple prior procedures and consequent vascular injury or thrombosis. Imaging of the vascular bed may be established by various modalities (ultrasound, computed tomography and magnetic resonance angiography) and should be considered by the operator when deemed appropriate. The use of a micropuncture kit with a 21-gauge needle and introducer can minimize potential trauma from inadvertent puncture of the carotid artery. Table 10.6 lists the advantages and disadvantages of different catheterization access sites.

While it is relatively easy to pass the catheter in to the RV and out to the PA from the right IJ, brachial or subclavian vein access, it may be challenging to do so via femoral access especially when the right-sided chambers are dilated. Figure 10.4 shows different techniques to pass the catheter into the PA via femoral access; individual operators may employ different and specific maneuvers to assist in passage through the right heart that include use of various shaped catheters and guidewires both within or external to the maneuvered catheter. Care must be taken at all times to avoid inadvertent contact and manipulation of intracardiac and intravascular structures that could result in arrhythmia or cardiac and vascular trauma.

Table 10.6 Access sites for right heart catheterization

Catheter site	Advantages	Disadvantages
Internal jugular vein	Easier access, lower complication rate, quicker discharge	Risk of carotid injury, difficult in obese with thick neck
Femoral vein	Easier catheter manipulation	Higher complication rate esp. bleeding, longer post procedure monitoring
Brachial vein	Easy access, less invasive	Catheter manipulation difficult

Catheter Choice

For adequate evaluation of pressures during the catheterization, large-bore catheters (e.g. 6 or 7 F) that yield high-quality hemodynamic data should be utilized. Of note, the internal catheter lumen diameter appears most important in this consideration. Thus, a large catheter with multiple ports (e.g., an 8 F catheter with RA, thermodilution, and PA ports) will generally produce tracings with lower frequency response than a single-port catheter of smaller bore but greater luminal diameter. The larger lumen diameter also allows the passage of conventional 0.035- and 0.038-in. diameter guidewires when necessary. Guidewire use inside large bore catheter may be required in cases where the PA is difficult to reach or when RHC is attempted from the femoral vein. Pre-shaped catheters such as coronary catheters can be used to help direct wire to a particular segment of the pulmonary artery (e.g. in cases of CTEPH, peripheral pulmonary arterial stenosis, or pulmonary venous obstruction, where selective PA segment access is required) and then exchanging for a balloon tipped end hole catheter.

End hole catheters are best adapted for use in obtaining wedge samples and pressures or when discerning pressures, gradients, or sampling within or over relatively small areas. Side hole catheters assist in avoidance of measures that may be dampened by inadvertent wedge positioning. The Swan-Ganz multi-port PA balloon end hole catheter has potential for thermodilution based measure of cardiac output, and is one of the most commonly used catheters for measuring right-heart pressures. This catheter's port system includes an end-hole, a side-hole 30 cm from the catheter tip, and a thermistor for measurement of cardiac output when using the thermodilution method. Simpler non-thermistor single and double-lumen balloon end-hole catheters exist and may have greater ease in manipulation through enlarged or distorted hearts and vascular structures.

Coronary angiography has evolved considerably to use the smallest-bore catheters, with many catheterization laboratories using 5 F or even 4 F catheters to decrease vascular complications. The radial artery is an increasingly used access site for coronary engagement and visualization, and is also used at the time of direct pressure measurement at the left cardiac chambers (such as direct left ventricular end diastolic pressure measurement). This approach allows immediate ambulation following the procedure, as well as improved coronary visualization (compared with smaller 4 F-diameter femoral catheters), and reduced bleeding complications (compared with femoral access). An Allen test should be performed to ensure that

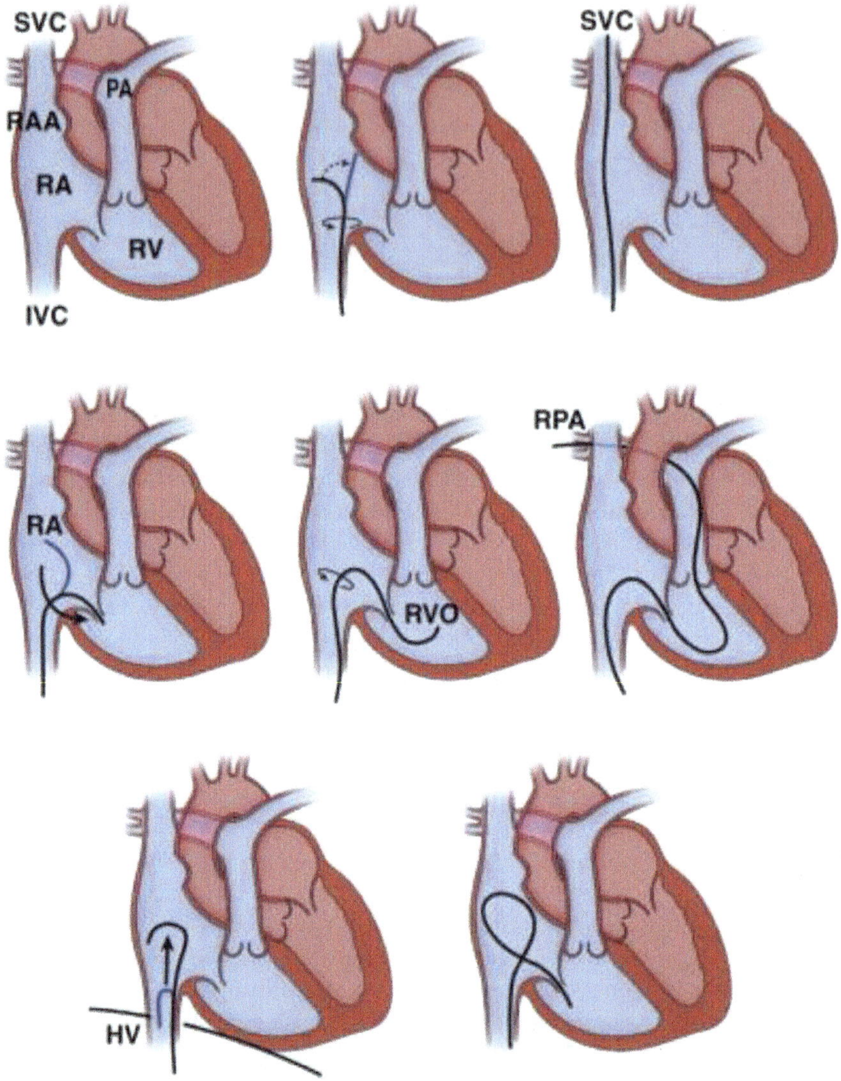

Fig. 10.4 Right-heart catheterization from the femoral vein, shown in cartoon form. *Top row*, the right-heart catheter is initially placed in the right atrium (RA) aimed at the lateral atrial wall. Counterclockwise rotation aims the catheter posteriorly and allows advancement into the superior vena cava (SVC). Although it is not evident in the figure, clockwise catheter rotation into an anterior orientation would lead to advancement into the right atrial appendage (RAA), precluding SVC catheterization. *Center row*, the catheter is then withdrawn back into the right atrium and aimed laterally. Clockwise rotation causes the catheter tip to sweep anteromedially and to cross the tricuspid valve. With the catheter tip in a horizontal orientation just beyond the spine, it is positioned below the right ventricular outflow (RVO) tract. Additional clockwise rotation causes the catheter to point straight up, allowing advancement into the main pulmonary artery and from there into the right pulmonary artery (RPA). *Bottom row*, two maneuvers useful in catheterization of a dilated right heart. A larger loop with a downward-directed tip may be required to reach the tricuspid valve and can be formed by catching the catheter tip in the hepatic vein (HV) and advancing the catheter

the ulnar artery is patent in the event of radial artery occlusion, though the true utility of this remains unclear and an abnormal Allen test does not preclude radial arterial access. However, it should be remembered that left heart catheterization although extremely safe, contributes to a higher risk of complications due to potential for bleeding, increased risk of renal complications because of contrast use and usually a higher radiation exposure (as well as adding a small but definable risk of stroke and death). Relative contraindications to cardiac catheterization are listed in Table 10.7 below.

Equipment Selection for the Hemodynamic Study

Most cardiac catheterization laboratories utilize fluid-filled transducers that are mounted on the catheterization table. Typically these pressure transducers are disposable and usually arrive pre-calibrated, but require initial confirmation and repeated "zeroing," a term that refers to the establishment of a reference point (typically the patient's mid-chest at the level of the second intercostal space, as an estimation of the patient's right atrium) for subsequent pressure measurements. Some laboratories choose to avoid hydrostatic errors in diastolic pressure measurement theorized to be present with such zeroing technique by using a transducer zero reference position of uppermost blood level of the chamber being sampled or measured, Regardless of method employed, failures to ensure appropriate zero reference account for some of the most common pressure measure errors. [67–69].

Table 10.7 Relative contraindications to diagnostic cardiac catheterization [66]

Acute gastrointestinal bleeding
Severe hypokalemia
Uncorrected digitalis toxicity
Anticoagulation with international normalized ratio >1.8 or severe coagulopathy
Previous anaphylactoid reaction to contrast media
Acute stroke
Acute renal failure or severe chronic non-dialysis-dependent kidney disease
Unexplained fever or untreated active infection
Severe anemia
Uncooperative patient

Fig. 10.4 (continued) quickly into the right atrium. The reverse loop technique (*bottom right*) gives the catheter tip an upward direction, aimed toward the outflow tract. *IVC* inferior vena cava, *PA* pulmonary artery, *RV* right ventricle (from Baim DS, Grossman W: Percutaneous approach, including transseptal and apical puncture. In Baim DS, Grossman W [eds]: Cardiac Catheterization, Angiography, and Intervention. 7th ed. Philadelphia, Lea & Febiger, 2006, p 86)

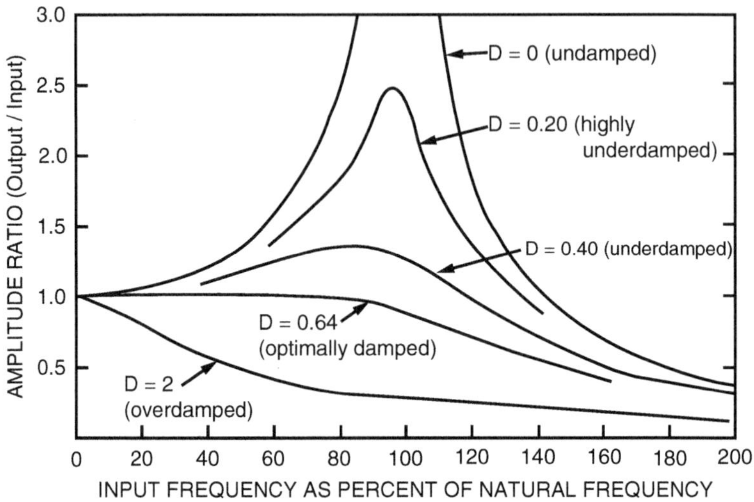

Fig. 10.5 Frequency response curves of a pressure measurement system, illustrating the importance of optimal damping. The amplitude of an input signal tends to be augmented as the frequency of that signal approaches the natural frequency of the sensing membrane. Optimal damping dissipates the energy of the oscillating sensing membrane gradually and thereby maintains a nearly flat natural frequency curve (constant output/input ratio) as it approaches the region of the pressure measurement system's natural frequency. *D* damping coefficient (from Baim, D.S. and W. Grossman, Grossman's cardiac catheterization, angiography, and intervention. 7th ed. 2006, Philadelphia: Lippincott Williams & Wilkins)

Choice of catheters (shortest, widest bore, non-compliant) and transmission fluid (low-density) used for pressure measurements, combined with elimination of air bubbles, as suggested earlier, optimizes effects of energy dissipation, or damping [70] (Fig. 10.5). Loss of high-frequency events with subsequent underestimation of the systolic pressure and overestimation of the diastolic pressure may occur with over-damping; narrow, sharp pressure wave upstrokes, or "ringing," can occur with under-damping.

Catheter whip artifact (motion of the tip of the catheter within the measured chamber) can be problematic in the accurate measurement of PA pressures. It has the potential to produce superimposed waves, typically of ±10 mmHg, but on occasion even greater deviation from true measure [71]. Catheter tip or luminal obstruction, at times due to catheter-vessel mismatch or internal thrombus formation, can cause significant changes in pressure contour. End-pressure artifact may occur when an end-hole catheter measures an artificially elevated pressure because of streaming or high velocity of the pressure wave. Another artifact similar to but distinct from whip artifact is catheter impact artifact, which can occur when walls of a cardiac chamber or valve hit the end of the measuring catheter. It can affect pressure measurements when a pigtail is used to measure LV pressures, and is impacted by mitral valve motion [70].

To avoid these artifacts, we strongly encourage the practice of taking multiple measurements, rebalancing the zero baseline during pressure evaluation at each chamber or vessel and intermittent catheter flushing with heparinized saline. The ability to "zero" prior to measurement of pressure in each chamber, assisted by visual confirmation of catheter placement in the appropriate chamber in catheterization laboratory is a distinct advantage compared to placement of Swanz-Ganz catheter in the ICU/stepdown setting.

Another way to measure intracardiac pressure besides the fluid filled system is via use of micromanometer catheters. Small transducers have been constructed that can fit on the distal tip of standard catheters and be used as intracardiac manometers. Micromanometer catheters are currently not routinely used during RHC, but rather they form the basis of the pressure wire used for measurement of intracoronary pressures and are usually used for hemodynamic measurements as part of more detailed research efforts.

Pressure Measurements and Cardiac Output Determination

Hemodynamic catheterization, a combined experience of pressure measurement, sampling, catheter advancement, and angiography, is an interactive procedure where data obtained from each chamber is compared to previously obtained data; the accuracy of measurements may require additional confirmation and additional tests may be added and performed to answer new questions that arise. As there can be multiple sources of error as discussed above, measurements should be repeated if a single value does not fit with the overall emerging picture. Frequent "zeroing," and looking for air bubbles in the catheter system and "flushing" all ensure most accurate measurements.

Based on the findings, further testing and interventions are considered; such may include nitric oxide (NO) or adenosine administration assessing pulmonary vasoreactivity (see below), oxygen supplementation as therapy for systemic arterial desaturation (when responsive to such), diuretic or nitrate therapy for isolated elevated LV end-diastolic pressures, limited angiography, and balloon-closure of a patent inter-chamber or intravascular communication (if seen or detected).

Right Atrial Pressures and Waveform

In normal RA pressure tracings (Fig. 10.6), the "a" wave (atrial systole) is higher than the "v" wave (passive filling of the RV, reflecting RA and RV compliance) in contrast to the LA. Elevated "v" waves on the RA tracing in a patient with PH may be caused by tricuspid regurgitation, RV failure with secondary lowering of compliance, or restrictive cardiomyopathy. Constrictive pericarditis and tamponade typically demonstrate equalization of the "a" and the "v" waves.

Normal RAP is 2–6 mmHg. The finding of elevated RAP at the time of the right heart study usually implies worse RV function. Elevated RAP has been shown in several studies to be an adverse prognostic factor in patients with PH [74, 75], whereas normal RAP during RHC is reassuring.

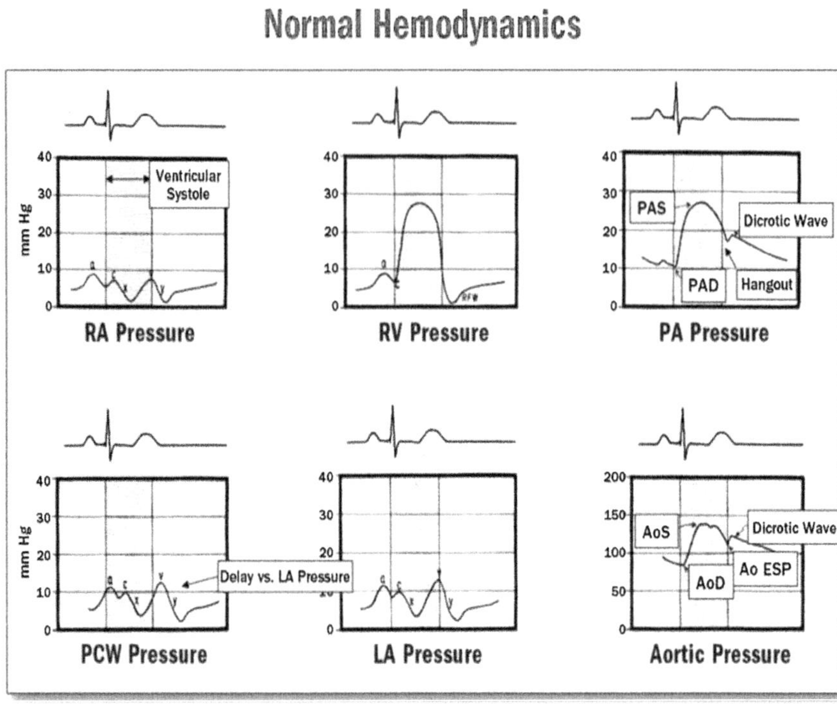

Fig. 10.6 Hemodynamic tracings of the cardiac chambers under normal conditions

Right Ventricle Pressure and Waveform

Normal RV systolic and end-diastolic pressures are 20–30 and 0–8 mmHg, respectively (Fig. 10.6). There may be a small (5 mmHg) systolic gradient between the RV and the PA. End-diastolic pressure is measured at the C point, which is the rise in ventricular pressure at the onset of isovolumic contraction. When the C point is not well seen, a line is drawn from the R wave on the simultaneous EKG recording to the ventricular pressure waveform.

Long-standing elevation of RV afterload leads to concentric RV hypertrophy and elevation of filling pressures, progressive tricuspid regurgitation (via annular dilation) and RV diastolic and eventually systolic dysfunction [76, 77]. These changes occur in a staged manner and should be interpreted with caution and never in isolation. Elevated RV systolic pressure or PA pressure by itself is not considered to be a prognostic factor for PH as a low or normal RVSP could signify a normal RV or a failing RV that cannot generate a high enough RVSP, depending on stage of the disease. In the early stages of disease when RV is able to mount a pressure response to afterload, RV pressure rise may be increased by up to ten times the normal value [78]. Occasionally, "a" waves will be present on the RV waveforms at this stage, indicating "restrictive physiology" with decreased compliance of the RA and RV. (Normally, the highly compliant RV is able to "accommodate" the contraction of the RA without a rise in pressure, making the "a" waves non-visible in a normal tracing.) In more severe forms of RV dysfunction, depressed upstroke and delayed relaxation may appear on the pressure tracings. Generally, RV end-diastolic pressure >12 mmHg, especially if accompanied by a mean RAP >8 mmHg, is suggestive of RV failure and carries poor prognosis [74].

Pulmonary Artery Pressure and Waveform

The resistance of the normal pulmonary circulation is relatively low, with little or no resting vascular tone. The PA tracing consists of a systolic wave, the incisura (indicating closure of the pulmonary valves), and a gradual decline in pressure until the following systole (Fig. 10.6). The determining factors of the mPAP are the hydrostatic pressure, the intra-alveolar pressure, LAP and alveolar gases. Normal sPAP is 20–30 mmHg and normal dPAP is 4–12 mmHg. If there is a systolic pressure difference between the RV and the PA, the possibilities of pulmonic valve stenosis or pulmonary artery (main or branch) stenosis or obstruction should be considered.

The PAP should be measured bilaterally and in multiple lobes, both proximally and distally to ensure absence of stenotic lesions and also because CTEPH may involve only certain lobar vessels. PA pressures should always be measured in the lower lobes (zone 3), as ventilation perfusion mismatch is least in lower lobe vessels. The diurnal variation of PAP is well known and it can be as much as 50–100 % with higher pressures often noted at night [79].

Pulmonary Capillary Wedge Pressure

Estimation of the pulmonary venous and pulmonary capillary pressure can be usually achieved via the wedge technique, accomplished on the basis of measuring the pulmonary wedge pressure. The PCWP waveform is similar to the LAP waveform, but is more damped and delayed as a result of transmission through the lungs (Fig. 10.6). Normally, dPAP is equal to mean PCWP as the pulmonary resistance is low. However, when PVR is elevated dPAP overestimates LAP.

Finessing the Wedge

There are several ways to confirm the appropriateness of catheter "wedging" and that the quality of PCWP measurement is high. The best way is to check either angiographic stability (reserved to personnel with experience in PA catheterization and angiography), or oxygen saturation within the wedge position. Oxygen saturation >90 % typically suggests an adequate wedge position [68]. Alternative is via *wedge angiography* [80], where 1–2 cc of contrast is hand injected distal to a "wedged" PAC to opacify the distal pulmonary vasculature. A satisfactory wedge position should have no evidence of contrast "washout" due to incompletely occluded proximal flow. (True wedge angiography can be performed with balloon deflation after injection, allowing contrast to flow through the pulmonary vasculature, thus outlining the physical appearance of the branch pulmonary arteries and revealing when present, the presence of distal pulmonary artery obstruction, pulmonary arteriovenous malformations, normal pulmonary venous drainage and possible evidence of pulmonary venous obstruction). Optimal PCWP is obtained with the measuring catheter positioned to ensure viewing of "a" and "v" waves without dampening or under wedging. Slow balloon inflation proximally and then advancing balloon catheter, or very slow distal inflation, or using a wire to obtain optimal distal placement, may help in accurate positioning of the catheter.

PCWP and PAOP (Pulmonary Artery Occlusion Pressure)

Elevated PAP can create difficulty in obtaining a true "wedge" with even small amounts of proximal flow around the balloon resulting in inaccurately high estimates of PCWP [81, 82]. When such error is suggested, the balloon can be deflated by 0.2–0.5 ml with slight forward pressure on the catheter, allowing the catheter and balloon to move forward within a smaller portion of the branch vessel thereby securing a better lodging and wedge.

Care must be taken to ensure measure of PCWP under conditions that sustain physiologic zone 3 (pulmonary venous pressure exceeding alveolar pressure). Wedging of the catheter can, in and of itself, lead to lack of distension of the effected distal vascular bed, leading to underestimating of true capillary pressure. In addition to positive pressure ventilation (as discussed earlier), both hypovolemia and advanced parenchymal lung disease can contribute to making alveolar pressure exceed pulmonary venous pressure, adding error to estimate of true pulmonary venous pressure.

On special occasion when subsegmental venous obstruction such as occurs in pulmonary veno-occlusive disease is suspected, occlusion of a larger, more proximal PA known as pulmonary artery occlusion pressure (PAOP) (Fig. 10.7) may provide a more accurate summed representation of more distal pulmonary venous and LAP. In this circumstance, PCWP has potential to reflect local or subsegmental pulmonary venous pressure (in the setting of increased local vascular resistance) rather than LAP [83]. Assessment of the curve of the decay from PAP to PAOP may be of assistance in determining the site of predominant increase in resistance (Fig. 10.8) [85].

Transpulmonary Gradient and Diastolic Pressure Gradient

The transpulmonary gradient (TPG) is calculated by subtracting the mean LAP (or PCWP, as a surrogate of post-capillary pressure) from the mPAP. TPG can be used to differentiate pre-capillary and post-capillary forms of PH [86]. A TPG of >12 mmHg

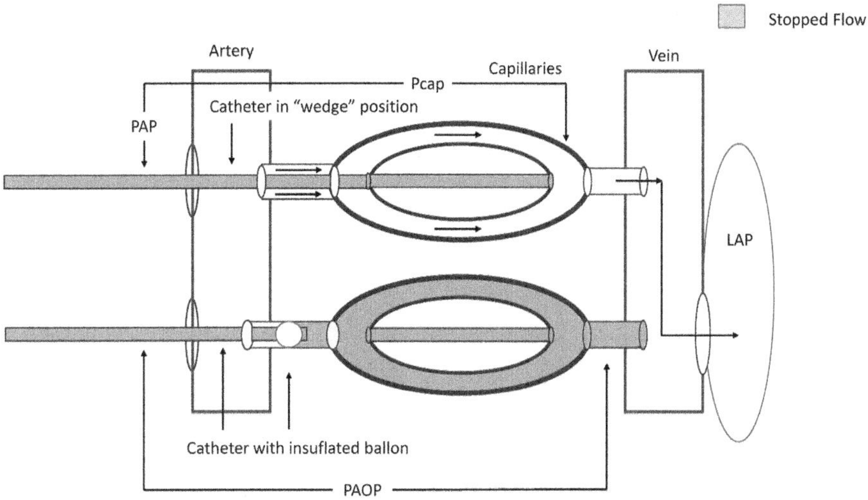

Fig. 10.7 Pulmonary artery occlusion pressure and pulmonary capillary wedge pressure

has been used classically to distinguish pre-capillary PH, which is the result of intrinsic pulmonary vascular disease, from post-capillary PH which is due to pulmonary venous or left atrial hypertension. Post-capillary PH may be expected to reverse when the cause of pulmonary venous hypertension is removed (such as seen in patients with mitral stenosis or diastolic heart failure). However, it is possible for diastolic heart failure or mitral stenosis to cause irreversible changes in PH and lead to pre-capillary hypertension as well.

A TPG value of 12 mmHg is considered to signify intrinsic pulmonary vascular disease, as this degree of PH is "out of proportion" to elevated pulmonary venous pressures. Some authors suggest that the diastolic gradient between dPAP and PCWP, or diastolic pressure gradient (DPG), is a better measure of "out of proportion" PH than TPG, as the TPG is affected by both stroke volume and also by the large v waves that can occur in the PCWP waveform (Fig. 10.9) [87].

Pulmonary Vascular Resistance (PVR)

Presence of PH does not delineate presence or absence of elevation of PVR. Definition of PAH requires additional hemodynamic criteria that include a PVR >3 Wood units and a PCWP <15 mm Hg. PVR is calculated using Ohm's Law in Wood units, as follows:

$$\text{PVR} = \frac{(\text{mPAP} - \text{PCWP})}{\text{Cardiac output}(\text{CO})} = \frac{(\text{TPG})}{\text{CO}}$$

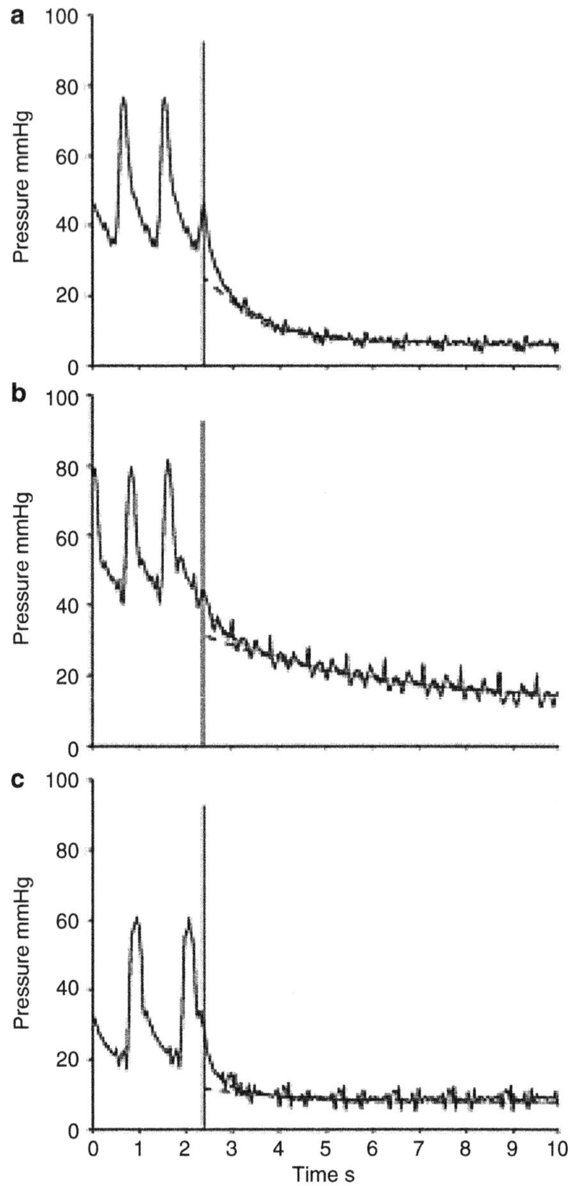

Fig. 10.8 Typical pulmonary artery occlusion recordings used to estimate pulmonary capillary pressure (P_c) in (**a**) a patient with a pulmonary arterial hypertension, (**b**) a patient with pulmonary veno-occlusive disease and (**c**) a patient with chronic thromboembolic pulmonary hypertension. The bi-exponential fittings are shown in *dotted lines*, and the evolution of P_c after occlusion (*vertical solid lines*) calculated with the three-compartment model of the pulmonary circulation in *dashed lines* [85] (from Single arterial occlusion to locate resistance in patients with pulmonary hypertension. Eur Respir J 2001)

Multiplying the resistance calculated in Wood units by 80 converts to the resistance units of dynes s/cm^5. A value of <200 dynes s/cm^5 (or 2.5 Wood units) is considered to be normal. Normal PVR at rest is age dependent, but PVR >2 WU can be considered elevated in all age populations.

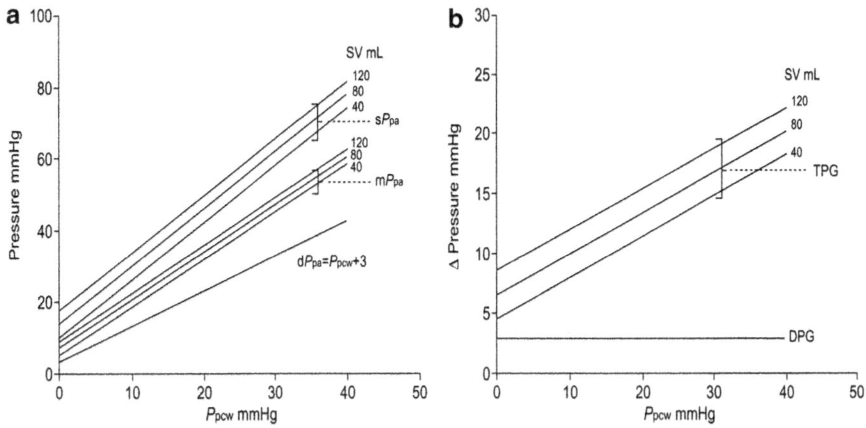

Fig. 10.9 Effects of pulmonary capillary wedge pressure (P_{pcw}) and stroke volume (SV) on systolic (s), diastolic (d), and mean (m) pulmonary arterial pressures (P_{pa}). If diastolic P_{pa} increases more than P_{pcw}, there is an out of proportion increase in systolic P_{pa} and mean P_{pa} that is a function of SV. The transpulmonary pressure gradient (TPG) increases, but the diastolic gradient (DPG) is independent of both pulmonary capillary wedge pressure (P_{pcw}) and SV

Pulmonary Vascular Resistance Index (PVRI)

It is generally recommended that PVR should be indexed to the patient's body size (PVRI) [88]. Using PVR instead of PVRI has been shown to be responsible for significant underestimation of PH in patients with high body mass index. PVRI is considered to mainly reflect the functional status of pulmonary vascular endothelium and smooth muscle cells and is positively related to blood viscosity and to changes in perivascular alveolar and pleural pressure. Unlike mPAP, PVRI increases with age: the upper limit for PVRI in normal subjects increases from about 2.8 indexed Wood units (6–10 years) to 3.2 (32–45 years) to 4.6 (60–83 years) indexed Wood units [1, 89–92].

Cardiac Output

There is no completely accurate method of measuring cardiac output in all patients. However, the two commonly used methods include the Fick and thermodilution techniques.

For comparison among patients, cardiac output should be corrected for the patient's body surface area and expressed as cardiac index (CI).

Fick Method

The basis of the Fick principle is that the rate of human oxygen consumption must equal the rate of oxygen addition to the body. This tenet also assumes a constancy of blood flow into and out of the lungs, free of shunt [93, 94]. This principle can be expressed as:

$$\text{Pulmonary blood flow}\left(1/\min\right) = \frac{O_2 \text{ consumption}\left(\text{ml}/\min\right)}{\left(\Delta O_2 \text{ concentration entering and leaving lungs}\right)}$$

or,

$$\text{Cardiac output}\left(1/\min\right) = \frac{\text{oxygen consumption}\left(\text{ml}/\min\right)}{\text{A}\quad VO_2 \times 1.36 \times \text{Hemoglobin}\left(\text{mg}/\text{dL}\right) \times 10}$$

where A-VO_2 is the arterial-venous oxygen saturation difference and the constant 1.36 is the oxygen-carrying capacity of hemoglobin (expressed in ml O_2/g Hgb). As contrasted to thermodilution methodology, the Fick calculation of cardiac output necessitates minimal waver in mean flow over time, and carries less error at lower measures of blood flow; therefore, it is typically utilized in patients with heart failure syndromes. Accuracy of measure falls away in subjects with inspiratory O_2 fractions larger than 60 %, and in those with significant mitral or aortic regurgitation [97].

Determination of cardiac output by catheterization based Fick method requires measure of the A-VO_2 content difference which requires knowledge of serum hemoglobin and determination of systemic arterial (as a surrogate for pulmonary vein) and mixed venous blood oxygen saturation (classically PA O_2 saturation, but SVC O_2 saturation is often used as a surrogate) as well as determination of oxygen consumption. All measurements should be collected as close in time to each other as possible, so as to avoid theoretic changes in ventilation, loading conditions and contractility. Steady state oxygen consumption, or uptake, should ideally be measured, via a fitting gas exchange mask that collects and measures the oxygen content of expired air, directly in the catheterization laboratory. Many catheterization laboratories use an "assumed" value (typically 125 ml/min/m^2 for most adult patients, and 110 ml/min/m^2 for elderly patients) for oxygen consumption. The use of the "assumed" rather than the directly measured O_2 consumption can be a major source of error in the Fick method, but when performed correctly, the total error indetermination of the cardiac output is about 10 % [95–97].

Thermodilution Method

The thermodilution method of estimation of cardiac output requires injection of an indicator substance such as a bolus of liquid (usually sterile normal saline) via the proximal port of a specially adapted multiport catheter. Cardiac output between two points along the catheter (injection and thermistor located more distally) is determined by knowing temperature at the origin and at the endpoint of measure, as well as assessing this change over time, as demonstrated in a thermodilution curve. The area under this curve, a function of temperature versus time, is inversely correlated with cardiac output, and is rapidly displayed in near real-time in most catheterization laboratories. Thermodilution methodology carries greatest risk of error at lower (and highest) cardiac output and in the presence of tricuspid regurgitation or irregular heart rhythm [100, 101], Nonetheless, due to ease of performance, thermodilution technique remains the most commonly used method for measure of cardiac output in most catheterization laboratories [98, 99].

Direct Measurement of Left-Sided Pressures

Possible conditions in which direct evaluation of the left-sided intracardiac pressures may be required include one or more of the following: (1) Uncertainty about a direct correlation between the PCWP and the LAP/LV end-diastolic pressure, such as in patients with suspected mitral stenosis, pulmonary vein obstruction or cor-triatriatum; (2) Clinical or imaging-based suspicion of restrictive or constrictive physiology, requiring concomitant measurement of RV and LV pressures.

Both constrictive pericarditis (CP) and restrictive cardiomyopathy (RCM) lead to impaired filling of left and right ventricles that result in decreased cardiac output. Both are characterized by initially normal systolic contractile function and are an important differential diagnosis for diastolic dysfunction due to left heart disease. In the cardiac catheterization laboratory concomitant measurement of LV and RV pressures helps in differentiating between these pathologic entities. In constrictive pericarditis (CP), as more blood enters the RV with inspiration, the intrapericardial pressure increases because of the limited space in the pericardium and LV filling is reduced. Hence in CP, RV systolic pressure rises with inspiration while LV systolic pressure decreases. The reverse happens during spontaneous expiration [102]. In contrast, LV and RV systolic pressures do not show discordance in variation with respiration, and will both increase during expiration and decrease during inspiration. Some of the clues that help distinguish between CP and RCM include (a) the persistence of higher left-sided filling pressures maintained in RCM and (b) the magnitude of pulmonary hypertension tends to be greater in RCM (RVSP is >3 times RVEDP) [103]. The "systolic area index" ratio which is calculated as the RV to LV systolic pressure-time area during inspiration versus expiration is shown to have a sensitivity of 97 % and a predictive accuracy of 100 % for the identification of patients with surgically documented CP (see Fig. 10.10) [104].

Suspicion or knowledge of significant left-sided valvular disease may require direct evaluation of the hemodynamics and pressure gradients across the involved valve(s). In these cases transseptal puncture and direct measurement of LAP may be required. If mitral stenosis is suspected and PCWP measurement is not reliable, direct LAP measurement should be performed. If underlying coronary artery disease is suspected to be the cause or contributor to diastolic dysfunction coronary angiography may be considered.

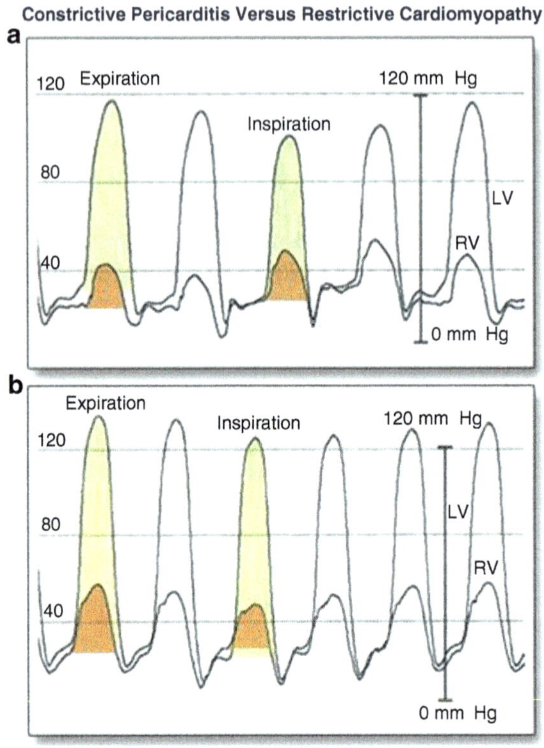

Fig. 10.10 LV and RV high-fidelity manometer pressure traces from two patients during expiration and inspiration. Note that both patients have early rapid filling and elevation and end-equalization of the left ventricular (LV) and right ventricular (RV) pressures at end expiration. (**a**) A patient with surgically documented constrictive pericarditis. During inspiration there is an increase in the area of the RV pressure curve (*orange shaded area*) compared with expiration. The area of the LV pressure curve (*yellow shaded area*) decreases during inspiration as compared with expiration. (**b**) A patient with restrictive myocardial disease documented by endomyocardial biopsy. During inspiration there is a decrease in the area of the RV pressure curve (*orange shaded area*) as compared with expiration. The area of the LV pressure curve (*yellow shaded area*) is unchanged during inspiration as compared with expiration (from Talreja DR, Nishimura RA, Oh JK, Holmes DR. Constrictive pericarditis in the modern era: novel criteria for diagnosis in the cardiac catheterization laboratory. J Am Coll Cardiol. 2008)

Volume Challenge to Unmask PH due to Diastolic Dysfunction

It has been shown in healthy individuals that administration of 1 l of saline over 6–8 min raises the PCWP by a maximum of 3 mm Hg, but not to >11 mmHg [1, 105]. In addition, in a population that is at elevated risk for diastolic dysfunction, administration of 500 ml of saline over 5 min can unmask patients in whom the PCWP increases to >15 mmHg [106]. Fluid volumes larger than 1 l, may cause the PCWP to rise even in healthy volunteers [107]. The diagnostic performance (sensitivity, specificity, and positive and negative predictive values) of fluid challenge has not yet been sufficiently evaluated nor has the safety of fluid challenge in patients with severe PH. However, when mild to moderate PH exists in the presence of modest suspicion of diastolic dysfunction, fluid challenge appears to be a reasonable test to perform.

Exercise Challenge During Right Heart Catheterization

Getting hemodynamic measurements during exercise can add to the information obtained from RHC done only at rest. For example, elevated PCWP during exercise can point towards diastolic dysfunction as a cause of PH. Borlaug and colleagues recently showed that during exercise, end-expiration PCWP rose to 32 ± 6 mmHg in patients with HFpEF compared with 13 ± 5 mmHg in controls [108]. Exercise hemodynamics may also be useful in distinguishing between PAH and PH associated with LV diastolic dysfunction in patients with the scleroderma (SSc) spectrum of disease [109]. In some patients mPAP may be only slightly elevated at rest, but exercise leads to symptoms and significant elevation in PAP and PVR, thus unmasking more severe PH [110]. Change in PAP during exercise along with symptoms can also be an important measure of response to treatment [110, 111] Exercise testing for PH during RHC is not yet standardized and at present is limited to centers with experience and expertise in interpreting pulmonary vascular responses to exercise [1]. In particular, change in PVR may be more important than the change in PAP and thus, measurement of cardiac output is usually needed to properly interpret pulmonary hemodynamic responses to exercise. Also, PCWP measured during exercise is unreliable due to multiple contributors such as changes in ventilatory pattern abdominal muscle contractions and differs from the recumbent to the upright position of the patient. Further discussion of this topic is presented in Chap. 11.

Pulmonary Angiography for CTEPH

It is quite safe to perform pulmonary angiography (typically isolated to particular PA segments or lobes) even in cases with severe PH, although the risk may be elevated in patients with severe decrease in cardiac output, elevation in RA or RV end diastolic pressure, or super-systemic RV pressures. While performing RHC in a patient with suspected PA or pulmonary vein obstructions, PA pressures should be measured bilaterally and in multiple lobes both proximally and distally. A preshaped catheter such as a coronary catheter can be used for the purpose of accessing specific lobes and then can be exchanged for balloon tipped end hole catheter for checking pressures. It should be kept in mind that there is a reflex rise in PAP and PVR after pulmonary angiography so pressures should be measured prior to performing this procedure. Pulmonary angiography should be performed in cases with suspected CTEPH, peripheral pulmonary artery stenosis, vasculitis, pulmonary AV malformations, or pulmonary venous obstruction [112].

Table 10.8 Agents for acute vasodilator testing (from McLaughlin VV et al, ACCF/AHA 2009 expert consensus document on pulmonary hypertension, Circulation 2009)

	Epoprostenol	Adenosine	Nitric oxide
Route of administration	Intravenous infusion	Intravenous infusion	Inhaled
Dose titration	2 ng/kg/min every 10–15 min	50 mcg/kg/min every 2 min	None
Dose range	2–10 ng/kg/min	50–250 mcg/kg/min	10–80 ppm
Side effects	Headache, nausea, lightheadedness	Dyspnea, chest pain, AV block	Increased left heart filling pressure in susceptible patients

AV atrioventricular

Vasoreactivity Testing

Vasoreactivity or vasodilator testing during RHC is beneficial as it may identify a subset of patients that respond to calcium channel blockers (CCB), or may assist in prognostic assessment. Acute vasoreactivity challenge should be performed with a short-acting pulmonary specific vasodilator that has no or very limited systemic hypotensive effects. The agent most commonly used is inhaled NO, while intravenous epoprostenol or adenosine can also be used as alternatives (with the caveat that they may cause systemic vasodilator effects) (Table 10.8) [1]. A positive acute response is defined as a reduction of mPAP by 10 mmHg *and* to an absolute value of ≤40 mmHg with an increased or unchanged cardiac output. Using these criteria, about 5–10 % of the patients with IPAH will have a positive pulmonary vasodilator response. Positive acute responders are likely to show a sustained response to long-term treatment with high doses of CCB. True vasodilator responders who demonstrate sustained response to CCB have an excellent prognosis, with up to a 95 % survival at 5 years [113]. In one study, however, 44 % of patients with IPAH who demonstrated an acute pulmonary vasodilator response showed no hemodynamic improvement after 1 year of therapy. Thus, the number of patients who can be treated with CCB alone is quite small [113].

References

1. Hoeper MM, et al. Definitions and diagnosis of pulmonary hypertension. J Am Coll Cardiol. 2013;62:D42–50.
2. McLaughlin VV, et al. ACCF/AHA 2009 expert consensus document on pulmonary hypertension: a report of the American College of Cardiology Foundation Task Force on Expert Consensus Documents and the American Heart Association: developed in collaboration with the American College of Chest Physicians, American Thoracic Society, Inc., and the Pulmonary Hypertension Association. Circulation. 2009;119:2250–94.
3. Galiè N, et al. Committee for Practice Guidelines (CPG). Guidelines for the diagnosis and treatment of pulmonary hypertension: the Task Force for the Diagnosis and Treatment of

Pulmonary Hypertension of the European Society of Cardiology (ESC) and the European Respiratory Society (ERS), endorsed by the International Society of Heart and Lung Transplantation (ISHLT). Eur Heart J. 2009;30:2493–537.
4. Levitzky MG. Chapter 4. Blood flow to the lung. In: Levitzky MG, editors. Pulmonary physiology, 8e. New York, NY: McGraw-Hill; 2013. http://accessmedicine.mhmedical.com/content.aspx?bookid=575&Sectionid=42512982. Accessed 8 Sept 2014.
5. Achilles J, et al. 12—Special circulations, In: Achilles J. editors. Cardiovascular physiology. 10th ed. Philadelphia; 2013. p. 237–62. ISBN 9780323086974, http://dx.doi.org/10.1016/B978-0-323-08697-4.00012-5. (http://www.sciencedirect.com/science/article/pii/B9780323086974000125)
6. Kovacs G, et al. Pulmonary vascular resistances during exercise in normal subjects: a systematic review. Eur Respir J. 2012;39:319–28.
7. Hughes JM, et al. Effect of lung volume on the distribution of pulmonary blood flow in man. Respir Physiol. 1968;4:58–72.
8. Glenny RW, Bernard S, Robertson HT, Hlastala MP. Gravity is an important but minor determinant of pulmonary blood flow heterogeneity in the baboon. FASEB J. 1997;11:1996.
9. Galvin I, Drummond GB, Nirmalan M. Distribution of blood flow and ventilation in the lung: gravity is not the only factor. Br J Anaesth. 2007;98:420–8.
10. Dumas JP, Bardou M, Goirand F, et al. Hypoxic pulmonary vasoconstriction. Gen Pharmacol. 1999;33:289–97.
11. Opotowsky AR, Ojeda J, Rogers F, Arkles J, Liu T, Forfia PR. Blood pressure response to the valsalva maneuver. A simple bedside test to determine the hemodynamic basis of pulmonary hypertension. J Am Coll Cardiol. 2010;56(16):1352–3.
12. Wiese J. The abdominojugular reflux sign. Am J Med. 2000;109(1):59–61.
13. Nath AR, Capel LH. Inspiratory crackles—early and late. Thorax. 1974;29(2):223–7.
14. Simon M, Sasahara AA, Cannilla JE. The radiology of pulmonary hypertension. Semin Roentgenol. 1967;2:368–88.
15. Rich S, Dantzker DR, Ayres SM, et al. Primary pulmonary hypertension. A national prospective study. Ann Intern Med. 1987;107(2):216–23.
16. Chetty KG, Brown SE, Light RW. Identification of pulmonary hypertension in chronic obstructive pulmonary disease from routine chest radiographs. Am Rev Respir Dis. 1982; 126(2):338–41.
17. Turner AF, Lau FY, Jacobson G. A method for the estimation of pulmonary venous and arterial pressures from the routine chest roentgenogram. AJR. 1972;116:97–106.
18. Milne EN. Physiological interpretation of the plain radiograph in mitral stenosis, including a review of criteria for the radiological estimation of pulmonary arterial and venous pressures. Br J Radiol. 1963;36:902–13.
19. Ng CS, Wells AU, Padley SP. A CT sign of chronic pulmonary arterial hypertension: the ratio of main pulmonary artery to aortic diameter. J Thorac Imaging. 1999;14(4):270–8.
20. Kuriyama K, Gamsu G, Stern RG, Cann CE, Herfkens RJ, Brundage BH. CT-determined pulmonary artery diameters in predicting pulmonary hypertension. Invest Radiol. 1984;19(1): 16–22.
21. Baque-Juston MC, Wells AU, Hansell DM. Pericardial thickening or effusion in patients with pulmonary artery hypertension: a CT study. AJR Am J Roentgenol. 1999;172(2):361–4.
22. Tan RT, Kuzo R, Goodman LR, et al. Utility of CT scan evaluation for predicting pulmonary hypertension in patients with parenchymal lung disease. Chest. 1998;113:1250–6.
23. Benza R, Biederman R, Murali S, Gupta H. Role of cardiac magnetic resonance imaging in the management of patients with pulmonary arterial hypertension. J Am Coll Cardiol. 2008;52(21):1683–92.
24. Kuehne T, Yilmaz S, Schulze-Neick I, et al. Magnetic resonance imaging guided catheterisation for assessment of pulmonary vascular resistance: in vivo validation and clinical application in patients with pulmonary hypertension. Heart. 2005;91:1064–9.
25. Henkens IR, Scherptong RW, Kralingen KW, Said SA, Vliegen HW. Pulmonary hypertension: the role of the electrocardiogram. Neth Heart J. 2008;16:250–4.

26. Rich S, Brundage BH. High-dose calcium channel-blocking therapy for primary pulmonary hypertension: evidence for long-term reduction in pulmonary arterial pressure and regression of right ventricular hypertrophy. Circulation. 1987;76(1):135–41.
27. Bossone E, Paciocco G, Iarussi D, Agretto A, Iacono A, Gillespie BW, Rubenfire M. The prognostic role of the ECG in primary pulmonary hypertension. Chest. 2002;121(2):513.
28. Rudski LG, Lai WW, Afilalo J, Hua L, Handschumacher MD, Chandrasekaran K, Solomon SD, Louie EK, Schiller NB. Guidelines for the echocardiographic assessment of the right heart in adults: a report from the American Society of Echocardiography endorsed by the European Association of Echocardiography, a registered branch of the European Society of Cardiology, and the Canadian Society of Echocardiography. J Am Soc Echocardiogr. 2010;23:685–713.
29. Fisher MR, Forfia PR, Chamera E, Housten-Harris T, Champion HC, Girgis RE, et al. Accuracy of Doppler echocardiography in the hemodynamic assessment of pulmonary hypertension. Am J Respir Crit Care Med. 2009;179:615–21.
30. McGoon M, Gutterman D, Steen V, Barst R, McCrory DC, Fortin TA, et al. Screening, early detection, and diagnosis of pulmonary arterial hypertension: ACCP evidence-based clinical practice guidelines. Chest. 2004;126:14S–34.
31. Skjaerpe T, Hatle L. Noninvasive estimation of systolic pressure in the right ventricle in patients with tricuspid regurgitation. Eur Heart J. 1986;7:704–10.
32. Abbas AE, Fortuin FD, Schiller NB, Appleton CP, Moreno CA, Lester SJ. Echocardiographic determination of mean pulmonary artery pressure. Am J Cardiol. 2003;92:1373–6.
33. Aduen JF, Castello R, Lozano MM, Hepler GN, Keller CA, Alvarez F, et al. An alternative echocardiographic method to estimate mean pulmonary artery pressure: diagnostic and clinical implications. J Am Soc Echocardiogr. 2009;22:814–9.
34. Lee RT, Lord CP, Plappert T, Sutton MS. Prospective Doppler echocardiographic evaluation of pulmonary artery diastolic pressure in the medical intensive care unit. Am J Cardiol. 1989;64:1366–70.
35. Reynolds DW, Bartelt N, Taepke R, Bennett TD. Measurement of pulmonary artery diastolic pressure from the right ventricle. J Am Coll Cardiol. 1995;25:1176–82.
36. Stephen B, Dalal P, Berger M, Schweitzer P, Hecht S. Noninvasive estimation of pulmonary artery diastolic pressure in patients with tricuspid regurgitation by Doppler echocardiography. Chest. 1999;116:73–7.
37. Abbas AE, Fortuin FD, Schiller NB, Appleton CP, Moreno CA, Lester SJ. A simple method for noninvasive estimation of pulmonary vascular resistance. J Am Coll Cardiol. 2003;41: 1021–7.
38. Haddad F, Zamanian R, Beraud AS, Schnittger I, Feinstein J, Peterson T, et al. A Novel noninvasive method of estimating pulmonary vascular resistance in patients with pulmonary arterial hypertension. J Am Soc Echocardiogr. 2009;22:523–9.
39. Addonizio LJ, Gersony WM, Robbins RC, Drusin RE, Smith CR, Reison DS, et al. Elevated pulmonary vascular resistance and cardiac transplantation. Circulation. 1987;76:V52–5.
40. Scapellato F, Temporelli PL, Eleuteri E, Corrá E, Imparato A, Giannuzzi P. Accurate noninvasive estimation of pulmonary vascular resistance by Doppler echocardiography in patients with chronic failure heart failure. J Am Coll Cardiol. 2001;37:1813–9.
41. Opotowsky AR, Clair M, Afilalo J, Landzberg MJ, Waxman AB, Moko L, Maron BA, Vaidya A, Forfia PR. A simple echocardiographic method to estimate pulmonary vascular resistance. Am J Cardiol. 2013;112:873–82.
42. Dabestani A, Mahan G, Gardin JM, Takenaka K, Burn C, Allfie A, et al. Evaluation of pulmonary artery pressure and resistance by pulsed Doppler echocardiography. Am J Cardiol. 1987;59:662–8.
43. Burgess MI, Bright-Thomas RJ, Ray SG. Echocardiographic evaluation of right ventricular function. Eur J Echocardiogr. 2002;3(4):252–62.
44. Arkles JS, Opotowsky AR, Ojeda J, Rogers F, Liu T, Prassana V, Marzec L, Palevsky HI, Ferrari VA, Forfia PR. Shape of the right ventricular Doppler envelope predicts hemodynamics and right heart function in pulmonary hypertension. Am J Respir Crit Care Med. 2011;183: 268–76.

45. Lai WW, Gauvreau K, Rivera ES, Saleeb S, Powell AJ, Geva T. Accuracy of guideline recommendations for two-dimensional quantification of the right ventricle by echocardiography. Int J Cardiovasc Imaging. 2008;24:691–8.
46. Anavekar NS, Gerson D, Skali H, Kwong RY, Yucel EK, Solomon SD. Two-dimensional assessment of right ventricular function: an echocardiographic-MRI correlative study. Echocardiography. 2007;24:452–6.
47. Forfia PR, Fisher MR, Mathai SC, Housten-Harris T, Hemnes AR, Borlaug BA, Chamera E, Corretti MC, Champion HC, Abraham TP, Girgis RE, Hassoun PM. Tricuspid annular displacement predicts survival in pulmonary hypertension. Am J Respir Crit Care Med. 2006;174(9):1034–41.
48. Badano LP, Ginghina C, Easaw J, Muraru D, Grillo MT, Lancellotti P, Pinamonti B, Coghlan G, Marra MP, Popescu BA, De Vita S. Right ventricle in pulmonary arterial hypertension: haemodynamics, structural changes, imaging, and proposal of a study protocol aimed to assess remodelling and treatment effects. Eur J Echocardiogr. 2010;11(1):27–37.
49. Tei C, Dujardin KS, Hodge DO, Bailey KR, McGoon MD, Tajik AJ, et al. Doppler echocardiographic index for assessment of global right ventricular function. J Am Soc Echocardiogr. 1996;9:838–47.
50. Meris A, Faletra F, Conca C, Klersy C, Regoli F, Klimusina J, et al. Timing and magnitude of regional right ventricular function: a speckle tracking derived strain study of normal subjects and patients with right ventricular dysfunction. J Am Soc Echocardiogr. 2010; 23:823–31.
51. Haddad F, et al. Right ventricular function in cardiovascular disease, part I: anatomy, physiology, aging, and functional assessment of the right ventricle. Circulation. 2008;117(11): 1436–48.
52. Ryan T, et al. An echocardiographic index for separation of right ventricular volume and pressure overload. J Am Coll Cardiol. 1985;5(4):918–27.
53. Hinderliter AL, et al. Frequency and prognostic significance of pericardial effusion in primary pulmonary hypertension. PPH Study Group. Primary pulmonary hypertension. Am J Cardiol. 1999;84(4):481. -4, A10.
54. Ranu H, Smith K, Nimako K, Sheth A, Madden BP. A retrospective review to evaluate the safety of right heart catheterization via the internal jugular vein in the assessment of pulmonary hypertension. Clin Cardiol. 2010;33:303–6.
55. Hoeper MM, Lee SH, Voswinckel R, et al. Complications of right heart catheterization procedures in patients with pulmonary hypertension in experienced centers. J Am Coll Cardiol. 2006;48:2546–52.
56. Massicotte A. A practice tool for the new oral anticoagulants. Can Pharm J (Ott). 2014; 147(1):25–32.
57. Francis GS, Cohn JN. The autonomic nervous system in congestive heart failure. Annu Rev Med. 1986;37:235–47.
58. Groeneveld AB, et al. Effect of the mechanical ventilatory cycle on thermodilution right ventricular volumes and cardiac output. J Appl Physiol (1985). 2000;89(1):89–96.
59. Couture P, et al. Effects of anesthetic induction in patients with diastolic dysfunction. Can J Anaesth. 2009;56(5):357–65.
60. Biondi JW, et al. The effect of incremental positive end-expiratory pressure on right ventricular hemodynamics and ejection fraction. Anesth Analg. 1988;67(2):144–51.
61. Theres H, et al. Phase-related changes in right ventricular cardiac output under volume-controlled mechanical ventilation with positive end-expiratory pressure. Crit Care Med. 1999;27(5):953–8.
62. Ragosta M. Normal waveforms, artifacts, and pitfalls. In: Textbook of clinical hemodynamics. Philadelphia: Saunders/Elsevier; 2008.
63. Summerhill EM, Baram M. Principles of pulmonary artery catheterization in the critically ill. Lung. 2005;183(3):209–19.
64. Dehmer GJ, Firth BG, Hillis LD. Oxygen consumption in adult patients during cardiac catheterization. Clin Cardiol. 1982;5(8):436–40.

65. Hemnes AR, Forfia PR, Champion HC. Assessment of pulmonary vasculature and right heart by invasive haemodynamics and echocardiography. Int J Clin Pract Suppl. 2009;162:4–19.
66. Bonow R, Mann D, Zipes D, Libby P. Technical aspects of cardiac catheterization. Braunwald's heart disease. http://www.r2library.com/Resource/Title/1437703984/ch0020s0569. (2012). Retrieved 8 Sept 2014.
67. Sabbah HN, Anbe DT, Stein PD. Negative intraventricular diastolic pressure in patients with mitral stenosis: evidence of left ventricular diastolic suction. Am J Cardiol. 1980;45(3): 562–6.
68. Paulus WJ, Vantrimpont PJ, Rousseau MF. Diastolic function of the nonfilling human left ventricle. J Am Coll Cardiol. 1992;20(7):1524–32.
69. Courtois M, et al. Anatomically and physiologically based reference level for measurement of intracardiac pressures. Circulation. 1995;92(7):1994–2000.
70. Baim DS, Grossman W. Grossman's cardiac catheterization, angiography, and intervention, 7th ed. Philadelphia: Lippincott Williams & Wilkins; 2006. xvii, 807 p.
71. Bonow R, Mann D, Zipes D, Libby P. Hemodynamic data. Braunwald's heart disease. http://www.r2library.com/Resource/Title/1437703984/ch0020s0577. (2012)Retrieved 8 Sept 2014.
72. Irvin CG, et al. Effect of breathing pattern on esophageal pressure gradients in humans. J Appl Physiol Respir Environ Exerc Physiol. 1984;57(1):168–75.
73. D'Alonzo GE, et al. Survival in patients with primary pulmonary hypertension. Results from a national prospective registry. Ann Intern Med. 1991;115(5):343–9.
74. Thenappan T, et al. Survival in pulmonary arterial hypertension: a reappraisal of the NIH risk stratification equation. Eur Respir J. 2010;35(5):1079–87.
75. Stein PD, et al. Performance of the failing and nonfailing right ventricle of patients with pulmonary hypertension. Am J Cardiol. 1979;44(6):1050–5.
76. Chemla D, et al. Haemodynamic evaluation of pulmonary hypertension. Eur Respir J. 2002;20(5):1314–31.
77. Fishman AP, Fisher AB, American Physiological Society. The respiratory system. Handbook of physiology 1985. Bethesda, MD: American Physiological Society; 1887. Distributed by Williams & Wilkins.
78. Gibbs JS, Cunningham D, Shapiro LM, Park A, Poole-Wilson PA, Fox KM. Diurnal variation of pulmonary artery pressure in chronic heart failure. Br Heart J. 1989;62:30–5.
79. Bell ALL, Shimomura S, Guthrie WJ, Hempel HF, Fitzpatrick HF, Begg CF. Wedge pulmonary arteriography. Its application in congenital and acquired heart disease. Radiology. 1959;73:566.
80. Zidulka A, Hakim TS. Wedge pressure in large vs. small pulmonary arteries to detect pulmonary venoconstriction. J Appl Physiol. 1985;59(4):1329–32.
81. Hellems HK, Haynes FW, Dexter L. Pulmonary capillary pressure in man. J Appl Physiol. 1949;2(1):24–9.
82. Kafi SA, et al. Partitioning of pulmonary vascular resistance in primary pulmonary hypertension. J Am Coll Cardiol. 1998;31(6):1372–6.
83. Fesler P, Pagnamenta A, Vachiery JL, Brimioulle S, Abdel Kafi S, Boonstra A, Delcroix M, Channick RN, Rubin LJ, Naeije R. Single arterial occlusion to locate resistance in patients with pulmonary hypertension. Eur Respir J. 2003;21:31–6.
84. Naeije R, Vachiery JL, Yerly P, et al. The transpulmonary pressure gradient for the diagnosis of pulmonary vascular disease. Eur Respir J. 2013;41:217–23.
85. Gerges C, Gerges M, Lang MB, et al. Diastolic pulmonary vascular pressure gradient. Chest. 2013;143(3):758–66.
86. McGregor M, Sniderman A. On pulmonary vascular resistance: the need for more precise definition. Am J Cardiol. 1985;55(1):217–21.
87. Tartulier MM, et al. Pulmonary arterial pressures in normal subjects. Effects of age and muscular exercise. Bull Physiopathol Respir (Nancy). 1972;8(6):1295–321.
88. Ehrsam RE, et al. Influence of age on pulmonary haemodynamics at rest and during supine exercise. Clin Sci (Lond). 1983;65(6):653–60.

89. Weir EK, Reeves JT. Pulmonary hypertension xiv. Mount Kisco, NY: Futura Pub. Co.; 1984, 442 p.
90. Lankhaar JW, Westerhof N, Faes TJ, et al. Quantification of right ventricular afterload in patients with and without pulmonary hypertension. Am J Physiol Heart Circ Physiol. 2006;291:H1731–7.
91. Cournand A, et al. Measurement of cardiac output in man using the technique of catheterization of the right auricle or ventricle. J Clin Invest. 1945;24(1):106–16.
92. Stead EA, et al. The cardiac output in male subjects as measured by the technique of right atrial catheterization. Normal values with observations on the effect of anxiety and tilting. J Clin Invest. 1945;24(3):326–31.
93. Kendrick AH, et al. Direct Fick cardiac output: are assumed values of oxygen consumption acceptable? Eur Heart J. 1988;9(3):337–42.
94. Fakler U, et al. Assumed oxygen consumption frequently results in large errors in the determination of cardiac output. J Thorac Cardiovasc Surg. 2005;130(2):272–6.
95. Ultman JS, Bursztein S. Analysis of error in the determination of respiratory gas exchange at varying FIO2. J Appl Physiol Respir Environ Exerc Physiol. 1981;50(1):210–6.
96. Moise SF, Sinclair CJ, Scott DH. Pulmonary artery blood temperature and the measurement of cardiac output by thermodilution. Anaesthesia. 2002;57(6):562–6.
97. Lehmann KG, Platt MS. Improved accuracy and precision of thermodilution cardiac output measurement using a dual thermistor catheter system. J Am Coll Cardiol. 1999;33(3): 883–91.
98. Hoeper MM, et al. Determination of cardiac output by the Fick method, thermodilution, and acetylene rebreathing in pulmonary hypertension. Am J Respir Crit Care Med. 1999;160(2): 535–41.
99. Hillis LD, Firth BG, Winniford MD. Analysis of factors affecting the variability of Fick versus indicator dilution measurements of cardiac output. Am J Cardiol. 1985;56(12): 764–8.
100. Hurrell DG, Nishimura RA, Higano ST, Appleton CP, Danielson GK, Holmes Jr DR, Tajik AJ. Value of dynamic respiratory changes in left and right ventricular pressures for the diagnosis of constrictive pericarditis. Circulation. 1996;93(11):2007.
101. Tyberg TI, Goodyer AV, Hurst 3rd VW, Alexander J, Langou RA. Left ventricular filling in differentiating restrictive amyloid cardiomyopathy and constrictive pericarditis. Am J Cardiol. 1981;47(4):791.
102. Talreja DR, Nishimura RA, Oh JK, Holmes DR. Constrictive pericarditis in the modern era: novel criteria for diagnosis in the cardiac catheterization laboratory. J Am Coll Cardiol. 2008;51(3):315.
103. Bush CA, Stang JM, Wooley CF, Kilman JW. Occult constrictive pericardial disease. Diagnosis by rapid volume expansion and correction by pericardiectomy. Circulation. 1977; 56:924–30.
104. Robbins IM, Newman JH, Johnson RF, et al. Association of the metabolic syndrome with pulmonary venous hypertension. Chest. 2009;136:31–6.
105. Fujimoto N, Borlaug BA, Lewis GD, et al. Hemodynamic responses to rapid saline loading: the impact of age, sex, and heart failure. Circulation. 2013;127:55–62.
106. Borlaug BA, Nishimura RA, Sorajja P, Lam CS, Redfield MM. Exercise hemodynamics enhance diagnosis of early heart failure with preserved ejection fraction. Circ Heart Fail. 2010;3:588–95.
107. Hager WD, Collins I, Tate JP, et al. Exercise during cardiac catheterization distinguishes between pulmonary and left ventricular causes of dyspnea in systemic sclerosis patients. Clin Respir J. 2013;7:227–36.
108. Tolle JT, Waxman AB, van Horn TL, et al. Exercise-induced pulmonary arterial hypertension. Circulation. 2008;118:2183–9.
109. Oudiz RJ, Rubin LJ. Exercise-induced pulmonary arterial hypertension. A new addition to the spectrum of pulmonary vascular diseases. Circulation. 2008;118:2120–1.

110. D'Alto M, Ghio S, D'Andrea A, et al. Inappropriate exercise-induced increase in pulmonary artery pressure in patients with systemic sclerosis. Heart. 2011;97:112–7.
111. Sitbon O, et al. Long-term response to calcium channel blockers in idiopathic pulmonary arterial hypertension. Circulation. 2005;111(23):3105–11.
112. Brennan JM, et al. Reappraisal of the use of inferior vena cava for estimating right atrial pressure. J Am Soc Echocardiogr. 2007;20(7):857–61.

Chapter 11
Cardiopulmonary Exercise Testing in Pulmonary Hypertension

David M. Systrom and Aaron B. Waxman

Abstract Early and accurate diagnosis of pulmonary vascular disease is important given the high mortality of untreated pulmonary hypertension. The development of cardiopulmonary exercise testing (CPET) has allowed an early diagnosis of PAH in "at risk" patients or those with suggestive clinical findings. CPET can quantify the degree of exercise impairment, and rule out a pulmonary mechanical limit to exercise. It can also be used to monitor disease progression and response to treatment. CPET generally consists of an incremental symptom-limited cycling or treadmill exercise test with measurements of ventilation and pulmonary gas exchange. Noninvasive testing is done with continuous 12-lead ECG, cuff blood pressure monitoring and pulse oximetry. Invasive CPET adds arterial and pulmonary artery catheters for blood gas, pH and pressure measurements. CPET when used in the context of a diagnostic algorithm, can confirm the diagnosis of exercise-induced PH, distinguish between pulmonary arterial and venous hypertension, and rule out confounders such as impaired systemic O_2 extraction. CPET may be used alone or combined with other modalities, such as transthoracic cardiac Doppler echo and MRI. Recent expert consensus statements suggest CPET is useful in the diagnosis, management and risk stratification of PH. This chapter provides an overview of the history of CPET, describes how measurements are obtained and interpreted, and discusses its use in diagnosis and monitoring of pulmonary hypertensive diseases including exercise-induced pulmonary hypertension and pulmonary hypertension associated heart and lung disease.

Keywords Cardiopulmonary exercise testing • Pulmonary arterial hypertension • Pulmonary hypertension

---

D.M. Systrom, M.D.
Pulmonary and Critical Care Medicine, Pulmonary Vascular Disease Program Director, Dyspnea and Performance Evaluation Program, Brigham and Women's Hospital Heart and Vascular, Center Assistant Professor of Medicine/Harvard Medical School, 75 Francis Street, PBB CA-3 Boston, MA 02115, USA

A.B. Waxman, M.D., Ph.D. (✉)
Pulmonary and Critical Care Medicine, Director, Pulmonary Vascular Disease Program, Executive Director, Center for Pulmonary-Heart Diseases, Brigham and Women's Hospital Heart and Vascular, Center Associate Professor of Medicine/Harvard Medical School, 75 Francis Street, PBB CA-3 Boston, MA 02115, USA
e-mail: abwaxman@partners.org

J.R. Klinger, R.P. Frantz (eds.), *Diagnosis and Management of Pulmonary Hypertension*, Respiratory Medicine 12, DOI 10.1007/978-1-4939-2636-7_11

Abbreviations

6MWT	6-min walk test
A-sDO_2	Alveolar–arterial oxygen tension difference
AT	Anaerobic threshold
BRI	Breathing reserve index
CaO_2	Oxygen content of arterial blood
CO	Cardiac output
CPET	Cardiopulmonary exercise test
CvO_2	Oxygen content of venous blood
DO_2	Oxygen delivery
DO_2max	Maximum systemic oxygen delivery
eiPAH	Exercise-induced pulmonary hypertension
EOV	Exercise oscillatory ventilation
HF	Heart failure
HFpEF	Heart failure with preserved ejection fraction
HFrEF	Heart failure with reduce ejection fraction
ITP	Intrathoracic pressure
IVS	Interventricular septum
LT	Lactate threshold
LV	Left ventricle
LVEF	Left ventricular ejection fraction
mPAP	Mean pulmonary artery pressure
MVV	Maximum voluntary ventilation
OUES	O_2 uptake efficiency slope
PAH	Pulmonary arterial hypertension
PAP	Pulmonary artery pressure
PASP	Pulmonary artery systolic pressure
PCWP	Pulmonary capillary wedge pressure
$PETCO_2$	End tidal PCO_2
PFO	Patent foramen ovale
PH	Pulmonary hypertension
PVD	Pulmonary vascular disease
PVL	Pulmonary vascular limit
PVR	Pulmonary vascular resistance
RA	Right atrium
RAP	Right atrial pressure
RER	Respiratory exchange ratio
RHC	Right heart catheterization
ROC	Receiver operating characteristic
RV	Right ventricle
RVSP	Right ventricular systolic pressure
SVR	Systemic vascular resistance
TPG	Transpulmonary gradient

ULN	Upper limit of normal
VAT	Ventilatory anaerobic threshold
VCO_2	Carbon dioxide production
VE	Minute ventilation
VEmax	Minute ventilation at peak exercise
VO_2	Oxygen uptake
VO_2max	Maximum oxygen uptake
VT	Tidal volume
WHO	World Health Organization

Introduction

The timely and accurate diagnosis of PH is important given the high mortality if left untreated [1, 2], the availability of increasingly effective medical therapies [3] and a long wait for a donor lung at most transplant centers [4]. The development of cardiopulmonary exercise testing (CPET) has allowed an early diagnosis of PH in "at risk" patients or those with subtle suggestive clinical findings, affording the opportunity to treat patients most likely to benefit and to monitor their response.

PH carries a poor prognosis, with a mortality of about 15 % in 1 year despite modern therapy. The diagnosis of PH is often delayed; the average time from onset of symptoms to diagnosis is approximately 2 years [2]. The delay is due, in part from the nonspecific signs and symptoms of the disease, and the complex, extensive workup necessary to determine a cause of elevated pulmonary artery pressure. Traditional evaluation of resting pulmonary function and gas exchange is insensitive [5, 6], and further contributes to the diagnostic delay. Early PH generally does not cause symptoms at rest and stressing pulmonary vasculature with exercise may be necessary to demonstrate abnormal structure and function [2, 7–10]. An appropriate analogy might be that of coronary artery disease; a resting left heart catheterization identifies severe disease, but milder hemodynamically significant disease requires a functional study for its diagnosis.

Cardiopulmonary exercise testing (CPET) is such a functional test that may elicit early [7] and reproducible [11, 12] abnormalities suggestive of PH. CPET generally consists of an incremental symptom-limited cycling or treadmill exercise test with measurements of ventilation and pulmonary gas exchange [13, 14]. The first CPET done was in the Harvard Fatigue Lab in the 1920s (Fig. 11.1) where many of the basic tenets of normal human exercise physiology were described using measurements of ventilation, pulmonary gas exchange, arterial blood gases and pH as well as noninvasive estimates of cardiac output.

Currently, CPET is subdivided into noninvasive testing (niCPET), done with continuous 12-lead ECG, cuff blood pressure monitoring and pulse oximetry, and invasive CPET (iCPET), which adds arterial and pulmonary artery catheters for blood gas, pH and pressure measurements. CPET may be used alone or combined with other modalities, such as transthoracic cardiac Doppler echo and MRI.

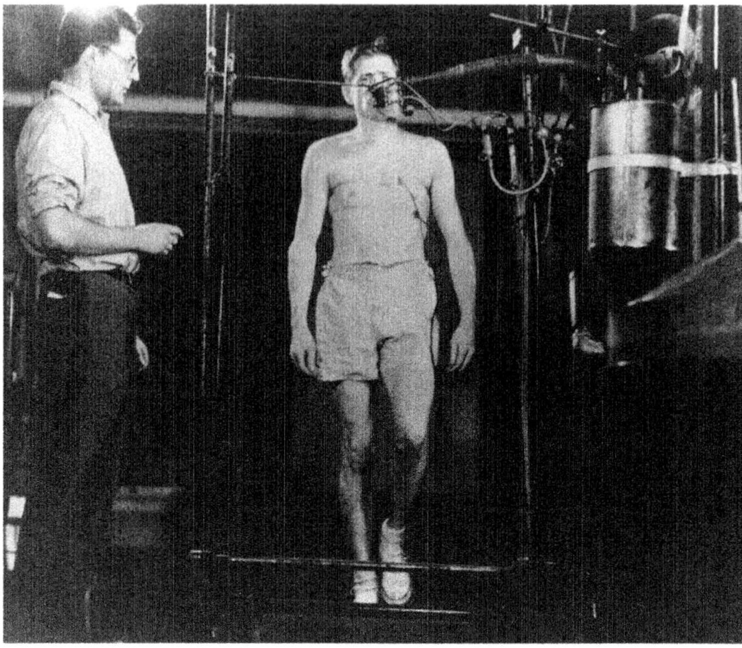

Fig. 11.1 The earliest known CPET was at the Harvard Fatigue Lab in the 1920s

There is a rapidly growing body of evidence supporting its utility in patients with suspected or confirmed PH. Recent expert consensus statements suggest CPET's is useful in the diagnosis, management and risk stratification of PH [15, 16]. CPET is safe even in established PH [17, 18] Severe PH with exertional syncopal episodes, cardiac arrhythmias, or acute right ventricular failure do, however, serve as contraindications to maximum exercise testing [13].

Noninvasive CPET

niCPET can be used as a screening test in the patient with unexplained exertional intolerance [14, 19] where a significant percentage of patients will ultimately be shown to have PH [7]. Such patients have generally undergone a time-honored history, physical examination, routine blood work, which are normal or, in the eyes of the clinician, show abnormalities insufficiently severe to explain symptoms. niCPET may also be appropriate in suspected PH, e.g., family members of Group 1 PH, or in "at risk" patients with for example connective tissue disease [20].

niCPET can quantify the degree of exercise impairment, rule in or out a pulmonary mechanical limit to exercise and suggest disorders manifested by abnormal O_2 delivery or subsequent uptake and utilization, including PH. niCPET variables that are useful in assessing the presence and severity of PH are shown in Table 11.1. These variables largely reflect PH-related impairment of O_2 delivery to the exercising

Table 11.1 Variables in niCPET useful in the assessment of PH

Maximum oxygen uptake
Ventilatory or gas exchange anaerobic threshold (AT)
Ventilatory reserve
Ventilatory efficiency
Arterial O_2 desaturation
$PETCO_2$ change
Exercise oscillatory ventilation
Oxygen uptake efficiency slope

muscle bed and ventilation-perfusion abnormalities in the lung [17, 21–25]. Additionally, niCPEt allows reproducible assessment of functional capacity and treatment efficacy in PH and can predict survival [11, 17, 22, 26–28].

Maximum Oxygen Uptake (VO_2max)

Overall fitness is generally assessed by the VO_2max, expressed as a percent of predicted for the patient's age, gender and estimate of lean body mass, derived from height [29] VO_2 increases linearly vs. work rate with a slope of approximately 10 mL/min/W in normal subjects [29]. This slope is not affected by age, gender, or training, but is shifted leftward in obese patients and may plateau in more severe heart failure (HF). In the obese patient, in the absence of pulmonary vascular disease, the VO_2 max may be surprisingly well-preserved, but the external work performed on the cycle ergometer is compromised. This results from the oxygen cost of moving heavy legs or respiratory muscle work.

In established PH, VO_2max decreases [7, 17, 23–25, 28, 30, 31]. Even milder exercise-induced PH depresses VO_2max compared to normal [7, 10]. VO_2max correlates inversely with resting pulmonary hemodynamics [17] and may improve with pulmonary vasodilator therapy [27, 32], but this is not uniformly observed [21], perhaps in part because of methodological concerns, but perhaps related to confounding deleterious effects of treatment.

VO_2max is a powerful predictor of mortality in PAH [33, 34] and a peak VO_2 below 10.4 mL/kg/min has been considered a key criterion for early mortality [22].

Ventilatory (VAT) or Gas Exchange "Anaerobic" Threshold (AT)

Heavy exercise increases blood lactate concentration, ventilation and VCO_2 relative to VO_2; the latter can be reliably detected noninvasively with CPET using an iterative least residual sum of the squares of a two-segment log–log plot [35]. For many years the lactic acidemia of exercise was assumed to be secondary to inadequate oxygen delivery to muscle with resultant increases in "anaerobic" glycolysis to produce ATP. However, skeletal muscle mitochondrial redox state is actually higher when working muscle is producing lactate than at rest, implying that oxygen supply is not the critical factor [36–38]. Likewise, the tight mechanistic link between LT and VAT has been under mined by the fact that the two may be uncoupled experimentally [39–41] and in McArdle's disease [42] where ventilatory patterns during incremental exercise are normal in the absence of lactic acidemia. Nonetheless, the AT varies with cardiovascular fitness, correlates well with human performance in the field, and remains a useful clinical index.

The VAT occurs at greater than 40 % of the predicted VO_2max in normal individuals, but earlier in cardiovascular disease including PH [17, 43, 44]. The AT correlates inversely with resting pulmonary hemodynamics [17] in established PH.

Ventilatory Reserve

Minute ventilation (VE) normally rises during incremental exercise as a result of a linear increase in breathing frequency and a hyperbolic increase in tidal volume (VT) [45]. VT reaches a plateau at approximately 50 % of the resting vital capacity, above which the elastic work of breathing is prohibitive [46]. The ratio of VE at peak exercise (VEmax) to the maximal voluntary ventilation (MVV) at rest has been termed the breathing reserve index [47]. A breathing reserve index of 0.70 can be sustained for 15 min in normal individuals, but values above 0.75 are usually not attained even at peak exercise [48].

Ventilation in patients with Group 1 PH may be excessive [49], but because the maximum voluntary ventilation is usually near-normal, relatively normal breathing reserve at peak exercise is usually found [17]. The niCPET can rule out a pulmonary mechanical limit to exercise by comparing VEmax to MVV. This is especially important in Group 3 PH where there are both pulmonary vascular and mechanical abnormalities limiting exercise. When an abnormal VAT precedes a BRI of 0.70, pulmonary vascular disease likely limits the patient's activities of daily living. Conversely, when a BRI of 0.70 precedes the AT, pulmonary mechanics are thought to be rate limiting.

Ventilatory Efficiency

Normally, CO_2 elimination by the lungs becomes more efficient during exercise [50]. Anatomic dead space increases because of a tethering effect on conducting airways at high VT. Conversely, during upright exercise, alveolar dead space decreases because of augmented blood flow to the lung apices, giving the net effect of a slight increase in total (physiologic) dead space (VD). However, this effect is more than offset by the increased VT, which produces a decrease in upright VD/VT from 0.45 at rest to less than 0.29 at maximum exercise [50]. Normally, the VE/ VCO_2 falls as a result to <37 at the ventilatory threshold [17].

Ventilatory inefficiency is one of the hallmarks of PH during exercise [7, 17, 23–25, 28, 30, 31, 51] and can be identified by an increased slope of the linear phase of VE/VCO_2 or its absolute value at the ventilatory threshold. It has been suggested that the latter is preferable as the slope may be artificially flattened by hyperventilation at rest in anticipation of exercise.

A high VE/VCO_2 during the submaximum domain of incremental exercise is explained by the alveolar ventilation equation:

$$VE / VCO2 = (k) / (PaCO2(1 - VD / VT)\text{. [17]}$$

Hyperventilation during low-level exercise is common in PH and usually ascribed to a combination of stretch receptors in the RV and pulmonary outflow track, J receptor stimulation (in HF and interstitial lung disease) and hypoxemic stimulation of arterial chemoreceptors [52]. In addition, alveolar dead space fails to fall normally [17, 53, 54] because of blunted pulmonary vascular distention and recruitment, and, perhaps, pulmonary vasospasm [55].

Thus, the combined influence of two invasively measured variables, VD/VT and $PaCO_2$ may make the noninvasive VE/VCO2 a powerful marker of the abnormal pulmonary vasculature. Using a stepwise regression model using PaCO2 and VD/ VT at anaerobic threshold as independent variables suggested that variability in VE/ VCO2 at anaerobic threshold was accounted for equally by both. In HFrEF we have demonstrated equal contributions of VD/VT and hyperventilation to ventilatory efficiency [56].

Reybrouck et al. [54] found that the VE/VCO2 slope was steeper in patients with PH than the slope in patients with normal mPAP, and a significant correlation between the slope and mPAP and the VD/VT. In PH, VE/VCO2 is inversely related to peak cardiac output [55], resting [17], and exercise [57] mPAP's and overall exercise capacity [54, 58] A sudden rise may suggest dynamic opening of a PFO and right to left shunting during exercise [23].

Ventilatory inefficiency can predict adverse events [59] and is likely a better predictor of survival than VO_2max [22, 34, 60]. Recent work suggests [60] ventilatory equivalent for carbon dioxide at anaerobic threshold >55 identifies patients with an over sevenfold increased risk of death within 24 months and better predicted the clinical outcome compared to $VO_2max < 10.4$ ml/min/kg.

Ventilatory efficiency improves after therapy, including pulmonary vasodilators [27, 61] and lung transplantation [49] Interestingly VE/VCO_2 slope's change after treatment does not appear to influence survival [62].

Arterial O_2 Desaturation

In the normal human during incremental exercise, arterial O_2 saturation remains normal and the A-aDO_2 widens due to hyperventilation and a rise in the RER. In PH, arterial O_2 desaturation and/or exaggerated widening of the $P(A-a)O_2$ is due both to V/Q mismatching and a diffusion defect induced by a rapid red cell transit time through a poorly compliant and recruitable pulmonary circulation. Prevalence of arterial O2 desaturation with exercise increases with PH severity [28].

Occasionally, a sudden fall in arterial oxygen saturation heralds the opening of a patent foramen ovale and increased right to left shunting due to elevation of right atrial pressure [23].

Exercise arterial O_2 desaturation is not generally a feature of ambulatory HFpEF or HFrEF. Recent work suggests severe O_2 desaturation is a negative prognosticator for PH [63].

End Tidal PCO_2 ($PETCO_2$)

The $PETCO_2$ normally rises at the AT, reflecting increased VCO_2 delivered to the pulmonary capillary which is disproportionately "sampled" at lower end-expiratory lung volumes. The negative Pa-$ETCO_2$ gradient is dependent on normal exercise induced pulmonary vascular recruitment and distension.

As with ventilatory efficiency, pulmonary vascular remodeling or dysfunction impairs this response and alveolar dead space fails to fall normally, diluting the end tidal breath with room air [24, 64]. When $PETCO_2$ at AT is <30 mmHg and especially <20 mmHg, in a patient with exertional dyspnea of unknown cause, PH should be considered as likely.

It has been shown that the $PETCO_2$ [28] transition from rest to AT can distinguish between PH and left ventricular dysfunction; $PETCO_2$ tends to decrease in PAH, whereas the $PETCO_2$ tends to increase in LVD [20, 64].

Like ventilatory inefficiency, disease severity and survival are predicted by the pattern of change [22]. Oudiz et al. have shown higher $PETCO_2$ at AT after treating PH after sildenafil [65].

O_2 Uptake Efficiency Slope (OUES)

In 1996, Baba et al. proposed a hybrid measurement of oxygen transport and ventilation during exercise as a surrogate for VO_2max in the pediatric population in whom the latter was difficult to reliably achieve [66]. The OUES is an objective, reproducible measure of cardiopulmonary reserve that does not require a maximal exercise effort. It integrates cardiovascular, musculoskeletal and respiratory function into a single index that is largely influenced by pulmonary dead space ventilation and exercise-induced lactic acidosis.

The OUES is derived from the relation between oxygen uptake ($\dot{V}O2$ [ml/min]) and minute ventilation ($\dot{V}E$ [l/min]) during incremental exercise and is determined by:

$\dot{V}O2 = a \log \dot{V}E + b,\quad \text{where } a = \text{OUES}$ (Fig. 11.2).

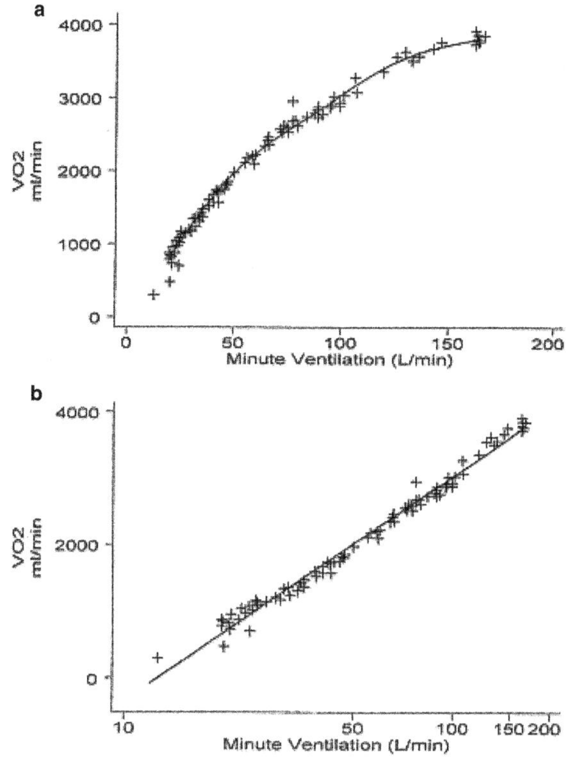

Fig. 11.2 O_2 uptake efficiency slope, derived from the semi-log plot (*panel* **b**) of the rectilinear plot (*panel* **a**) of VO_2 vs. VE during submaximum exercise [67]

Major factors that influence the OUES are: CO_2 output (derived from muscle aerobic metabolism as well as from the pH buffering function of bicarbonate), arterial pCO_2 set-point, and VD/VT.

A low OUES predicts poor survival in HF [68] and worse outcome in PH [69]. Ramos et al. performed an ROC curve analysis in PH (area under the curve = 0.688 [0.542–0.833], $p < 0.01$), indicating a best OUES cutoff for prognostication of 0.56 L/min/log.

Exercise Oscillatory Ventilation (EOV)

Cyclic fluctuations in minute ventilation during exercise, called exercise oscillatory ventilation (EOV), have been observed in 19–51 % of patients with HF [70–75]. Exercise oscillatory ventilation is a noninvasive parameter that is easily measurable (Fig. 11.3) during submaximum exercise.

We recently examined iCPET data for EOV in 56 patients with HFrEF (mean ± SEM age, 59 ± 2 years; left ventricular ejection fraction, 30 ± 1 %) and 19 age-matched control subjects were studied with incremental cardiopulmonary exercise

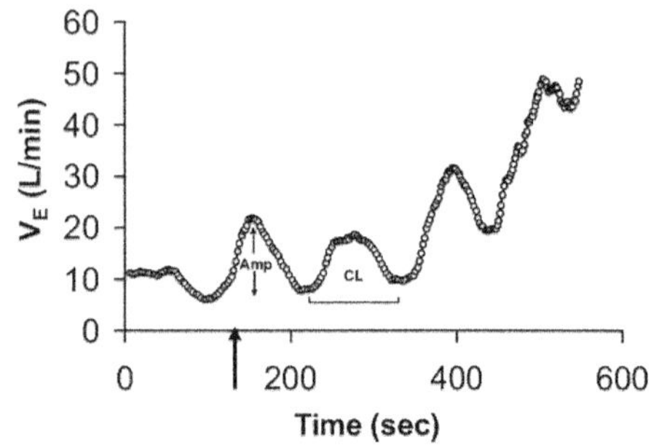

Fig. 11.3 Exercise oscillatory ventilation defined as ≥3 cyclic fluctuations of minute ventilation ($\dot{V}E$) during exercise with an amplitude >25 % of the mean trough-to-trough $\dot{V}E$ during that interval. *CL* cycle length; *Amp* amplitude [76]

testing. We detected EOV in 45 % of HF (HF+EOV) patients and in none of the control subjects. The HF+EOV group did not differ from the HF patients without EOV (HF−EOV) in age, sex, body mass index, left ventricular ejection fraction, or origin of HF. Univariate predictors of the presence of EOV in HF, among measurements performed during exercise, included higher right atrial pressure and pulmonary capillary wedge pressure and lower cardiac index (CI) but not $PACO_2$ or PAO_2. Multivariate logistic regression identified that low exercise CI is the strongest predictor of EOV (odds ratio, 1.39 for each 1.0-L/min/m^2 decrement in CI; 95 % confidence interval, 1.14–1.70; $P=0.001$). Among HF patients with EOV, exercise CI was inversely related to EOV cycle length ($R=-0.71$) and amplitude ($R=-0.60$; both $P<0.001$). In 11 HF+EOV subjects treated with 12 weeks of sildenafil, EOV cycle length and amplitude decreased proportionately to increases in CI. We conclude EOV is closely related to reduced CI, elevated filling pressures and impaired RV contractility (Fig. 11.4) during exercise and may be an important surrogate for exercise-induced hemodynamic impairment in HF patients.

Exercise oscillatory ventilation has emerged as a potent independent risk factor for adverse prognosis in HF [70, 72, 77]. To our knowledge this has not yet been determined for PAH and PH Groups 3–5.

Noninvasive CPET Diagnostic Algorithms for PH

When used together, patterns of CPET variable changes may increase sensitivity and specificity of exercise testing for the diagnosis of PH [78–81]. Our laboratory validated a classic noninvasive CPET diagnostic algorithm for PH in a population of unexplained dyspnea with direct central hemodynamic measurements [26]. We evaluated 130 consecutive, clinically indicated iCPET's whose phenotyping (see below) was performed to determine if PH were present at maximum exercise and limited exercise tolerance (pulmonary vascular limit (PVL) defined as a PVRmax >120 dyn s cm^{-5} and a maximum systemic oxygen delivery (DO_2max) <80 % of predicted, in the absence of limiting abnormal pulmonary mechanics or poor effort). We evaluated the accuracy of a published diagnostic algorithm [78] (Fig. 11.5) and sequentially altered branch-point threshold values to maximize accuracy in

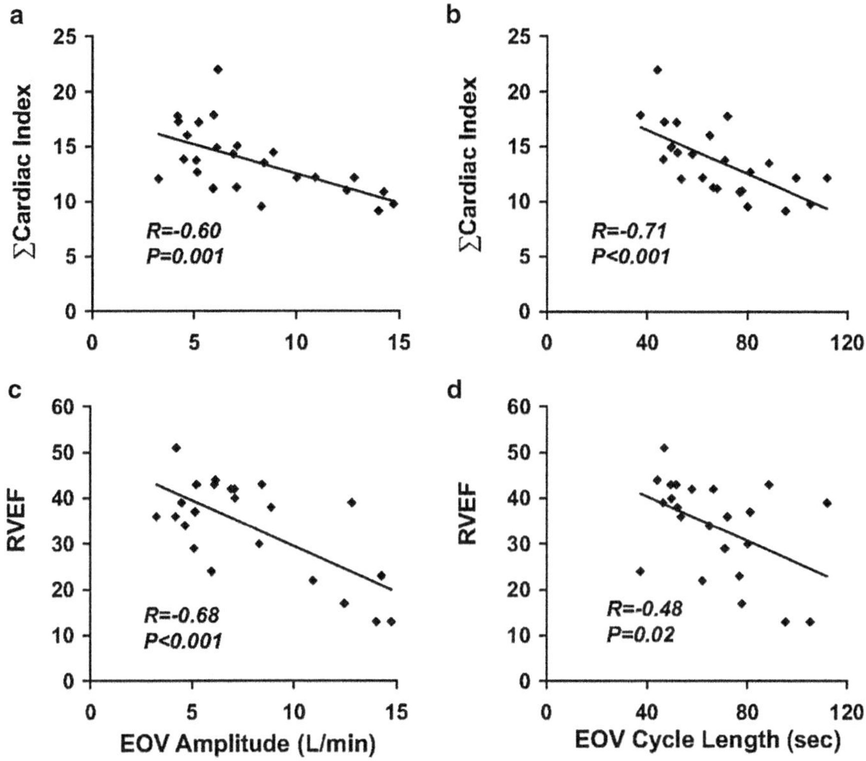

Fig. 11.4 Correlations between exercise oscillatory ventilation (EOV) parameters and cardiac performance; EOV amplitude is inversely related to cumulative cardiac index during exercise (Σcardiac index; **a**) and right ventricular ejection fraction (RVEF; **c**). In addition, EOV cycle length is inversely related to cumulative cardiac index during exercise (**b**) and RVEF (**d**)

diagnosing PVL. We based threshold values used at each branch point on the 95 % confidence intervals for healthy individuals during exercise [78]. Thus, for the diagnosis of PVL, branch-point values were adjusted in the following order: % predicted VO_2max, anaerobic threshold as % predicted VO_2max, breathing reserve maximum, and VE/VCO_2 and anaerobic threshold.

Figure 11.6 shows the changing sensitivity, specificity, and accuracy for PVL when a representative branch point (VE/VCO_2 at anaerobic threshold) was altered systematically. If consecutive branch-point values resulted in identical accuracy, we chose the median value.

In an identical fashion, we determined the utility of isolated peak exercise measurements of VD/V˙T and PA-aO_2 for PVL. We used upper limit of normal values for peak exercise VD/VT and PA-aO_2 of 0.28 and 35 mmHg, respectively [78].

The sensitivity of the isolated peak exercise VD/VT for PVL was 20 %, with specificity of 85 % and accuracy of 56 %. Similarly, the isolated peak exercise PA-aO_2 had sensitivity for PVL of 24 %, specificity of 92 %, and accuracy of 60 %.

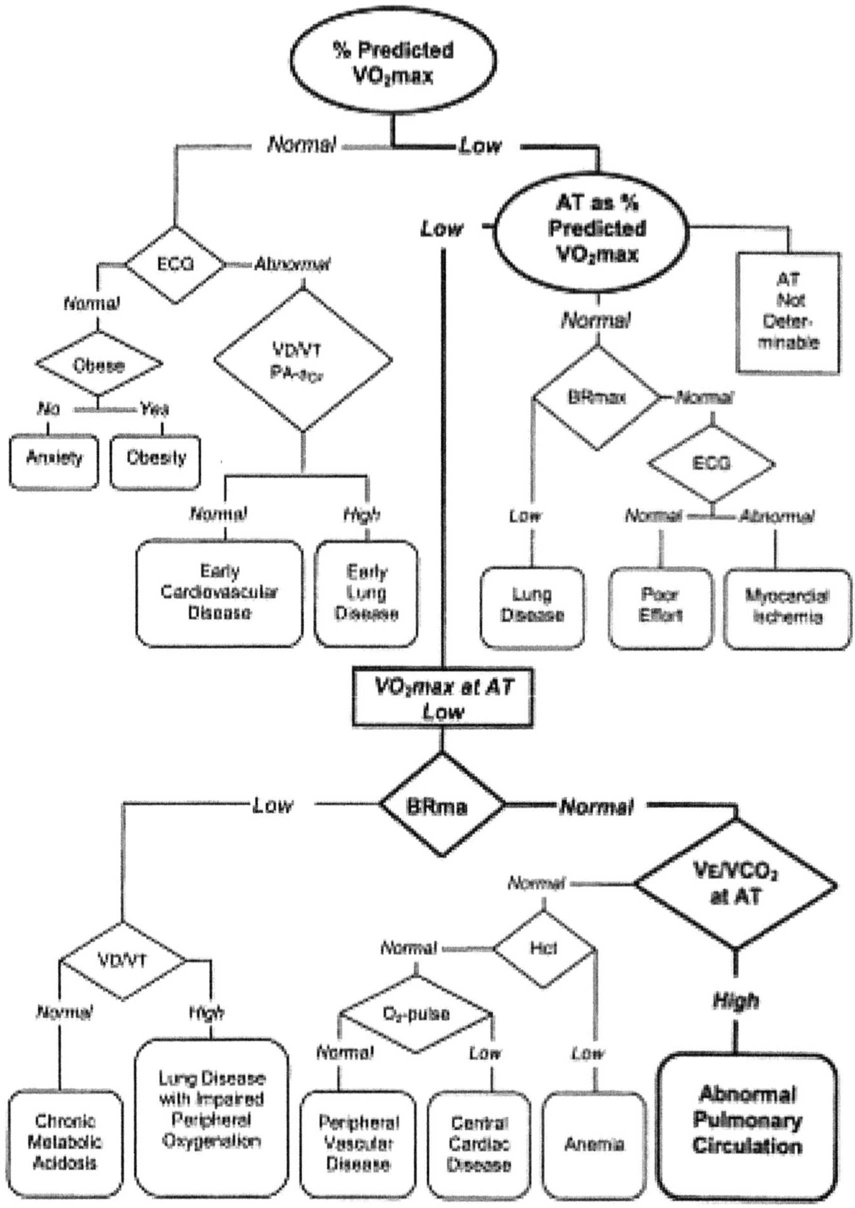

Fig. 11.5 A popular noninvasive CPET diagnostic algorithm with key branch points for PH in *bold*

The noninvasive algorithm's sensitivity for PVL was 79 %, specificity was 75 %, and accuracy was 76 % ($n=93$). Systematic alteration of branch-point values improved the algorithm's specificity and accuracy to 88 % and 85 %, respectively. The greatest improvement in sensitivity for detecting pulmonary vascular limit

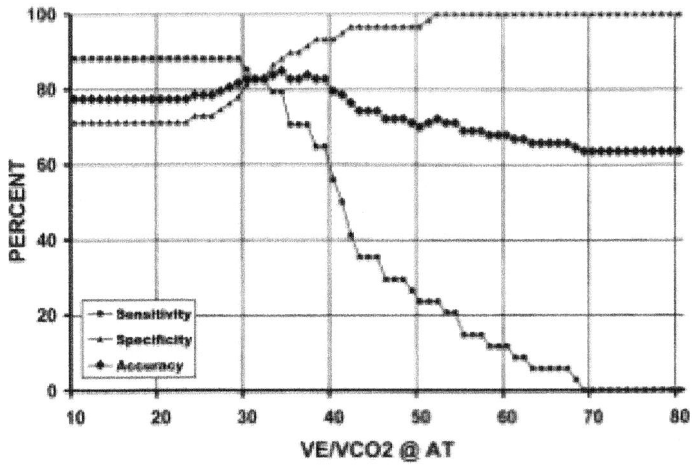

Fig. 11.6 Improvement of accuracy of a noninvasive CPET diagnostic algorithm by adjusting a key branch point (VE/VCO_2) cutoff value

resulted from a decrease in the threshold value for VE/VCO_2 at anaerobic threshold; we applied a stepwise linear regression model to this branch point. When $PaCO_2$ and VD/VT at anaerobic threshold were denoted as independent variables, the model assigned equal weight to both (standard coefficients = 0.59 and 0.57, respectively, $p < 0.0001$).

A recent study by [20] confirms the utility of a niCPEt algorithm for early detection of pulmonary vascular disease in an at risk population. The authors further suggest that one can distinguish right from left sided disease by the addition of $PETCO_2$ changes from rest to AT.

A suggested niCPET for the diagnosis of PH is suggested (Fig. 11.7).

In summary, niCPET is a useful diagnostic modality that can suggest early or mild PH in at-risk patients or those with unexplained exertional intolerance. Confirmation of PH is almost always necessary through right heart catheterization. The remainder of this chapter focuses on combining CPET with RHC hemodynamic measurements.

Invasive CPET

Measurement of central hemodynamics during exercise has been performed for many years [82–84], but only more recently combined with CPET [85]. In our hands, an iCPET refers to niCPET with the addition of pulmonary and radial artery catheters for pressure measurements and blood sampling.

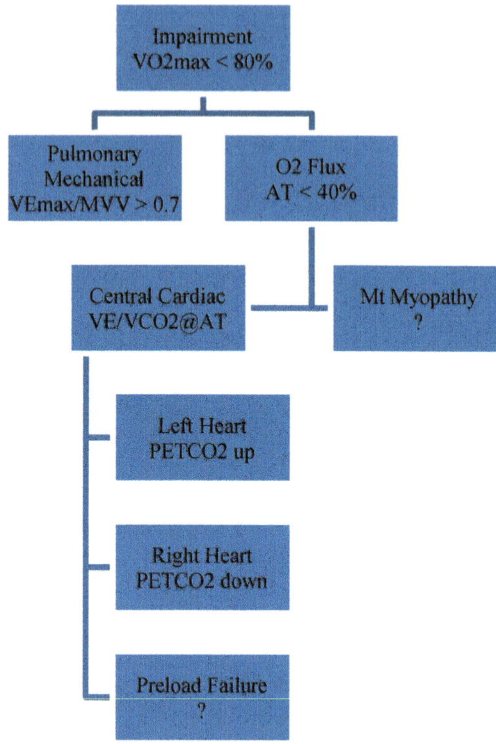

Fig. 11.7 A suggested noninvasive CPET diagnostic algorithm. PH may be suggested by a decreased VO_2max, early AT, ventilatory efficiency and decreased $PETCO_2$'s

Methods

A detailed description of methods utilized in the BWH Advanced Cardiopulmonary Exercise Testing Facility has recently been published [86].

iCPET (Fig. 11.8) is best performed using a cycle ergometer to minimize upper body motion and a continuous ramp protocol to ensure a linear increment in work rate and resulting VO_2. Upright positioning most closely mimics normal physical activity but either upright or supine exercise can be utilized to derive Ppa–flow relationships [87]. Radial arterial line placement allows precise systemic blood pressure measurement, as well as serial arterial blood gases, to assess important indicators of pulmonary vascular function, including dead space volume/tidal volume, alveolar–arterial gradient and direct Fick cardiac outputs when coupled with assessment of oxygen uptake and mixed venous saturation.

We use an ultrasound-guided internal jugular approach to PAC placement so cycling exercise is unimpeded. The optimal zero reference point for central pressures (approximating the right atrium) has recently been reviewed for supine RHC [88]. It has been suggested that in the upright position mid right atrial ZRP is well approximated by the fourth intercostal space at the junction with the sternum and is used by our laboratory. Pulmonary capillary wedge pressure (PCWP) should be verified

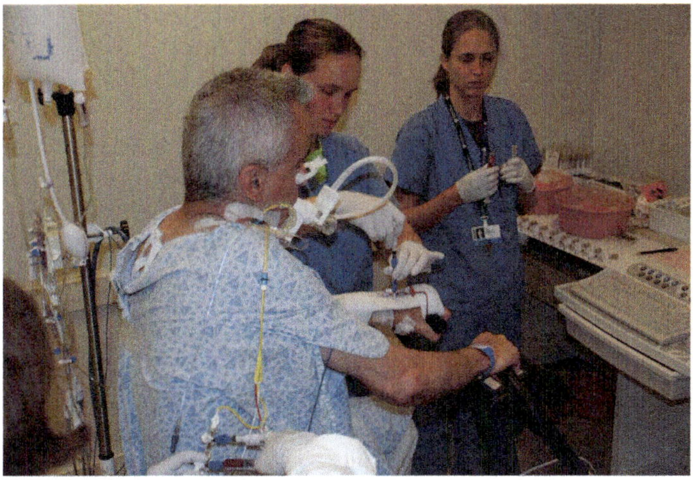

Fig. 11.8 iCPET setup at BWH. Non invasive CPET with breath-by breath measurement of pulmonary gas exchange and ventilation is combined with simultaneous radial and pulmonary arterial blood gas and pH sampling every minute at rest and incremental maximum exercise

based on characteristic waveforms, systemic oxygen saturation, and/or appearance on fluoroscopy. The critical extravascular closure pressure imposed by the lung parenchyma that contains the pulmonary vasculature is typically below that of the PCWP during exercise [89], and therefore PCWP can be used as the downstream pressure in order to determine transpulmonary pressure gradients (TPG = mPAP-PCWP) and pulmonary vascular resistance (PVR = TPG/CO). Care should be taken to maintain consistent upright posture relative to the leveled transducers throughout exercise. Serial measurements of mPAP, PCWP, and CO should be performed at regular intervals (i.e., every minute) during incremental exercise to characterize pressure–flow relationships.

Pleural pressure swings and their influence on pulmonary artery input and outflow pressures and beat-to-beat stroke volume deserve special discussion. For instance, the exaggerated end expiratory pressures seen in the obese patient and in COPD do likely contribute dynamically increased right heart afterload by compression of alveolar vessels, which may in turn contribute to the patient's exertional intolerance. If, however, one assumes iCPET's clinical role is in the detection of early pulmonary vasculopathy or HFpEF, one might wish to eliminate the confounding effects of respiratory pressure swings. The classic approach to the problem was to ignore it and take a mean PAP or PCWP through the respiratory cycle. In the 1980s, end-expiratory measures came into vogue, largely in the mechanically ventilated patient, when it was assumed zero airway flow at end expiration would result in the least contamination of PAC derived pressures and this has recently been recommended for supine, resting RHC [90] and utilized during exercise [91, 92].

When measuring hemodynamics during exercise in COPD, subtracting esophageal pressure (Pes), in order to acquire the true intra-cavitary and thereby deriving actual transmural pressure which is critical in the detection of pulmonary vascular disease, is preferable [93]. The usefulness of the RAP waveform to estimate the pressure surrounding the heart was shown by Tyberg et al. [94]. This method assumes that pressure in the very compliant right atrium is predominantly dependent on pressure surrounding the heart (pericardial pressure, or in our case ITP), rather than by right atrial volume. We showed that this method was useful during exercise in COPD-patients, as long as the lowest point of the RAP during expiration was used. This is explained by the fact that during the right atrial contraction dissociation between RAP and ITP is created. Therefore, only the pressure of an empty and relaxing right atrium is useful to estimate ITP. We found a small bias with mPAPtm and PCWPtm when RAPnadir was used to correct expiratory mPAP and PCWP, with a very reasonable 95 % CI. This method may not be useful in patients with more pronounced right heart failure, as this causes RAP to rise, even during relaxation.

We have recently examined the worst case scenario: moderate to severe COPD referred for evaluation of suspected PH with exercise [95]. Central hemodynamics were measured simultaneously with esophageal pressure during exercise in 30 COPD patients. mPAP and PCWP were assessed in four different manners:

1. At end-expiration.
2. Averaged over the respiratory cycle.
3. Corrected from the right atrial pressure (RAP) nadir.
4. Corrected from the RAP respiratory swing and compared with the "gold standard" transmural mPAP and PCWP.

An example of a severe COPD patient's PAP's during exercise with and without correction for ITP is shown in Fig. 11.9. Maximum exercise cardiac output was 10.9 ± 3.8 L/min. The large swings in Peso were transduced into all central pressure; on average responsible for a difference between inspiratory values and expiratory values of about 20 mmHg. The expiratory Peso at maximal exercise ranged from +3 to + 25 mmHg. The mPAP/Q slope decreased from 6.4 ± 3.7–4.4 ± 3.2 mmHg/L

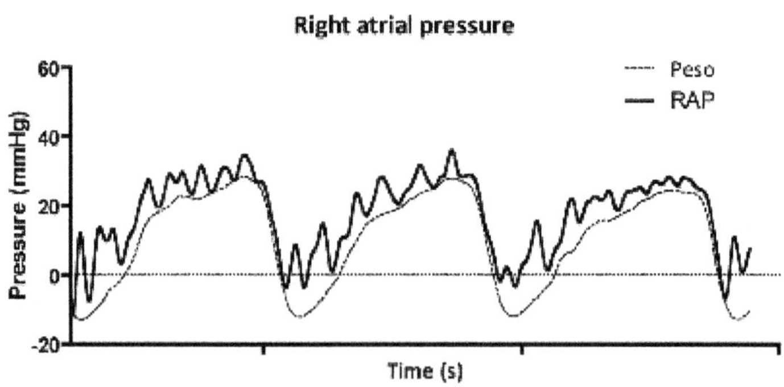

Fig. 11.9 Simultaneous measurement of RAP and esophageal pressure (Peso) at maximal exercise in the same patient as shown in Fig. 11.1. RAPnadir is the lowest point in RAP during expiration, which represents RAP during relaxation. Note that RAP falls towards Peso during relaxation. RAPswing was determined as the difference between inspiratory RAP and expiratory RAP [95]

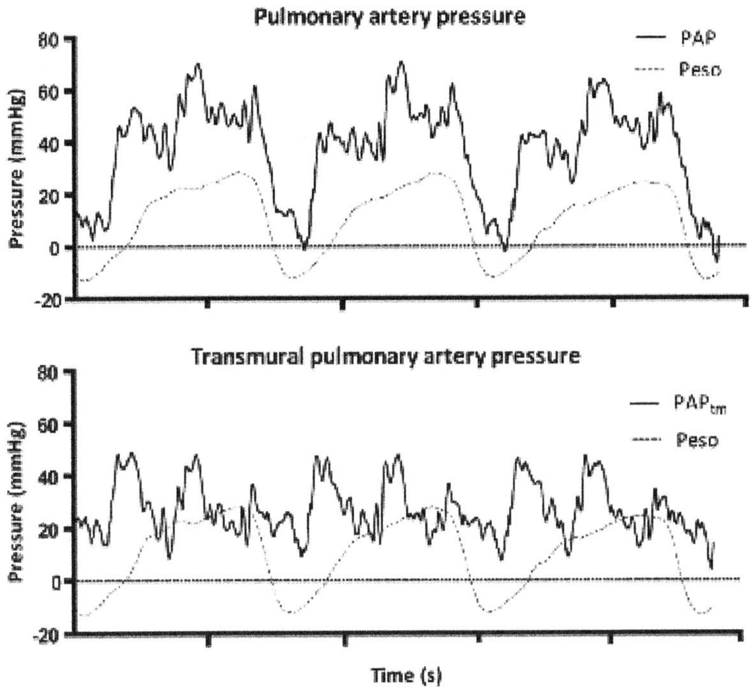

Fig. 11.10 Example of pulmonary artery pressure before (PAP) and after (PAPtm) continuous correction for esophageal pressure (Peso) at maximal exercise in a patient with severe COPD (FEV1: 30 % of predicted) [95]

($p<0.001$) after correction for ITP. Seven patients had a mPAP/Q slope >3 mmHg before correction which decreased to <3 mmHg after correction for the ITP. Twenty-two patients had a PCWP recording. Nineteen patients of the 22 had a PCWP >20 mmHg with exercise without correction for ITP. Seven patients a had PCPWtm>20; in three of them PCPWtm was between 20 and 25 mmHg.

"Gold standard" mPAPtm and PCWPtm at maximum exercise were 47 ± 15 and 17 ± 8 mmHg respectively (Fig. 11.10). The average mPAP values at maximal exercise of the four methods were; $mPAP_{end\text{-}exp}$: 59 ± 14, $mPAP_{averaged}$: 50 ± 14, $mPAP_{rap\text{-}nadir}$: 44 ± 15, and $mPAP_{rap\_swing}$: 38 ± 15 mmHg. The average PCWP values at maximum exercise of the four methods were; $PCWP_{end\text{-}exp}$: 27 ± 9, $PCWP_{averaged}$: 20 ± 8, $PCWP_{rap\text{-}nadir}$: 15 ± 7, and $PCWP_{swing}$: 11 ± 8 mmHg.

Bland-Altman analyses showed the best agreement of mPAP (Fig. 11.11) averaged over the respiratory cycle (bias: 2.5 mmHg, limits-of-agreement (−6.0 to 11.8) and when corrected with the nadir of RAP (bias: −3.6 mmHg, limits: −11.2 to 3.9). Measuring mPAP at end-expiration (bias: 10.3 mmHg, limits: 0.5–20.3) and mPAP corrected with the RAP-swing (bias: −9.3 mmHg, limits: −19.8 to 2.1) resulted in lower levels of agreement (Fig. 11.12). Bland-Altman plots of the four methods of PCWP measurements during exercise were similar and are shown in Fig. 11.13; both are summarized in Table 11.2.

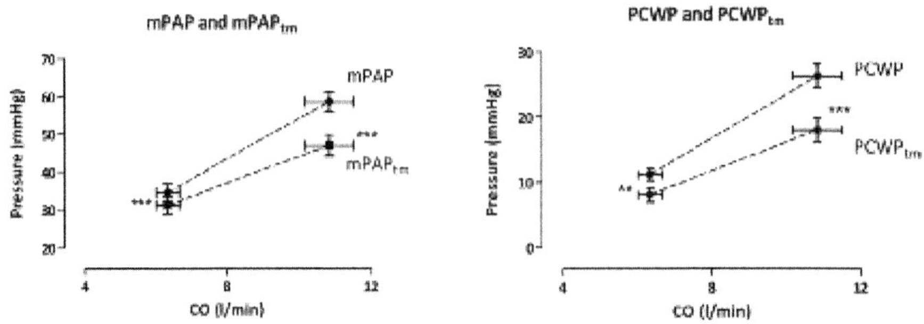

Fig. 11.11 Average pressure flow relations before and after correction for esophageal pressure. *mPAP* mean pulmonary artery pressure, *mPAPtm* transmural mPAP (calculated as mPAP-Peso), *PCWP* pulmonary capillary wedge pressure, *PCWPtm* transmural PCWP (calculated as PCWP-Peso). $^{**}p<0.01$, $^{***}p>0.001$ [95]

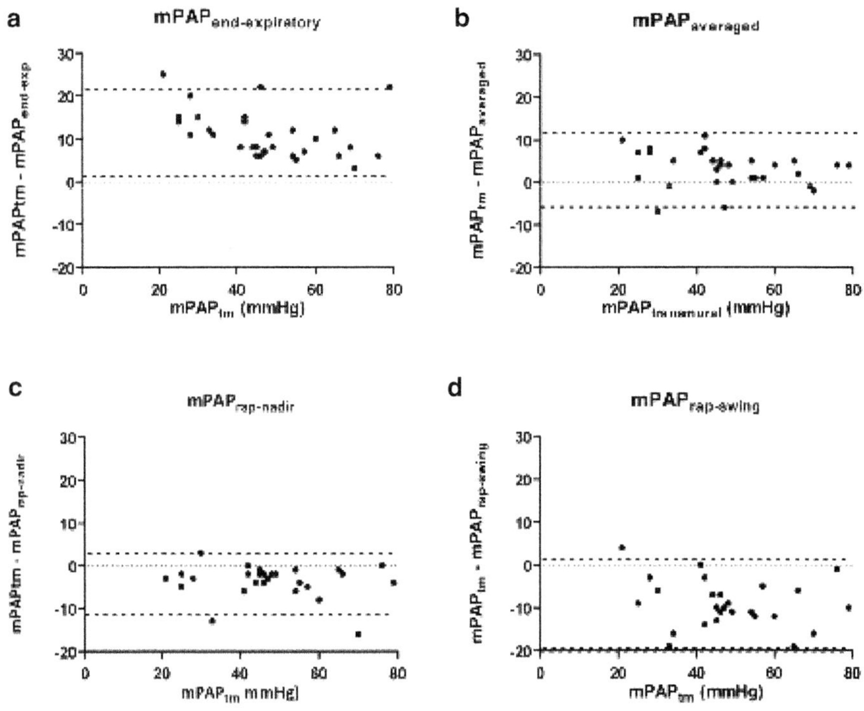

Fig. 11.12 Bland-Altman analyses of the difference between pulmonary artery pressure (mPAP) and transmural mean pulmonary artery pressure (mPAPtm) plotted vs. the mPAPtm. (**a**) mPAP measured at end expiration, (**b**) mPAP averaged over the respiratory cycle (**c**) mPAP corrected with the lowest point of RAP during expiration (RAP-nadir) and (**d**) mPAP corrected with the swing in RAP (RAP-swing). *Dotted lines* represent the 95 % coincidence intervals [95]

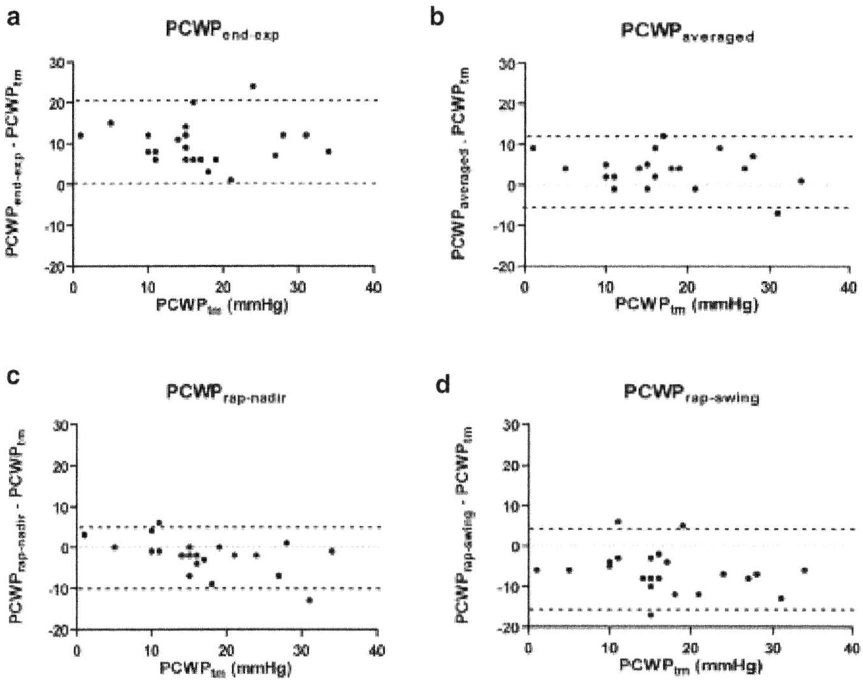

Fig. 11.13 Bland-Altman analyses of the difference between pulmonary capillary wedge pressure (PCWP) and transmural pulmonary capillary wedge pressure (PCWPtm) plotted vs. the PCWPtm. (**a**) PCWP measured at end expiration, (**b**) PCWP averaged over the respiratory cycle (**c**) PCWP corrected with the lowest point of RAP during expiration (RAP-nadir) and (**d**) PCWP corrected with the swing in RAP (RAP-swing). *Dotted lines* represent the 95 % coincidence intervals [95]

Table 11.2 Effect of ITP swings on PCWP, mPAP, and RAP {Boerrigter [95] #1813}

95 % limits of agreement (mmHg)					
	Number	r^2	Bias ± SD (mmHg)	From	To
$mPAP_{end\ expiratory}$	30	0.86	10.3 ± 5.9	0.5	20.3
$mPAP_{averaged}$	30	0.92	2.5 ± 4.4	−6.0	11.8
$mPAP_{rap\_nadir}$	30	0.94	−3.6 ± 3.8	−11.2	3.9
$mPAP_{rap\_swing}$	30	0.86	−9.3 ± 5.9	−19.8	2.1
$PCWP_{end\ expiratory}$	22	0.69	9.9 ± 5.3	−0.5	20.3
PCWPAVERAGED	22	0.75	3.2 ± 4.4	−5.3	11.8
$PCWP_{rap\_nadir}$	22	0.73	−2.0 ± 42	−2.0	4.2
$PCWP_{rap\_swing}$	22	0.64	−6.3 ± 5.3	−16.6	4.0

Our findings support the use of mPAP and PCWP averaged over 2–3 respiratory cycles in order to acquire more accurate assessment of the transmural values of mPAP and PCWP during exercise in COPD-patients. The patients in the present study showed a wide range of expiratory Peso at exercise, reaching to as high as

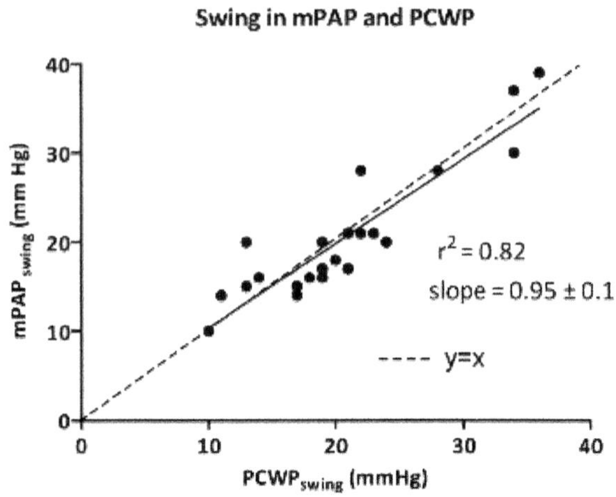

Fig. 11.14 Illustrates the relation between mPAPswing and PWCPswing. The swing in mPAP and PCWP did not differ (mean difference 0.9 mmHg, $p = 0.35$). There was a strict relation between RAPswing and PCWPswing ($r^2 = 0.9$, $p < 0.001$) with a slope 1.02 and no significant difference between RAPswing and PCWPswing (mean difference 0.7 mmHg, $p = 0.28$) [95]

25 mmHg, which is consistent with previous studies on pulmonary mechanics. In these studies, as well as the present study, the positive excursion of Peso during expiration is at least as large as the negative excursion during inspiration. It is therefore not surprising that mPAP averaged over the respiratory cycle is a more realistic measure of intravascular pressure. Albeit more accurate than $mPAP_{end\text{-}exp}$, $mPAP_{averaged}$ was still a slight overestimation, which can be explained by the increased expiratory time.

Lastly, we showed that the swings in mPAP, PCWP and RAP were similar ($r^2 = 0.82$, slope: 0.95 ± 0.1) (Fig. 11.14). This has several convenient implications. The consequence of an identical effect of ITP swing on mPAP and PCWP is that the difference between the two, the transpulmonary pressure gradient is unaffected by the swing in ITP. This only holds when both the mPAP and PCWP being recorded at the same time point in the respiratory cycle. So, although individually, mPAP and PCWP are overestimations of intravascular pressure, the $mPAP_{end\text{-}expand}$ $PCWP_{end\text{-}exp}$ combined lead to the correct transpulmonary pressure gradient or PVR (transpulmonary gradient/CO). It underscores the importance of PVR as part of the suggested definition of exercise induced pulmonary arterial hypertension [7], as it prevents patients being diagnosed simply because of an increased ITP.

The similar effect of ITP swings in RAP and PCWP also has a potential implication in evaluating exercise hemodynamics. The increase in PCWP calculated as a ratio to the increase in RAP (ΔPCWP/ΔRAP), as previously suggested [25, 96], is unaffected by ITP swings. This ratio might therefore be of potential help in the difficult situation of a high PCWP with exercise in the presence of ITP- swings. This would be especially helpful in diagnosing exercise-induced HFpEF [97].

We conclude central hemodynamics measured at end-expiration leads to an overestimation of intravascular pressures in exercising COPD-patients. More reliable data are generated by averaging pressures over the respiratory cycle or using the RAP waveform to correct for intrathoracic pressure. Assessment of the pulmonary gradient is unaffected by respiratory swings. The patients in the study of Boerrigter et al. had at least moderate airflow limitation, likely a worst-case scenario for the

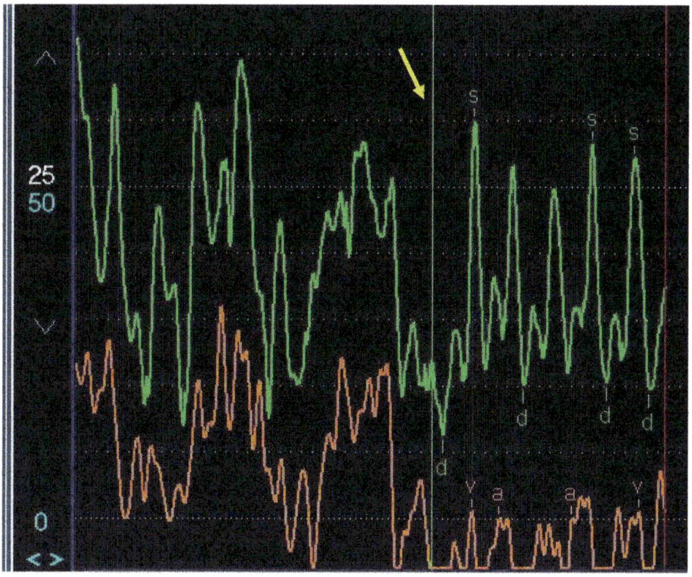

Fig. 11.15 Effects of relaxed exhalation to FRC on PAP's during moderate exercise

influence of ITP on central pressure measurements. We can only speculated to what extent our findings can be extrapolated to patients with less severe airflow limitation such as PH. Pulmonary vascular pressure therefore should be averaged over 2–3 respiratory cycles not only in COPD [7, 8, 28] but also healthy subjects [98, 99]. Whether an averaged mPAP is a more accurate estimate of the intravascular pressure at maximal exercise in PH without parenchymal lung disease remains unknown and depends on the amplitude and the length of the inspiratory and expiratory excursions in ITP.

We have recently adopted a slow-breathing maneuver to avoid respirophasic change in pulmonary vascular pressures. Fig. 11.15 shows respirophasic change of PAP during moderate exercise; at the arrow, the patient is asked to "relax and miss a breath or two". Over 90 % of our patients coached in this manner, with a brief practice while at rest on cycle ergometer, can successfully perform the maneuver. The same maneuver results in a stable PCWP measurement (Fig. 11.16).

iCPET Variables

In a manner similar to niCPET, certain variables (Table 11.3) obtained by niCPET plus radial or arterial catheter pressure and blood gas measurements help confirm the presence of PH and differentiate PH with a TPG vs Group 2 without (pulmonary arterial vs. venous hypertension).

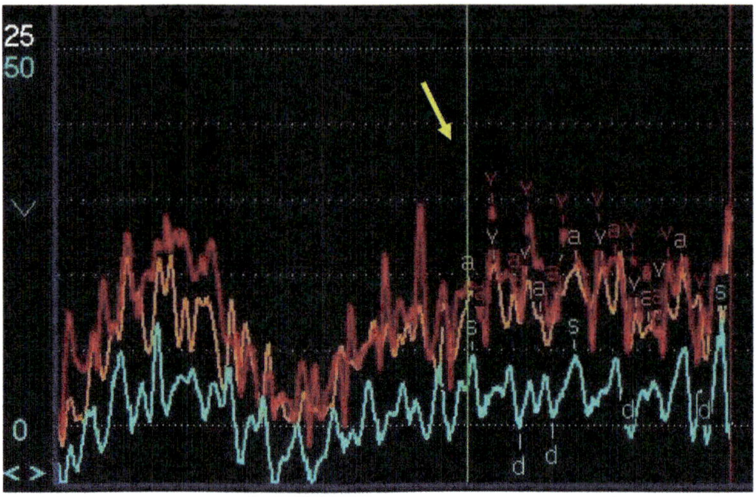

Fig. 11.16 Effects of relaxed exhalation to indicate that the red tracing is the PCWP

Table 11.3 iCPET characteristics of PH

Decreased VO_2max
Decreased AT
Qt < 80 % predicted
Blunted VD/VT fall >0.30
Arterial O_2 desaturation or widened P(A-a) O_2 > 30 mmHg
PAP > 30 mmHg
PVR > 120 dyn s cm^{-5}
PCWP/RAP slope < 1.4
mPAP vs. Qt slope > 3.0

Cardiac Output (Qt)

The Fick Principle and conservation of mass dictate that in the steady-state, $VO_2 = Qt \times (CaO_2 - CvO_2)$ where Qt = cardiac output and $(CaO_2 - CvO_2)$ is the difference in O_2 content (ml/L) between arterial and mixed venous blood. Thus during iCPET continuous breath-by breath measurement of VO_2 and simultaneous blood gas sampling from the distal PA port and radial artery catheter every minute allow the calculation of a Direct Fick cardiac output. Dividing predicted absolute VO_2max (ml/min) for a given patient by an expected peak $(Ca - vO_2(ml/L)) = [Hb] \times 10$ yields an estimated Qtmax predicted.

Cardiac output generally limits VO_2max in healthy adults. Maximal cardiac output, which facilitates transport of oxygen from the alveolus to skeletal muscle, determines the maximal oxygen uptake and aerobic capacity to a large degree. Maintenance of CaO_2 and depression of CvO_2 during exercise are also circulatory functions, requiring exquisite matching of blood flow to ventilation and tissue metabolism, respectively. Cardiac output normally increases by approximately 5 mL/min for every 1 mL/min increase in VO_2 [100]. This slope is not altered by training, but maximum cardiac output improves with conditioning to four to five times resting values (up to levels of approximately 25 L/min in a young healthy individual). Maximum cardiac outputs above 40 L/min have been reported in elite athletes, and elite athletes may exhaust their breathing reserve before attaining maximal cardiac output [101].

Stroke volume (SV) increases in a hyperbolic fashion vs. VO_2, and maximum values can be augmented by up to 50 % with training [100, 102, 103]. The rise in SV during exercise is mediated in part by increased contractility, reflected by a 0.10 increase in left ventricular ejection fraction (LVEF) from rest to peak exercise [104]. Left ventricular end-diastolic volume (LVEDV) also increases by 20–40 %, augmenting SV by the Frank-Starling mechanism [105]. LV filling is enhanced during exercise by capacitance venoconstriction, greater negative intrathoracic pressures, and the pumping action of exercising limbs [106]. In a heart with normal lusitropic properties, LV end-diastolic pressure increases to approximately 20 mmHg at maximum exercise [87]. In PH, variable contributions of increased right heart afterload and decreased contractility blunt Qtmax and, in turn, VO_2max [7].

Pulmonary Artery Pressure

Pulmonary arterial pressure responses to exercise were first characterized over 60 years ago [82]. Pulmonary hypertension was previously defined in United States and European guidelines as a mean PAP (mPAP) >25 mmHg at rest or >30 mmHg during exercise [107, 108]. In 2008, the Working Group on Diagnosis and Assessment of Pulmonary Arterial Hypertension from the Fourth World Symposium on PH (Dana Point, CA) concluded that mPAP >30 mmHg should be abandoned as a diagnostic criteria for PH whose decision has remained controversial [8, 9, 109, 110]. This decision was based on the age-dependent nature of exercise mPAP and limited data on normal subjects derived from heterogeneous levels, types, and postures during exercise testing [111]. The key paper was a meta-analysis of 47 studies describing 72 populations of healthy volunteers who underwent RHC with invasive measurement of mPAP at rest and during exercise [112]. Data were stratified by gender, age, type of exercise (i.e., cycle ergometry, treadmill exercise), body position (upright vs supine), and exercise levels (slight, submaximal, and maximal). For all subjects at maximal exercise, the ULN was 37 (supine) and 35 mmHg (upright). However, during supine exercise Ppa was significantly higher in subjects aged >50 years (29.4 + 8.4 mmHg) compared to those aged 30–50 years (20.0 + 4.7 mmHg) and 30 years (18.2 + 5.1 mmHg). The upper limit of normal for mPAP in subjects aged <50 years was 29.0 mmHg vs. 46.2 mmHg in subjects aged >50 years. Of note this analysis included TM exercise which is associated with mPAP 8–13 % higher than cycle ergometry and did not report how respiratory pressure swings were controlled for. Moreover, the PCWP and upper limit of PVR were not analyzed.

Pulmonary Vascular Resistance

In the normal human increases in cardiac output exceed the increase in TPG and PVR falls. The PVR fall during exercise is a consequence of both passive distention of a compliant circulation and active vasodilation mediated in part by NO [113]. Pulmonary capillary wedge pressure increases about 1.4 mmHg for every 1.0 mmHg increase in right atrial pressure, suggesting interdependence of right and left ventricular filling [7, 96].

The upper limit for PVRmax in healthy humans remains poorly defined. Reeves et al. [87] calculated that in young, healthy subjects, the upper limit of a normal PVRmax is 56 dyn s cm^{-5} (O.7 Wood units). Granath et al. [98] studied 27 healthy, older men (aged 71+6 years) and found an upper 95 % confidence interval for PVRmax of 120 dyn s cm^{-5} (1.5 Wood units). Kovacs et al. recently described the changes in PVR in healthy individuals primarily during supine exercise. The data were stratified by sex, age, type of exercise (i.e., cycle ergometry and treadmill exercise), body position (upright vs. supine), and exercise level (slight, submaximum and maximum). The authors concluded that a decline in PVR is seen during the exercise response in healthy normal subjects. A limitation of the study was the paucity of individuals aged >50 years; subjects aged 51–69 years were limited to only 13 and 4 patients in supine and upright positions, respectively. Of these, PVR was available for only 8 (47 %) subjects. Kovacs focused on changes of PVR from rest to exercise, but did not emphasize absolute exercise values. Of note for those subjects ages 51–70 who performed two levels of (supine) exercise, $mPAP_{ex}$ was 28.0 ± 7.6 mmHg and PVRex 57 + 27 dyn s cm^{-5}. If one calculates an ULN for both $mPAP_{ex}$ is 43.4 mmHg but PVRex is only 111 dyn s cm^{-5}. The latter is in accord with the ULN for PVRmax described by Granath et al. [98]. We suggest a dual definition of exercise PH include both an ULN of $mPAP_{max}$ and an ULN for PVRmax. Until further studies are done in the aged population, 120 dyn s cm^{-5} represents a reasonable ULN for PVRmax.

Pressure–Flow Relationships

It has recently been suggested that patterns of change of mPAP vs. cardiac output (ΔmPAP/ΔQt) during exercise may identify a pulmonary vasculopathy without maximally stressing the patient. Reeves et al. [87] performed exercise measurements in 63 healthy young adults at rest and at least two levels of exercise and determined average ΔmPAP/ΔQt <1 mmHg/min/L. Kovacs et al. {Kovacs, 2012 #1942} reported a normal ΔmPAP/ΔQt <1.06 mmHg/min/L. Our 16 normals showed a ΔPpa/ΔQt of 1.4 [7]. ΔmPAP/ΔQt increases as a function of age with an ULN of about 3.0 [9].

A steep ΔmPAP/ΔQt relation is seen in Groups 1 and 2 PH. Fig. 11.17 shows ΔmPAP/ΔQt in scleroderma, PAH compared to the normal.

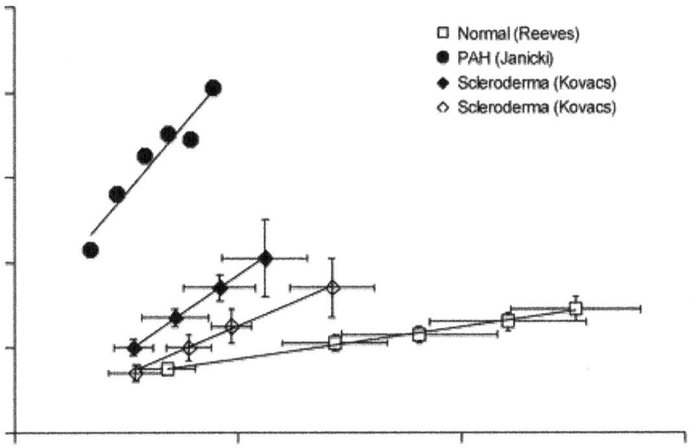

Fig. 11.17 Normal subjects (*open square*), patients with scleroderma with resting mPAP in the lower normal range (*open diamond*) and upper normal range (*filled diamond*), and patients with resting PAH (*filled circle*) demonstrate approximately linear pressure–flow responses during exercise

It can be concluded that the compliant pulmonary vasculature can accommodate large increases in blood flow during exercise with a proportionate modest increment in mPAP and a fall in PVR. When assessing mPAP, it is critical to account for Qt augmentation; therefore, determination of ΔmPAP/ΔQt or PVR is preferable to mPAP alone.

iCPET Diagnostic Algorithms

Once a central cardiac limit is established based on a low VO_2max, early AT, and a depressed Qtmax, left heart disease can be differentiated from the right using PAC-derived hemodynamics. This allows a direct Fick cardiac output ($VO_2 = Qt \times (CaO_2 - CvO_2)$) and one can determine whether VO_2max is decreased because of a blunted peak cardiac output (a true cardiac limit) or failure to systemically extract O_2 (e.g., a Mt myopathy). iCPET can be used as an initial test where PH is strongly suspected, when resting RHC numbers are borderline or when the noninvasive test is either suggestive of PH or unrevealing in a symptomatic patient. It is useful to differentiate a pulmonary mechanical from a pulmonary vascular limit in a patient with suspected Group 3 PH [64].

Patients with exercise-induced PAH, which is discussed further below, have normal cardiopulmonary hemodynamics at rest, but on iCPET demonstrate increased mean pulmonary artery pressure >30 mmHg and pulmonary vascular resistance >80–120 dyn s cm^5 [7, 96, 98]. In patients with normal biventricular function, an increased mean PCWP >20 mmHg [96] at peak exercise in the absence

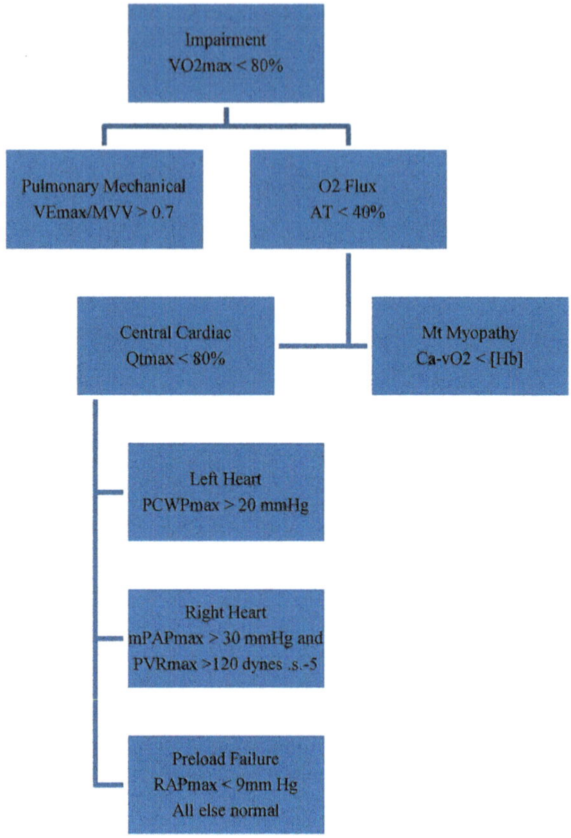

Fig. 11.18 iCPET diagnostic algorithm

of elevations to pulmonary vascular resistance suggests exercise-induced HFpEF. Exertional intolerance may be associated with preload-dependent limitations to stroke volume and cardiac output [114]. In this patient population, failure to augment right atrial pressure on exercise is observed despite abnormally decreased cardiac output. Finally, impaired systemic O_2 extraction ($Ca\text{-}vO_2 < [Hb]$) indicates left to right shunting or a Mt myopathy [115].

An iCPET diagnostic algorithm is suggested Fig. 11.18. Using this approach we recently reviewed the iCPET diagnoses made at one institution over a 1-year period (Fig. 11.19).

Exercise Induced Pulmonary Arterial Hypertension (eiPAH)

Our group has studied a subset of patients with unexplained exertional intolerance, and depressed VO_2max whose sole explanation is an abnormal rise in mPAP and blunted fall of PVR during incremental exercise. An example is shown in Fig. 11.20.

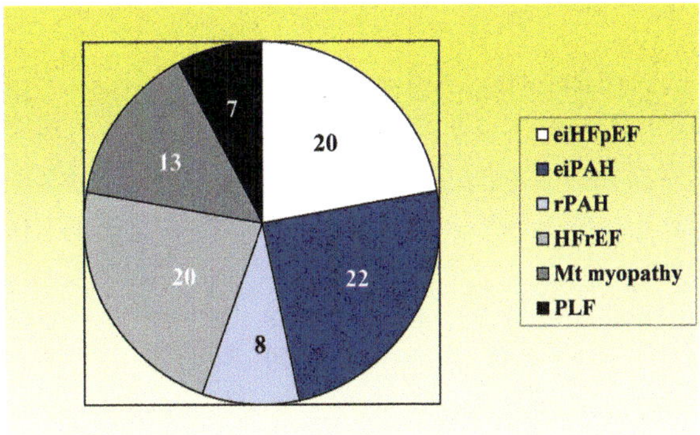

Fig. 11.19 iCPET diagnoses over a 1-year period at one institution (%)

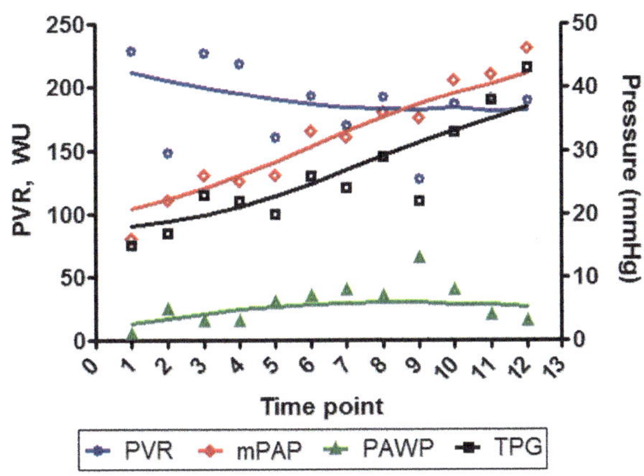

Fig. 11.20 Central hemodynamics in representative symptomatic eiPH patient

We systematically reviewed results of 406 sequential patients undergoing iCPET to evaluate dyspnea "eiPAH" was defined as resting mPAP <25 mmHg coupled with exercise mPAP >30 mmHg, and PVR >80 dyn s cm^{-5} and PCWP <20 mmHg [7]. Patients with eiPAH (n=78) were compared to patients with normal exercise capacity and hemodynamics (n=16) and patients with resting PAH (mPAP >25 mmHg, PCWP <15 mmHg, n=15). We found VO_2max % predicted was lowest in resting PAH (55.8±20.3 %), intermediate in eiPAH (66.5±16.3 %), and highest in normals (91.7±13.7 %), whereas peak mPAP (48±11 vs. 37±6 vs. 27+4 mmHg) and PVR (294±158 vs. 161±60 vs. 62±20 dyn s cm^{-5}, respectively; all P<0.05) followed an opposite pattern [7].

Within the eiPAH group, mPAP response to exercise followed one of two patterns. eiPAH patients with "takeoff" physiology demonstrate significantly higher VO_2max and Qtmax than "plateau" eiPAH (Fig. 11.21). The "takeoff" physiology seen in the exercise induced PAH patients resemble normal/detrained "takeoff" physiology while the "plateau" physiology resembles the physiology seen in

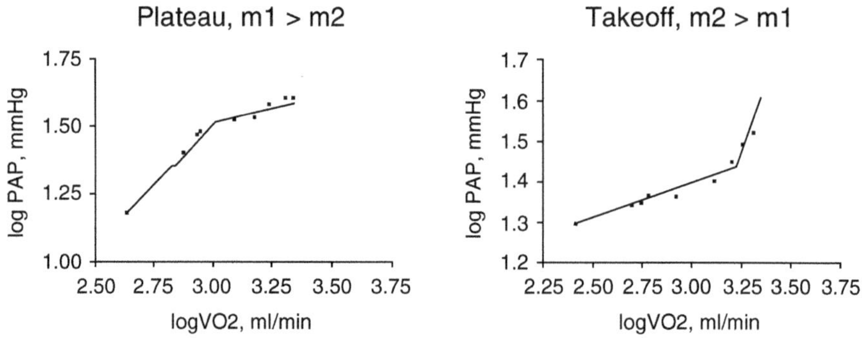

Fig. 11.21 *Left panel*: Representative plateau pattern of log–log plot of mPAP vs. VO_2 in eiPAH. *Right*: Representative "take-off" pattern of log–log plot of mPAP vs. VO_2 in eiPAH

those with resting PAH. These data suggest that eiPAH is an intermediate exercise phenotype between normal subjects and those with resting PAH and that abnormal central hemodynamics during exercise substantively contribute to exertional symptoms and impairment.

Subsequent studies have provided further evidence of the functional significance of exercise-induced elevations in PAP in "at-risk populations" for PAH [10, 116–118]. Fowler et al. [10] described 17 subjects eiPAH patients with reduced VO_2max (1.2±0.4 vs. 1.7±0.5 L min, $P<0.05$), in turn related to decreased peak exercise cardiac output (72±19 % predicted). She and her colleagues also demonstrated elevated ventilatory equivalent for carbon dioxide (41.0±7.3 vs. 31.0±2.9, $P<0.05$) and reduced end-tidal carbon dioxide tension (32.6±3.6 vs. 39.4±2.7 mmHg, $P<0.05$) at the anaerobic threshold. Kovacs et al. showed that a higher exercise mPAP and PVR in patients with "borderline" resting mPAP was associated with reduced 6-min walk distance and reduced peak workload [117].

Whyte et al. [119], examined the hemodynamic response to exercise in "at risk" patients aged <50 years with normal resting mPAP. They showed that individuals who increased mPAP >30 mmHg (24 out of 38) tended to have a higher resting mPAP and PVR. In particular, 88 % of patients with "borderline" resting mPAP of 21–24 mmHg developed mPAP >30 mmHg on mild-to-moderate exercise tended to have a lower 6-min walk test compared to the remaining 14 patients.

Whether exercise-induced elevations in mPAP and PVR provide a window into the diagnosis of early, potentially more treatable forms of PAH is uncertain [108, 120, 121]. Tolle et al. [7] described five subjects with eiPAH who underwent a repeat clinically indicated iCPET. The time to retest was 29.8+10.7 months. Both underlying diagnoses and treatment regimens were heterogeneous. At peak exercise, there was a nonsignificant decrease in VO_2max (69.8+20.2 to 61.2+21.9 % predicted) that was associated with a similar change in Qtmax (86.4+25.6 to 80.0+23.8 % predicted, $p>0.05$ for both), but with no change in central hemodynamics (mPAP: 38.4+4.3 to 37.2+7.5 mmHg; PVR: 175+79 to 131+29 dyn s/cm^5,

$p > 0.05$ for both). Saggar et al. described 3/11 eiPAH SSc patients developing resting PAH over 24 weeks of open label ambrisentan [122]. Condliffe et al. found that 19 % of patients with scleroderma with eiPAH develop resting pulmonary hypertension after 2.3 years [123]. Long-term follow-up is needed, preferably as part of RCT's.

We conclude eiPAH is a clinically relevant entity whose abnormal central hemodynamics cause symptoms and substantively impair exercise tolerance. A standardized approach to its diagnosis and definition is needed. Long term prognosis, relationship to resting PH and optimal treatment need to be better defined.

Exercise-Induced HFpEF

niCPET has been used extensively in the diagnosis and management of HFpEF [124, 125] quantifying the exercise impairment and ruling out a pulmonary mechanical limit. Guazzi et al. has also shown that niCPET variables such as peak VO_2, VE/VCO_2 slope, rest and peak end tidal CO_2 ($PETCO_2$) are correlated with diastolic function in HFpEF patients [125]. Although VO_2max is an important prognostic factor in HFrEF, this association is not as clearly established for HFpEF patients [125].

iCPET has been used to investigate the central hemodynamics [126] and relative contributions of Qt and systemic O_2 extraction in HFpEF [97, 127, 128] iCPET has been suggested as a useful diagnostic modality in the diagnosis of eiHFpEF [129]. Borlaug et al. [97, 130] reported hemodynamic responses to exercise in 55 patients with exertional dyspnea and normal resting hemodynamic measurements. Exercise-induced changes in PCWP and PAP in patients with HFpEF were significantly higher than those in patients with noncardiac dyspnea. Kitzman et al. similarly found that compensated outpatients with HFpEF had normal resting PCWP but marked increases in exercise PCWP, suggesting that HFpEF may initially manifest with only intermittent elevations in cardiac filling pressures [130].

In HFpEF peak oxygen uptake may be additionally affected by impaired systemic O_2 extraction [131, 132] as demonstrated by a reduced peak arterial–venous oxygen during iCPET.

Mixed eiPH

A significant percentage of HFpEF patients demonstrate a reactive increase in pulmonary vascular resistance (PVR) which is recognized at resting RHC, which is likely associated with worse outcome [133]. Tailored therapy of exercise-induced mixed PH, phenotyped by iCPET, shows more promise than larger clinical trials of heterogeneous, noninvasively defined HFpEF patients.

iCPET in Established Heart and Lung Disease

Pulmonary Arterial Hypertension

While exercise hemodynamic measurements are not necessary to confirm the diagnosis of established resting PH, they may aid in probing the compensatory capacity of the RV-pulmonary vascular unit. mPAP usually worsens during exercise when compared to rest [134]. With increased temporal resolution (e.g., q 1-min Fick Qt determinations), established PH shows a plateau in mPAP relative VO_2 during maximum incremental exercise [7, 135] which may be indicative of dynamic RV dysfunction.

HFrEF

Likewise, iCPET is not necessary for the diagnosis of decompensated HF, but the pulmonary vascular response to exercise yields important mechanistic and prognostic information. For instance, Lam et al. [136] studied 60 consecutive patients with HFrEF (age 60 ± 12 years, left ventricular ejection fraction 0.31 ± 0.07, mean ± SD) and 19 controls with iCPET. During low-level exercise (30 W), LVSD subjects, compared with controls, had greater augmentation in mean PAPs (15 ± 1 vs. 5 ± 1 mmHg), transpulmonary gradients (5 ± 1 vs. 1 ± 1 mmHg), and effective pulmonary artery elastance (0.05 ± 0.02 vs. −0.03 ± 0.01 mmHg/mL, $P < 0.0001$ for all). A linear increment in PAP relative to work (0.28 ± 0.12 mmHg/W) was observed in 65 % of LVSD patients, which exceeded that observed in controls (0.07 ± 0.02 mmHg/W, $P < 0.0001$). Exercise capacity and survival was worse in patients with a PAP/W slope above the median than in patients with a lower slope. In the remaining 35 % of LVSD patients, exercise induced a steep initial increment in PAP (0.41 ± 0.16 mmHg/W) followed by a plateau. The plateau pattern, compared with a linear pattern, was associated with reduced VO_2max (10.6 ± 2.6 vs. 13.1 ± 4.0 mL/kg/min, $P = 0.005$), lower right ventricular stroke work index augmentation with exercise (5.7 ± 3.8 vs. 9.7 ± 5.0 g/m^2, $P = 0.002$), and increased mortality (hazard ratio 8.1, 95 % CI 2.7–23.8, $P < 0.001$).A steep increment in PAP during exercise and failure to augment PAP throughout exercise are associated with decreased exercise capacity and survival in patients with LVSD, and may therefore represent therapeutic targets (Fig. 11.22).

Chronic Obstructive Pulmonary Disease

As noted above niCPET can differentiate between a pulmonary vascular and mechanical limit to exercise. iCPET can confirm resting or eiPH in chronic obstructive pulmonary disease (COPD). Per the discussion above [95], care must be taken

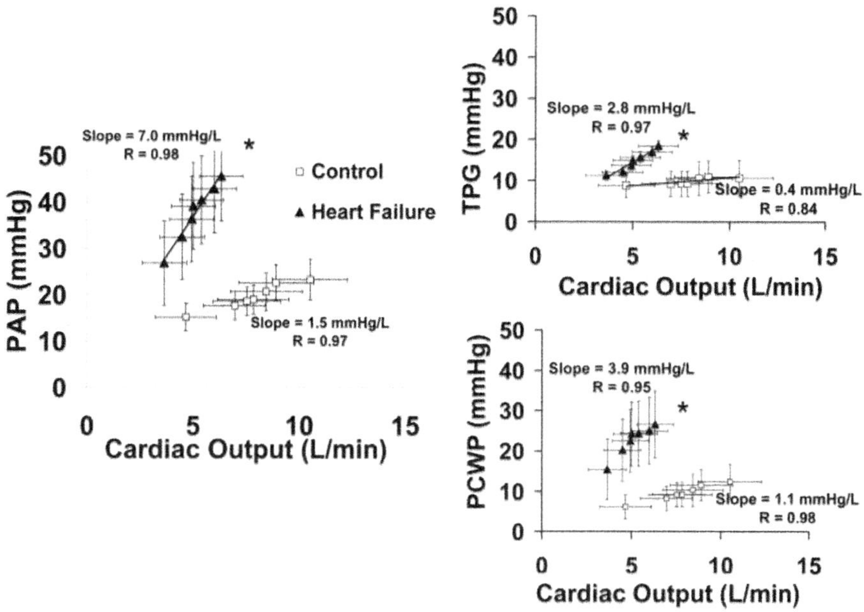

Fig. 11.22 (*Left panel*) Mean pulmonary arterial pressures (PAP) relative to cardiac outputs during incremental exercise in patients with LVSD. (*Right panels*) Transpulmonary gradient (TPG) and pulmonary capillary wedge pressure (PCWP) responses to exercise relative to cardiac output augmentation in patients with LVSD. *$P<0.005$ for the comparison of pressure changes in patients with LVSD with pressure changes in controls [136]

to average input and outflow pressures through several respiratory cycles and to measure mPAP and PCWP for TPG at the same point of the respiratory cycle. Exercise stroke volume appears to be limited by PH in COPD [137] A recent study suggested a high prevalence of eiPH in COPD [92]. We have used iCPET to determine the relative contributions of cardiac output and systemic O_2 extraction to the exercise limit in COPD [138, 139].

Conclusions

Cardiopulmonary exercise testing is an important diagnostic tool in the evaluation of the patient with suspected PH. Noninvasive testing is an appropriate screening test for unexplained exertional intolerance or the patient "at risk" for PH. It and can quantify the degree of impairment, and rule out a pulmonary mechanical limit to exercise. Noninvasive parameters, especially ventilatory inefficiency and $PETCO_2$ changes with exercise, especially when used in the context of a niCPET diagnostic algorithm, show reasonable diagnostic accuracy. niCPET can confirm the diagnosis of exercise-induced PH, distinguish between pulmonary arterial and venous hypertension, and rule out confounders such as impaired systemic O_2 extraction.

References

1. Thenappan T, et al. A USA-based registry for pulmonary arterial hypertension: 1982–2006. Eur Respir J. 2007;30(6):1103–10.
2. Whyte K. Towards early detection of pulmonary hypertension: a call to arms. Eur Respir J. 2014;43(1):16–9.
3. Pullamsetti SS, et al. Novel and emerging therapies for pulmonary hypertension. Am J Respir Crit Care Med. 2014;189(4):394–400.
4. Norfolk SG, Lederer DJ, Tapson VF. Lung transplantation and atrial septostomy in pulmonary arterial hypertension. Clin Chest Med. 2013;34(4):857–65.
5. Moser KM, et al. Chronic thromboembolic pulmonary hypertension: clinical picture and surgical treatment. Eur Respir J. 1992;5(3):334–42.
6. Mohsenifar Z, et al. Lack of sensitivity of measurements of Vd/Vt at rest and during exercise in detection of hemodynamically significant pulmonary vascular abnormalities in collagen vascular disease. Am Rev Respir Dis. 1981;123(5):508–12.
7. Tolle JJ, et al. Exercise-induced pulmonary arterial hypertension. Circulation. 2008;118(21): 2183–9.
8. Saggar R, et al. Pulmonary vascular responses to exercise: a haemodynamic observation. Eur Respir J. 2012;39(2):231–4.
9. Naeije R, et al. Exercise-induced pulmonary hypertension: physiological basis and methodological concerns. Am J Respir Crit Care Med. 2013;187(6):576–83.
10. Fowler RM, et al. Implications of exercise-induced pulmonary arterial hypertension. Med Sci Sports Exerc. 2011;43(6):983–9.
11. Hansen JE, et al. Reproducibility of cardiopulmonary exercise measurements in patients with pulmonary arterial hypertension. Chest. 2004;126(3):816–24.
12. Barron A, et al. Test-retest repeatability of cardiopulmonary exercise test variables in patients with cardiac or respiratory disease. Eur J Prev Cardiol. 2014;7:7.
13. American Thoracic Society. ATS/ACCP Statement on cardiopulmonary exercise testing. Am J Respir Crit Care Med. 2003;167(2):211–77.
14. Balady GJ, et al. Clinician's guide to cardiopulmonary exercise testing in adults: a scientific statement from the American Heart Association. Circulation. 2010;122(2):191–225.
15. Grünig E, et al. Non-invasive diagnosis of pulmonary hypertension: ESC/ERS Guidelines with Updated Commentary of the Cologne Consensus Conference 2011. Int J Cardiol. 2011;154 Suppl 1:S3–12.
16. Committee W, et al. Clinical recommendations for cardiopulmonary exercise testing data assessment in specific patient populations. Eur Heart J. 2012;33(23):2917–27.
17. Sun XG, et al. Exercise pathophysiology in patients with primary pulmonary hypertension. Circulation. 2001;104(4):429–35.
18. Smith G, et al. Safety of maximal cardiopulmonary exercise testing in pediatric patients with pulmonary hypertension. Chest. 2009;135(5):1209–14.
19. Arena R, et al. Cardiopulmonary exercise testing in the assessment of pulmonary hypertension. Expert Rev Respir Med. 2011;5(2):281–93.
20. Dumitrescu D, et al. Developing pulmonary vasculopathy in systemic sclerosis, detected with non-invasive cardiopulmonary exercise testing. PLoS One. 2010;5(12):e14293.
21. Oudiz R, Barst R, Hansen J. Cardiopulmonary exercise testing and six-minute walk correlations in pulmonary arterial hypertension. Am J Cardiol. 2006;97:123–6.
22. Wensel R, Opitz C, Anker S. Assessment of survival in patients with primary pulmonary hypertension. Importance of cardiopulmonary exercise testing. Circulation. 2002;106: 319–24.
23. Sun X, et al. Gas exchange detection of exercise-induced right-to-left shunt in patients with primary pulmonary hypertension. Circulation. 2002;105:54–60.
24. Riley M, et al. Gas exchange responses to continuous incremental cycle ergometry exercise in primary pulmonary hypertension in humans. Eur J Appl Physiol. 2000;83:63–70.

25. Miyamoto S, Nagaya N, Satoh T. Clinical correlates and prognostic significance of six-minute walk test in patients with primary pulmonary hypertension. Comparison with cardio-pulmonary exercise testing. Am J Respir Crit Care Med. 2000;161:487–92.
26. Markowitz DH, Systrom DM. Diagnosis of pulmonary vascular limit to exercise by cardio-pulmonary exercise testing. J Heart Lung Transplant. 2004;23(1):88–95.
27. Nagaya N, Shimizu Y, Satoh T. Oral beraprost sodium improves exercise capacity and ventilatory efficiency in patients with primary or thromboembolic pulmonary hypertension. Heart. 2002;87:340–5.
28. Yasunobu Y, et al. End-tidal pco2 abnormality and exercise limitation in patients with primary pulmonary hypertension. Chest. 2005;127(5):1637–46.
29. Hansen JE, Sue DY, Wasserman K. Predicted values for clinical exercise testing. Am Rev Respir Dis. 1984;129(2 Pt 2):S49–55.
30. D'Alonzo GE, et al. Comparison of progressive exercise performance of normal subjects and patients with primary pulmonary hypertension. Chest. 1987;92(1):57–62.
31. Gläser S, et al. Impact of pulmonary hypertension on gas exchange and exercise capacity in patients with pulmonary fibrosis. Respir Med. 2009;103(2):317–24.
32. Wax D, Garofano R, Barst RJ. Effects of long-term infusion of prostacyclin on exercise performance in patients with primary pulmonary hypertension. Chest. 1999;116(4):914–20.
33. Humbert M, McLaughlin V. Proceedings of the 4th World Symposium on Pulmonary Hypertension. J Am Coll Cardiol. 2009;54:S1–116.
34. Groepenhoff H, et al. Exercise testing to estimate survival in pulmonary hypertension. Med Sci Sports Exerc. 2008;40(10):1725–32.
35. Beaver WL, Wasserman K, Whipp BJ. A new method for detecting anaerobic threshold by gas exchange. J Appl Physiol. 1986;60(6):2020–7.
36. Putman CT, et al. Skeletal muscle pyruvate dehydrogenase activity during maximal exercise in humans. Am J Physiol. 1995;269(3 Pt 1):E458–68.
37. Stainsby WN, et al. Oxidation/reduction state of cytochrome oxidase during repetitive contractions. J Appl Physiol. 1989;67(5):2158–62.
38. Graham TE, Saltin B. Estimation of the mitochondrial redox state in human skeletal muscle during exercise. J Appl Physiol. 1989;66:561–6.
39. Poole DC, Gaesser GA. Response of ventilatory and lactate thresholds to continuous and interval training. J Appl Physiol. 1985;58:1115–21.
40. Gaesser GA, Poole DC. Lactate and ventilatory thresholds: disparity in time course of adaptations to training. J Appl Physiol. 1986;61:99–1004.
41. Phillips SM, et al. Effects of training duration on substrate turnover and oxidation during exercise. J Appl Physiol. 1996;81(5):2182–91.
42. Hagberg JM, et al. Exercise and recovery ventilatory and VO2 responses of patients with McArdle's disease. J Appl Physiol. 1990;68:1393–8.
43. Sue DY, Hansen JE. Normal values in adults during exercise testing. Clin Chest Med. 1984;5:89–98.
44. Wasserman K, McIlroy MB. Detecting the threshold of anaerobic metabolism in cardiac patients during exercise. Am J Cardiol. 1964;14:844–52.
45. Wasserman K, Whipp BJ. Exercise physiology in health and disease. Am Rev Respir Dis. 1975;112:219–49.
46. Hey EN, et al. Effects of various respiratory stimuli on the depth and frequency of breathing in man. Respir Physiol. 1966;1:193–205.
47. Medoff BD, et al. Breathing reserve at the lactate threshold to differentiate a pulmonary mechanical from cardiovascular limit to exercise. Chest. 1998;113(4):913–8.
48. Rochester DF. Tests of respiratory muscle function. Clin Chest Med. 1988;9:249–61.
49. Theodore J, et al. Augmented ventilatory response to exercise in pulmonary hypertension. Chest. 1986;89(1):39–44.
50. Jones NL. Normal values for pulmonary gas exchange during exercise. Am Rev Respir Dis. 1984;129(Suppl):S44–6.

51. Kleber FX, et al. Impairment of ventilatory efficiency in heart failure: prognostic impact. Circulation. 2000;101(24):2803–9.
52. Habedank D, et al. Ventilatory efficiency and exercise tolerance in 101 healthy volunteers. Eur J Appl Physiol. 1998;77:412–26.
53. Fukuchi K, Hayashida K, Nakanishi N. Quantitative analysis of lung perfusion in patients with primary pulmonary hypertension. J Nucl Med. 2002;43:757–61.
54. Reybrouck T, Mertens L, Schulze-Neick I. Ventilatory inefficiency for carbon dioxide during exercise in patients with pulmonary hypertension. Clin Physiol. 2008;28:337–44.
55. Reindl I, Wernecke K, Opitz C. Impaired ventilatory efficiency in chronic heart failure: possible role of pulmonary vasoconstriction. Am Heart J. 1998;136:778–85.
56. Lewis GD, et al. Determinants of ventilatory efficiency in heart failure: the role of right ventricular performance and pulmonary vascular tone. Circ Heart Fail. 2008;1(4):227–33.
57. Raeside DA, et al. Pulmonary artery pressure measurement during exercise testing in patients with suspected pulmonary hypertension. Eur Respir J. 2000;16(2):282–7.
58. Mitani R, Haraguchi M, Takata S. Excessive ventilatory response during exercise in patients with non-hypoxic pulmonary hypertension. Circ J. 2002;66:453–6.
59. Yetman AT, et al. Utility of cardiopulmonary stress testing in assessing disease severity in children with pulmonary arterial hypertension. Am J Cardiol. 2005;95(5):697–9.
60. Schwaiblmair M, et al. Ventilatory efficiency testing as prognostic value in patients with pulmonary hypertension. BMC Pulm Med. 2012;12(1):23.
61. Wensel R, et al. Effects of iloprost inhalation on exercise capacity and ventilatory efficiency in patients with primary pulmonary hypertension. Circulation. 2000;101(20):2388–92.
62. Groepenhoff H, et al. Prognostic relevance of changes in exercise test variables in pulmonary arterial hypertension. PLoS One. 2013;8(9):e72013.
63. Paciocco G, et al. Oxygen desaturation on the six-minute walk test and mortality in untreated primary pulmonary hypertension. Eur Respir J. 2001;17(4):647–52.
64. Hansen JE, et al. Mixed-expired and end-tidal CO2 distinguish between ventilation and perfusion defects during exercise testing in patients with lung and heart diseases. Chest. 2007;132(3):977–83.
65. Oudiz RJ, et al. Effect of sildenafil on ventilatory efficiency and exercise tolerance in pulmonary hypertension. Eur J Heart Fail. 2007;9(9):917–21.
66. Baba R, et al. Oxygen uptake efficiency slope: a new index of cardiorespiratory functional reserve derived from the relation between oxygen uptake and minute ventilation during incremental exercise. J Am Coll Cardiol. 1996;28(6):1567–72.
67. Hollenberg M, Tager IB. Oxygen uptake efficiency slope: an index of exercise performance and cardiopulmonary reserve requiring only submaximal exercise. J Am Coll Cardiol. 2000;36(1):194–201.
68. Sun XG, Hansen JE, Stringer WW. Oxygen uptake efficiency plateau best predicts early death in heart failure. Chest. 2012;141(5):1284–94.
69. Ramos RP, et al. Exercise oxygen uptake efficiency slope independently predicts poor outcome in PAH. Eur Respir J. 2013;5:5.
70. Corra U, et al. Sleep and exertional periodic breathing in chronic heart failure: prognostic importance and interdependence. Circulation. 2006;113(1):44–50.
71. Kremser CB, O'Toole MF, Leff AR. Oscillatory hyperventilation in severe congestive heart failure secondary to idiopathic dilated cardiomyopathy or to ischemic cardiomyopathy. Am J Cardiol. 1987;59(8):900–5.
72. Sun XG, et al. Oscillatory breathing and exercise gas exchange abnormalities prognosticate early mortality and morbidity in heart failure. J Am Coll Cardiol. 2010;55(17):1814–23.
73. Guazzi M, Raimondo R, Vicenzi M. Exercise oscillatory ventilation may predict sudden cardiac death in heart failure patients. J Am Coll Cardiol. 2007;50:299–308.
74. Guazzi M, et al. Exercise oscillatory breathing in diastolic heart failure: prevalence and prognostic insights. Eur Heart J. 2008;29(22):2751–9.
75. Arena R, et al. Prognostic value of timing and duration characteristics of exercise oscillatory ventilation in patients with heart failure. J Heart Lung Transplant. 2008;27(3):341–7.

76. Murphy RM, et al. Exercise oscillatory ventilation in systolic heart failure: an indicator of impaired hemodynamic response to exercise. Circulation. 2011;124(13):1442–51.
77. Leite JJ, et al. Periodic breathing during incremental exercise predicts mortality in patients with chronic heart failure evaluated for cardiac transplantation. J Am Coll Cardiol. 2003;41(12):2175–81.
78. Wasserman K, Hansen JE, Sue DY, Casaburi R, Whipp BJ. Principles of exercise testing and interpretation. 3rd ed. Baltimore, MD: Lipincott Williams & Wilkins; 1999. p. 193.
79. Weisman IM, Zeballos RJ. An integrated approach to the interpretation of cardiopulmonary exercise testing. Clin Chest Med. 1994;15(2):421–45.
80. Eschenbacher WL, Mannina A. An algorithm for the interpretation of cardiopulmonary exercise tests. Chest. 1990;97(2):263–7.
81. Ramos RP, et al. Clinical usefulness of response profiles to rapidly incremental cardiopulmonary exercise testing. Pulm Med. 2013;359021(10):12.
82. Hickam JB, Cargill WH. Effect of exercise on cardiac output and pulmonary arterial pressure in normal persons and in patients with cardiovascular disease and pulmonary emphysema. J Clin Invest. 1948;27(1):10–23.
83. Slonim NB, et al. The effect of mild exercise in the supine position on the pulmonary arterial pressure of five normal human subjects. J Clin Invest. 1954;33(7):1022–30.
84. Damato AN, Galante JG, Smith WM. Hemodynamic response to treadmill exercise in normal subjects. J Appl Physiol. 1966;21(3):959–66.
85. Janicki JS, et al. The pressure-flow response of the pulmonary circulation in patients with heart failure and pulmonary vascular disease. Circulation. 1985;72(6):1270–8.
86. Maron BA, et al. The Invasive Cardiopulmonary Exercise Test. Circulation. 2013;127(10): 1157–64.
87. Reeves JT, et al. Increased wedge pressure facilitates decreased lung vascular resistance during upright exercise. Chest. 1988;93(Suppl):97S–9.
88. Kovacs G, et al. Zero reference level for right heart catheterisation. Eur Respir J. 2013; 42(6):1586–94.
89. Fowler NO. The normal pulmonary arterial pressure-flow relationships during exercise. Am J Med. 1969;47(1):1–6.
90. Champion HC, Michelakis ED, Hassoun PM. Comprehensive invasive and noninvasive approach to the right ventricle-pulmonary circulation unit: state of the art and clinical and research implications. Circulation. 2009;120(11):992–1007.
91. Blanco I, et al. Hemodynamic and gas exchange effects of sildenafil in patients with chronic obstructive pulmonary disease and pulmonary hypertension. Am J Respir Crit Care Med. 2010;181(3):270–8.
92. Hilde JM, et al. Haemodynamic responses to exercise in patients with COPD. Eur Respir J. 2013;41(5):1031–41.
93. Lockhart A, et al. Elevated pulmonary artery wedge pressure at rest and during exercise in chronic bronchitis: fact or fancy. Clin Sci. 1969;37(2):503–17.
94. Tyberg JV, et al. The relationship between pericardial pressure and right atrial pressure: an intraoperative study. Circulation. 1986;73(3):428–32.
95. Boerrigter BG, et al. Measuring central pulmonary pressures during exercise in COPD: how to cope with respiratory effects? Eur Respir J. 2013;43(5):1316–25.
96. Reeves JT, et al. Operation Everest II: cardiac filling pressures during cycle exercise at sea level. Respir Physiol. 1990;80:147–54.
97. Borlaug BA, et al. Exercise hemodynamics enhance diagnosis of early heart failure with preserved ejection fraction. Circ Heart Fail. 2010;3(5):588–95.
98. Granath A, Jonsson B, Strandell T. Circulation in healthy old men, studied by right heart catheterization at rest and during exercise in supine and sitting position. Acta Med Scand. 1964;176:425–46.
99. Groves BM, et al. Operation Everest II: elevated high-altitude pulmonary resistance unresponsive to oxygen. J Appl Physiol. 1987;63(2):521–30.

100. Weber KT, Janicki JS. Cardiopulmonary exercise testing: physiologic principles and clinical applications. Philadelphia: WB Saunders; 1986.
101. Dempsey JA. Is the lung built for exercise? Med Sci Sports Exerc. 1986;18:143–55.
102. Weber KT, Janicki JS. Cardiopulmonary exercise testing for evaluation of chronic cardiac failure. Am J Cardiol. 1985;55:22A–31.
103. Blomqvist CG, Saltin B. Cardiovascular adaptations to physical training. Annu Rev Physiol. 1983;45:169–89.
104. Mahler DA, et al. Volumetric responses of right and left ventricles during upright exercise in normal subjects. J Appl Physiol. 1985;58:1818–22.
105. Manyari DE, Kostuk WJ. Left and right ventricular function at rest and during bicycle exercise in the supine and sitting positions in normal subjects and patients with coronary artery disease: assessment by radionuclide ventriculography. Am J Cardiol. 1983;51:36–42.
106. Shepherd JT. Circulatory response to exercise in health. Circulation. 1987;76(Suppl V):VI3–10.
107. Galie N, et al. Guidelines on diagnosis and treatment of pulmonary arterial hypertension. The Task Force on Diagnosis and Treatment of Pulmonary Arterial Hypertension of the European Society of Cardiology. Eur Heart J. 2004;25(24):2243–78.
108. McGoon M, et al. Screening, early detection, and diagnosis of pulmonary arterial hypertension: ACCP Evidence-Based Clinical Practice Guidelines. Chest. 2004;126(1_suppl):14S–34.
109. Hoeper MM, et al. Definitions and diagnosis of pulmonary hypertension. J Am Coll Cardiol. 2013;62(25, Suppl):D42–50.
110. Lewis GD, et al. Pulmonary vascular hemodynamic response to exercise in cardiopulmonary diseases. Circulation. 2013;128(13):1470–9.
111. Badesch DB, et al. Diagnosis and assessment of pulmonary arterial hypertension. J Am Coll Cardiol. 2009;54(1 Suppl):S55–66.
112. Kovacs G, et al. Pulmonary arterial pressure during rest and exercise in healthy subjects: a systematic review. Eur Respir J. 2009;34(4):888–94.
113. Kane DW, et al. Exercise-induced pulmonary vasoconstriction during combined blockade of nitric oxide synthase and beta adrenergic receptors. J Clin Investig. 1994;93(2):677–83.
114. Fu Q, et al. Cardiac origins of the postural orthostatic tachycardia syndrome. J Am Coll Cardiol. 2010;55(25):2858–68.
115. Taivassalo T, et al. The spectrum of exercise tolerance in mitochondrial myopathies: a study of 40 patients. Brain. 2003;126(2):413–23.
116. Fowler RM, Gain KR, Gabbay E. Exercise intolerance in pulmonary arterial hypertension. Pulm Med. 2012;2012:359204.
117. Kovacs G, et al. Borderline pulmonary arterial pressure is associated with decreased exercise capacity in scleroderma. Am J Respir Crit Care Med. 2009;180(9):881–6.
118. Steen V, et al. Exercise induced pulmonary arterial hypertension in patients with systemic sclerosis. Chest. 2008;134(1):146–51.
119. Whyte K, et al. The association between resting and mild-to-moderate exercise pulmonary artery pressure. Eur Respir J. 2012;39(2):313–8.
120. Proudman SM, et al. Pulmonary arterial hypertension in systemic sclerosis: the need for early detection and treatment. Intern Med J. 2007;37(7):485–94.
121. Raeside DA, et al. Pulmonary artery pressure variation in patients with connective tissue disease: 24 hour ambulatory pulmonary artery pressure monitoring. Thorax. 1998;53(10): 857–62.
122. Saggar R, et al. Brief report: effect of ambrisentan treatment on exercise-induced pulmonary hypertension in systemic sclerosis: a prospective single-center, open-label pilot study. Arthritis Rheum. 2012;64(12):4072–7.
123. Condliffe R, et al. Connective tissue disease-associated pulmonary arterial hypertension in the modern treatment era. Am J Respir Crit Care Med. 2009;179(2):151–7.
124. Guazzi M, Cahalin LP, Arena R. Cardiopulmonary exercise testing as a diagnostic tool for the detection of left-sided pulmonary hypertension in heart failure. J Card Fail. 2013;19(7): 461–7.

125. Guazzi M, Myers J, Arena R. Cardiopulmonary exercise testing in the clinical and prognostic assessment of diastolic heart failure. J Am Coll Cardiol. 2005;46(10):1883–90.
126. Bhella PS, et al. Abnormal haemodynamic response to exercise in heart failure with preserved ejection fraction. Eur J Heart Fail. 2011;13(12):1296–304.
127. Borlaug BA. Mechanisms of exercise intolerance in heart failure with preserved ejection fraction. Circ J. 2013;78(1):20–32.
128. Abudiab MM, et al. Cardiac output response to exercise in relation to metabolic demand in heart failure with preserved ejection fraction. Eur J Heart Fail. 2013;15(7):776–85.
129. van Empel VPM, Kaye DM. Integration of exercise evaluation into the algorithm for evaluation of patients with suspected heart failure with preserved ejection fraction. Int J Cardiol. 2013;168(2):716–22.
130. Kitzman DW, et al. Exercise intolerance in patients with heart failure and preserved left ventricular systolic function: failure of the Frank-Starling mechanism. J Am Coll Cardiol. 1991;17(5):1065–72.
131. Tolle J, Waxman A, Systrom D. Impaired systemic oxygen extraction at maximum exercise in pulmonary hypertension. Med Sci Sports Exerc. 2008;40(1):3–8.
132. Haykowsky MJ, et al. Determinants of exercise intolerance in elderly heart failure patients with preserved ejection fraction. J Am Coll Cardiol. 2011;58(3):265–74.
133. Lam CS, et al. Pulmonary hypertension in heart failure with preserved ejection fraction: a community-based study. J Am Coll Cardiol. 2009;53(13):1119–26.
134. Laskey WK, et al. Pulmonary artery hemodynamics in primary pulmonary hypertension. J Am Coll Cardiol. 1993;21(2):406–12.
135. Wonisch M, et al. Continuous haemodynamic monitoring during exercise in patients with pulmonary hypertension. Int J Cardiol. 2005;101(3):415–20.
136. Lewis GD, et al. Pulmonary vascular response patterns during exercise in left ventricular systolic dysfunction predict exercise capacity and outcomes. Circ Heart Fail. 2011;4(3): 276–85.
137. Holverda S, et al. Stroke volume increase to exercise in chronic obstructive pulmonary disease is limited by increased pulmonary artery pressure. Heart. 2009;95(2):137–41.
138. Oelberg DA, et al. Ventilatory and cardiovascular responses to inspired He-O2 during exercise in chronic obstructive pulmonary disease. Am J Respir Crit Care Med. 1998;158(6): 1876–82.
139. Oelberg DA, et al. Systemic oxygen extraction during incremental exercise in patients with severe chronic obstructive pulmonary disease. Eur J Appl Physiol Occup Physiol. 1998;78(3): 201–7.

Chapter 12
Adjunct Therapy and Calcium Channel Blockers

Terence K. Trow

Abstract Before the era of pulmonary arterial hypertension (PAH)-specific therapies, clinicians treating patients with pulmonary hypertension (PH) employed nonspecific, time-honored treatments in an effort to help these unfortunate patients. While the role of these therapies has not been rigorously studied they are still commonly used as adjuncts to PAH-specific therapies. This chapter outlines the logic and rationale behind the use of digoxin therapy, anticoagulation, oxygen therapy, diuretic therapy, and high-dose calcium channel blocker therapy and reviews the limited data supporting the use of these therapies in patients with PAH.

Keywords Pulmonary hypertension • Digoxin • Anticoagulation • Oxygen therapy • Diuretic therapy • Vasodilator responsiveness • Vasoreactivity testing • Calcium channel blockers

Abbreviations

ACCP	American College of Chest Physicians
ACE	Angiotensin-converting enzyme
APAH	Associated pulmonary arterial hypertension
CCB	Calcium channel blocker
CHD	Congenital heart disease
CO	Cardiac output
COPD	Chronic obstructive pulmonary disease
CPAP	Continuous positive airway pressure
HIF-1	Hypoxia-inducible factor-1
iNO	Inhaled nitric oxide
INR	International normalized ratio
IPAH	Idiopathic pulmonary arterial hypertension

T.K. Trow, M.D. (✉)
Director, Yale Pulmonary Vascular Disease Program, Section of Pulmonary, Critical Care, and Sleep Medicine, Department of Internal Medicine, Yale University School of Medicine, New Haven, CT, USA
e-mail: Terence.trow@yale.edu

J.R. Klinger, R.P. Frantz (eds.), *Diagnosis and Management of Pulmonary Hypertension*, Respiratory Medicine 12, DOI 10.1007/978-1-4939-2636-7_12

LA	Left atrium
LAP	Left atrial pressure
LV	Left ventricle
LVEF	Left ventricular ejection fractions
mPAP	Mean pulmonary artery pressure
OSA	Obstructive sleep apnea
PA	Pulmonary artery
PAH	Pulmonary arterial hypertension
PASMC	Pulmonary artery smooth muscle cells
PAWP	Pulmonary artery wedge pressure
PH	Pulmonary hypertension
PVR	Pulmonary vascular resistance
RA	Right atrial
RHF	Right heart failure (RHF)
RV	Right ventricle
RVEF	Right ventricular ejection fraction
SSc	Systemic sclerosis
WHO	World Health Organization

Introduction

Until the development of pulmonary arterial hypertension (PAH)-specific therapy two decades ago, clinicians relied on nonspecific therapies such as oxygen, diuretics, digoxin, and anticoagulation therapy to relieve symptoms in patients with this dreaded disorder. While these therapeutic approaches did not prove to impact meaningfully on survival [1], most experts feel that these adjunctive therapies have beneficial effects for pulmonary hypertension (PH) patients [2–4] despite the lack of robust, randomized, placebo-controlled data to support these interventions. Their use has been based largely on concepts originating from physiologic observations and experience with these treatments in other cardiac and pulmonary disease states that share symptoms and similar clinical features [4]. While it is unlikely that large, prospective, clinical trials of these standard adjunctive therapies will ever be conducted, their use in conjunction with PAH-specific therapies is well established in the day-to-day clinical management of these patients. This chapter discusses current recommendations regarding these therapies as well as the current role of high-dose calcium channel blocker (CCB) therapy in a subset of PAH patients.

Digoxin Therapy

The use of cardiac glycosides dates back to Sir William Withering's 1785 description of the use of foxglove in the management of "dropsy" and other diseases [5]. Once a mainstay in the treatment of heart failure and atrial fibrillation, their use has lessened over the years as newer therapies such as vasodilators, angiotensin-converting enzyme (ACE) inhibitors, and newer inotropic agents emerged [6]. Nonetheless, these generally inexpensive and well-tolerated agents still have a role in the management of heart failure [6, 7].

Cardiac glycosides such as digoxin exert a number of potentially beneficial cardiac effects. Digoxin binds to the membrane-bound α subunit of the sodium-potassium ATPase, promoting sodium-calcium exchange which in turn increases the intracellular calcium concentration available to contractile proteins [6–8], with resultant positive inotropic effects. In dogs this positive inotropic effect is obtained with little oxygen wasting making it a metabolically efficient drug [9]. Digitalis preparations have no effect on cardiac output in normal control subjects [6, 10, 11] but significantly improve left ventricular ejection fraction in those with systolic heart failure [12–15]. Aside from their positive inotropic effects digitalis preparations have salutary effects on the neurohormonal activation known to be important in systolic heart failure [16–20].

Numerous double-blinded studies examining the effect of digoxin have demonstrated improvement in clinical status [13, 17, 21–24]. Digoxin reduced the incidence of hospitalizations and the number of emergency room visits for heart failure in the Captopril-Digoxin Multicenter Trial of 300 patients with mild to moderate heart failure [13] and increased the exercise time while reducing both plasma norepinephrine concentrations and renin activity at 6 months of therapy in the Dutch Ibopamine Multicenter Trial [17]. In studies examining the effects of withdrawing digoxin therapy, patients who remained on digoxin maintained their exercise ability whereas those randomized to placebo but continuing on ACE inhibitors and diuretics [21] or diuretics alone [23] had a deterioration in their exercise capacity. In the study by Packer et al. patients withdrawn from digoxin had a sixfold increase in worsening of heart failure as reflected in heart failure-related hospitalizations, emergency care visits for heart failure, or the need for concomitant heart failure therapy [21]. In the largest trial of digoxin therapy to date, 7,788 patients were randomized to 0.25 mg of digoxin daily or placebo in the setting of background ACE inhibitor and diuretic therapy [25]. Although this study showed no difference in all-cause mortality between the placebo and digoxin groups, there was a 25 % reduction in the number of hospitalizations for worsening heart failure in the digoxin-treated group and total hospitalizations were reduced 65 % in the digoxin-treated group [25].

The abundance of data supporting digoxin use for patients with left heart failure resulted in extrapolation to patients with PAH and right heart failure (RHF). Rich et al. studied the effects of a single dose of digoxin in 17 consecutive patients with severe PAH and right heart failure and normal left ventricular function [26]. After 2 h, cardiac output increased from 3.49 + 1.2 L/min to 3.81 L/min + 1.2 L ($p=0.028$) suggesting modest inotropic effect. Neurohormonal samples in this study also revealed a significant fall in norepinephrine levels (680 + 89 to 580 + 85 pg/ml; $p=0.013$) and significant and unexpected increases in atrial natriuretic peptide (311 + 44 to 421 + 9 pg/ml; $p=0.010$) following digoxin administration. Plasma renin activity decreased but not significantly so (0.085 + 1.2 to 0.59 + 1.21 ng/ml/h; $p=0.07$).

It is of interest in this study that as pulmonary vascular resistance decreased with nitroprusside administration no effect of digoxin on pulmonary artery pressure was noted [26]. Others have suggested a role for digoxin in those with chronic obstructive pulmonary disease (COPD) and associated PAH [World Health Organization (WHO) Class III PAH]. Recent animal data suggests that digoxin may inhibit hypoxia-inducible factor-1 (HIF-1) transcriptional activity in the chronic hypoxia murine model of PH [27]. Mice injected daily with digoxin had attenuated right ventricular (RV) hypertrophy, pulmonary vascular remodeling, and RV pressure compared to saline-treated mice exposed to the same degree of chronic hypoxia [27]. Furthermore, when digoxin was given after PH was already established in these mice, RV pressures and pulmonary artery smooth muscle cell (PASMC) intracellular calcium increases were attenuated as well [27]. Furthermore, early work on digitalis glycosides did demonstrate inotropic effects on the right ventricle [28]. This work has provided theoretical grounds for the use of digoxin in patients with COPD-associated PH. In a study of 15 patients with COPD and RHF, Mathur et al. showed that after 8 weeks of digoxin therapy RV ejection fraction (RVEF) as measured by radionuclide angiography improved in the 4 patients that had reduced left ventricular ejection fractions (LVEF) at the study outset but did not change in the remaining 11 patients who had normal LVEF to begin with [29].

Based on this limited human data, use of digoxin in patients with PAH is controversial. If its use is elected, prescribers should be highly mindful of the potential for toxicity [4, 30, 31]. Since many patients will be on concomitant diuretic therapy, monitoring of serum potassium and magnesium is mandatory [4, 6, 7] as hypokalemia and hypomagnesemia increase automaticity and promote sodium pump inhibition by digoxin with resulting arrhythmogenic effects [6, 33]. Digoxin is renally cleared and should be used with caution in those with impaired renal function and a reduced starting dose is more appropriate in these patients [4, 34]. A recent study of digoxin levels revealed that an increased mortality rate existed for those patients with higher serum digoxin levels with optimum outcomes seen in serum digoxin levels of 0.5–0.8 ng/ml [32]. Mortality risk also seems increased in those with active myocardial ischemia [6, 25, 31] and digoxin should not be used in this setting. The prescriber must also be aware of interactions with agents such as macrolides, cyclosporine, amiodarone, itraconazole, and many other drugs which can increase digoxin levels increasing the potential for toxicity [4, 34, 35].

Anticoagulation

Many factors increase the tendency for patients with PAH to form clot in the pulmonary vascular bed. Many PAH patients lead a more sedentary existence increasing the risk of venous thrombosis. Venous engorgement and stasis also occur due to elevated right atrial (RA) pressures. Advancing disease results in poor flow through the pulmonary circulation as a result of declining cardiac output [4]. Structural remodeling leads to altered interactions between circulating platelets and the

Table 12.1 Prothrombotic abnormalities in pulmonary arterial hypertension

Abnormalities	Subjects	Reference
Platelet aggregation related		
Increased urinary thromboxane metabolite (11 dehydroxy TxB2)	IPAH	[41]
Decreased urinary PGI2 metabolite (PGI-M)	IPAH	[41]
Decreased nitric oxide (exhaled or urinary excretion)	IPAH, APAH	[57]
Increased circulating platelet aggregates	APAH	[48]
Increased thromboxane A2	IPAH	[41]
Decreased prostacyclin	IPAH	[41]
Increased circulating platelet aggregates	APAH	[48]
Increased plasma serotonin and decreased platelet serotonin	IPAH	[53, 54]
Increased plasma-P selectin	IPAH	[64]
Decreased thrombomodulin	IPAH	[42, 49, 64]
Endothelial function related		
Decreased NO synthase	IPAH	[56]
Decreased prostacyclin synthase expression	IPAH	[36]
Decreased PGI2 metabolite (PGI-M)	IPAH	[41]
Increased urinary thromboxane metabolite (11 dehydroxy TxB2)	IPAH	[41]
Decreased thrombomodulin	IPAH	[42, 49, 64]
Increased von Willebrand factor	IPAH, APAH	[42, 43]
Increased fibrinogen inhibitor plasminogen activator 1	IPAH	[42, 59]
Coagulation and fibrinolytic related		
Increased prevalence of antiphospholipid Ab/lupus anticoagulant	IPAH, CTEPH	[58]
Increased von Willebrand factor antigen level	IPAH	[42, 43]
Increased fibrinogen inhibitor plasminogen activator 1	IPAH	[42, 59]
Increased euglobulin lysis time	IPAH	[42]
Increased fibrinogen level	APAH	[42]

Modified with permission from Alam S, Palevesky HI. Clin Chest Med 2007; 28:91–115

pulmonary arterial endothelium [36, 37] with potential for in situ clot formation [36, 38–40]. In addition a number of human studies have revealed idiopathic PAH (IPAH) to be a prothrombotic state [41–57] (see Table 12.1). Interestingly this prothrombotic state does not appear to be the result of inherited thrombophilias [58–60] but rather a dysregulation of the normal balance between thrombin formation and the prevention of clot formation at least in part due to endothelial cell dysfunction [36, 37, 42, 43, 46, 49, 56, 57, 59, 61, 70], in part due to platelet activation [37, 41, 42, 48, 46, 49, 52–54, 57], and in part due to proteins related to coagulation and fibrinolysis [42, 43, 55, 58, 59]. Some of these abnormalities appear reversible with the use of PAH-specific therapies [62–65]. While these observations are supportive of a role for thrombotic arteriopathy in patients with PAH, it is unclear from the current literature if this is a cause or consequence of IPAH or associated forms of

PAH (APAH) [57, 61]. Irrespective, thrombotic arteriopathy may alter the disease course and prognosis in IPAH and APAH.

To date, three retrospective [66–68] and one non-blinded, non-placebo-controlled prospective study [69] have suggested a survival advantage to those patients with IPAH treated with anticoagulation in the form of warfarin. In the single-center retrospective study by Fuster et al., the course of 120 IPAH patients pulmonary hypertension was examined. In a multivariate analysis of a number of variables only pulmonary arterial oxygen saturation and use of anticoagulant therapy emerged as prognosticators of survival [66]. In the 56 patients with autopsy lung specimens, 18 had plexogenic arteriopathy and in 32 the major histologic feature was chronic thrombus. To further investigate the role of anticoagulation 78 additional patients treated with anticoagulation were compared to 37 receiving no anticoagulation. This analysis showed a more favorable survivorship in the warfarin-treated group [66]. Of note, from a study design standpoint the numbers were too small to reach statistical significance. Additionally, the criteria used to decide when not to anticoagulate were not clear leaving the potential for selection bias.

In the study by Frank et al., 173 patients with PAH (104 who took aminorex and 69 with PH of unexplained etiology) were retrospectively reviewed [67]. Fifty-six of the 104 aminorex induced PAH and 24 of the 69 patients with IPAH received warfarin therapy. Patients with aminorex APAH fared better than those with IPAH (7.5 years vs. 3.9 years; $p = <0.001$) and the best survival times occurred in those aminorex APAH who were anticoagulated (8.3 years vs. 6.1 years). In addition, those receiving anticoagulation therapy early after onset of symptoms had a better prognosis (10.9 year survival) than those commencing anticoagulation therapy 2 years or longer after symptomatic presentation [67]. Of note, no differences in survival were seen in the first 5 years of follow-up but some survival advantage was seen in the IPAH group in the subsequent 5 years that did not reach statistical significance.

In a more contemporary retrospective study during an era of PAH-specific therapy, Kawut et al. reviewed patients with PAH that was idiopathic, familial, or associated with anorexigen use [68]. The primary combined end point was death or lung transplantation. Eighty-four patients with newly diagnosed PAH were included. Interestingly, their analysis demonstrated that warfarin use was associated with increased survival in their cohort while the use of other PAH-specific medications were not [68]. Once again, the criteria for deciding who not to anticoagulate was not defined raising concern for potential selection bias.

In the only single-center, prospective trial of warfarin therapy in IPAH, no control group existed and the authors used a historical control group from the National Institute of Health Primary Pulmonary Hypertension Registry. Sixty-four patients were assessed for response to high-dose CCB therapy [69]. Twenty-six % ($n = 17$) responded (defined as a > 20 % decrease in mean pulmonary artery pressure or a 20 % or more decrease in pulmonary vascular resistance) and were maintained on high-dose CCB for 5 years. Warfarin therapy was given to 55 % of all patients as concurrent therapy. Warfarin therapy was associated with increased survival in the group as a whole, and particularly in patients who were nonresponders to high-dose CCB.

The decision to put patients on warfarin therapy was based on the finding of nonuniform perfusion on a ventilation-perfusion (V/Q) scan [69].

Based on the biological rationale offered earlier and on the results of these four studies the current expert recommendation is to treat IPAH patients with warfarin anticoagulation in the absence of contraindications [2, 3] and to consider warfarin therapy in APAH patients with more advanced disease such as those on continuous intravenous therapy, in the absence of contraindications [3]. Since little data exist in the APAH subgroup the presumption that anticoagulation will have beneficial effects on survival remains speculative. The recommended anticoagulation dose of warfarin is that which achieves an international normalized ratio (INR) of 1.5–2.5 [3, 7] though some experts in Europe recommend achieving INRs between 2.0 and 3.0 [4]. A decision to anticoagulate APAH subgroups must be weighed against the risk for potential bleeding complications [71–73] especially in those with systemic sclerosis (SSc) APAH where a high risk of gastrointestinal bleeding can be expected [73]. Indeed, a recent retrospective study of 275 patients with SSc-APAH and 155 patients with IPAH used Bayesian propensity scores to adjust for baseline differences between patients exposed and not exposed to warfarin. In a matched cohort of SSc-APAH ($n=98$; 49 treated with warfarin) the median hazard ratio was 1.06 while in a matched cohort of IPAH patients [$n=66$; 33 treated with warfarin] the median hazard ratio was 1.07. This analysis suggested that there was a 70 % probability that warfarin provided no significant benefit or was harmful [74]. The authors concluded that SSc-APAH should not receive warfarin therapy. Likewise in portopulmonary APAH, experts advise that anticoagulation should probably be avoided due to the risk of bleeding [2]. In addition, consideration of the other medications being used may influence the decision to anticoagulate as concerning drug-drug interactions can occur [75]. The finding of an increased incidence of subarachnoid hemorrhage in the imatinib-treated patients who were also receiving warfarin in the IMPRES study underscores the need for careful consideration of context in the use of anticoagulation [76]. Anticoagulation is an irrefutable part of the treatment of chronic thromboembolic PAH [77].

While warfarin therapy is the recommended form of anticoagulation, it is not clear that other forms of anticoagulation should not be considered. In fact, numerous animal studies have suggested that heparin may have some advantages in PAH. In a murine model of PH induced by chronic hypoxia, high-dose heparin therapy partially but significantly reduced RV systolic pressures and remodeling of distal small pulmonary arteries [78]. A similar finding has been reported in a guinea pig chronic hypoxia model where PH and total pulmonary resistance were partially reversed with the continuous infusion of heparin [79]. When heparin and warfarin treatment were compared in the same guinea pig model, only heparin showed partial reversal of PH once established [80]. The mechanism for this effect of heparin is unclear but inhibition of platelet-derived growth factor (PDGF) [78] and inhibition of smooth muscle growth in the pulmonary artery perhaps by alterations in the regulation of cyclin-dependent kinase [81] and/or the guanine nucleotide exchange factor –H1/Rho A/Rho kinase/p27 pathway [82] have been suggested. Heparin has not been studied in humans with PAH. Other forms of anticoagulation have not been studied adequately in PAH though a double-blind, placebo-controlled, crossover study of 19 IPAH patients (9 on intravenous (IV) epoprostenol) assessed the effect of aspirin and clopidogrel [83]. The authors noted a reduction in measures of platelet aggregability and aspirin was noted to reduce thromboxane metabolite production without affecting prostaglandin I_2 metabolite synthesis [83]. Recently, the direct factor Xa inhibitor rivaroxaban was compared with warfarin and enoxaparin in a monocrotaline rat model of PAH [84]. Rivaroxaban reduced systolic and end-diastolic RV pressure increases and RV hypertrophy while warfarin reduced RV pressure increases only. Enoxaparin had no effect on either RV pressure or RV hypertrophy [83]. Neither of these agents have been studied in humans with PAH.

Oxygen Therapy

The role of oxygen therapy has not been specifically studied in PAH, but recommendations for its use [2, 3] have been extrapolated from data in hypoxemic patients with COPD. It is well known that hypoxemia is a strong stimulus for pulmonary vasoconstriction, possibly through a reactive oxygen species and induced superoxide dismutase pathway [85], and that this occurs as an attempt to match lung perfusion with ventilation. Two landmark trials established the benefit of oxygen therapy in hypoxemic patients with COPD [86, 87], with both studies showing long-term improvements in survival in patients treated with 15 h/day or more of oxygen therapy. Interestingly, oxygen therapy does not correct or even near-correct PH in patients with COPD though it does improve it and the noted improved survival in COPD patients treated with oxygen is not felt to be due to the modest reduction in pulmonary artery pressure (PAP) [88]. In fact, in the Nocturnal Oxygen Therapy in Hypoxemic Chronic Obstructive Lung Disease Trial (NOTT), it was patients with low baseline pulmonary vascular resistance (PVR) that had improved mortality on continuous oxygen supplementation, whereas patients with high PVR did not experience a survival benefit [86]. Those with the largest drop in PVR at right-heart catheterization at 6 months in fact had the greatest mortality again suggesting that alteration of the PH per se did not confer the survival benefit [4, 86].

Many patients with PAH have hypoxemia at rest or intermittently with exercise and sleep, and it is important for practitioners to know that as many as 60 % of PAH patients who do not desaturate with exercise in the office evaluations will do so during sleep even in the absence of sleep apnea [89]. Intermittent worsening of oxygen saturation during exercise is often seen as a consequence of increased right-to-left shunting through a patent foramen ovale. Currently, it is recommended that patients with PAH whose partial pressure of arterial oxygen is consistently less than or equal to 55 mmHg or whose oxyhemoglobin saturation is less than or equal to 88 % at rest, during sleep, or with ambulation receive oxygen therapy [2–4]. In addition, patients with evidence of chronic hypoxemia such as polycythemia (hematocrit >55), signs of cor pulmonale, or suggestion of right heart failure on an electrocardiogram or echocardiography should receive oxygen therapy if the oxyhemoglobin saturation is less than or equal to 89 % or if the PaO_2 is less than 60 mmHg [4, 90]. In addition, all patients with a diffusion of carbon monoxide impairment of moderate-to-severe nature warrant testing of oxyhemoglobin desaturation [91, 92]. These recommendations are based solely on expert opinion in patients with IPAH or APAH as no direct evidence exists to support these recommendations (with the exception of COPD-APAH).

The role of oxygen therapy in congenital heart disease (CHD) APAH is controversial. Nocturnal administration of oxygen in children with CHD-APAH has been shown to slow the rate of progression of polycythemia and to improve symptoms [93, 94]. Whether or not oxygen therapy improves survival is not clear. One small study of 15 patients with CHD-APAH studied oxygen supplementation (15 or more h/day) over 5 years. Nine patients received oxygen therapy and six did not. A mortality benefit was seen with 9/9 alive in the oxygen therapy group and 1/6 alive in the untreated group at the 5-year time point [93]. However, a recent well-designed, prospective, randomized, controlled study of 23 adult patients with CHD-APAH and Eisenmenger's syndrome showed no survival benefit with nocturnal oxygen administration [94]. In addition, no improvement in 6-min walk distances, hematocrit levels, or quality of life were seen in the oxygen-treated group [94].

Patients with obstructive sleep apnea (OSA) will generally have mild-to-moderate PH [95–98] in anywhere from 17 to 53 % of the time [96, 97]. Moderate-to-severe PH should not be attributed to sleep-disordered breathing in these patients and other causes such as pulmonary venous hypertension from obesity cardiomyopathy or concurrent COPD should be looked for. In OSA-related PH continuous positive airway pressure (CPAP) combined with oxygen therapy (when needed) will result in a more pronounced decrease in mean PAP and PVR than that seen in patients treated with oxygen alone. Full resolution of PH in this setting is not expected with even the most compliant of CPAP use [99–101]. Patients with the obesity hypoventilation syndrome, however, can develop severe PAH and RHF and treatment requires noninvasive positive pressure ventilation or bilevel positive pressure ventilation which can reverse hypercapnea and signs of RHF within months [102–104]. In patients who cannot tolerate such therapy tracheostomy with chronic outpatient mechanical ventilation at night should be offered [4] and has the potential to be life saving [105, 106].

Oxygen therapy carries with it a number of logistic and social stigma issues that need to be addressed with its recipients. The inconvenience of ambulatory systems, limitations of time that portable systems allow, danger of falls over long cords and tubing, and stigma some patients feel when seen in public may all negatively impact on the patients' self-concept and the perception that others have of them. These issues need to be discussed frankly with patients before oxygen therapy is prescribed.

Diuretics

Diuretics are a mainstay in the management of left heart failure [107], and while never systematically studied are universally accepted in the management of peripheral edema in RHF [2–4]. The short-term effects of diuretics in patients with RHF from PH are usually obvious, and their effect on symptoms likewise usually transparent [4]. In fact, the benefit of diuretics is so intuitively obvious that a randomized, double-blinded, controlled, prospective trial is not likely to occur.

Theoretic basis for their use in RHF includes improvement in RV-LV interdependency with reduced paradoxical septal bowing which causes attendant encroachment on LV stroke volume [108] and impairment of LV diastolic function [109, 110]. Aldosterone antagonism has been shown to reduce both morbidity and mortality in patients with severe left heart failure with New York Heart Association class III or IV functional status [111]. In this study a low dose of spironolactone was added to ACE inhibitor therapy and furosemide diuretic therapy. An impressive 35 % decrease in need for subsequent hospitalization was observed and the 2-year mortality was 35 % for the spironolactone group compared to 46 % in controls [111]. No such trial of the effects of aldosterone antagonists has been performed in patients with PAH and RHF. Extreme caution should be used with these agents in patients with RHF who have concurrent renal failure and/or diabetes [4], and in patients using ACE inhibitors or nonsteroidal anti-inflammatory agents [106]. Careful modification of potassium supplements and follow-up of electrolytes are critical when aldosterone antagonists are prescribed.

Amiloride, a potassium-sparing diuretic, has been shown to reduce PASMC proliferation and significantly reduces PAP and total pulmonary resistance compared to controls in a hypoxia-induced rat model of PH [112]. The clinical relevance of this observation to PAH patients is speculative as no clinical studies with these agents in PAH exist.

The use of diuretics in patients with PAH requires careful monitoring. Maintenance of potassium concentration above 4.0 mmol/L is important, especially in patients on digoxin therapy to avoid arrhythmias. Rapid, large-volume diuresis should be avoided except when frank cardiogenic pulmonary edema and/or worsening hypoxemia is present as the very preload-dependent RV may react to underfilling with hypotension [4]. Orthostatic dizziness should be addressed with dose adjustments accordingly to avoid hypotension, but underdosing in the setting of low blood pressure that these patients often have can result in overall clinical worsening, worsening hepatic congestion, or bowel wall edema with symptoms of early satiety [4, 68]. Optimal volume status represents a narrow window requiring frequent evaluations by the practitioner. Patients with RHF often require salt and fluid restriction, leg elevation when not ambulating, and compressive stockings to control their edema in conjunction with judicious diuretic use [4].

Calcium Channel Blockers

Vasoconstriction is a component of the elevated PVR seen in patients with PAH. In an earlier era, this was felt to be the major component to the aberrant vascular bed in these patients and as such numerous attempts at reversing vasoconstriction with medications originally designed for systemic hypertension ensued [112–115]. As our understanding of the pathogenesis of PAH evolved it became clearer that vasoconstriction was only a part of the story and that dysregulated endothelial cell function with attendant PASMC proliferation, vascular inflammation [36, 116, 117], and in situ thrombosis [38–40, 66] all play pivotal roles in elevating the PVR. As such it is now recognized that only a minority of IPAH patients have primary aberrant vasoconstriction as their phenotype [69, 118, 119] and that when present this corresponds to a truly different genetic subgroup that do not have bone morphogenic receptor protein gene mutations [120]. In fact, by earlier definitions of a positive pulmonary vasodilator response (defined as a drop in mPAP or PVR by >20 %) 26 % of a cohort of IPAH patients demonstrated this phenomena and seemed to do remarkably well during a 5-year follow-up period when treated with high-dose CCB [69]. More recent retrospective evaluation of vasoresponders meeting this earlier criteria revealed that a significant portion of them did not have sustained responses to high-dose CCB [119] resulting in a more stringent definition of a "vasoresponder" [119]. Using these new criteria of a positive pulmonary vasodilator response (drop in mPAP by 10 mmHg or more to an absolute value of 40 or less with no change or an improvement in cardiac output) only 6.8 % of IPAH patients were deemed vasoresponders who might do well with high-dose CCB therapy [119]. These criteria are now the recommended American College of Chest Physicians (ACCP) criteria for diagnosing a positive pulmonary vasodilator response in IPAH patients during right-heart catheterization testing that would predict sustained benefit from high-dose CCB therapy. An acute pulmonary vasodilator response occurs even less often in patients with APAH [121, 122]. The role of acute vasoreactivity testing in APAH and the role of high-dose CCB in these patients are not known, though the report of the French experience by Montani et al. would suggest that they do not have a role in HIV-APAH, connective-tissue disease APAH, or CHD-APAH [122]. There may be a role for high-dose CCB in anorexigen-APAH who meet the ACCP criteria for acute vasoresponders [122]. Pragmatically, acute vasoreactivity testing is still routinely done in many forms of APAH if only to appease insurance companies and third-party payers that cheaper CCB therapy is not appropriate in these patients.

The choice of agent used for acute vasodilator testing has also evolved over time. Use of titrated administration of CCB agents [69] should no longer be used in the current era as these agents are longer acting than current alternatives and they may precipitate systemic hypotension and worsening hypoxemia [4]. Inhaled nitric oxide (iNO), intravenous (IV) prostacyclin, or IV adenosine are all acceptable agents for acute testing [2, 123]. Few head-to-head comparisons of these agents exist but in a recent study comparing IV adenosine to iNO in acute pulmonary vasoreactivity testing, 6 of 39 (15 %) with IPAH were found to be responders by the current ACCP criteria to iNO while none of these patients demonstrated a vasodilator response to adenosine, perhaps due to side effect limitations in reaching the maximal adenosine dose [124]. Regardless of the agent selected, caution must be used in certain situations. Vasodilator testing should not be done in patients with severely depressed cardiac function (e.g., cardiac index < 2.0) as undesirable drops in systemic blood pressure may occur [4]. It should be done with extreme caution in patients with pulmonary artery wedge pressures (PAWP) > 15 mmHg and in the event of sudden worsening of the oxyhemoglobin saturation the trial should be aborted and intravenous morphine, nitroglycerin, and diuretics administered if needed. Reports of acute pulmonary edema development during acute vasodilator testing exist [125–128] and death from such pulmonary edema has occurred in the context of occult pulmonary venoocclusive disease [129]. In patients with elevated PAWP, the use of nitroprusside as an acute vasodilator has been advocated [130]. It should be emphasized that failure to respond acutely to vasodilator testing does not exclude improvement with long-term use of prostacyclin or other PAH-specific therapies [128, 131–133].

Only when patients meet the ACCP criteria for vasoresponsiveness should high-dose CCB therapy be prescribed. This can occur in an inpatient setting with a PA catheter in place or slowly by oral titration as an outpatient [4]. In general, nifedipine should be used in those with heart rates <100 while many advocate diltiazem for those with heart rates >100 [4, 69, 119, 134]. Amlodipine is also an acceptable agent in vasoreactive patients [4]. Close follow-up is essential as nearly half of the patients meeting acute vasodilator criteria will not have durable response and may require other PAH-specific therapies [119]. Empiric use of CCB is never indicated and may be fatal [4]. The studies of high-dose CCB properly applied in the proper subgroup suggest excellent survivals compared with nonresponders [69, 119]. A small observational study of seven patients initially shown to be nonresponders appeared to develop a vasodilator response several months after treatment with epoprostenol [134]. The clinical significance of this and its implication for CCB use in this subgroup of patients are unknown.

Summary

In an era of PAH-specific therapies, adjunctive use of digoxin, anticoagulation, oxygen, and diuretics is still advised in IPAH patients on the basis of retrospective, uncontrolled studies or on assumptions from data in other similar disease states [2, 3]. Their use in APAH remains speculative but common. In the absence of better randomized, controlled studies a low threshold should exist for discontinuation should side effects or tolerability issues emerge. Acute vasoreactivity testing defines a small subset of IPAH patients in whom high-dose CCB monotherapy can be effective. These patients generally have a better prognosis and greater survival times but still require close monitoring for durability of response as many will ultimately require addition of other PAH-specific therapies.

References

1. D'Alonzo GE, Barst RJ, Ayres SM, Bergofsky EH, Brundage BH, et al. Survival in patients with primary pulmonary hypertension. Results from a national prospective registry. Ann Intern Med. 1991;115:343–9.
2. Badesch DB, Abman SH, Ahearn GS, Barst RJ, McCrory DC, Simonneau G, et al. Medical therapy for pulmonary hypertension. ACCP evidence-based clinical practice guidelines. Chest. 2004;126:S35–62.
3. ACCF/AHA 2009 Expert Consensus Document on Pulmonary Hypertension. J Am Coll Cardiol. 2009;53:1573–619.
4. Alam S, Palevsky HI. Standard therapies for pulmonary arterial hypertension. Clin Chest Med. 2007;28:91–115.
5. Withering W. An account of the foxglove and some of its medical uses, with practical remarks on dropsy, and other diseases. In: Willis FA, Keys TE, editors. Classics of cardiology, vol. 1. New York: Henry Schuman, Dover Publications; 1941. p. 231–52.
6. Eichhorn EJ, Gheorghiade M. Digoxin. Prog Cardiovasc Dis. 2002;44:251–66.
7. Dec GW. Digoxin remains useful in the management of chronic heart failure. Med Clin N Am. 2003;87:317–37.
8. Little WC, Rassi A, Freeman GL. Comparison of effects of dobuatmine and ouabaing on left ventricular contraction and relaxation in closed-chest dogs. J Clin Invest. 1987;80:613–20.
9. Li PC, Hos CS, Swaminathan R. The chronic effects of long-term digoxin administration on Na^+/K^+-ATPase activity in rat tissues. Int J Cardiol. 1993;40:95–100.
10. Hasenfuss G, Mulieri LA, Allen PD, Just H, Alpert NR. Influence of isoproterenol and ouabain on excitation-contraction coupling, cross-bridge function, and energetics in failing human myocardium. Circulation. 1996;94:S3155–60.
11. Braunwald E. Effects of digitalis on the normal and the failing heart. J Am Coll Cardiol. 1985;5:S51A–9.
12. Mason DT, Braunwald E. Studies on digitalis. IX. Effects of oubain on the nonfailing human heart. J Clin Invest. 1963;42:1105–11.
13. The Captopril-Digoxin Multicenter Research Group. Comparative effects of therapy with captopril and digoxin in patients with mild to moderate heart failure. JAMA. 1988;259: 539–44.
14. Gheorghiade M, Hall V, Lakier JB, Goldstein S. Comparative hemodynamic and neurohormonal effects of intravenous captopril and digoxin and their combinations in patients with severe heart failure. J Am Coll Cardiol. 1989;13:134–42.
15. Davies RF, Beanland DS, Nadeau C, Phanefu D, Morris A, Parker JO, et al. Enalapril versus digoxin in patients with congestive heart failure: a multicenter study. Canadian enalapril versus digoxin study group. J Am Coll Cardiol. 1991;18:1602–9.
16. Gheorghiade M, Ferguson D. Digoxin. A neurohormonal modulator in heart failure? Circulation. 1991;84:2181–6.
17. Van Veldhusien DJ, Man int'Veld AJ, Dunselman PHJM, Lok DJA, Dohmen HJM, Poortersmans JC, et al. Double-blind placebo-controlled study of Ibopamine and digoxin in patients with mild to moderate heart failure: results of the Dutch ibopamine multicenter trial (DIMT). J Am Coll Cardiol. 1993;22:1564–73.
18. Krum H, Bigger JT, Goldsmith RL, Packer M. Effect of long-term digoxin therapy on autonomic function in patients with chronic heart failure. J Am Coll Cardiol. 1995;25:289–94.
19. Newton GE, Tong JH, Schofield AM, Baines AD, Floras JS, Parker JD. Digoxin reduces cardiac sympathetic activity in severe congestive heart failure. J Am Coll Cardiol. 1996; 28:155–61.
20. Ferguson DW, Berg WJ, Sanders JS, Roach PJ, Kempf JS, Kienzle MG. Sympathoinhibitory responses to digitalis glycosides in heart failure patients. Direct evidence from sympathetic neural recordings. Circulation. 1989;80:65–77.

21. Packer M, Gheorghiade M, Young JB, Costantini PJ, Adams KF, Cody RJ, et al. Withdrawal of digoxin from patients with chronic heart failure treated with angiotensin –converting-enzyme inhibitors. N Engl J Med. 1993;329:1–7.
22. DiBianco R, Shabetai R, Kostuk W, Moran J, Schlant RC, Wright R. A comparison of oral milrionoe, digoxin, and their combination in the treatment of patients with chronic heart failure. N Engl J Med. 1989;320:677–83.
23. Uretsky BF, Young JB, Shahidi FE, Yellen LG, Harrison MC, Jolly MK. Randomized study assessing the effect of digoxin withdrawal in patients with mild to moderate chronic congestive heart failure: results of the PROVED trial. J Am Coll Cardiol. 1993;22:955–62.
24. Gheorghiade M, Zarowitz BJ. Review of randomized trials of digoxin therapy in patients with chronic heart failure. Am J Cardiol. 1992;69:S48G–63.
25. The Digitalis Investigation Group. The effect of digoxin on mortality in patients with heart failure. N Engl J Med. 1997;336:525–33.
26. Rich S, Seidlitz M, Dodin E, Osimani D, Judd D, Genthner D, et al. Chest. 1998; 114:787–92.
27. Abud EM, Undem C, Punjab A, Zaiman AL, Myers AC, Semenza GL, et al. Digoxin inhibits development of hypoxic pulmonary hypertension in mice. PNAS. 2012;109:1239–44.
28. Cattell M, Gold H. The influence of digitalis glycosides on the force of contraction of mammalian cardiac muscle. J Pharmacol Exp Ther. 1938;62:116–25.
29. Mathur PN, Powles P, Pugsley SO, McEwan MP, Campell EJM. Effect of digoxin on right ventricular function in severe chronic airflow obstruction. Ann Intern Med. 1981;95:283–8.
30. Marik PE, Fromm L. A case series of hospitalized patients with elevated digoxin levels. Am J Med. 1998;105:110–5.
31. Leor J, Goldbout U, Rabinowitz B, Reicher-Ross H, Boyko V, Kaplinsky E, et al. Digoxin and increased mortality among patients recovering from acute myocardial infarction: importance of digoxin dose. Cardiovasc Drugs Ther. 1995;9:723–9.
32. Rathore SS, Curtis JP, Wang Y, Bristow MR, Krumholz HM. Association of serum digoxin concentration and outcomes in patients with heart failure. JAMA. 2003;289:871–8.
33. Smith TW, Antman EM, Friedman PL, Blatt CM, Marsh JD. Digitalis glycosides: mechanisms and manifestations of toxicity. Prog Cardiovasc Dis. 1984;27(1):21–56.
34. Jelliffe RW, Brooker G. A nomogram for digoxin therapy. Am J Med. 1974;57:63–8.
35. Juurlink DN, Mamdani M, Kopp A, Laupacis A, Redelmeir DA. Drug-drug interactions among elderly patients hospitalized for drug toxicity. JAMA. 2003;289:1652–8.
36. Humbert M, Morrell NW, Archer SL, Stenmark KR, MacLean MR, Lang IM, et al. Cellular and molecular pathobiology of pulmonary arterial hypertension. J Am Coll Cardiol. 2004;43:S13–24.
37. Johnson SR, Granton JT, Mehta S. Thrombotic arteriopathy and anticoagulation in pulmonary hypertension. Chest. 2006;130:545–52.
38. Wagenvoort CA. Lung biopsy specimens in the evaluation of pulmonary vascular disease. Chest. 1980;77:614–25.
39. Bjornsson J, Edwards WD. Primary pulmonary hypertension: a histopathological study of 80 cases. Mayo Clin Proc. 1985;60:16–25.
40. Pietra GG, Edwards WD, Kay JM, Rich S, Kernis J, Schloo B, et al. Histopathology of primary pulmonary hypertension. A qualitative and quantitative study of pulmonary vessels from 58 patients in the National Heart, Lung, and Blood Institute Primary Pulmonary Hypertension Registry. Circulation. 1989;80:1198–206.
41. Christman BW, McPherson CD, Newman JH, King GA, Bernard BR, Groves BM, et al. An imbalance between the excretion of thromboxane and prostacyclin metabolites in pulmonary hypertension. N Engl J Med. 1992;327:70–5.
42. Welsh CH, Hassell KL, Badesch DB, Kressin DC, Marlar RA. Coagulation and fibrinolytic profiles in patients with severe pulmonary hypertension. Chest. 1996;110:710–7.
43. Collados MR, Sandoval J, Lopez S, Masso FA, Paez A, Borbolla JR, Monatano LF. Characterization of von Willebrand factor in primary pulmonary hypertension. Heart Vessels. 1999;14:246–52.

44. Lopes AA, Maeda NY. Circulating von Willebrand factor antigen as a predictor of short-term prognosis in pulmonary hypertension. Chest. 1998;114:1276–82.
45. Lopes AA, Maeda NY, Aiello VD, Bydlowski SP. Abnormal multimeric and oligomeric composition is associated with enhanced endothelial expression of von Willebrand factor in pulmonary hypertension. Chest. 1993;104:1455–60.
46. Geggel RL, Carvalho AC, Hoyer LW, Reid LM. von Willebrand factor abnormalities in primary pulmonary hypertension. Am Rev Respir Dis. 1987;135:294–9.
47. Huber K, Beckman R, Frank H, Kneussl M, Mlczoch J, Binder BR. Am J Respir Crit Care Med. 1994;150:929–33.
48. Lopes AA, Maeda NY, Almeida A, Jaeger R, Ebaid M, Charmone DF. Circulating platelet aggregates indicative of in vivo platelet activation in pulmonary hypertension. Angiology. 1993;44:701–6.
49. Cacoub P, Karmochkine M, Dorent R, Nataf P, Piette JC, Godeau P, et al. Plasma levels of thrombomodulin in pulmonary hypertension. Am J Med. 1996;101:160–4.
50. Eisenberg PR, Lucore C, Kaufman L, Sobel BE, Jaffe AS, Rich S. Circulation. 1990;82:841–7.
51. Can MM, Tanboga IH, Demircan HC, Ozkan A, Koca F, Keles N, et al. Enhanced hemostatic indices in patients with pulmonary arterial hypertension: an observational study. Thromb Res. 2010;126:280–2.
52. Herve P, Droute L, Dosquet C, Launa JM, Rain B, Simonneau G, et al. Primary pulmonary hypertension in a patient with a familial platelet storage pool disease: role of serotonin. Am J Med. 1990;89:117–20.
53. Herve P, Launau JM, Scrobohaci M, Brenot F, Simonneau G, Petipretz P, et al. Increased plasma serotonin in primary pulmonary hypertension. Am J Med. 1995;99:249–54.
54. Kerveur A, Callebert J, Humbert M, Herve P, Simonneau J, Launay JM, Drouet L. High plasma serotonin levels in primary pulmonary hypertension. Effect of long-term epoprostenol(prostacyclin) therapy. Arterioscler Thromb Vasc Biol. 2000;20:2233–9.
55. Langleben D, Moroz LA, McGregor M, Lisbona R. Decreased half-life of fibrinogen in primary pulmonary hypertension. Thromb Res. 1985;40:577–80.
56. Giaid A, Saleh D. Reduced expression of endothelial nitric oxide synthase in the lungs of patients with pulmonary hypertension. N Engl J Med. 1995;333:214–21.
57. Archer SL, Djaballah K, Humbert M, Weir EK, Fartoukh M, Dallava-santucci J, et al. Am J Respir Crit Care Med. 1998;158:1061–7.
58. Wolf M, Boyer-Neumann C, Parent F, Eschwege V, Jaillet H, Meyer D, et al. Thrombotic risk factors in pulmonary hypertension. Eur Respir J. 2000;15:395–9.
59. Hoeper MM, Sosada M, Fabel H. Plasma coagulation profiles in patients with severe primary pulmonary hypertension. Eur Respir J. 1998;12:1446–9.
60. Lang IM, Klepeko W, Pabinger I. No increased prevalence of factor V Leiden mutation in chronic major vessel thromboembolic pulmonary hypertension (CTEPH). Thromb Haemost. 1996;76:476–7.
61. Chaouat A, Weitzenblum E, Higenbottom T. The role of thrombosis in severe pulmonary hypertension. Eur Respir J. 1996;9:356–63.
62. Girgis RE, Champion HC, Diette GB, Johns RA, Permutt S, Sylvester JT. Am J Respir Crit Care Med. 2005;172:352–7.
63. Veyradier A, Nishikubo T, Humbert M, Wolf M, Sitbon O, Simonneau G, et al. Improvement of von Willebrand factor proteolysis after prostacyclin infusion in severe pulmonary arterial hypertension. Circulation. 2000;102:2460–2.
64. Sakamaki F, Kyotani S, Nagaya N, Sato N, Oya H, Satoh T, et al. Increased plasma p-selectin and decreased thrombomodulin in pulmonary arterial hypertension were improved by continuous prostacyclin therapy. Circulation. 2000;102:2720–5.
65. Boyer-Neumann C, Brenot F, Wolf M, Peynaud-Debayle E, Duroux P, Meyer D, et al. Continuous infusion of prostacyclin decreases plasma levels of tPA and PAI-1 in pulmonary hypertension. Thromb Haemost. 1995;73:735–6.

66. Fuster V, Steele PM, Edwards WD, Gersh BJ, McGoon M, Frye RL. Primary pulmonary hypertension: natural history and importance of thrombosis. Circulation. 1984;70:580–7.
67. Frank H, Mlczoch J, Huber K, Schuster E, Gurtner P, Kneusl M. Chest. 1997;112:714–21.
68. Kawut SM, Horn EM, Berekashvili KK, Garofano RP, Goldsmith RL, Widliz AC, et al. New predictors of outcomes in idiopathic pulmonary arterial hypertension. Am J Cardiol. 2005; 95:199–203.
69. Rich S, Kaufman E, Levy PS. The effect of high doses of calcium-channel blockers on survival in primary pulmonary hypertension. N Engl J Med. 1992;327:76–81.
70. Hrachovinova JP, Ambroz D, Maresova J, Polacek P, Simkova I, Linhart A, et al. Effect of warfarin anticoagulation on thrombin generation in patients with idiopathic pulmonary arterial hypertension. Bratisi Lek Listy. 2010;111:595–8.
71. Levine MN, Raskob G, Beyth RJ, Keron C, Schulman S. Hermorrhagic complications of anticoagulant treatment: the seventh ACCP conference on antithrombotic and thrombolytic therapy. Chest. 2004;126:S287–310.
72. Optiz CF, Mueller EA, Pittrow D. Bleeding events in pulmonary arterial hypertension. Eur J Clin Invest. 2009;39:68–73.
73. Duchini A, Sessoms SL. Gastrointestinal hemorrhage in patients with systemic sclerosis and CREST syndrome. Am J Gastroenterol. 1998;1998(93):1453–6.
74. Johnson SR, Granton JT, Tomlinson GA, Grosbein HA, Le T, Lee P, et al. Warfarin in systemic sclerosis-associated and idiopathic pulmonary arterial hypertension. A Bayesian approach to evaluation treatment for uncommon disease. J Rheumatol. 2012;39:276–85.
75. Spangler ML, Saxean S. Warfarin and bosentan interactions in a patient with pulmonary hypertension secondary to bilateral pulmonary emboli. Clin Ther. 2010;32:53–6.
76. Hoeper MM, Barst RJ, Bourge RC, Feldman J, Frost AE, Galié N, Gómez-Sánchez MA, Grimminger F, Grünig E, Hassoun PM, Morrell NW, Peacock AJ, Satoh T, Simonneau G, Tapson VF, Torres F, Lawrence D, Quinn DA, Ghofrani HA. Imatinib mesylate as add-on therapy for pulmonary arterial hypertension: results of the randomized IMPRES study. Circulation. 2013;127(10):1128–38.
77. Poli D, Miniati M. The incidence of recurrent venous thromboembolism and chronic thromboembolic hypertension following a first episode of pulmonary embolism. Curr Opin Pulm Med. 2011;17:392–7.
78. Hales CA, Kradin RL, Brandstetter RD, Zhu YJ. Impairment of hypoxic pulmonary artery remodeling by heparin in mice. Am Rev Respir Dis. 1983;128:747–51.
79. Hassoun PM, Thompson BT, Hales CA. Partial reversal of hypoxic pulmonary hypertension by heparin. Am Rev Respir Dis. 1992;145:193–6.
80. Hassoun PM, Thompson BT, Steigman D, Hales CA. Effect of heparin and warfarin on chronic hypoxic pulmonary hypertension and vascular remodeling in the guinea pig. Am Rev Respir Dis. 1989;139:763–8.
81. Yu L, Quinn DA, Garg HG, Hales CA. Gene expression of cyclin-dependent kinase inhibitors and effect of heparin on their expression in mice with hypoxia-induced pulmonary hypertension. Biochem Biophys Res Commun. 2006;345:1565–72.
82. Yu L, Quinn DA, Garg HG, Hale CA. Heparin inhibits pulmonary artery smooth muscle cell proliferation through guanine nucleotide exchange factor-H1/RhoA/Rho kinase/p27. Am J Respir Crit Care Med. 2011;44:524–30.
83. Robbins IM, Kawut SM, Yung D, Reilly MP, Loyd W, Cunningham G, et al. A study of aspirin and clopidogrel in idiopathic pulmonary hypertension. Eur Respir J. 2006;27:578–84.
84. Delbeck M, Nickel KF, Perzborn E, Ellinghaus P, Strassburger J, Kast R, et al. A role for coagulation factor Xa in experimental pulmonary hypertension. Cardiovasc Res. 2011; 92:159–68.
85. Weissman N, Tadic A, Hanze J, Rose F, Winterhalder S, Nollen M, et al. Hypoxic vasoconstriction in intact lungs: a role for NADPH oxidase-derived H_2O_2? Am J Physiol Lung Cell Mol Physiol. 2000;279:L683–90.
86. Nocturnal Oxygen Therapy Trial Group. Continuous or nocturnal oxygen therapy in hypoxemic chronic obstructive lung disease. Ann Intern Med. 1980;93:391–8.

87. Long term domiciliary oxygen therapy in chronic hypoxic cor pulmonale complicating chronic bronchitis and emphysema: report of the Medical Research Council Working Party. Lancet 1981;1:681-6.
88. Timms RM, Khaja FU, Williams GW, Nocturnal Oxygen Therapy Trial Group. Hemodynamic response to oxygen therapy in chronic obstructive pulmonary disease. Ann Intern Med. 1985;102:29–36.
89. Minai O, Pandya C, Golish JA, Avecillas JF, McCarthy K, Marlow S, et al. Predictors of nocturnal oxygen desaturation in pulmonary artery hypertension. Chest. 2007;131:109–17.
90. Global strategy for the diagnosis, management, and prevention of chronic obstructive pulmonary disease: NHLBI/WHO workshop report. In: Global initiative for chronic obstructive pulmonary lung disease. Bethesda, MD: National Heart, Lung and Blood Institute; 2005 Available at http://www.goldcopd.com/Guidelineitem.asp?11=2&12=1&intID=989. Accessed October 7, 2012.
91. Owens GR, Rogers RM, Pennock B, Levin D. The diffusing capacity as a predictor of arterial oxygen desaturation during exercise in patients with chronic obstructive pulmonary disease. N Engl J Med. 1984;310:1218–21.
92. Kelley MA, Panettieri RA, Krupinski AV. Resting single-breath diffusion capacity as aw screening test for exercise-induced hypoxemia. Am J Med. 1986;80:807–12.
93. Bowyer JJ, Bust CM, Denison DM, Shinebourne EA. Effect of long term oxygen treatment at home in children with pulmonary vascular disease. Br Heart J. 1986;55:385–90.
94. Widlitz A, Barst RJ. Pulmonary artery hypertension in children. Eur Respir J. 2003;21: 155–76.
95. Sandoval J, Aguirre JS, Pulido T, Martinez-guerra L, Santos E, Avlarado P, et al. Nocturnal oxygen therapy in patients with the Eisenmenger syndrome. Am J Respir Crit Care Med. 2001;164:1682–7.
96. Koo KW, Sax DS, Snider G. Arterial blood gases and pH during sleep in chronic obstructive pulmonary disease. Am J Med. 1975;58:663–70.
97. Atwood CW, McCrory D, Garcia JG, Abman SH, Ahearn GS. Pulmonary artery hypertension and sleep-disordered breathing: ACCP evidence-based clinical practice guidelines. Chest. 2004;126:S72–7.
98. Podszus T, Bauer W, Mayer J, Penzel T, Peter JH, von Wichert P. Sleep apnea and pulmonary hypertension. Klin Wochenschr. 1986;64:131–4.
99. Alchanatis M, Tourkhhoriti G, Kakaouros S, Kosmas E, Podaras S, Jordanoglou JB. Daytime pulmonary hypertension in patients with obstructive sleep apnea. The effect of continuous positive airway pressure on pulmonary hemodynamics. Respiration. 2001;68:566–72.
100. Sakjov D, Saunders NA, Bune AJ, McEvoy RD. Continuous positive airway pressure treatment improves pulmonary hemodynamics in patients with obstructive sleep apnea. Am J Respir Crit Care Med. 2002;165:152–8.
101. Arias M, Garcia-Rio F, Alonso-Fernandes A, Martinez I, Viallamor J. Pulmonary hypertension in obstructive sleep apnoea: effects of continuous positive airway pressure: a randomized, controlled cross-over study. Eur Heart J. 2006;27:106–13.
102. Littleton SW, Mokhlesi B. The Pickwickian syndrome – obesity hypoventilation syndrome. Clin Chest Med. 2009;30:467–78.
103. Kessler R, Chaouat A, Schinkewitch P, Faller M, Casel S, Krieger J, et al. The obesity-hypoventilation syndrome revisited. A prospective study of 34 consecutive cases. Chest. 2001;120:369–76.
104. Masa JF, Celli BR, Riesco JA, Hernandez M, Sanches de Cos J, Disdier C. The obesity hypoventilation syndrome can be treated with mechanical ventilation. Chest. 2001;119: 1102–7.
105. Nowbar S, Burkart KM, Gonzales R, Fedorowicz A, Gozansky WS, Gaudio JC, et al. Obesity-associated hypoventilation in hospitalized patients: prevalence, effects, and outcome. Am J Med. 2004;116:1–7.

106. Budweiser S, Riedi SG, Jorres RA, Heinemann F, Pfeifer M. Mortality and prognostic factors in patients with obesity-hypoventilation syndrome undergoing noninvasive ventilation. J Intern Med. 2007;261:375–83.
107. ACC/AHA 2005 guideline update for the diagnosis and management of chronic heart failure in the adult. A report of the American College of Cardiology/American Heart Association Task Force for Practice Guidelines (Writing Committee to update the 2001 Guidelines for the Evaluation and Management of Heart Failure) ACC-www.acc.org; AHA-www.american-heart.org 2005; e1-e82.
108. Gan CTJ, Lankhaar JWS, Marcus T, Westerhof N, Marques KM, Bronzwaer JGF, et al. Impaired left ventricular filling due to right-to-left ventricular interaction in patients with pulmonary arterial hypertension. Am J Physiol Heart Circ Physiol. 2006;290:H1528–33.
109. Dittrich HC, Chow LC, Nicod PH. Early improvement in left ventricular diastolic function after relief of chronic right ventricular pressure overload. Circulation. 1989;80:823–30.
110. Krayenbuehl HP, Turina J, Hess O. Left ventricular function in chronic pulmonary hypertension. Am J Cardiol. 1978;41:1150–8.
111. Pitt B, Zannad F, Remme WJ, Cody R, Castaigne A, Perez A, et al. The effect of spironolactone on morbidity and mortality in patients with severe left heart failure. N Engl J Med. 1999;341:709–17.
112. Quinn DA, Du HK, Thompson BT, Hales CA. Amiloride analogs inhibit chronic hypoxic pulmonary hypertension. Am J Respir Crit Care Med. 1998;157:1263–8.
113. Rubin LJ, Peter RH. Oral hydralazine therapy for primary pulmonary hypertension. N Engl J Med. 1980;302:69–73.
114. Carmerini F, Alberti E, Klugmann S, Salvi A. Primary pulmonary hypertension: effects of nifedipine. Br Heart J. 1980;44:352–6.
115. Packer M, Greenberg B, Massie B, Dash H. Deleterious effects of hydralazine in patients with pulmonary hypertension. N Engl J Med. 1982;306:1326–31.
116. McLaughlini VV, McGoon MD. Pulmonary arterial hypertension. Circulation. 2006;114(13): 1417–31.
117. Newman JH, Phillips JA, Loyd JE. Narrative review: the enigma of pulmonary arterial hypertension: new insights from genetic studies. Ann Intern Med. 2008;148:278–83.
118. Rich S, Kaufmann E. High dose titration of calcium channel blocking agents for primary pulmonary hypertension: guidelines for short-term testing. J Am Coll Cardiol. 1991;18: 1323–7.
119. Sitbon O, Humbert M, Jais X, Ioos V, Hamid AM, Provencher S, et al. Long-term response to calcium channel blockers in idiopathic pulmonary hypertension. Circulation. 2005;111: 3105–11.
120. Elliot CG, Glissmeyer EW, Gavlena GT, Carlquist J, McKinney JT, McGoon MD, et al. Relationship of BMPR2 mutations to vasoreactivity in pulmonary arterial hypertension. Circulation. 2006;113:2509–15.
121. Humbert M, Sitbon O, Chaouat A, Bertocchi M, Habib G, Gressin V, et al. Pulmonary arterial hypertension in France. Results from a national registry. Am J Respir Crit Care Med. 2006;173:1023–30.
122. Montani D, Savale L, Natali D, Jais X, Herve P, Garcia G, et al. Long-term response to calcium-channel blockers in non-idiopathic pulmonary arterial hypertension. Eur Heart J. 2010;31:1898–907.
123. Guidelines of diagnosis and treatment of pulmonary arterial hypertension. The Task Force on Diagnosis and Treatment of Pulmonary Arterial Hypertension of the European Society of Cardiology. Eur Heart J. 2004;25:2243–78.
124. Oliveira EC, Ribeiro ALP, Amaral CFS. Adenosine for vasoreactivity testing in pulmonary hypertension: a head-to-head comparison with inhaled nitric oxide. Respir Med. 2010;104: 606–11.
125. Preston IR, Klinger JR, Houtchens J, Nelson D, Mehta S, Hill NS. Pulmonary edema caused by inhaled nitric oxide therapy in two patients with pulmonary hypertension associated with CREST syndrome. Chest. 2002;121:656–9.

126. Farber HW, Graven KK, Kokolski G, Korn JH. Pulmonary edema during acute infusion of epoprostenol in a patient with pulmonary hypertension and limited scleroderma. J Rheumatol. 1999;26:1195–6.
127. Strange C, Bolster M, Mazur J, Taylor M, Gossage JR, Silver R. Chest. Hemodynamic effects of epoprostenol in patients with systemic sclerosis and pulmonary hypertension. 2000;118:1077–82.
128. Rubin LJ, Mendoza J, Hood M, McGoon M, Barst R, Williams WB, et al. Treatment of primary pulmonary hypertension with continuous intravenous prostacyclin (epoprostenol). Results of a randomized trial. Ann Intern Med. 1990;112:485–91.
129. Palmer SM, Robinson LJ, Wang A, Gossage JR, Bashore T, Tapson VF. Massive pulmonary edema and death after prostacyclin infusion in a patient with pulmonary veno-occlusive disease. Chest. 1998;113:237–40.
130. Zakliczynski M, Zebik T, Maruszewski M, Swierad M, Zembala M. Usefulness of pulmonary hypertension reversibility test with sodium nitroprusside in stratification of early death risk after orthotopic heart transplantation. Transplant Proc. 2005;37:1346–8.
131. Barst RJ, Rubin LJ, McGoon MD, Caldwell EJ, Long WA, Levy PS. Survival in primary pulmonary hypertension with long-term continuous intravenous prostacyclin. Ann Intern Med. 1994;121:409–15.
132. Barst RJ, Rubin LJ, Long WA, McGoon MD, Rich S, Badesch DB, et al. A comparison of continous intravenous epoprostenol(prostacylin) with conventional therapy for primary pulmonary hypertension. N Engl J Med. 1996;334:296–301.
133. Rich S, Brundage BH. High-dose calcium channel-blocking therapy for primary pulmonary hypertension: evidence for long-term reduction in pulmonary arterial pressure and regression of right ventricular hypertrophy. Circulation. 1987;76(1):135–41.
134. Ziesche R, Petkov V, Wittman K, Kopatschka J, Striebellehner L, Schenk P, et al. Treatment with epoprostenol reverts nitric oxide non-responsiveness in patients with primary pulmonary hypertension. Heart. 2000;83:406–9.

Chapter 13
Prostacyclin Therapy for Pulmonary Arterial Hypertension

Ioana R. Preston

Abstract Prostacyclins are the first class of agents that showed efficacy in the treatment of pulmonary arterial hypertension (PAH) in a clinical trial and, for a long time, the only treatment specifically approved for this devastating disease. As new therapies have emerged for PAH in recent years, the class of prostacyclins has also evolved and several formulations of different prostacyclin analogs, using various routes of delivery, have been tested and shown to be efficacious in PAH. This chapter reviews the pharmacology of prostacyclins and the results of pivotal clinical trials testing various formulations. Lastly, it examines practical aspects of dosing, management of side effects, and expectations of treatment goals.

Keywords Prostacyclin • Epoprostenol • Treprostinil • Iloprost • Pulmonary hypertension

Abbreviations

6MWD	6 min walk distance
cAMP	Cyclic AMP
HETE	Hydroxyeicotetraenoic acid
HIV	Human immunodeficiency virus
IPAH	Idiopathic pulmonary arterial hypertension
LOX	Lipoxygenase
mPAP	Mean pulmonary artery pressure
NIH	National Institutes of Health
NYHA	New York Heart Association
PAH	Pulmonary arterial hypertension
PG	Prostaglandin

I.R. Preston, M.D. (✉)
Pulmonary, Critical Care and Sleep Division, Tufts Medical Center,
800 Washington Street, Box #257, Boston, MA, USA
e-mail: ipreston@tuftsmedicalcenter.org

J.R. Klinger, R.P. Frantz (eds.), *Diagnosis and Management of Pulmonary Hypertension*, Respiratory Medicine 12, DOI 10.1007/978-1-4939-2636-7_13

PGI_2	Prostacyclin
PH	Pulmonary hypertension
PVR	Pulmonary vascular resistance
TXA_2	Thromboxane A_2

Prostacyclin, Prostacyclin Receptors and Signaling

Prostaglandins (PGs) are products that are enzymatically derived from arachidonic acid and act as autocrine and paracrine effectors to regulate pulmonary vascular tone. The conversion of arachidonic acid into various PGs is achieved in a highly regulated manner and many arachidonic acid derivatives have been linked to a variety of pulmonary diseases. PGs elicit their molecular, pharmacologic, and biochemical effects through binding and activation of specific receptor sites [1]. The current nomenclature classifies prostanoid receptors as: IP, EP_1, EP_2, EP_3, EP_4, DP_1, FP, and TP receptors. The IP, EP_2, EP_4, and DP_1 receptors are classically known to be Gs-coupled receptors, linked to cyclic AMP (cAMP) generation. On the other hand, EP_1, FP, and TP couple with calcium mobilization pathways through Gq and Gi proteins [2].

Prostacyclin (PGI_2) was first described in 1976 by the Nobel prize-winning group led by Sir John Vane [3] as a product of arachidonic metabolism and is the major PG generated by the endothelium of pulmonary arteries. Prostacyclin is produced via the action of prostacyclin synthase and IP is its natural receptor. Nevertheless, the biology of prostacyclin signaling is more complex, since prostacyclin appears to have functionally relevant effects at other prostanoid receptors [4]. In fact, it is believed that the off-target effects of prostacyclin administration, such as gastrointestinal side effects (nausea, diarrhea), are due to the nonselective activation of prostanoid receptors [5, 6].

Prostacyclin has vasodilator properties and helps to maintain the low resistance of the pulmonary circuit [7]. In addition to its vasodilator effects, prostacyclin has antiplatelet activity via release of cAMP, as well as anti-inflammatory, antiproliferative, and antimitogenic actions [8–10].

Imbalance of Vasoactive Arachidonic Acid Mediators in PAH

Prostacyclin/Thromboxane A_2 Imbalance in the Pathogenesis of PAH

Thromboxane A_2 (TXA_2) is produced from arachidonic acid via the action of thromboxane synthase and opposes the actions of prostacyclin by promoting vasoconstriction, platelet aggregation, and smooth muscle cell proliferation [11]. In pulmonary arterial hypertension (PAH), the balance between these two molecules is shifted toward TXA_2. Using a rat model, Rabinovitch et al. [12] showed that induction of prostacyclin release prevents hypoxic pulmonary hypertension (PH) and vascular remodeling. Conversely, mice overexpressing prostacyclin synthase are protected against the development of hypoxic PH [13]. The abnormalities in prostacyclin/TXA_2 described in experimental models of PH were also found in human disease [14]. Lung expression of prostacyclin synthase is decreased in PAH patients [15] and this translates to a decrease in urinary levels of 2,3-dinor-6-keto-prostaglandin F1α, a metabolite of prostacyclin, and an increase in urinary levels of 11-dehydro-thromboxane B_2, a metabolite of TXA_2 [16].

Abnormal Hydroxyeicosatetraenoic Acid (HETE) Metabolism in PAH

In addition to PGI_2 and TXA_2, lung vasculature synthesizes various hydroxyeicotetraenoic acids (HETEs) from arachidonic acid and several reports suggest that they participate in vascular remodeling of experimental PH [17–22]. HETEs are produced enzymatically via a group of enzymes called lipoxygenases (LOX), cytochrome P450 isoenzymes, and cyclooxygenases [23]. Several reports suggest that the three major LOXs (5-, 12-, and 15-LOX) participate in vascular remodeling in PH [17–19]. 5-LOX inhibitors attenuate the growth of human pulmonary artery endothelial cells in culture, while 5-LOX overexpression in rat lungs worsens the severity of PH in the monocrotaline model. Conversely, 5-LOX inhibitors prevent the development of the disease [20]. Similarly, 12-LOX gene expression is increased and 12-LOX protein is upregulated in the lungs of hypoxic rats and 12-HETE, the major product of 12-LOX, stimulates proliferation of pulmonary artery smooth muscle cells through a MAPK-dependent mechanism [19]. 15-HETE mediates hypoxic pulmonary vasoconstriction [21, 22] and displays antiapoptotic effects in pulmonary artery smooth muscle cells [24].

Early Trials of Prostacyclin Infusion

In the early to mid 1980s, individual experience and small-scale registries showed that continuous infusion of the prostacyclin analog epoprostenol produced improvement in symptoms and hemodynamics in selected patients with advanced PAH [25–30]. At the same time, investigators began testing acute vasodilatory response to epoprostenol in PAH during right heart catheterization because it was unclear whether only patients with an acute hemodynamic improvement (drop in pulmonary artery pressure, increased cardiac output) benefited from prostacyclin therapy. Hemodynamic measurements performed at baseline and after acute PGI_2 administration demonstrated benefits in lowering pulmonary artery pressure (PAP) and pulmonary vascular resistance (PVR). Interestingly, subjects lacking an acute hemodynamic response to vasodilatory testing still appeared to benefit from long-term treatment [31].

Clinical Trials with Epoprostenol in PAH

The encouraging initial experience with epoprostenol was followed by positive results from the first randomized trial in 18 patients with PAH in which epoprostenol improved pulmonary hemodynamics, exercise capacity, and symptoms [31]. The open-label extension trial also reported improvements in hemodynamics and exercise capacity, as measured by the 6 min walk distance (6MWD) [32]. Although significant adverse events including sepsis, two deaths and a rapid deterioration were reported, most were attributed to the infusion system causing thrombus, sepsis, and pump malfunction. This trial supported prior evidence that epoprostenol is effective in PAH. The pivotal, prospective controlled trial randomized 81 idiopathic PAH (IPAH) patients with New York Heart Association (NYHA) functional class 3 and 4 symptoms who had failed calcium channel blocker therapy to receive either epoprostenol in addition to standard of care or standard of care alone for 12 weeks [33]. Epoprostenol was gradually uptitrated and at the end of the study the average dose was 9.2 ng/kg/min. The primary endpoint, 6MWD, improved significantly in the treatment group from a median of 315 to 362 m, while the standard of care group worsened from a median of 270 to 204 m ($p<0.002$). Hemodynamic improvement was evidenced by a significant decrease in mean PAP of 8 % and PVR of 21 % in the epoprostenol group versus an increase of 3 % and 9 %, respectively in the conventional group. Eight patients died during the 12-week trial, all in the conventional therapy group, conferring a significant survival benefit in the treated group ($p<0.003$) (Fig. 13.1). Nonfatal adverse events in the treatment group included four episodes of sepsis and one episode of thromboembolism. This pivotal study, which is the only study to date to show an improvement in survival in PAH, led to the

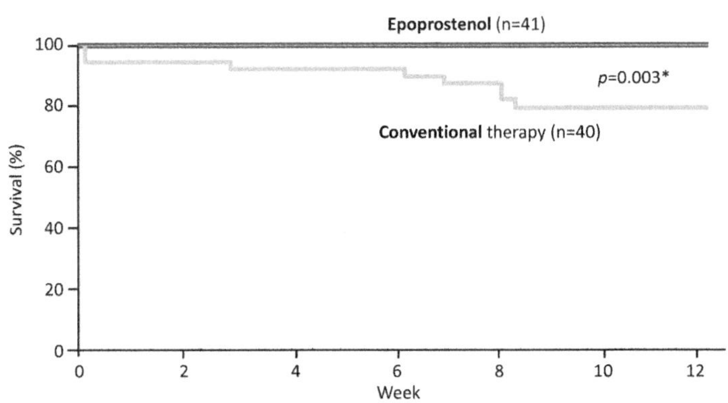

Fig. 13.1 Survival among the 41 patients treated with epoprostenol and the 40 patients receiving conventional therapy. Data on patients who underwent transplantation during the 12-week study were censored at the time of transplantation. Estimates were made by the Kaplan–Meier product-limit method. The two-sided p value from the log-rank test was 0.003. Survival analysis with data on patients receiving transplants not censored at transplantation resulted in the same level of significance (two-sided $p=0.003$ by the log-rank test). From [33]

approval of epoprostenol by the FDA as the first drug indicated for the treatment of PAH in December 1995.

A second prospective randomized controlled trial of epoprostenol was conducted in patients with PAH associated with scleroderma [34]. One hundred and twenty-one symptomatic patients in NYHA functional class 3 or 4 were randomized 1:1 to epoprostenol versus standard of care. At the end of the 12-week period, patients randomized to epoprostenol were receiving an average of 11.2 ng/kg/min of epoprostenol. The main outcome, 6MWD, improved from a median of 270 to 316 m in the treated group, while the group assigned to standard of care declined from a median of 240 to 192 m ($p<0.001$). Similarly, significant improvements in functional class and pulmonary hemodynamics were noted in the treated arm, while mortality was not different.

Initial Dose and Titration Strategy

Epoprostenol continuous infusion is usually initiated at a dose of 2 ng/kg/min and the dose is gradually uptitrated over the next several months. Although the frequency of titration and the average dose used varies from center to center and from country to country, the general rule is to uptitrate once or twice a week by a few ng/kg/min in the first month, until side effects occur. Thereafter, uptitration is performed at a slower pace over the following months to improve exercise capacity, functional class, and hemodynamics, while minimizing side effects. The side effect profile of epoprostenol is usually well tolerated in most subjects. These include flushing, headache, nausea, loose stools, jaw discomfort with "first bite," and foot pain with prolonged standing or walking (Table 13.1) [35–37].

Experience with Epoprostenol Infusion in PAH

In an open-label trial of 18 patients with IPAH, Kaplan–Meier estimates of 1-, 2- and 3-year survival were 86.9 %, 72.4 %, and 63.3 %, respectively, compared with 77.4 %, 51.6 %, and 40.6 % observed prior to the development of epoprostenol [38]. Cohort analyses in Europe and in the United States have provided convincing evidence of the long-term benefits of epoprostenol infusion. One year of epoprostenol therapy in 162 IPAH patients from France was associated with improvements in clinical function and hemodynamics [35]. Similarly, 178 IPAH patients treated in the US had improved survival compared with that observed in the NIH registry which was conducted before epoprostenol was developed and used as a historical control [36]. The survival rate at 1 year was 85 % vs. 58 %, 2 years 70 % vs. 43 %, 3 years 63 % vs. 33 %, and at 5 years 55 % vs. 28 % ($p<0.001$). Adverse prognostic factors included a clinical history of right heart failure, advanced functional class, and hemodynamic parameters such as an elevated right atrial pressure and depressed cardiac index.

Table 13.1 Side effects and complications of parenteral and inhaled prostacyclins

	Route of administration
Side effects	
Headache	Intravenous, subcutaneous, inhaled
Jaw pain with first bite	Intravenous, subcutaneous, inhaled
Nausea, vomiting	Intravenous, subcutaneous, inhaled
Diarrhea	Intravenous, subcutaneous, inhaled
Leg pain	Intravenous, subcutaneous, inhaled
Flushing, rash	Intravenous, subcutaneous, inhaled
Restlessness	Intravenous, subcutaneous, inhaled
Cough	Inhaled
Site pain	Subcutaneous
Complications	
Line infection	Intravenous
Bloodstream infection, sepsis	Intravenous
Catheter breakage, occlusion	Intravenous, subcutaneous
Pump malfunction	Intravenous, subcutaneous
Hemorrhage from the site	Intravenous, subcutaneous
Syncope	Intravenous, subcutaneous, inhaled
Paradoxical embolism	Intravenous
Thrombocytopenia	Intravenous, subcutaneous

Long-term administration of PG requires a permanent central venous catheter and a portable infusion pump [37]. The complex delivery system requires education regarding sterile technique, operation of the pump, and care of the catheter. The original formulation of epoprostenol (Flolan®) needs to be prepared daily and requires that the drug cassette be kept cool with ice packs due to limited stability of the drug at room temperature (approximately 8 h at room temperature). A strong support system, and a "partner" who is willing to learn how to mix and deliver the drug is strongly recommended to obviate problems if the subject is too ill or unable to prepare medication on a given day. Serious complications include infection (exit site and/or bacteremia) thrombosis of the catheter, and risk of temporary interruption of the infusion because of iatrogenic "switching" or pump malfunction (Table 13.1) [39]. The incidence of catheter-related sepsis ranges from 0.1 to 0.6 cases per patient-year [26, 39].

Evidence also supports epoprostenol use in PAH from associated etiologies. Similar improvements in exercise functional capacity and functional class have been seen in subjects with PAH associated with congenital left-to-right cardiac shunts [40], portal hypertension [41], and human immunodeficiency virus (HIV) infection [42].

Generic epoprostenol sodium was approved by the FDA in April 2008 as a therapeutic equivalent to branded epoprostenol (Flolan®), based on pharmacologic bioequivalence. Generic epoprostenol was available in the US for a brief period of time after its approval, although its production was interrupted due to manufacturer-related problems. In addition to generic epoprostenol, FDA approved epoprostenol-ES (Veletri®) in 2010, a new epoprostenol formulation that has greater drug stability at room temperature. After reconstituting as directed, epoprostenol-ES is stable for up to 5 days when refrigerated (36–46 F; 2–8 °C), or up to 48 h at room temperature (77 F; 25 °C), which makes the use of frozen gel packs unnecessary and allows more drug to be prepared in advance for convenient storage [43]. Recent experience supports the safety and efficacy of epoprostenol-ES as new therapy and as a transition from epoprostenol [44, 45].

Parenteral Prostacyclin Analogs

Treprostinil is a tricyclic benzidene prostacyclin analog that shares pharmacologic actions similar to epoprostenol, including antiproliferative activity on human pulmonary arterial smooth muscle cells [46]. Treprostinil differs from epoprostenol in that it is highly chemically stable at room temperature and neutral pH and has a longer half-life (3–4 h) [47]. The improved stability of this compound and its solubility at physiologic pH enables subcutaneous infusion, thereby avoiding the potential complications of the intravenous delivery system used for epoprostenol administration. The bioavailability of subcutaneous treprostinil is excellent, as demonstrated in healthy volunteers [47].

Subcutaneous treprostinil was approved in 2002 for the treatment of PAH patients of NYHA class II–IV. A 12-week multicenter, randomized, double-blind trial that enrolled patients with idiopathic PAH, PAH related to congenital heart defects or connective tissue disease, compared treprostinil to placebo in 470 patients [48]. Treprostinil significantly improved the main outcome, 6MWD, as well as dyspnea, fatigue, and signs and symptoms of pulmonary hypertension. At 12 weeks, there was also an improvement in hemodynamic parameters, including right atrial pressure, mean PAP, PVR and cardiac output. Although the 6MWD improvement in the treatment arm was minimal (a median difference of 16 m, compared with the placebo group), there was a clear dose–response relationship, with patients receiving more than 13.8 ng/kg/min increasing their walk distance by 36 m, while those receiving less than 10 ng/kg/min showing no improvement (Fig. 13.2). In a subset analysis from the subcutaneous trials, patients who had PAH related to connective tissue disease also experienced improvement in exercise capacity, symptoms of PAH, and pulmonary hemodynamics [49].

Subcutaneous infusion of treprostinil does not require daily mixing and preparation of the infusion. The drug comes premixed and the pump reservoir holds enough drug for approximately 72 h of infusion. There is no need for ice packs, or intravenous catheter care. The infusion site can be changed every 3–4 days, although some patients use the same site for 3–6 weeks, as long as the site is clean and pain at the site of infusion is tolerable. The most common side effect is pain at the site of infusion, which responds usually to a combination of local anesthetic solutions, nonsteroidal anti-inflammatories, gabapentins, or low-dose narcotics (Table 13.1) [50].

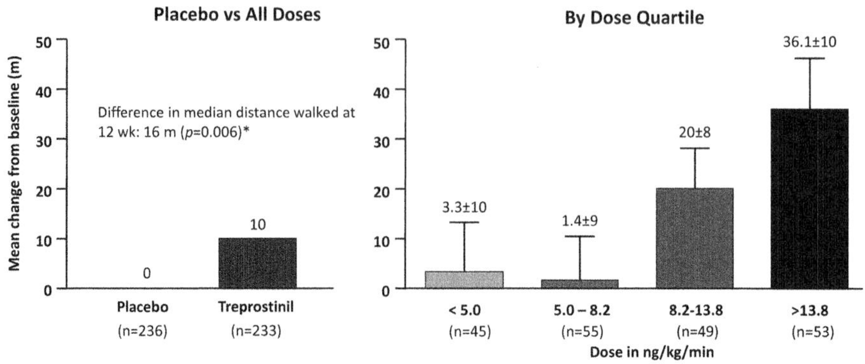

Fig. 13.2 Mean change in the 6-min walk distance from baseline to week 12 versus week 12 treprostinil dose quartile. From [48]

Usually the pain subsides within 48 h after the start of a new site. The most common site of infusion is the abdomen, although some patients prefer the flank, thigh, or shoulder area.

The FDA has also approved the use of intravenous treprostinil based on bioequivalence to its subcutaneous formulation [47]. The advantage over intravenous epoprostenol is that the cassette is changed every other day and, unlike the original form of epoprostenol (Flolan) but same as the newer form (Veletri) it does not require ice packs. The longer half-life of intravenous treprostinil may also decrease the risk of cardiovascular collapse in case of inadvertent temporary interruption of the infusion. In a prospective, open-label study, 31 PAH patients stable on intravenous epoprostenol were transitioned to intravenous treprostinil [51]. Twenty-seven patients completed the 12-week protocol and four patients transitioned back to epoprostenol. Treprostinil was dosed to minimize side effects, while avoiding symptom worsening. Overall, patients maintained their walks and functional class, although pulmonary hemodynamics worsened slightly, suggesting that treprostinil is an alternative to intravenous epoprostenol in selected patients who are being followed very closely. It is important to note that treprostinil is less potent than epoprostenol on a per ng basis, so higher doses may be required. Long-term experience with intravenous treprostinil was reported in a 48-week prospective, multicenter, open-label trial in 16 PAH patients on no prior PAH-specific therapy and in 31 patients transitioned from intravenous epoprostenol [52]. In de novo patients, intravenous treprostinil increased the 6MWD by a mean of 125 m and improved secondary endpoints, while 23 of the transitioned patients maintained their walks and functional class. Five patients died during the trial of causes not related to the therapy and seven discontinued due to adverse events. Lastly, a 12-week multicenter, randomized, double-blind, placebo-controlled trial was conducted in India [53]. Forty-four patients were enrolled before the study was terminated early due to safety concerns. A high number of adverse events related to catheter placement and sepsis were seen in both the placebo and treprostinil treatment arms. The end of the study analysis showed that treprostinil increased 6MWD by a placebo-corrected median of 83 m ($p=0.008$) and improved functional class and dyspnea score.

As intravenous treprostinil requires the same delivery system as epoprostenol, concerns over catheter-related complications are also present. An early report to Center of Disease Control and Prevention showed higher bloodstream infections with treprostinil compared with epoprostenol, especially with gram-negative water-born bacteria [54]. Subsequent modifications in the delivery system to a closed hub system, as well as using Flolan diluent that has a higher pH than the normal saline diluent designed for use with treprostinil, showed a decrease in the risk of bloodstream infections [55, 56].

Inhaled Prostacyclins

The rationale of using the inhaled route for prostacyclin delivery came from the notion that local distribution would avoid systemic side effects and complications associated with parenteral administration. Iloprost is a prostacyclin analog that has been used intravenously in some countries in Europe. Early trials demonstrated acute and chronic (3 months) pulmonary vasodilator properties of iloprost [57]. Its acute effect lasted 90 min. Subsequently, the pivotal randomized placebo-controlled trial of inhaled iloprost enrolled 203 patients with IPAH, PAH associated with connective tissue disease, drugs and toxins, or chronic thromboembolic disease in NYHA functional class 3 and 4 [58]. Patients averaged 7.5 inhalation treatments a day. When compared with the placebo arm, significantly more patients receiving iloprost reached the primary endpoint, defined as the combination of functional class improvement and increase in 6MWD of at least 10 % in the absence of deterioration or death. In addition, significant improvements were recorded in dyspnea and quality of life scores, as well as in post-inhalational hemodynamic parameters (Fig. 13.3).

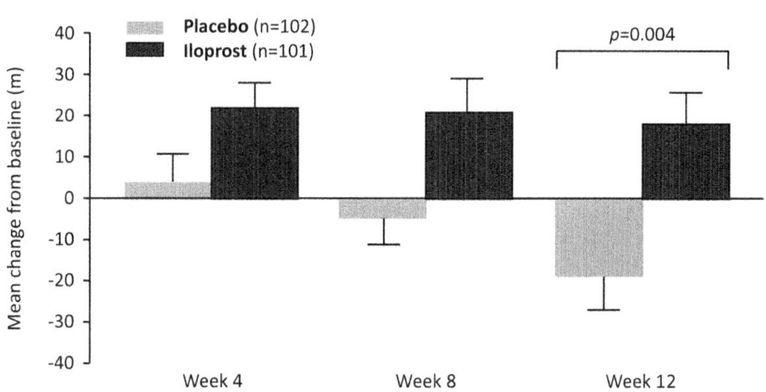

Fig. 13.3 Effect of inhaled iloprost and placebo on the mean (±SE) change from baseline in the distance walked in 6 min, according to an intention-to-treat analysis. The *p* value was obtained with Wilcoxon's test for two independent samples. From [58]

There was a trend toward more syncopal events in the treatment arm. Subsequently, long-term experience with inhaled iloprost was reported in 24 patients treated for at least 1 year [59]. Nevertheless, the limitations of efficacy of inhaled iloprost when compared with parenteral prostacyclins were described in selected patients who deteriorated on the inhaled therapy and were rescued by transitioning to intravenous epoprostenol or intravenous iloprost [60], suggesting the possibility that the total dose delivered and/or the short half-life (20 min) are limiting factors in achieving efficacy. Another application for inhaled iloprost has been in combination therapy for PAH. STEP II trial (iloprost inhalation solution Safety and pilot efficacy Trial in combination with bosentan for Evaluation in Pulmonary arterial hypertension) randomized 65 patients to add inhaled iloprost or placebo to bosentan [61]. Twelve weeks of combination therapy improved NYHA functional class, pulmonary hemodynamics, and time to clinical worsening compared to placebo. As a result of these trials, inhaled iloprost is approved by the FDA as monotherapy, or in combination with bosentan for PAH patients in functional class III or IV. The drug is administered via a dedicated aerosolization device at least six times a day. Mild symptoms of prostacyclin overdose such as headache, jaw pain, as well as cough have been reported. Although the current device is easy to use, has batteries and is light, the main drawback of inhaled iloprost is the frequency of administration (6–9 times a day), which makes compliance a major issue.

The second inhaled prostacyclin available is inhaled treprostinil. In a cross-over study comparing acute effects of inhaled treprostinil with inhaled iloprost, both agents produced similar improvement in PVR [62]. However, the peak effect occurred later and the duration of effect lasted longer with inhaled treprostinil, suggesting the need for less frequent administration with inhaled treprostinil. Based on initial results as well as pilot studies in patients with PAH, a randomized, placebo-controlled study was conducted to evaluate the safety and efficacy of inhaled treprostinil in PAH patients on background oral therapies. TRIUMPH-I (Treprostinil Sodium Inhalation Used in the Management of Pulmonary Arterial Hypertension) randomized 235 patients who were stable on bosentan or sildenafil to receive placebo or inhaled treprostinil at a dose of nine inhalations four times a day. At 12 weeks, the placebo-corrected median increase in 6MWD was significantly greater in the treatment arm compared with placebo [63]. Although dyspnea score, NYHA functional class and time to clinical worsening were not significantly better in patients who received inhaled treprostinil, quality of life scores and plasma NT-pro-BNP levels were improved. Inhaled treprostinil is delivered four times a day via an OptiNeb ultrasonic nebulizer (NebuTec, Germany). Overall, inhaled treprostinil is well tolerated, with adverse effects consistent with prostacyclin effects, as well as cough.

Oral Prostacyclin Analogs

Given the cumbersome administration of parenteral prostacyclins and the limitations of inhaled therapies, oral prostacyclin analogs have been tested for their ease of administration. Beraprost is an oral prostacyclin analog available in Japan.

A randomized trial conducted in Japan found improved survival with beraprost compared with conventional treatment (76 % versus 44 %, respectively) [64]. A 3-month randomized trial conducted in Europe showed significant improvements in 6MWD and functional class with beraprost, although hemodynamics did not improve [35]. A subsequent 12-month multicenter trial failed to show sustained benefit in the treatment arm, although there were significant improvements in 6MWD at 3 and 6 months [65]. For this reason, beraprost has not been approved in the US for the treatment of PAH. Most recently, the oral formulation of treprostinil was studied in three multicenter, randomized placebo-controlled trials. FREEDOM-C was a multicenter, double-blind, placebo-controlled trial that randomized 350 patients on background oral therapies (endothelin receptor antagonists and/or phosphodiesterase 5 inhibitors) [66]. Placebo-corrected median improvement in 6MWD was 11 m and not significantly greater than in controls ($p = 0.07$), although there were significant improvements in dyspnea score and in the combined 6MWD and dyspnea score. The increase from baseline in 6MWD was 4 m for patients who achieved a dose of <1 mg twice daily or discontinued due to side effects, 18 m for patients who achieved a week-16 dose of 1.25–3.25 mg twice daily and 34 m for patients who were on a dose of 3.5–16 mg twice daily, suggesting a dose-related efficacy. In the FREEDOM-C2 trial, 310 patients stable on endothelin receptor antagonists and/or phosphodiesterase 5 inhibitors were randomized to receive placebo or active drug over 16 weeks [67]. At the initiation of study drug, the first dose was lower than in the initial FREEDOM-C trial and the drug was better tolerated. The mean dose was 3.1 ± 1.9 mg twice a day. However, the placebo-corrected median difference in 6MWD did not achieve statistical significance (10 m, $p = 0.089$), nor did secondary endpoints. Lastly, FREEDOM-M was a multicenter, placebo-controlled double-blind study which evaluated oral treprostinil as monotherapy for PAH [68]. Three hundred and forty-nine patients were randomized over 12 weeks to receive active drug or placebo. There were significant improvements in the primary outcome, 6MWD, compared with placebo. In the intention-to-treat analysis, the improvement was 26 m ($p = 0.0001$) at peak and 17 m ($p = 0.0025$) at trough plasma study concentrations (Fig. 13.4). Secondary endpoints did not achieve statistical significance. The side effects most commonly encountered in the three studies were headache, diarrhea, nausea, flushing, and jaw pain. As a result of the FREEDOM studies in conjunction with recognition of the effectiveness of the previously approved non-oral formulations of treprostinil, oral treprostinil became the first oral prostacyclin analog approved by the FDA for the treatment of PAH. Oral treprostinil can be given twice or three times a day and should be administered with food to minimize gastrointestinal side effects. Three times daily dosing seems to be better tolerated than twice daily dosing, reflecting fewer swings in plasma levels. The dose is titrated as tolerated to achieve improvement in symptoms and exercise capacity. Caution needs to be exercised when patients cannot take oral medications, such as those undergoing surgical procedures, as long interruptions may necessitate its reintroduction at a lower dose and/or temporary use of parenteral prostacyclin replacement therapy.

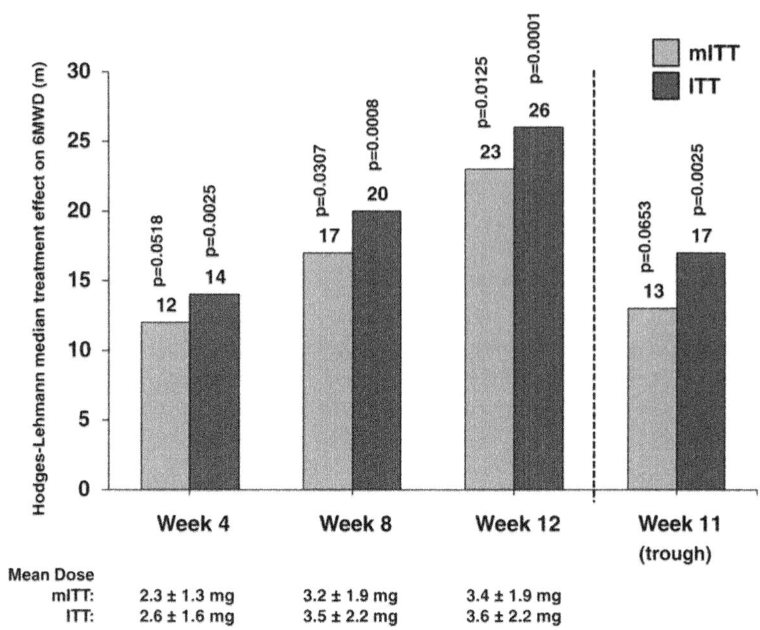

Fig. 13.4 Change in 6-min walk distance (6MWD). 6MWD at weeks 4, 8, and 12 was recorded at estimated peak plasma study drug concentrations; week 11 was recorded at estimated trough plasma study drug concentrations. For the modified intent-to-treat (mITT) population at week 12, there was a median treatment effect of 23 m ($p = 0.0125$). Results presented as placebo-corrected Hodges-Lehmann between-treatment median difference for the mITT and intent-to-treat (ITT) populations. Mean ± SD oral treprostinil dose (twice daily) included for completers at each study time point. From [67], with permission

Investigational Prostacyclins

Selexipag is a derivative of 4,5-diphenyloxazole, an oral pro-drug that is hydrolyzed to the active metabolite, a selective IP receptor agonist with high affinity for the IP receptor. In a phase 2 study, Simonneau et al. reported data on 43 symptomatic PAH patients stable on an endothelin receptor antagonist and/or phosphodiesterase 5 inhibitor who were randomized to active drug or placebo [69]. The dose was uptitrated from 200 μg twice a day to maximum 800 μg twice a day as tolerated. There was a significant decrease in PVR as the primary outcome (30.3 % reduction in geometric mean PVR, $p = 0.0045$) with good safety and tolerability profile (Fig. 13.5). A large multicenter, placebo-controlled, double-blind, event-driven study enrolling 1,156 PAH patients on background endothelin receptor antagonist and/or phosphodiesterase 5 inhibitor has recently been completed. The primary outcome was time to first clinical worsening and the results should be forthcoming [70].

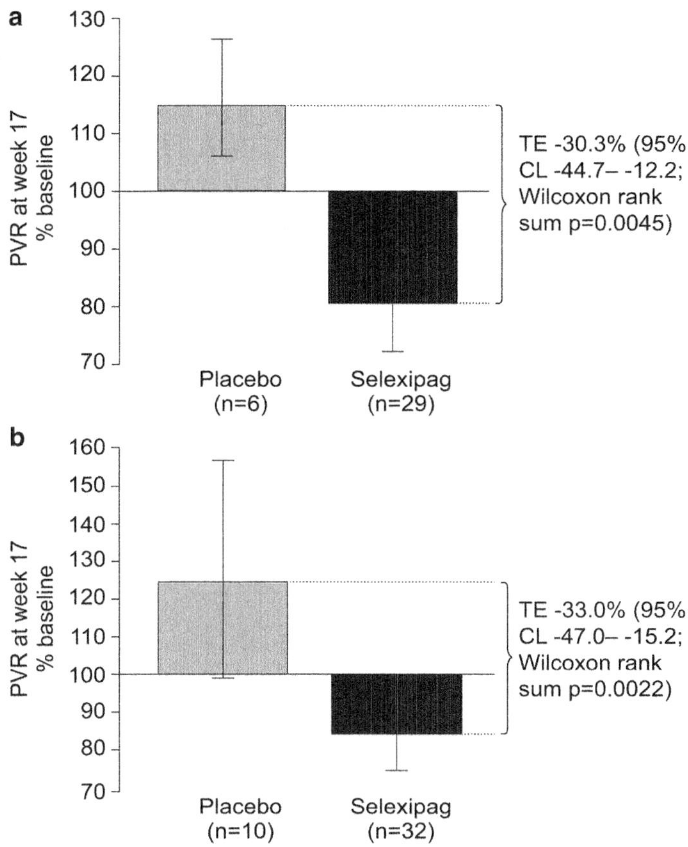

Fig. 13.5 Change in pulmonary vascular resistance (PVR) from baseline to week 17. (**a**) Per protocol set and (**b**) all-treated set. Data are presented as means and error bars represent 95 % confidence limits (CL). Baseline PVR values (mean ± SD) for per protocol population for selexipag were 951.9 ± 434.5 dyn s cm^{-5} and for placebo were 826.8 ± 195.8 dyn s cm^{-5}. Baseline PVR values (mean ± SD) for the all-treated population for selexipag were 948.6 ± 428.0 dyn s cm^{-5} and for placebo were 867.2 ± 379.38 dyn s cm^{-5}. *TE* treatment effect. From [68]

Lastly, novel delivery systems for intravenous prostacyclins are being investigated with the goal to increase patient convenience and decrease the risk of bloodstream infections or catheter failure. For this purpose, implantable pump delivery systems are being studied for intravenous treprostinil. The Lenus Pro™ pump has been used for this purpose, though lacks the option of adjusting pump infusion rate, necessitating changing the concentration of the treprostinil in order to change the dose [71]. The purpose of the DellVery trial (Device Implantable Intravascular Catheter to deliver Remodulin in PAH) is to assess the safety of the Model 10642 Implantable intravascular catheter used in combination with the SynchroMed II implantable infusion system to deliver treprostinil intravenously [72]. The study has enrolled patients stable on intravenous treprostinil and the primary endpoint is the rate of catheter-related complications per 1,000 patient days. While the SynchroMed II has been approved for delivery of other therapies, such as cancer treatments, it has not been approved to deliver treprostinil. If proven to be safe, this mode of delivery will most likely improve the quality of life of PAH patients requiring intravenous treprostinil.

Conclusions

There are currently multiple formulations and routes of administration of prostacyclin analogs and more are under investigation. The intravenous and subcutaneous prostacyclins have been available for many years and there is a fair amount of experience in clinical practice. The inhaled prostacyclins are being used increasingly due to their convenience over the parenteral systems and milder systemic side effects. The first oral formulation has been only recently approved and clinical experience is limited. Presently available data do not suggest that the various forms of prostacyclin therapy have equivalent efficacy. Current treatment guidelines recommend the use of intravenous epoprostenol over other forms of prostacyclin for PAH patients with advanced disease (NYHA functional class IV). The choice of therapy for individual patient should take into consideration the severity of the disease, the patient's capability of handling complex systems, individual preference, and goals of therapy. Regardless of the therapy chosen, patients need to be monitored closely for adequate titration of the drug in order to achieve the specific goals and to avoid serious adverse effects and complications.

References

1. Hirata T, Narumiya S. Prostanoid receptors. Chem Rev. 2011;111:6209–30.
2. Coleman RA, Smith WL, Narumiya S. International Union of Pharmacology classification of prostanoid receptors: properties, distribution, and structure of the receptors and their subtypes. Pharmacol Rev. 1994;46:205–29.
3. Moncada S, Gryglewski R, Bunting S, Vane JR. An enzyme isolated from arteries transforms prostaglandin endoperoxides to an unstable substance that inhibits platelet aggregation. Nature. 1976;263:663–5.
4. Orie NN, Clapp LH. Role of prostanoid IP and EP receptors in mediating vasorelaxant responses to PGI2 analogues in rat tail artery: evidence for Gi/o modulation via EP3 receptors. Eur J Pharmacol. 2011;654:258–65.
5. Kiriyama M, Ushikubi F, Kobayashi T, Hirata M, Sugimoto Y, Narumiya S. Ligand binding specificities of the eight types and subtypes of the mouse prostanoid receptors expressed in Chinese hamster ovary cells. Br J Pharmacol. 1997;122:217–24.
6. Narumiya S, Sugimoto Y, Ushikubi F. Prostanoid receptors: structures, properties, and functions. Physiol Rev. 1999;79:1193–226.
7. Moncada S, Radomski MW, Palmer RM. Endothelium-derived relaxing factor. Identification as nitric oxide and role in the control of vascular tone and platelet function. Biochem Pharmacol. 1988;37:2495–501.

8. Lovgren AK, Jania LA, Hartney JM, et al. COX-2-derived prostacyclin protects against bleomycin-induced pulmonary fibrosis. Am J Physiol Lung Cell Mol Physiol. 2006;291: L144–56.
9. Sinzinger H, Silberbauer K, Winter M, Auerswald W. Is human arterial smooth muscle cell proliferation regulated by prostacyclin? Exp Pathol. 1979;17:354–6.
10. Vane JR, Botting RM. Pharmacodynamic profile of prostacyclin. Am J Cardiol. 1995;75: 3A–10.
11. Sachinidis A, Flesch M, Ko Y, et al. Thromboxane A2 and vascular smooth muscle cell proliferation. Hypertension. 1995;26:771–80.
12. Rabinovitch M, Mullen M, Rosenberg HC, Maruyama K, O'Brodovich H, Olley PM. Angiotensin II prevents hypoxic pulmonary hypertension and vascular changes in rat. Am J Physiol. 1988;254:H500–8.
13. Geraci MW, Gao B, Shepherd DC, et al. Pulmonary prostacyclin synthase overexpression in transgenic mice protects against development of hypoxic pulmonary hypertension. J Clin Invest. 1999;103:1509–15.
14. Christman BW. Lipid mediator dysregulation in primary pulmonary hypertension. Chest. 1998;114:205S–7.
15. Tuder RM, Cool CD, Geraci MW, et al. Prostacyclin synthase expression is decreased in lungs from patients with severe pulmonary hypertension. Am J Respir Crit Care Med. 1999;159: 1925–32.
16. Christman BW, McPherson CD, Newman JH, et al. An imbalance between the excretion of thromboxane and prostacyclin metabolites in pulmonary hypertension. N Engl J Med. 1992;327:70–5.
17. Casey LC, Fletcher JR, Zmudka MI, Ramwell PW. Prevention of endotoxin-induced pulmonary hypertension in primates by the use of a selective thromboxane synthetase inhibitor, OKY 1581. J Pharmacol Exp Ther. 1982;222:441–6.
18. Dusting GJ, Moncada S, Vane JR. Prostaglandins, their intermediates and precursors: cardiovascular actions and regulatory roles in normal and abnormal circulatory systems. Prog Cardiovasc Dis. 1979;21:405–30.
19. Preston IR, Hill NS, Warburton RR, Fanburg BL. Role of 12-lipoxygenase in hypoxia-induced rat pulmonary artery smooth muscle cell proliferation. Am J Physiol Lung Cell Mol Physiol. 2006;290:L367–74.
20. Jones JE, Walker JL, Song Y, et al. Effect of 5-lipoxygenase on the development of pulmonary hypertension in rats. Am J Physiol Heart Circ Physiol. 2004;286:H1775–84.
21. Li S, Ran Y, Zheng X, et al. 15-HETE mediates sub-acute hypoxia-induced TRPC1 expression and enhanced capacitative calcium entry in rat distal pulmonary arterial myocytes. Prostaglandins Other Lipid Mediat. 2010;93:60–74.
22. Zhu D, Medhora M, Campbell WB, Spitzbarth N, Baker JE, Jacobs ER. Chronic hypoxia activates lung 15-lipoxygenase, which catalyzes production of 15-HETE and enhances constriction in neonatal rabbit pulmonary arteries. Circ Res. 2003;92:992–1000.
23. Funk CD. Prostaglandins and leukotrienes: advances in eicosanoid biology. Science. 2001; 294:1871–5.
24. Nie X, Song S, Zhang L, et al. 15-Hydroxyeicosatetraenoic acid (15-HETE) protects pulmonary artery smooth muscle cells from apoptosis via inducible nitric oxide synthase (iNOS) pathway. Prostaglandins Other Lipid Mediat. 2012;97:50–9.
25. Reeves JT, Groves BM, Turkevich D. The case for treatment of selected patients with primary pulmonary hypertension. Am Rev Respir Dis. 1986;134:342–6.
26. Sitbon O, Humbert M, Nunes H, et al. Long-term intravenous epoprostenol infusion in primary pulmonary hypertension: prognostic factors and survival. J Am Coll Cardiol. 2002;40:780–8.
27. Rubin LJ, Groves BM, Reeves JT, Frosolono M, Handel F, Cato AE. Prostacyclin-induced acute pulmonary vasodilation in primary pulmonary hypertension. Circulation. 1982;66:334–8.
28. Weir EK, Rubin LJ, Ayres SM, et al. The acute administration of vasodilators in primary pulmonary hypertension. Experience from the National Institutes of Health Registry on Primary Pulmonary Hypertension. Am Rev Respir Dis. 1989;140:1623–30.

29. Higenbottam T, Wheeldon D, Wells F, Wallwork J. Long-term treatment of primary pulmonary hypertension with continuous intravenous epoprostenol (prostacyclin). Lancet. 1984;1: 1046–7.
30. Jones DK, Higenbottam TW, Wallwork J. Treatment of primary pulmonary hypertension intravenous epoprostenol (prostacyclin). Br Heart J. 1987;57:270–8.
31. Rubin LJ, Mendoza J, Hood M, et al. Treatment of primary pulmonary hypertension with continuous intravenous prostacyclin (epoprostenol). Results of a randomized trial. Ann Intern Med. 1990;112:485–91.
32. Barst RJ, Rubin LJ, McGoon MD, Caldwell EJ, Long WA, Levy PS. Survival in primary pulmonary hypertension with long-term continuous intravenous prostacyclin. Ann Intern Med. 1994;121:409–15.
33. Barst RJ, Rubin LJ, Long WA, et al. A comparison of continuous intravenous epoprostenol (prostacyclin) with conventional therapy for primary pulmonary hypertension. The Primary Pulmonary Hypertension Study Group. N Engl J Med. 1996;334:296–302.
34. Badesch DB, Tapson VF, McGoon MD, et al. Continuous intravenous epoprostenol for pulmonary hypertension due to the scleroderma spectrum of disease. A randomized, controlled trial. [see comment]. Ann Intern Med. 2000;132:425–34.
35. Galie N, Humbert M, Vachiery JL, et al. Effects of beraprost sodium, an oral prostacyclin analogue, in patients with pulmonary arterial hypertension: a randomized, double-blind, placebo-controlled trial. J Am Coll Cardiol. 2002;39:1496–502.
36. McLaughlin VV, Shillington A, Rich S. Survival in primary pulmonary hypertension: the impact of epoprostenol therapy. Circulation. 2002;106:1477–82.
37. Barst RJ. Diagnosis and treatment of pulmonary artery hypertension. Curr Opin Pediatr. 1996;8:512–9.
38. Barst RJ, Galie N, Naeije R, et al. Long-term outcome in pulmonary arterial hypertension patients treated with subcutaneous treprostinil. Eur Respir J. 2006;28:1195–203.
39. Humbert M, Sanchez O, Fartoukh M, et al. Short-term and long-term epoprostenol (prostacyclin) therapy in pulmonary hypertension secondary to connective tissue diseases: results of a pilot study. Eur Respir J. 1999;13:1351–6.
40. Rosenzweig EB, Kerstein D, Barst RJ. Long-term prostacyclin for pulmonary hypertension with associated congenital heart defects. Circulation. 1999;99:1858–65.
41. Kuo PC, Johnson LB, Plotkin JS, Howell CD, Bartlett ST, Rubin LJ. Continuous intravenous infusion of epoprostenol for the treatment of portopulmonary hypertension. Transplantation. 1997;63:604–6.
42. Nunes H, Humbert M, Sitbon O, et al. Prognostic factors for survival in human immunodeficiency virus-associated pulmonary arterial hypertension. Am J Respir Crit Care Med. 2003;167:1433–9.
43. Fuentes A, Coralic A, Dawson KL. A new epoprostenol formulation for the treatment of pulmonary arterial hypertension. Am J Health Syst Pharm. 2012;69:1389–93.
44. Chin KM, Badesch DB, Robbins IM, et al. Two formulations of epoprostenol sodium in the treatment of pulmonary arterial hypertension: EPITOME-1 (epoprostenol for injection in pulmonary arterial hypertension), a phase IV, open-label, randomized study. Am Heart J. 2014;167:218–25.
45. Sitbon O, Delcroix M, Bergot E, et al. EPITOME-2: an open-label study assessing the transition to a new formulation of intravenous epoprostenol in patients with pulmonary arterial hypertension. Am Heart J. 2014;167:210–7.
46. Clapp LH, Finney P, Turcato S, Tran S, Rubin LJ, Tinker A. Differential effects of stable prostacyclin analogs on smooth muscle proliferation and cyclic AMP generation in human pulmonary artery. Am J Respir Cell Mol Biol. 2002;26:194–201.
47. Laliberte K, Arneson C, Jeffs R, Hunt T, Wade M. Pharmacokinetics and steady-state bioequivalence of treprostinil sodium (Remodulin) administered by the intravenous and subcutaneous route to normal volunteers. J Cardiovasc Pharmacol. 2004;44:209–14.
48. Simonneau G, Barst RJ, Galie N, et al. Continuous subcutaneous infusion of treprostinil, a prostacyclin analogue, in patients with pulmonary arterial hypertension: a double-blind, randomized, placebo-controlled trial. Am J Respir Crit Care Med. 2002;165:800–4.

49. Oudiz RJ, Schilz RJ, Barst RJ, et al. Treprostinil, a prostacyclin analogue, in pulmonary arterial hypertension associated with connective tissue disease. Chest. 2004;126:420–7.
50. White RJ, Levin Y, Wessman K, Heininger A, Frutiger K. Subcutaneous treprostinil is well tolerated with infrequent site changes and analgesics. Pulm Circ. 2013;3:611–21.
51. Gomberg-Maitland M, Tapson VF, Benza RL, et al. Transition from intravenous epoprostenol to intravenous treprostinil in pulmonary hypertension. Am J Respir Crit Care Med. 2005;172:1586–9.
52. Benza RL, Tapson VF, Gomberg-Maitland M, Poms A, Barst RJ, McLaughlin VV. One-year experience with intravenous treprostinil for pulmonary arterial hypertension. J Heart Lung Transplant. 2013;32:889–96.
53. Hiremath J, Thanikachalam S, Parikh K, et al. Exercise improvement and plasma biomarker changes with intravenous treprostinil therapy for pulmonary arterial hypertension: a placebo-controlled trial. J Heart Lung Transplant. 2010;29:137–49.
54. Centers for Disease Control and Prevention (CDC). Bloodstream infections among patients treated with intravenous epoprostenol or intravenous treprostinil for pulmonary arterial hypertension–seven sites, United States, 2003-2006. MMWR Morb Mortal Wkly Rep. 2007;56:170–2.
55. Ivy DD, Calderbank M, Wagner BD, et al. Closed-hub systems with protected connections and the reduction of risk of catheter-related bloodstream infection in pediatric patients receiving intravenous prostanoid therapy for pulmonary hypertension. Infect Control Hosp Epidemiol. 2009;30:823–9.
56. Rich JD, Glassner C, Wade M, et al. The effect of diluent pH on bloodstream infection rates in patients receiving IV treprostinil for pulmonary arterial hypertension. Chest. 2012;141:36–42.
57. Olschewski H, Walmrath D, Schermuly R, Ghofrani A, Grimminger F, Seeger W. Aerosolized prostacyclin and iloprost in severe pulmonary hypertension. Ann Intern Med. 1996;124:820–4.
58. Olschewski H, Simonneau G, Galie N, et al. Inhaled iloprost for severe pulmonary hypertension. N Engl J Med. 2002;347:322–9.
59. Hoeper MM, Schwarze M, Ehlerding S, Adler-Schuermeyer A, Spiekerkoetter E, Niedermeyer J, Hamm M, Fabel H. Long-term treatment of primary pulmonary hypertension with aerosolized iloprost, a prostacyclin analogue. N Engl J Med. 2000;342(25):1866–70.
60. Schenk P, Petkov V, Madl C, et al. Aerosolized iloprost therapy could not replace long-term IV epoprostenol (prostacyclin) administration in severe pulmonary hypertension. Chest. 2001;119:296–300.
61. McLaughlin VV, Gaine SP, Barst RJ, et al. Efficacy and safety of treprostinil: an epoprostenol analog for primary pulmonary hypertension. J Cardiovasc Pharmacol. 2003;41:293–9.
62. Voswinckel R, Enke B, Reichenberger F, et al. Favorable effects of inhaled treprostinil in severe pulmonary hypertension: results from randomized controlled pilot studies. J Am Coll Cardiol. 2006;48:1672–81.
63. McLaughlin VV, Benza RL, Rubin LJ, et al. Addition of inhaled treprostinil to oral therapy for pulmonary arterial hypertension: a randomized controlled clinical trial. J Am Coll Cardiol. 2010;55:1915–22.
64. Nagaya N, Uematsu M, Okano Y, et al. Effect of orally active prostacyclin analogue on survival of outpatients with primary pulmonary hypertension. J Am Coll Cardiol. 1999;34:1188–92.
65. Barst RJ, McGoon M, McLaughlin V, et al. Beraprost therapy for pulmonary arterial hypertension. J Am Coll Cardiol. 2003;41:2119–25.
66. Tapson VF, Torres F, Kermeen F, et al. Oral treprostinil for the treatment of pulmonary arterial hypertension in patients on background endothelin receptor antagonist and/or phosphodiesterase type 5 inhibitor therapy (the FREEDOM-C study): a randomized controlled trial. Chest. 2012;142:1383–90.
67. Tapson VF, Jing ZC, Xu KF, et al. Oral treprostinil for the treatment of pulmonary arterial hypertension in patients receiving background endothelin receptor antagonist and

phosphodiesterase type 5 inhibitor therapy (the FREEDOM-C2 study): a randomized controlled trial. Chest. 2013;144:952–8.
68. Jing ZC, Parikh K, Pulido T, et al. Efficacy and safety of oral treprostinil monotherapy for the treatment of pulmonary arterial hypertension: a randomized, controlled trial. Circulation. 2013;127:624–33.
69. Simonneau G, Torbicki A, Hoeper MM, et al. Selexipag: an oral, selective prostacyclin receptor agonist for the treatment of pulmonary arterial hypertension. Eur Respir J. 2012;40: 874–80.
70. Ewert R, Halank M, Bruch L, Ghofrani HA. Am J Respir Crit Care Med. 2012;186:1196–8.
71. Selexipag (ACT-293987) in Pulmonary Arterial Hypertension, GRIPHON Trial. 2010. 2014. Available at http://www.clinicaltrials.gov/ct2/show/NCT01106014?term=selexipag&rank=2
72. DellVery for Pulmonary Arterial Hypertension (PAH). 2011. Accessed July 18, 2014, at http://www.clinicaltrials.gov/ct2/show/NCT01321073?term=treprostinil&rank=60

Chapter 14
Endothelin Receptor Antagonists

Josanna Rodriguez-Lopez and Richard N. Channick

Abstract Endothelin-1 (ET-1) is a potent vasoconstrictor and mitogen that is secreted by the endothelium. Pulmonary vascular expression of endothelin is increased in pulmonary hypertension and plasma levels correlate with the severity of disease. Several endothelin receptor antagonists (ERAs) have been developed and are available for the treatment of pulmonary arterial hypertension (PAH). These drugs have been shown to be effective at improving functional capacity, decreasing pulmonary vascular resistance and delaying the time to clinical worsening and play an important role in the management of PAH. This chapter briefly reviews how the endothelin signaling pathway modulates pulmonary vascular function and describes its role in the pathogenesis of PAH. The major clinical trials responsible for the currently available ERAs are presented along with their findings and limitations. Recently, adopted treatment guidelines for the use of ERAs in the treatment of pulmonary hypertensive disease are discussed along with potential side effects and adverse reactions associated with the use of these drugs.

Keywords Endothelin • Endothelin-1 • Endothelin receptor • Endothelin receptor antagonist • Pulmonary hypertension • Pulmonary arterial hypertension

Abbreviations

6MWD	6-min Walk distance
CTEPH	Chronic thromboembolic pulmonary hypertension
ERA	Endothelin receptor antagonist
ET-1	Endothelin-1
ET-2	Endothelin-2
ET-3	Endothelin-3
ET_A	Endothelin receptor A
ET_B	Endothelin receptor B

J. Rodriguez-Lopez, M.D. • R.N. Channick, M.D. (✉)
Pulmonary and Critical Care Division, Massachusetts General Hospital, Harvard Medical School, 55 Fruit Street, Boston, MA 02114-2696, USA
e-mail: RCHANNICK@mgh.harvard.edu

J.R. Klinger, R.P. Frantz (eds.), *Diagnosis and Management of Pulmonary Hypertension*, Respiratory Medicine 12, DOI 10.1007/978-1-4939-2636-7_14

IPAH	Idiopathic pulmonary arterial hypertension
mPAP	Mean pulmonary artery pressure
NO	Nitric oxide
PAH	Pulmonary arterial hypertension
PPET-1	Preproendothelin
PVR	Pulmonary vascular resistance
TPR	Total pulmonary resistance

Endothelin

The endothelins are a family of 21-amino acid peptides that play a key role in the regulation of vascular tone. The first member of this family to be identified was endothelin-1 (ET-1), a 2,492 Da peptide with potent vasoconstrictor properties, isolated in 1988 by Yanagisawa et al. [1]. Two additional endothelin isopeptides, endothelin-2 (ET-2) and endothelin-3 (ET-3), were subsequently discovered [2].

Vascular endothelial cells are the major source of endothelin production in humans. However, endothelin is also produced in a wide range of additional cell types including bronchial epithelium, macrophages, cardiac myocytes, glomerular mesangial cells and glial cells, among others [3–6].

The discovery that endothelin-1 is expressed in pulmonary artery endothelial cells and its receptors are expressed in pulmonary artery smooth muscle cells, led to the development of endothelin receptor antagonists as a therapy for pulmonary arterial hypertension (PAH).

Endothelin Receptors

There are two distinct receptors for the endothelin family of peptides, endothelin receptor A (ETA) and endothelin receptor B (ETB). The endothelin receptors belong to the family of receptors connected to guanine nucleotide-binding (G) proteins [7]. ETA receptors are expressed on pulmonary vascular smooth muscle cells while ETB receptors are located on both pulmonary vascular endothelial cells and smooth muscle cells. When activated, the ETA receptor mediates vasoconstriction. The mechanism is thought to occur via G-protein-induced phospholipase C activation; 1,4,5-inositol triphosphate (IP3) formation; and the consequent release of Ca^{2+} from intracellular stores [7]. In addition to mediating vasoconstriction, ET-1 is known to be a potent mitogen, with the ability to induce proliferation in a number of cell types, including vascular smooth muscle cells [8]. It has been shown that the mitogenic actions of ET-1 are mediated by both the ETA and ETB receptors [9]. ETB receptors on endothelial cells mediate vasodilation via increased production of nitric oxide (NO) and prostacyclin [10]. In addition to its pulmonary vasodilation properties, there are data suggesting that the ETB receptor may actually mediate a vasoconstrictive effect through a population of ETB receptors located on vascular smooth muscle cells [11]. The vasoconstrictive actions of ETB receptors may become more pronounced in the pathologic setting of pulmonary hypertension than in the normal pulmonary vasculature [12].

In humans with pulmonary hypertension, the roles of abnormal endothelin production and receptor-mediated effects have been well demonstrated. Patients with idiopathic pulmonary arterial hypertension (IPAH) demonstrate higher serum levels of ET-1 than control subjects. Lung specimens from patients with IPAH, when compared to those from patients without pulmonary hypertension, exhibit increased ET-1 staining of the muscular pulmonary arteries and increased expression of preproendothelin-1 (PPET-1) in the endothelial cells of the same vessels [13]. Similarly, elevated ET-1 levels have been seen in patients with PAH associated with congenital heart disease [14] and chronic thromboembolic pulmonary hypertension (CTEPH).

Currently Available Endothelin Receptor Antagonists

The discovery, testing, and approval of oral endothelin receptor antagonists (ERA) exemplifies true translational research, that is, insights into the vascular pathobiology of PAH coupled with systematic clinical trials and drug development. This coupling of academia and the pharmaceutical industry led directly to breakthroughs in the treatment of a life-threatening disease, and has led to dramatic improvements in patients' lives and outcomes.

Bosentan

Bosentan is a dual ERA and ERB antagonist that became the first orally active drug for the treatment of PAH when it received Food and Drug Administration (FDA) approval in November 2001. It is indicated for the treatment of WHO group 1 PAH patients in WHO functional class III or IV PAH. The first double-blind, placebo-controlled trial randomized 32 patients with IPAH (84 %) or PAH associated with scleroderma, functional class III, to bosentan or placebo for 12 weeks [15]. The primary endpoint was the placebo-corrected change in 6-min walk distance (6-MWT), with secondary endpoints including change in pulmonary hemodynamics, WHO functional class, Borg dyspnea index, and clinical worsening. The placebo-corrected improvement in 6-MWT was 76 m in favor of the bosentan group. In addition, cardiac index and pulmonary vascular resistance (PVR) were significantly improved with bosentan. There were asymptomatic increases in liver aminotransferases in two patients on bosentan, but these returned to baseline without discontinuing or changing the dose.

The subsequent BREATHE-1 (bosentan randomized trial of endothelin antagonist therapy) trial randomized 213 patients with IPAH (70 %) and pulmonary hypertension associated with connective tissue disease who were WHO functional classes

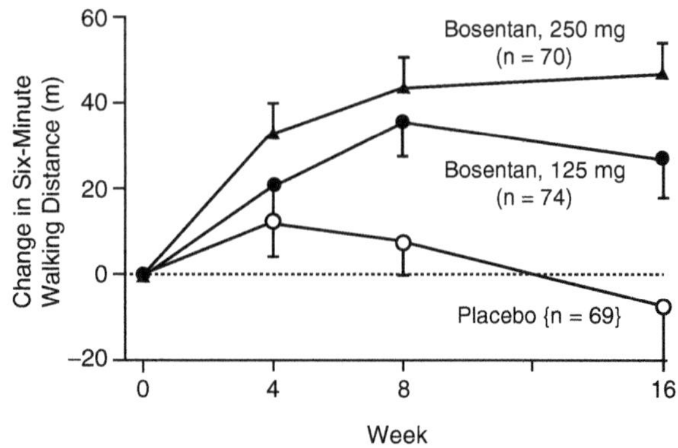

Fig. 14.1 Effect of bosentan on the primary endpoint of change in 6-min walk distance at week 16 from the BREATHE-1 trial. Based on a placebo-corrected improvement in walk distance of 44 m, and its safety profile, bosentan was approved at a dose of 125 mg twice daily (From [16])

III and IV to placebo or bosentan at a dose of 125 or 250 mg twice daily. At 16 weeks, the bosentan group had a placebo-corrected 6MWD improvement of 44 m ($p<0.001$) (Fig. 14.1) [16]. In addition, there were improvements in the Borg dyspnea score and time to clinical worsening in both bosentan groups. Increases in liver aminotransferases greater than eight times upper limit of normal were again noted in the bosentan group and were dose-dependent with two patients in the 125 mg group and five patients in the 250 mg group.

In addition to the above "registration" trials of bosentan, a randomized controlled trial of bosentan in PAH patients less functionally impaired (WHO class II), the EARLY trial, demonstrated a benefit in reducing PVR and preventing clinical worsening at 6 months. No statistically significant effect on 6MWD was seen, although baseline walk distance was greater than 400 m, confirming that this cohort had better baseline exercise capacity [17].

Long-term survival data in patients on bosentan, although uncontrolled, have been published. Of the 169 IPAH patients enrolled in the two pivotal trials of bosentan, estimated survival at 1 year and 2 years was 96 % and 89 % respectively, as compared to the predicted survival of 69 % and 57 % [18] (based on a validated NIH equation calculating predicted survival from baseline hemodynamics). It should be acknowledged that there are no prospective controlled survival data with the newer agents, given obvious ethical concerns about such trials in the era of existing therapy.

Bosentan is primarily metabolized in the liver through the P450 enzyme system. Clinical trials have shown that bosentan can precipitate hepatocellular injury, in particular when given at higher doses. Combined data from multiple trials have shown that there is a greater incidence in hepatic injury in patients treated with bosentan when compared to placebo. Greater than threefold elevations in aminotransferases were seen in 11 % of bosentan-treated patients ($n=658$) compared with 2 % of patients treated with placebo ($n=280$).

In the BREATHE-1 study, increases in hepatic aminotransferases occurred in 10 % of the patients and were found to be dose-dependent (more frequent in the

250 mg group), and reversible with dose reductions or upon stopping the drug. Based on these findings, the recommended dose of bosentan is 125 mg twice daily. Patients on bosentan must undergo baseline monitoring of liver function tests prior to initiation of the drug, and monthly thereafter.

Bosentan in Other Types of Pulmonary Hypertension

The initial bosentan trials only included adult patients with IPAH and associated PAH, predominantly scleroderma or connective tissue-related PAH. Data regarding the use of bosentan in other classes of PAH are limited. BREATHE-4 was a small, uncontrolled, prospective study of 16 patients with class III and IV HIV-associated PAH. The study found that HIV-associated PAH patients treated with bosentan had similar safety and efficacy profiles to prior groups studied [19]. At 16 weeks there were significant improvements in 6MWD, echocardiographic parameters, and quality of life scores. However, there was no comparison placebo arm. There was also an improvement in functional class, with 14 out of the 16 patients improving at least one class when compared to baseline. Treatment with bosentan did not have a negative impact on control of HIV infection. In this small study, bosentan had similar hepatic tolerability to that found in other patients with PAH, despite several patients being co-infected with either hepatitis B or C virus. In patients with hepatitis co-infection, bosentan should be used with caution and frequent monitoring of liver function tests.

BREATHE-5 was a randomized, placebo-controlled trial that evaluated the effect of bosentan in patients with Eisenmenger's syndrome due to congenital heart disease and functional class III PAH [20]. Fifty-four patients were randomized in a 2:1 fashion to bosentan ($n = 37$) or placebo ($n = 17$) for 16 weeks. Bosentan treatment did not reduce systemic arterial blood oxygen saturation, and showed significant improvement in hemodynamics (PVR, mPAP) and exercise capacity, with a treatment effect of +53 m in 6MWD. An open-label extension of this study revealed improvement in functional class in 24 out of the 37 patients. A subgroup analysis comparing atrial septal defect to ventricular septal defect patients receiving bosentan did not show any significant difference between the two groups [21]. This suggests the location of septal defects is not an important determinant of treatment response with bosentan.

The Bosentan Effects in iNopErable Forms of chronic Thromboembolic pulmonary hypertension (BENEFiT) trial investigated bosentan use in CTEPH [22]. One hundred and fifty-seven patients with CTEPH, who had either inoperable disease or persistent pulmonary hypertension 6 months after pulmonary endarterectomy, were enrolled. A statistically significant treatment effect of −24.1 % reduction in PVR was demonstrated in patients treated with bosentan over placebo. There was an improvement in 6MWD, but it did not reach statistical significance.

Ambrisentan

Ambrisentan is a specific ETA receptor antagonist approved for PAH, functional classes II and III at doses of 5 or 10 mg once daily. Following a Phase 2, dosing study showing improvement in pulmonary hemodynamics [23], two randomized controlled trials, ARIES 1 and ARIES 2 (ARIES 1: 5 mg, 10 mg, placebo; ARIES 2: 2.5 mg, 5 mg, placebo) were conducted, enrolling a total of 394 patients [24]. Both trials demonstrated improvement in the primary endpoint of placebo-corrected 6MWD (Fig. 14.2). In ARIES-2, there was a significant improvement in time to clinical worsening in the treatment group as compared with placebo. There was a trend toward improvement in time to clinical worsening in the ARIES-1 study, but it was not statistically significant ($p = 0.307$). World Health Organization

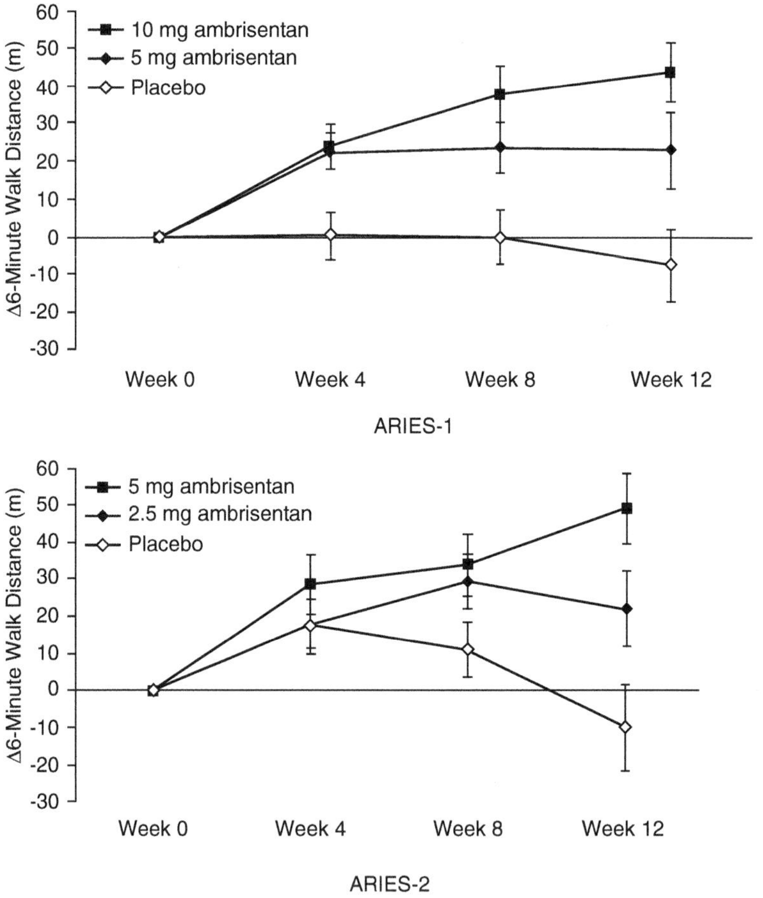

Fig. 14.2 Effect of ambrisentan on the primary endpoint of change in 6-min walk distance at week 12, from the ARIES-1 and ARIES-2 trials. Based on this finding, ambrisentan was approved at doses of 5 mg daily and 10 mg daily (From [24])

(WHO) functional class improvement was significant in ARIES-1 and there was trend toward improvement in ARIES-2 but did not reach statistical significance ($p = 0.117$). Two hundred and ninety-eight patients were enrolled and followed in a long-term extension study over 48 weeks. Eighteen patients required additional therapies (prostanoids or phosphodiesterase type-5 [PDE-5] inhibitors). Of the 280 patients continued on ambrisentan monotherapy, the improvement in 6MWD at 12 weeks was 40 m and maintained at 39 m. Although there were no patients with elevations in serum aminotransferases >3 times upper limit of normal while on ambrisentan, in the trials, long-term follow-up has revealed cases of transaminase elevations which resolve upon discontinuation of ambrisentan. However, because post-marketing surveillance suggested a minimal risk of drug-induced liver toxicity, the FDA removed the black box warning and requirement for monthly liver function monitoring. However, regular monitoring of pregnancy tests and hemoglobin is still required.

Macitentan

Macitentan is a novel dual ERA that was developed by modifying the chemical structure of bosentan to produce a drug with high oral efficacy and lipophilicity. This led to discovery of several alkyl sulfamide-substituted pyrimidines, including macitentan. Chemically, macitentan is *N*-[5-(4-bromophenyl)-6-[2-[(5-bromo-2-pyrimidinyl)oxy]ethoxy]-4-pyrimidinyl]-*N*′-propylsulfamide [25].

Compared with bosentan and ambrisentan, macitentan has a higher pKa and distribution coefficient, resulting in a higher percentage of nonionized drug at physiologic pH and favoring distribution across the phospholipid bilayer of the cell membrane. Compared to bosentan, macitentan also has improved receptor association and dissociation kinetics with more sustained receptor binding [26]. In human pulmonary artery smooth muscle cells, this leads to insurmountable antagonism and suggests that macitentan may have the ability to block endothelin more effectively in the setting of variable endothelin levels.

Macitentan: Initial Phase 1 and 2 Clinical Trials

Macitentan was first studied in healthy subjects in single dose followed by ascending multiple dose studies of 1–30 mg of macitentan versus placebo [27]. In these studies, macitentan was well tolerated and pharmacokinetics were supportive of once daily dosing with a maximal effect on endothelin levels at a dose of 10 mg. The half-life of macitentan was 14–18 h, while the half-life of ACT-132577, an active but less potent metabolite, was approximately 48 h. Drug elimination and formation of the active metabolite is catalyzed by cytochrome (CYP) P450, predominantly CYP3A4 and CYP2C19.

Macitentan: Phase 3 Clinical Trial

The landmark Phase 3 clinical trial that led to approval of macitentan in the U.S. and several other countries was the SERAPHIN (Study with an Endothelin Receptor Antagonist in Pulmonary arterial Hypertension to Improve cliNical outcomes) trial [28]. The study was designed as an event-driven morbidity and mortality trial. In this study, 742 patients with symptomatic PAH (52 % FC II, 46 % FC III and 2 % FC IV) were randomized 1:1:1 to receive placebo ($n = 250$), macitentan 3 mg ($n = 250$), or macitentan 10 mg ($n = 242$) and were followed for a median duration of 115 weeks. The study cohort included patients with idiopathic and heritable PAH (57 %), PAH associated with connective tissue disease (31 %), PAH associated with congenital heart disease (8 %), and PAH associated with HIV or drug/toxin exposure (4 %). Sixty-four percent of patients were on stable background PAH therapy with phosphodiesterase inhibitors or oral or inhaled prostanoids which they were allowed to continue throughout the study.

The primary endpoint was time from initiation of treatment to the first occurrence of a morbidity event related to PAH or death from any cause in an intention-to-treat analysis. The components of the morbidity/mortality event endpoint included death, atrial septostomy, lung transplantation, initiation of intravenous or subcutaneous prostanoids, or a composite endpoint for worsening of PAH.

The primary endpoint occurred in 46.4 ($n = 116$), 38 ($n = 95$), and 31.4 % ($n = 76$) of patients treated with placebo, macitentan 3 mg and macitentan 10 mg, respectively, with a hazard ratio of 0.70 (97.5 % CI, 0.52–0.96; $p = 0.01$) for macitentan 3 mg versus placebo and a hazard ratio of 0.55 (97.5 % CI 0.39–0.76; $p < 0.001$) for macitentan 10 mg versus placebo (Fig. 14.3). Worsening of PAH was the most frequent first event, which is not unexpected since worsening of PAH often precedes other components of the endpoint, such as initiation of prostanoids or mortality.

A prespecified secondary endpoint, death or hospitalization due to PAH, occurred in 33.6 % of the placebo group, 26 % of the macitentan 3 mg group and 20.7 % of the macitentan 10 mg group with a hazard ratio of 0.67 (97.5 % CI, 0.46–0.97, $p = 0.01$) for macitentan 3 mg versus placebo and a hazard ratio of 0.50 (97.5 % CI 0.34–0.75, $p < 0.001$) for macitentan 10 mg versus placebo (Fig. 14.3). Hospitalization accounted for the majority of these events, and there was no statistically significant difference in mortality between the groups. The study, however, was not designed or powered to show an effect on the endpoint of mortality alone.

The benefit of macitentan was observed irrespective of background therapy for PAH; macitentan 10 mg reduced the risk of the primary endpoint by 38 % (95 % CI 11–57 %) in the presence of background PAH therapy and 55 % (95 % CI 28–72 %) in the absence of PAH background therapy. Macitentan also demonstrated an improvement in secondary endpoints, including functional class and exercise capacity. In a subset of 145 patients who had right heart catheterizations and pulmonary hemodynamics reported at baseline and month 6, patients in both macitentan groups also had significant decreases in PVR (66.4 % [95 % CI 56.6–77.8 %] and 61.5 %

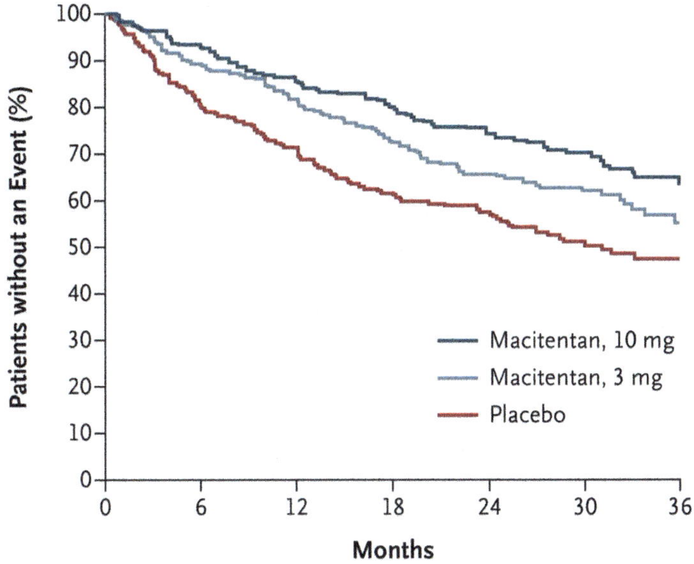

No. at Risk							
Placebo	250	188	160	135	122	64	23
Macitentan, 3 mg	250	213	188	166	147	80	32
Macitentan, 10 mg	242	208	187	171	155	91	41

Fig. 14.3 Effects of macitentan compared to placebo on time to first morbidity/mortality event. The hazard ratio for macitentan 10 mg daily compared to placebo was 0.55 (relative risk reduction of 45 % over the course of the study). Based on this finding, macitentan was approved at 10 mg daily (From [28])

[95 % CI 62.4–81.4 %] of placebo-corrected change from baseline for 3 mg and 10 mg macitentan, respectively) and an increase in cardiac index (0.69 L/min/m^2 [95 % CI 0.40–0.97] and 0.63 L/min/m^2 [95 % CI 0.28–0.97] placebo-corrected change from baseline for 3 mg and 10 mg macitentan, respectively).

SERAPHIN was the first event-driven study ever done in PAH. Compared to other clinical trials that led to drug approval for ambrisentan and bosentan in which patients were only exposed to therapy for 12–16 weeks [15, 16, 24], the treated patients in SERAPHIN had a median drug exposure of 115 weeks. Additionally, compared to other studies that have predominantly evaluated PAH monotherapy versus placebo, this study also included patients on background PAH therapy and demonstrated a beneficial effect of macitentan as monotherapy or in combination with other PAH medications. It is also important to note that even in patients on background PAH therapy, there was a significant incidence of morbidity/mortality over the course of the study, which was decreased with macitentan.

In SERAPHIN, the occurrence of aminotransferase elevation or edema and the number of people discontinuing treatment due to adverse effects were similar in placebo and active treatment groups. There was a small, dose-related decrease in hemoglobin from macitentan. Based on the results of SERAPHIN, macitentan (Opsumit, Actelion Pharmaceuticals) was approved by the United States FDA in October 2013 for the treatment of patients with Group 1 PAH and functional class II–IV symptoms at a recommended dose of 10 mg daily. It became commercially available for use in the United States in November 2013. Similar to ambrisentan, there is no required monthly liver function test monitoring for macitentan.

Comparing ERAs to Other PAH Therapy

ERAs have rarely been compared to other PAH therapies in head-to-head trials. The Sildenafil versus Endothelin Receptor Antagonist for Pulmonary Hypertension (SERAPH) trial directly compared bosentan to sildenafil. Twenty-six patients with class III PAH (IPAH and associated with connective tissue disease) were randomized to receive either sildenafil (50 mg b.i.d. for 4 weeks followed by 50 mg t.i.d.) or bosentan (62.5 mg b.i.d. for 4 weeks followed by 125 mg b.i.d.) as initial PAH monotherapy [29]. After 16 weeks, there was not a significant difference between the two groups in 6MWD, right ventricular mass, cardiac function, brain natriuretic peptide, or Borg dyspnea score.

A retrospective analysis compared 139 class III IPAH patients initially treated with bosentan monotherapy, to a historical cohort of 346 class III IPAH patients who were initially treated with intravenous epoprostenol [30]. Survival estimates up to 36 months were not significantly different in those initially treated with bosentan compared with those initially treated with epoprostenol. This suggests that initial treatment with oral bosentan in class III idiopathic PAH patients, followed by or with the addition of other treatment if necessary, does not adversely affect the long-term outcome compared with initial intravenous epoprostenol therapy. A pilot study was then conducted to see if PAH patients stable on prostacyclin therapy could be transitioned to oral bosentan therapy [31]. This was an open-label trial of 22 PAH patients who were clinically stable on intravenous epoprostenol or subcutaneous treprostinil for at least 3 months. The patients were observed closely while bosentan was added and prostracyclin therapy was titrated down. Ten out of the 22 patients were transitioned off prostacyclin therapy after a mean duration of 6 months. Seven out of those ten patients remained stable off of prostacyclin, for a mean duration of 18 months. Three patients who were titrated off required re-initiation of prostacyclin therapy given clinical deterioration, with two of these resulting in death. Of the 12 patients who did not tolerate off-titration of prostacyclin, 2 subsequently died. Those who transitioned successfully were on a lower baseline prostacyclin dose and had lower mPAPs than those who failed.

The guidelines, as developed at the 5th World Symposium on PH, give all three available ERAs a Grade 1 recommendation for PAH patients who are Functional Class II or III, and Grade 2 recommendation for PAH patients who are Functional Class IV [32].

Combination Therapy with ERAs

ERAs are commonly used in combination with other PAH therapies. The current World Symposium guidelines support this approach, based on emerging data [32]. This combination approach has generally been studied in a sequential, add-on fashion, with ERAs often being the first-line agents.

The effect of bosentan as add-on therapy to prostacyclins was studied in a prospective trial of 20 patients with IPAH who were either on inhaled iloprost ($n=9$) or oral beraprost ($n=11$) [33]. Combination therapy was tolerated by all patients. After 3 months of combination therapy, exercise tolerance increased by 58 m, and maximal oxygen consumption (measured by cardiopulmonary stress test) increased from 11 to 13.8 ml/kg/min, when compared to baseline. Another small prospective study added bosentan 62.5 mg twice daily to eight IPAH patients who were already on high-dose intravenous epoprostenol [34]. The addition of bosentan was well tolerated and seven out of eight patients had a reduction in the epoprostenol dose from an average of 99.6 ng/kg/min down to 82.8 ng/kg/min. Treatment effects were maintained for a total of 1 year and only two patients had progression of disease. A retrospective study on PAH patients receiving subcutaneous treprostinil found that 19 out of 38 patients had received add-on therapy with bosentan because they remained functional class III on treprostinil monotherapy. The patients who received add-on bosentan therapy showed significant improvement in pulmonary pressures, 6MWT distance, and Borg dyspnea score [35].

The BREATHE-2 trial was a double-blind, placebo-controlled, prospective study which looked at combination upfront therapy with IV epoprostenol and bosentan [36]. Thirty-three patients with class III or IV PAH were randomized in a 2:1 ratio to receive bosentan 62.5 mg twice daily for 4 weeks followed by 125 mg twice daily or placebo, 2 days after starting IV epoprostenol. At 16 weeks, both groups had a decrease in the primary outcome of total pulmonary resistance (TPR). There was a trend toward a greater decrease from baseline TPR in the bosentan/epoprostenol group, which was not statistically significant.

Adverse Effects Associated with ERAs

Several potentially serious adverse reactions can occur with the use of ERAs. All ERAs presently available for the treatment of PAH are teratogenic and woman of child-bearing potential need to be counseled about the potential of severe birth defects to their child if they become pregnant while taking these medications. Women who are sexually active should use two reliable forms of birth control. Serum pregnancy test is required prior to starting therapy and monthly thereafter.

Elevation of liver transaminases can occur in patients taking ERAs, particularly with bosentan. As a result, the FDA has mandated monthly liver function testing (LFT) for all patients who are treated with bosentan as long as they are receiving drug. Extended LFT monitoring after drug discontinuation is not needed. Drug should be stopped if there is an elevation of AST or ALT greater than five times the upper limit of normal or elevation in total bilirubin greater than two times the upper limit of normal. Bosentan therapy can be continued at a reduced dose if AST or ALT rises between three and five times the upper limit of normal, but LFTs should be monitored more frequently thereafter. Although elevation of transaminases is seen less frequently with the other ERAs and monitoring of LFTs is not mandatory, it is recommended that LFTs be measured prior to starting therapy with ambrisentan or macitentan and quarterly thereafter or at the discretion of the practitioner.

Other common adverse effects associated with ERA use include drug interactions, peripheral edema, and low-grade anemia. The ERAs are metabolized primarily in the liver by cytochrome p450 isoenzymes CYP2C9, CYP3A4 and to a lesser extent CYP2C19. Use of the ERAs in conjunction with other medications that induce or inhibit this pathway have potential to cause significant interactions. Drugs that inhibit these isoenzymes such as ketoconazole, cyclosporine A or ritonavir, increase plasma levels of ERAs and should be avoided or used with caution. The incidence of LFT abnormalities is also increased when bosentan is taken with glyburide. At the same time, bosentan has been shown to decrease plasma levels of warfarin and oral hypoglycemic agents and the dose of these drugs may need to be adjusted if given with bosentan. Peripheral edema is usually controlled with low-dose diuretics, but in some patients may be unmanageable and necessitate switching to another drug. Patients should always be evaluated for other causes of increasing edema such as heart and renal failure. The anemia that has been associated with ERA use is usually mild with the average decrease in hemoglobin about 1 g/dl, but decreases greater than 15 % from baseline have also been reported. The decrease in hemoglobin usually occurs within the first month and remains fairly stable thereafter. Blood counts should be measured prior to the start of ERA therapy and a month later and then at the discretion of the practitioner.

Due to the number of potential adverse events associated with the use of ERAs, these drugs are only available through specialty pharmacies and patients are required to sign a consent form acknowledging potential adverse effects prior to starting therapy.

Summary

The treatment of PAH remains complex with an increasing number of therapeutic options. Treatment should be individualized and guided by the patient's clinical status and hemodynamic testing. There are now evidence-based treatment algorithms for the initial treatment of PAH [32, 37]. Expert guidelines recommend the use of ERA in PAH patients who are functional class II and III. In patients treated with bosentan, monthly liver function tests should be monitored. If after 2–3 months of therapy there is not an improvement in functional class or exercise capacity, or if there is clinical decline, addition of prostanoids or phosphodiesterase inhibitors should be considered.

References

1. Yanagisawa M, Kurihara H, Kimura S, et al. A novel potent vasoconstrictor peptide produced by vascular endothelial cells. Nature. 1988;332(6163):411–5.
2. Luscher TF, Barton M. Endothelins and endothelin receptor antagonists: therapeutic considerations for a novel class of cardiovascular drugs. Circulation. 2000;102(19):2434–40.
3. Firth JD, Ratcliffe PJ. Organ distribution of the three rat endothelin messenger RNAs and the effects of ischemia on renal gene expression. J Clin Invest. 1992;90(3):1023–31.
4. Masaki T, Kimura S, Yanagisawa M, Goto K. Molecular and cellular mechanism of endothelin regulation. implications for vascular function. Circulation. 1991;84(4):1457–68.
5. Markewitz BA, Farrukh IS, Chen Y, Li Y, Michael JR. Regulation of endothelin-1 synthesis in human pulmonary arterial smooth muscle cells. Effects of transforming growth factor-beta and hypoxia. Cardiovasc Res. 2001;49(1):200–6.
6. Shi-Wen X, Chen Y, Denton CP, et al. Endothelin-1 promotes myofibroblast induction through the ETA receptor via a rac/phosphoinositide 3-kinase/Akt-dependent pathway and is essential for the enhanced contractile phenotype of fibrotic fibroblasts. Mol Biol Cell. 2004;15(6): 2707–19.
7. Dupuis J, Stewart DJ, Cernacek P, Gosselin G. Human pulmonary circulation is an important site for both clearance and production of endothelin-1. Circulation. 1996;94(7):1578–84.
8. Wagner OF, Christ G, Wojta J, et al. Polar secretion of endothelin-1 by cultured endothelial cells. J Biol Chem. 1992;267(23):16066–8.
9. Dupuis J, Hoeper MM. Endothelin receptor antagonists in pulmonary arterial hypertension. Eur Respir J. 2008;31(2):407–15.
10. Boulanger C, Luscher TF. Release of endothelin from the porcine aorta. inhibition by endothelium-derived nitric oxide. J Clin Invest. 1990;85(2):587–90.
11. Morey AK, Razandi M, Pedram A, Hu RM, Prins BA, Levin ER. Oestrogen and progesterone inhibit the stimulated production of endothelin-1. Biochem J. 1998;330(Pt 3):1097–105.
12. Davie N, Haleen SJ, Upton PD, et al. ET(A) and ET(B) receptors modulate the proliferation of human pulmonary artery smooth muscle cells. Am J Respir Crit Care Med. 2002;165(3): 398–405.
13. Chua BH, Krebs CJ, Chua CC, Diglio CA. Endothelin stimulates protein synthesis in smooth muscle cells. Am J Physiol. 1992;262(4 Pt 1):E412–6.
14. Hofman FM, Chen P, Jeyaseelan R, Incardona F, Fisher M, Zidovetzki R. Endothelin-1 induces production of the neutrophil chemotactic factor interleukin-8 by human brain-derived endothelial cells. Blood. 1998;92(9):3064–72.
15. Channick RN, Simonneau G, Sitbon O, et al. Effects of the dual endothelin-receptor antagonist bosentan in patients with pulmonary hypertension: a randomised placebo-controlled study. Lancet. 2001;358(9288):1119–23.
16. Rubin LJ, Badesch DB, Barst RJ, et al. Bosentan therapy for pulmonary arterial hypertension. N Engl J Med. 2002;346(12):896–903.
17. Galie N, Rubin L, Hoeper M, et al. Treatment of patients with mildly symptomatic pulmonary arterial hypertension with bosentan (EARLY study): a double-blind, randomised controlled trial. Lancet. 2008;371(9630):2093–100.
18. Sitbon O, Badesch DB, Channick RN, et al. Effects of the dual endothelin receptor antagonist bosentan in patients with pulmonary arterial hypertension: a 1-year follow-up study. Chest. 2003;124(1):247–54.
19. Sitbon O, Gressin V, Speich R, et al. Bosentan for the treatment of human immunodeficiency virus-associated pulmonary arterial hypertension. Am J Respir Crit Care Med. 2004;170(11): 1212–7.
20. Galie N, Beghetti M, Gatzoulis MA, et al. Bosentan therapy in patients with Eisenmenger syndrome: a multicenter, double-blind, randomized, placebo-controlled study. Circulation. 2006;114(1):48–54.

21. Berger RM, Beghetti M, Galie N, et al. Atrial septal defects versus ventricular septal defects in BREATHE-5, a placebo-controlled study of pulmonary arterial hypertension related to Eisenmenger's syndrome: a subgroup analysis. Int J Cardiol. 2010;144(3):373–8.
22. Jais X, D'Armini AM, Jansa P, et al. Bosentan for treatment of inoperable chronic thromboembolic pulmonary hypertension: BENEFiT (bosentan effects in iNopErable forms of chronIc thromboembolic pulmonary hypertension), a randomized, placebo-controlled trial. J Am Coll Cardiol. 2008;52(25):2127–34.
23. Galie N, Badesch D, Oudiz R, et al. Ambrisentan therapy for pulmonary arterial hypertension. J Am Coll Cardiol. 2005;46(3):529–35.
24. Galie N, Olschewski H, Oudiz RJ, et al. Ambrisentan for the treatment of pulmonary arterial hypertension: results of the ambrisentan in pulmonary arterial hypertension, randomized, double-blind, placebo-controlled, multicenter, efficacy (ARIES) study 1 and 2. Circulation. 2008;117(23):3010–9.
25. Bolli MH, Boss C, Binkert C, et al. The discovery of a N-[5-(4-bromophenyl)-6-[2-[(5-bromo-2-pyrimidinyl)oxy]ethoxy]-4-pyrimidinyl]-N′-propylsulfamide (Macitentan), an orally active, potent, dual endothelin receptor antagonist. J Med Chem. 2012;55(17):7849–61.
26. Gatfield J, Grandjean CM, Sasse T, Clozel M, Nayler O. Slow receptor dissociation kinetics differentiate macitentan from other endothelin receptor antagonists in pulmonary arterial smooth muscle cells. PLoS One. 2012;7(10):1–11.
27. Giersbergen PL, Dingemanse J. Safety, tolerability, pharmacokinetics and pharmacodynamics of macitentan, an endothelin receptor antagonist, in an ascending multiple dose study in healthy subjects. J Clin Pharmacol. 2013;53(11):1131–8.
28. Pulido T, Adzerikho I, Channick RN, et al. Macitentan and morbidity and mortality in pulmonary arterial hypertension. N Engl J Med. 2013;369:809–18.
29. Wilkins MR, Paul GA, Strange JW, et al. Sildenafil versus endothelin receptor antagonist for pulmonary hypertension (SERAPH) study. Am J Respir Crit Care Med. 2005;171(11):1292–7.
30. Sitbon O, McLaughlin VV, Badesch DB, et al. Survival in patients with class III idiopathic pulmonary arterial hypertension treated with first line oral bosentan compared with an historical cohort of patients started on intravenous epoprostenol. Thorax. 2005;60(12):1025–30.
31. Steiner MK, Preston IR, Klinger JR, et al. Conversion to bosentan from prostacyclin infusion therapy in pulmonary arterial hypertension: a pilot study. Chest. 2006;130(5):1471–80.
32. Galiè N, Corris PA, Frost A, Girgis RE, Granton J, Jing ZC, Klepetko W, McGoon MD, McLaughlin VV, Preston IR, Rubin LJ, Sandoval J, Seeger W, Keogh A. Updated treatment algorithm of pulmonary arterial hypertension. J Am Coll Cardiol. 2013;62(25 Suppl):D60–72.
33. Hoeper MM, Taha N, Bekjarova A, Gatzke R, Spiekerkoetter E. Bosentan treatment in patients with primary pulmonary hypertension receiving nonparenteral prostanoids. Eur Respir J. 2003;22(2):330–4.
34. Akagi S, Matsubara H, Miyaji K, et al. Additional effects of bosentan in patients with idiopathic pulmonary arterial hypertension already treated with high-dose epoprostenol. Circ J. 2008;72(7):1142–6.
35. Benza RL, Rayburn BK, Tallaj JA, Pamboukian SV, Bourge RC. Treprostinil-based therapy in the treatment of moderate-to-severe pulmonary arterial hypertension: long-term efficacy and combination with bosentan. Chest. 2008;134(1):139–45.
36. Humbert M, Barst RJ, Robbins IM, et al. Combination of bosentan with epoprostenol in pulmonary arterial hypertension: BREATHE-2. Eur Respir J. 2004;24(3):353–9.
37. Taichman DB, Ornelas J, Chung L, Klinger JR, Lewis S, Mandel J, Palevsky HI, Rich S, Sood N, Rosenzweig EB, Trow TK, Yung R, Elliott CG, Badesch DB. Pharmacologic therapy for pulmonary arterial hypertension in adults: CHEST guideline and expert panel report. Chest. 2014;146(2):449–75.

Chapter 15
Modulation of cGMP Synthesis and Metabolism

Kristen J. Bubb, Adrian J. Hobbs, and James R. Klinger

Abstract The cyclic nucleotide cGMP acts as the secondary messenger for nitric oxide (NO) and natriuretic peptides (NP). It is synthesised by the activation of soluble or particulate guanylate cyclase by NO or NP, respectively. The primary downstream target of cGMP is cGMP-dependent kinase (PKG) which acts at a variety of intracellular sites to inhibit vasoconstriction, proliferation and hypertrophic responses and phosphodiesterases that are responsible for its metabolism. cGMP-mediated pulmonary vasodilation plays a critical role in maintaining normal pulmonary vascular pressure, and a growing body of evidence suggests that decreased cGMP synthesis or increased cGMP metabolism may contribute to the pathogenesis of pulmonary vascular disease. Several medications that target deficiencies in NO and cGMP signalling have recently been approved for the treatment of pulmonary arterial hypertension. This chapter will discuss the NO and NP/cGMP signalling pathways as they pertain to modulation of pulmonary vascular function and will review the efficacy and safety of the phosphodiesterase inhibitors and soluble guanylate cyclase stimulators that have been developed for the treatment of PAH. Alternative approaches to enhancing cGMP signalling that may be useful in developing new therapies for PAH will also be presented.

Keywords Cyclic guanosine monophosphate • cGMP • Nitric oxide • Natriuretic peptide • Guanylate cyclase • Pulmonary arterial hypertension • Nitric oxide synthase • Phosphodiesterase

K.J. Bubb • A.J. Hobbs
William Harvey Research Institute, Barts and The London Medical School, London, UK

J.R. Klinger, M.D. (✉)
Division of Pulmonary, Sleep and Critical Care Medicine, Rhode Island Hospital, Alpert Medical School of Brown University, 593 Eddy Street, Providence, RI 02903, USA
e-mail: James_Klinger@brown.edu

J.R. Klinger, R.P. Frantz (eds.), *Diagnosis and Management of Pulmonary Hypertension*, Respiratory Medicine 12, DOI 10.1007/978-1-4939-2636-7_15

Abbreviations

ANP	Atrial natriuretic peptide
BH_4	Tetrahydrobiopterin
BNP	Brain natriuretic peptide
cAMP	Cyclic adenosine-3′,5′-monophosphate
cGMP	Cyclic guanosine-3′,5′-monophosphate
CHF	Congestive heart failure
CNP	C-type natriuretic peptide
eNOS	Endothelial nitric oxide synthase
GC	Guanylatecyclase
GTP	Guanosine triphosphate
iNOS	Inducible nitric oxide synthase
NEP	Neutral endopeptidase
nNOS	Neuronal nitric oxide synthase
NO	Nitric oxide
NPR-A	Natriuretic peptide receptor-A
NPR-B	Natriuretic peptide receptor-B
NPR-C	Natriuretic peptide receptor-C
PDE	Phosphodiesterase
PDE5i	Phosphodiesterase type 5 inhibitor
pGC	Particulate guanylatecyclase
PH	Pulmonary hypertension
PKG	cGMP-dependent protein kinase
Ppm	Parts per million
sGC	Soluble guanylatecyclase
V/Q	Ventilation/perfusion

Introduction

Cyclic guanosine-3′,5′-monophosphate (cGMP) is a pivotal intracellular second-messenger in a variety of cell types. In vascular smooth muscle cells, cGMP is a major signalling molecule in the complex pathway that results in smooth muscle relaxation and therefore vasodilation. Within the cardiovascular system, cGMP also inhibits smooth muscle cell proliferation and platelet aggregation, and is vital for vascular endothelial cell and cardiomyocyte function. cGMP is synthesised from its precursor, guanosine triphosphate (GTP), by a family of enzymes termed guanylate cyclases (GCs) and can activate a variety of biological targets. The major effector protein within vascular smooth muscle cells is cGMP-dependent protein kinase, or protein kinase G (PKG); activation of which brings about the majority of the functional effects of cGMP via phosphorylation of specific target molecules. In vascular smooth muscle, for example, PKG causes vasodilation predominantly by decreasing intracellular calcium concentration and/or reducing calcium sensitivity. This is achieved by removal of calcium through ion pumps and by decreased calcium entry; the latter can occur through inhibition of both transmembrane voltage-gated calcium channels and receptor/G-protein coupling [50]. Furthermore, calcium-activated potassium channels, when stimulated by increased intracellular calcium, cause cell membrane hyperpolarisation, which, in turn, inhibits voltage-gated calcium channels and produces smooth muscle relaxation. In addition, PKG-dependent phosphorylation of the receptor for inositol 1,4,5-triphosphate (IP3) decreases calcium release from the sarcoplasmic reticulum (for review see [50]).

It is now well established that cGMP is important in maintaining normal pulmonary vascular hemodynamics and that drugs that increase intracellular cGMP levels are effective treatments for pulmonary hypertension (PH). This is exemplified by the development of phosphodiesterase (PDE) 5 inhibitors (PDE5i) that blunt the metabolism of cGMP and soluble GC stimulators that enhance cGMP synthesis as therapy for pulmonary vascular disease. In this chapter, the major pathways responsible for cGMP synthesis and metabolism in the pulmonary circulation will be discussed as well as how these pathways have been targeted to develop modern treatments for PAH.

cGMP Synthesis

The synthesis of cGMP is triggered by activation of GC enzymes, which are designated according to their localisation. Soluble guanylate cyclase (sGC) is a cytoplasmic protein which acts as the target for the ubiquitous vasoprotective signalling molecule nitric oxide (NO), whereas particulate guanylate cyclase (pGC) is a membrane-bound protein that is activated by a family of cardiac- and endothelium-derived mediators, the natriuretic peptides. Figure 15.1 shows a basic overview of cGMP synthesis, indicating pharmacological interventions modulating these processes.

Nitric Oxide

Within blood vessels, NO is synthesised in endothelial cells from the substrate L-arginine [66] via an enzyme known as endothelial NO synthase (eNOS, or NOS-3). There are two further isoforms of NOS, both of which are expressed in various vascular and non-vascular locations (see [84]); neuronal (nNOS, NOS-1) and inducible (iNOS, NOS-2) NOS. The production of NO from L-arginine involves a two-step oxidation reaction, utilising both NADPH and molecular oxygen to form L-citrulline and NO [3]. Endothelial NOS, like all NOS isoforms, is a homodimer consisting of a C-terminal reductase domain and an N-terminal oxygenase domain. The reductase domain contains binding sites for NADPH, which donates electrons

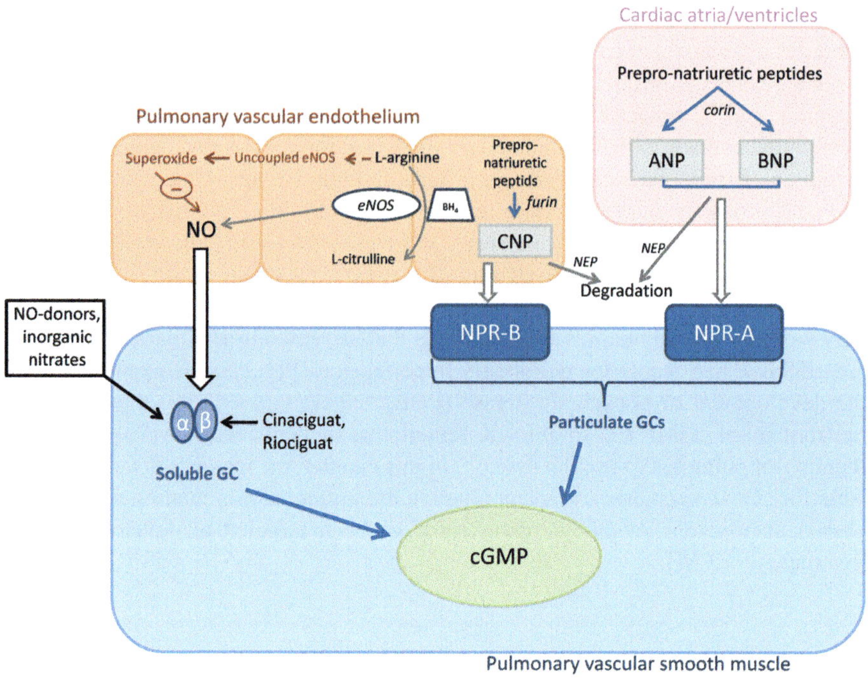

Fig. 15.1 Vascular synthesis of cGMP. Cyclic GMP can be synthesised by two distinct mechanisms: NO-stimulated sGC activity and natriuretic peptide-triggered pGC turnover. Therapeutically, sGC-mediated cGMP generation can be recapitulated by NO-donors, inorganic nitrate, and sGC stimulators/activators such as cinaciguat and riociguat. Neutral endopeptidase (NEP) is responsible for the degradation of natriuretic peptides, and inhibition of this enzyme can be used therapeutically to raise endogenous natriuretic peptide bioactivity

for the reaction, and FAD/FMN which act as electron conduits. The oxygenase domain contains a heme group and also binding sites for the essential cofactor tetrahydrobiopterin (BH_4), and substrate L-arginine. Electrons transfer from NADPH bound at the C-terminal of the reductase domain, to the heme in the oxygenase domain (of the opposite monomer), resulting in the reduction and activation of oxygen, oxidation of L-arginine to L-citrulline and NO generation (reviewed in [19]). In healthy arteries, the major stimulus for eNOS is increased intracellular calcium, which triggers binding of calmodulin to the oxygenase domain, increasing the rate of NADPH-derived electron transfer between the domains. Calcium increases in endothelial cells occur in response to many endothelium-dependent dilators, including bradykinin and substance P. Phosphorylation of eNOS, in response to shear stress, oestrogen, vascular endothelial growth factor, and insulin, also stimulates enzyme activity and NO generation; this is facilitated by non-calmodulin-dependent pathways, such as protein kinase A, Akt and AMP-activated protein kinase [20]. However, in certain cardiovascular diseases, including PH, it is thought that eNOS may exist in an 'uncoupled state', in which substrate L-arginine or BH_4 become rate-limiting; in this scenario, eNOS transfers electrons to molecular oxygen, rather than oxidising L-arginine, thereby forming superoxide, a species thought to precipitate vascular dysfunction [89]. Thus, it is not only the amount of substrate available for NO production but also the correct coupling of NOS that is important for sufficient NO bioavailability.

Alterations in the synthesis of NO occur in patients with PH and in pre-clinical models of the disease [55]. Endothelial dysfunction is considered to be one of the early events leading to PH, and this is associated with reduced NO synthesis [59]. Interestingly, eNOS expression in the pulmonary vasculature has been shown to decrease in patients with PH [29], whereas other studies report higher levels [95]. These conflicting findings most likely reflect differential mechanisms causing PH, as a third study suggests slow eNOS expression in the pulmonary arterioles of PH patients, but high eNOS levels in the diseased plexiform lesions that occur in pulmonary vessels of PH sufferers [53]. This uncertainty is mirrored in animal models of PH, with a reported increase [48, 71, 85], decrease [77] or no change [59] in eNOS expression shown in various model systems. Furthermore, in eNOS knockout (KO) mice (in which the eNOS gene has been deleted), basal pulmonary resistance is increased [11], but in response to chronic hypoxia, PH disease severity may be worsened [82], unchanged [18] or ameliorated (Johns) compared with wild-type mice. One explanation for these differences in eNOS expression found in PH patients and disease models is the uncoupling of the enzyme (as mentioned above). Thus, whilst lower enzyme expression and activity (i.e. NO production) can contribute to pulmonary vasoconstriction, higher levels of eNOS protein may not necessarily be beneficial if uncoupling of the enzyme leads to superoxide production (rather than NO) and thereby exacerbates the disease. This thesis is supported in *hph1* mice, which have an inherent BH_4 deficiency. Exaggerated responses to hypoxia-induced PH as a result of eNOS uncoupling are found in these animals [64]. A recent report has also highlighted a novel mechanism whereby eNOS-mediated oxidative stress impairs PKG phosphorylation [102]. Under normal conditions eNOS is inhibited by coupling to caveolin-1, however when caveolin-1 expression is decreased eNOS can become abnormally hyperactive and influence superoxide production. Thus, the level of eNOS activity per se is not necessarily as important as the products and downstream signalling that it evokes.

NO-Based Therapeutics

The balance between eNOS-driven NO production and enzyme uncoupling has been targeted as a potential therapeutic avenue for PH. Supplementation with the eNOS cofactor, BH_4, or a more stable analogue, has been investigated and can effectively normalise eNOS expression and endothelial function [46]; such an approach may prove to be effective in PH [4]. However, BH_4 supplementation for 4 weeks prior to coronary artery bypass did not improve endothelial function in patients with coronary artery disease, thought to be because of oxidation of BH_4 to BH_2 [14]. This oxidation may have been due to the oral administration of the drug, thus, modification of the route of administration may still uncover an effective treatment. Another drug, cicletanine, which is presumed to work by coupling eNOS/BH_4 activity to promote NO (rather than superoxide) production is beneficial in animal models of PH [36] and decreases pulmonary resistance in PH patients [73], although these effects may also be attributed to natriuretic peptides or cAMP. Unfortunately, clinical trials did not find cicletanine to be effective in the treatment of PAH and further development of the drug for this indication is unlikely.

In some cases, NO production may be limited by the substrate, L-arginine, and increasing this may be useful in enhancing NO synthesis. L-arginine administration attenuates PH in both hypoxic and monocrotaline-treated rats [57] and acutely decreases pulmonary vascular resistance in PH patients [54]. Short-term administration of oral L-arginine has been reported to improve pulmonary hemodynamics in patients with PH [58, 63]. However, no extended clinical trials have been undertaken in patients with PAH and the effectiveness of this approach is yet to be determined.

In general, PH is associated with reduced bioavailability of NO. Thus, attempts have been made to simply increase its level in the pulmonary circulation by having patients inhale it. Inhalation of just trace amounts of NO, in the range of 1–20 parts per million (ppm) have been shown to have an acute pulmonary vasodilator effect. Inhaled NO has been developed and approved for treatment of infants with persistent pulmonary hypertension of the newborn and is presently undergoing clinical trial in adult patients with PAH.

Inhaled NO has the advantage of being delivered directly to pulmonary vessels and thus largely avoids the systemic vasodilation associated with other modes of delivery [81]. This method of delivery also results in better ventilation/perfusion (V/Q) matching since more NO is delivered to better ventilated areas of the lung. However, the use of inhaled NO to treat patients with PAH has been hampered by its extremely short half-life resulting in the need for near continuous inhalation and uncertainty regarding potential for pulmonary hypertensive rebound response if inhalation is abruptly interrupted. In addition, inhaled NO therapy is plagued by the need for a cumbersome and expensive delivery device [4, 55, 81]. In an attempt to bypass some of these problems, NO donors have been developed that provide longer-lasting NO release. Nebulised NONOates [31, 87] and inhaled glycerol trinitrate [30] are both effective in reducing pulmonary vascular resistance; however, there are still concerns about the lack of pulmonary specificity with these drugs [4]. An alternative 'NO-donor' therapy may be to enhance endogenous NO production by administering inorganic nitrite and/or nitrate. A study from our own laboratory has shown that in animal models of PH, induced by either chronic hypoxia or secondary to bleomycin-induced lung fibrosis, several disease parameters are reversed by oral therapy with either of these compounds [5]. This strategy relies on a recently discovered phenomenon where inorganic nitrite is converted to NO and O_2 by a variety of heme-based enzymes including haemoglobin and myoglobin especially under conditions of hypoxia and acidosis [37, 86]. The advantage of this approach is that production of NO is maximised in the lung in models of PH, suggesting it should represent a more pulmonary-specific strategy. Moreover, inorganic nitrates can be derived from natural dietary sources such as beetroot and green leafy vegetables, intimating this may be a cost-effective treatment regimen. Clinical evaluation of inorganic nitrite and nitrate administration in PH patients is on-going.

Soluble Guanylate Cyclase

Soluble GC is a heterodimer formed of alpha and beta subunits, and both subunits are required for catalytic activity. In addition, a prosthetic heme group is essential for sGC activation by NO, as NO-triggered enzyme turnover is abolished when the heme group is removed and restored when the heme group is reconstituted (for review see [22]). Activation of sGC by NO involves the uncharged NO radical binding a reduced Fe^{2+} heme moiety. NO binding to this prosthetic group results in a conformational change which activates the enzyme, increasing the V_{max} more than 200-fold. Due to this heme-dependency for NO-mediated activation, changes to the redox state of sGC, which may occur in cardiovascular disease, including PH, can result in down-regulation of activity and/or expression [69]. Importantly, from a therapeutic perspective, sGC can be activated by synthetic compounds even when it is in an inactive state. In PH the expression and activity of sGC is up-regulated, probably as a compensatory mechanism to adapt to reduced NO bioavailability [4] and sGC-null mice showed an exaggerated response to hypoxia-induced PH [90]. Therefore, sGC has proven to be an important candidate target for PH therapy.

Soluble GC activators, such as cinaciguat (BAY 58-2667), can stimulate sGC when it is in an oxidised or heme-free state, whereas sGC stimulators (e.g. riociguat; BAY 63-2521) can induce sGC activation and stabilise the enzyme in its active configuration via allosteric binding. Thus, sGC stimulators have synergistic effects with NO because they act directly on sGC to induce cGMP synthesis while enhancing the ability of sGC to respond to NO. For example, BAY 41-2272 alone increases sGC activity by ~20-fold but in combination with subthreshold concentrations of NO, sGC activity is increased 200-fold [80]. In comparison, sGC activators only cause additive effects when combined with NO. In rodent models of PH, treatment with either sGC activators such as cinaciguat or sGC stimulators, such as BAY 41-2272 [15] or riociguat [47] attenuates disease severity. The reliance on an intact NO generating system is evident as treatment effects of BAY 41-2272 are abolished in eNOS KO mice [15]. The sGC stimulators have also been shown to attenuate PH in a wide range of other animal studies (summarised in [80]).

The efficacy of sGC stimulation observed in animal models of PH led to the development of riociguat for the treatment of PAH [26]. Following the successful completion of a phase II trial in patients with PAH, 2 large randomised, placebo-controlled studies were conducted to evaluate the efficacy of riociguat for treatment of PAH and chronic thromboembolic disease [27, 28]. In both studies, riociguat improved 6-min walk distance, pulmonary hemodynamics and delayed time to clinical worsening (Fig. 15.2a, b). These studies led to the approval of riociguat for treatment of PAH and CTEPH in 2013.

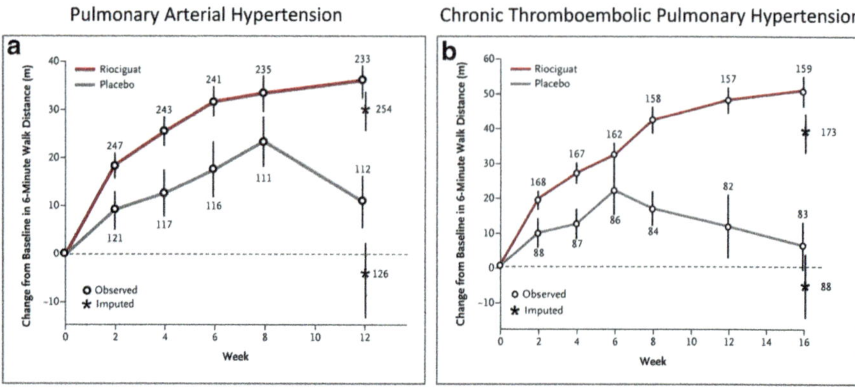

Fig. 15.2 Effect of soluble guanylate cyclase stimulator on 6-min walking distance (**a**) Mean (±SE) changes from baseline in the 6-min walk distance over 12 weeks in the PATENT-1 study where patients with pulmonary arterial hypertension received riociguat at a dose up to 2.5 mg or placebo three times daily (From [27]). (**b**) Mean (±SE) changes from baseline in the 6-min walk distance over 16 weeks in the CHEST study where patients with chronic thromboembolic pulmonary hypertension were treated with riociguat or placebo (From [28]). For both (**a**) and (**b**), the number at each data point indicates the number of patients included in the assessment at that time point

Natriuretic Peptides

There are three structurally similar vasoactive members of the natriuretic peptide family: atrial, brain and C-type natriuretic peptide (ANP, BNP, CNP). These peptides are generated after enzymatic cleavage of precursor pre-propeptides facilitated by the endopeptidases, corin, in the case of ANP/BNP [96], and furin for CNP [94]. ANP and BNP act in an endocrine fashion and are primarily released in response to hypervolemia. These hormones, as their names suggest, are responsible for regulating salt (natriuresis) and fluid (diuresis) homeostasis. ANP and BNP are stored in granules in the cardiac atria and released in response to atrial wall stretch in response to increased intravascular volume and are then distributed to target tissues such as the kidneys and systemic vasculature. BNP is also synthesised and released from the cardiac ventricles (the name refers to its original site of identification) particularly in pathological situations. The plasma levels of ANP and BNP rise sharply in patients with congestive heart failure (CHF) and PH, and correlate with disease severity and survival. Thus, these peptides are often used as biomarkers; this is particularly true of BNP or its N-terminal inactive fragment, NT-proBNP [62, 67].

A third member of the natriuretic peptide family, CNP, is highly expressed in the brain, chondrocytes and vascular endothelial cells and is secreted from the latter cell type at an increased rate in response to inflammation and shear stress.

The natriuretic peptides increase intracellular cGMP levels by binding to cell surface GC-linked receptors, commonly referred to as particular guanylate cyclases (pGC) (Fig. 15.1). The natriuretic peptide receptors A and B (NPR-A and NPR-B) are transmembrane receptors which contain a ligand-binding extracellular domain, an intracellular protein kinase-like domain and a C-terminal GC catalytic region. The protein kinase like domain binds ATP, which leads to increased NP-induced GC stimulation. Conversely, the receptor can become desensitised by dephosphorylation at this region [56]. NPR-A is highly expressed in renal, vascular smooth muscle, heart and lung tissue and is most sensitive to ANP, followed by BNP and, at high (pharmacological) concentrations, CNP [67]. Evidence of NPR-A being solely responsible for the natriuretic/diuretic actions of ANP has been shown in NPR-A knockout mice, where these mechanisms were completely lost [40]. NPR-B is the major receptor for CNP, and essential for normal bone growth (loss-of-function mutants of NPR-B have severe bone deformities and dwarfism) [10]. A third NPR, NPR-C, is known as the natriuretic peptide clearance receptor. This protein is particularly abundant in the vasculature; indeed it is the most highly expressed of the NPRs, but it is not linked to a GC domain. As its name suggests, NPR-C plays an important role in removing all three NPs from the circulation. Upon binding to NPR-C, natriuretic peptides are rapidly internalised within the cell and degradation of the peptides occur by lysosomes, before the receptor is returned to the cell surface [51]. Under normal circumstances, the affinity of all three natriuretic peptides for NPR-C is similar; however, a pathophysiological environment can result in alterations in NPR-C affinity and expression. As an example, under conditions of acute or chronic hypoxia, NPR-C expression can be down-regulated [41, 49], presumably as a compensatory response to maintain higher levels of protective natriuretic peptides.

The physiological effects of increasing concentrations of ANP or BNP include direct vasodilatation due to cGMP-mediated smooth muscle relaxation, increased glomerular filtration, reduced salt and water reabsorption, lower renin secretion and aldosterone synthesis, all of which reduce blood volume, and subsequently blood pressure. ANP and BNP also have direct effects on the heart, and are involved in reducing hypertrophic growth (ANP) and fibrosis (BNP). Importantly, ANP and BNP have been shown to blunt the development of pulmonary hypertension in animals and mice lacking NPR-A have increased pulmonary vascular remodelling and right ventricular mass and develop more severe pulmonary hypertension when exposed to chronic hypoxia [45, 99]. These findings suggest that ANP and/or BNP are important in the regulation of pulmonary vascular tone and right heart hypertrophy.

The majority of the effects of CNP are mediated via a different pGC, NPR-B. Ligand binding to NPR-B induces cGMP synthesis causing local vasodilation, rather than an endocrine effect on blood volume and pressure. However, recent evidence also suggests cGMP-independent vasodilation by CNP which is mediated via NPR-C (a non-guanylate cyclase-coupled receptor) [2]. Whether CNP has a role in PH remains uncertain. Infusion of exogenous CNP does not show efficacy in two well characterised models of PH; either chronic hypoxia alone or in combination with SU5416 (a vascular endothelial growth factor receptor inhibitor). However, exogenous CNP was shown to reduce monocrotaline-induced PH and increase survival [34]. Further work is required to establish any function of endogenous CNP in the pathogenesis of PH.

Natriuretic Peptide-Based Therapy

Exogenously administered natriuretic peptides have shown promise as treatments for PH. Treatment with ANP [35] and BNP [44] attenuates right ventricular hypertrophy and pulmonary vascular remodelling in rats with hypoxia-induced PH. In humans exposed to acute hypoxemia, BNP infusion significantly reduced pulmonary vascular resistance compared with placebo [9]; whilst ANP was not effective in this study, in a small cohort of patients with PH secondary to chronic obstructive pulmonary disease, ANP infusion lowered pulmonary vascular resistance by a third and dose-dependently reduced pulmonary artery pressure [1]. BNP was also found to lower mPAP in patients with PAH when combined with a phosphodiesterase inhibitor [43]. Thus, ANP and or BNP might be considered treatment options for PH. However, these peptides have short plasma half-lives (e.g. ANP has a half-life of <1 min in rats [61] and <3 min in humans [97]) and they are not amenable to oral administration, making them poor candidates. An alternative strategy is to enhance endogenously produced natriuretic peptides by preventing their clearance or degradation. As NPR-C is involved in the clearance of natriuretic peptides, blockade of NPR-C can increase the bioavailability and therefore the biological effects of ANP and BNP. Thus, antagonists at this receptor, which have been developed [88] could increase bioavailability of natriuretic peptides, making this a useful therapeutic target [5]. A second mechanism by which bioavailability of natriuretic peptides can be enhanced is by inhibiting their degradation. Neutral endopeptidase (NEP) metabolises natriuretic peptides by cleavage and inactivation; thus NEP inhibitors, such as ecadotril, can boost endogenous natriuretic peptides. NEPs are not selective for natriuretic peptides, they metabolise a vast array of peptides, many of which are involved in regulation of vascular tone, including angiotensin II, bradykinin, endothelin-1 and substance P. Thus, the use of NEP inhibitors to enhance natriuretic peptides may be offset by enhancement of vasoconstrictor peptides (for review see [52]). Nevertheless, the relative specificity of natriuretic peptides for the pulmonary circulation results in a beneficial effect of NEP inhibition for the treatment of PH [6, 42]. Moreover, inhibition of NEP appears to specifically enhance natriuretic peptide activity in the pulmonary circulation, entailing a relatively pulmonary-selective activity.

cGMP Metabolism

The balance between the synthesis of cGMP (discussed above) and the breakdown by phosphodiesterase enzymes largely determines the dynamic, local concentrations of cGMP available for downstream signalling. There is also a role for ATP-dependent multidrug resistance transporter proteins in exporting cGMP from smooth muscle cells; however, this effect is reported to be small compared to the role of PDEs in regulation of cGMP [21]. Nonetheless, pharmacological inhibition or genetic deletion of MRP activity has been shown to ameliorate experimental PH. Figure 15.3 shows an overview of cGMP signalling in the vasculature, including the role of PDE isozymes.

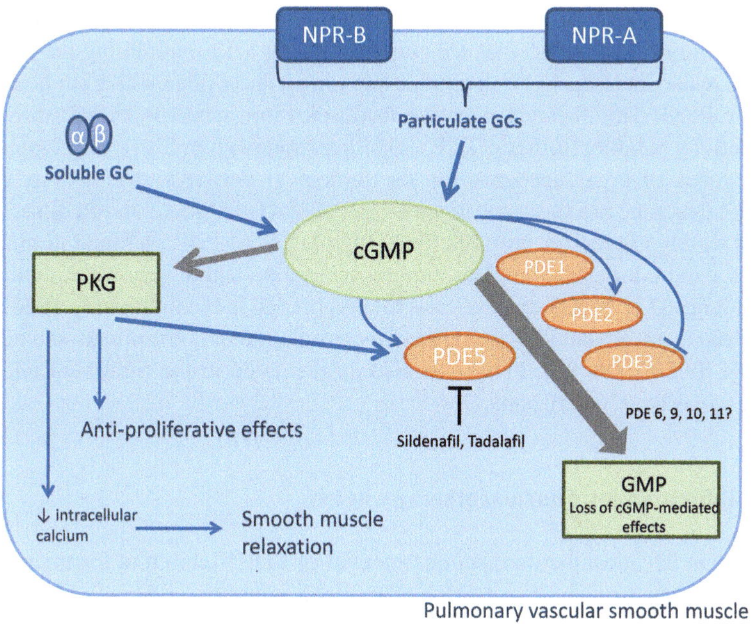

Fig. 15.3 Metabolism and action of vascular-derived cGMP. The major actions of cGMP in vascular smooth muscle are relaxation and anti-proliferation, mediated by protein kinase G (PKG). The bioavailability of cGMP can be reduced by phosphodiesterase (PDE)-mediated hydrolysis. Within vascular tissue, PDE5 is the best characterised cGMP-specific PDE, and is the primary target to enhance cGMP bioavailability therapeutically. Sildenafil and tadalafil are PDE5 inhibitors licensed for use in PH. Other PDEs that hydrolyse cGMP may be involved in pulmonary vascular hemodynamics and the pathogenesis of PH

PDE-Dependent Hydrolysis of cGMP

Cyclic GMP is degraded to inactive GMP by PDEs thereby reducing the substrate available for PKG activation. There are 11 known families of PDEs [1–12], each of which contain 1–4 gene-related isozymes/splice variants, encoding, in total, more than 100 different PDE proteins [39]. These enzymes can metabolise either cGMP, cAMP or both. PDEs 4, 7 and 8 have no, or minimal, cGMP hydrolysing activity and are not discussed further in this chapter. Of the remaining PDEs, all hydrolyse cGMP to varying degrees. To date, PDE5 is the most well characterised cGMP metabolising PDE and is thought to be the most active cGMP hydrolysing PDE in smooth muscle under basal conditions [72].

PDE5 is a homodimer, with both monomers containing a regulatory and a catalytic domain. The regulatory domain contains two GAF cGMP binding sites, GAF-A and GAF-B. PDE5 binds to cGMP at a high affinity at the GAF-A binding site. Cyclic AMP can also bind to this GAF site, however PDE5 is ~100-fold less selective for cAMP over cGMP. Upon binding, catalytic activity is enhanced whereas when this GAF-A binding site is blocked, inhibition of enzyme activity occurs. Inhibitors of PDE5 that are currently in use act by inhibiting the catalytic domain. Adjacent to the GAF-A binding site is a serine residue which is phosphorylated by PKG. This forms a negative feedback loop, whereby cGMP-stimulated PKG activity inhibits further cGMP signalling (reviewed in [38]). Expression of a single gene, PDE5A, accounts for the biological activity attributed to PDE5, although this gene has three splice variants, PDE5A1, PDE5A2 and PDE5A3. This gene is widely expressed, with relatively high levels of PDE5A found in platelets, kidneys, cerebellum, and pancreas, but it is most abundant in vascular smooth muscle and lungs [12]. PDE5 expression is relatively high in the pulmonary circulation, and indeed is up-regulated in the pulmonary circulation of both animals and patients with PH [60, 75, 76, 92]. PDE5A is also up-regulated in the right ventricle after pressure-overload hypertrophy.

PDE5 Inhibition for Pharmacotherapy in PH

Over recent decades, the therapeutic potential of PDE5 inhibitors for treatment of PH has been vigorously investigated. The PDE5 inhibitor, sildenafil, was initially trialled as anti-angina medication, and it was by serendipitous observations that the beneficial effect on penile erection was discovered, which led to the widespread use of sildenafil, marketed as Viagra, for the treated of erectile dysfunction. It was found that PDE5 expression was particularly high in the smooth muscle cells of the corpus cavernosum of the penis, which explained why smooth muscle relaxation, which is required to increase blood volume within the penis, was stimulated at this site [70].

After this discovery, the use of sildenafil in other regions with high PDE5 expression was considered. Following promising results from several small clinical trials, a large randomised placebo-controlled trial of sildenafil for treatment of PAH was conducted [25]. Sildenafil was given at a dose of 20, 40 or 80 mg three times daily. After 12 weeks of treatment, 6-min walking distance and pulmonary hemodynamics were significantly better in patients in any of the sildenafil treatment groups compared to placebo (Fig. 15.4a). Sildenafil was subsequently approved at the lowest of the three doses (20 mg three times daily) for the treatment of PAH in 2005.

Adult patients with PAH have similar acute pulmonary vasodilator responses to any of the three presently available PDE5 inhibitors that are presently available to treat erectile dysfunction. In addition to sildenafil, vardenafil and tadalafil have been shown to improve PAH in adults. Vardenafil is not approved for the treatment of PAH in the US, but tadalafil was approved for this indication in the US in 2009 following the completion of a randomised controlled trial of 2.5, 10, 20 or 40 mg tadalafil given once daily compared to placebo [23]. In that study, only the 40 mg dose was successful as defined a priori as improvement in placebo-adjusted 6-min walk test after 16 weeks of treatment at pre-specified significance level of $P>0.01$ (Fig. 15.4b). Of the PDE5 inhibitors licensed for use in PH, tadalafil is longer lasting and more specific to PDE5 relative to PDE1-4 than sildenafil [39]. Importantly, in humans with PH both sildenafil [25] and tadalafil [23] are effective in improving symptoms and outcomes.

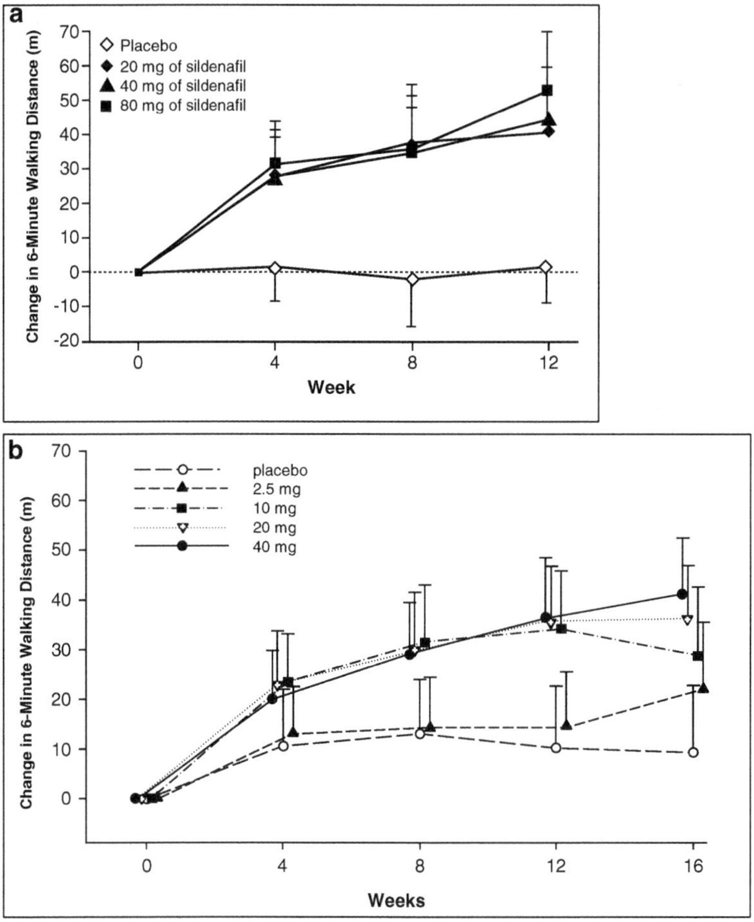

Fig. 15.4 Effect of phosphodiesterase-5 inhibitors on 6-min walking distance (**a**) Mean changes from baseline, with 95 % confidence intervals, in the 6-min walking distance over 12 weeks in the SUPER study where patients received sildenafil of placebo three times daily (From [25]). (**b**) Mean changes from baseline, with 95 % CIs, in the 6-min walking distance over 16 weeks in the PHIRST study where patient received tadalafil or placebo once daily (From [23])

Pre-clinical studies have provided insight into the therapeutic mechanisms of PDE5 inhibitors. It was established that sildenafil is effective in inhibiting PH in chronically hypoxic mice [100], in monocrotaline-treated rats [74], and in acutely hypoxic neonatal lambs [91] and pigs [78]. In fact, a plethora of experimental evidence exists supporting the thesis that PDE5 inhibition can improve PH in animal models [81]. However, as with patient responses to sildenafil (~45 % patients do not respond favourably), there is still significant room for improvement in treatment options. Therefore investigators, both pre-clinical and clinical, are now focussing on combination therapies. It is clear that targeting one element of cGMP signalling alone may not substantially increase cGMP, or at least be maximally efficacious. For example, reducing the degradation of cGMP may be ineffective if there is not sufficient substrate for cGMP generation. Thus, an improved efficacy may be apparent by employing a strategy based on increasing cGMP production at the same time as reducing degradation. In this regard, mice lacking NPR-A are less responsive to chronic sildenafil treatment in models of PH [101] suggesting that natriuretic peptides are essential for PDE5 inhibition to succeed. In accord, the beneficial effects of sildenafil to reduce right ventricular pressure in rats exposed to acute hypoxia are augmented by concomitant infusion of ANP [68]. Further still, treatment with the NEP inhibitor ecadotril (to enhance endogenous natriuretic peptides) and sildenafil results in a synergistic reduction in right ventricular pressure and hypertrophy in chronically pulmonary hypertensive rats [6]. Further still, in humans, BNP alone does not reduce pulmonary artery pressure acutely, but enhances the benefits of sildenafil [43]. Together, the studies described above demonstrate that the generation of cGMP due to increased natriuretic peptide bioactivity underpins the benefit of PDE5 inhibition in PH. In accord, it is therefore conceivable that NO therapy would produce a similar result. Thus, it has recently been shown that combined treatment with an sGC stimulator (BAY 41-8453) and a PDE5 inhibitor (zaprinast) results in prolonged pulmonary vasodilation in a model of PH [17]. In addition, in response to chronic hypoxia, sildenafil treatment is more effective in reducing PH in wild-type compared with eNOS knockout mice [100]. However, the use of PDE5 inhibitors in combination with nitrovasodilators is contraindicated (due to the development of life-threatening systemic hypotension), due to a lack of pulmonary specificity. In addition, combined use of riociguat and sildenafil or tadalafil is contra-indicated due to risk of symptomatic hypotension [24]. Therefore, combination therapy targeting natriuretic peptide-stimulated cGMP is likely to offer a superior, pulmonary-specific approach.

PDE1

PDE1 is thought to become the most predominant in hydrolysing cGMP under conditions of high calcium, such as occurs during smooth muscle contraction [72]. Unlike PDE5, PDE1 is expressed at low levels in the pulmonary tissues. However, PDE1 is substantially up-regulated in pulmonary vasculature undergoing proliferation. In both patients with PH and in monocrotaline-treated rats, PDE1 expression is greater in pulmonary arteries and smooth muscle cells compared with basal expression. Furthermore, inhibition of PDE1 reduces right ventricular pressure and pulmonary resistance [75]. PH induced by chronic exposure to cold temperature in rats is also reversed by PDE1 inhibition [13]. Likewise, PDE1 inhibition enhances the vasodilator response to NO in an acute hypoxia PH model in lambs [16]. These data advocate PDE1 as a therapeutic target for PH.

PDE2

PDE2 metabolises cGMP and cAMP to similar degrees. PDE2 is considered a cGMP-stimulated PDE. PDE2 has similar GAF binding domains as PDE5, and cGMP can bind to the regulatory domain, causing a feedback loop whereby cGMP stimulation causes increased cyclic nucleotide hydrolysis. PDE2 is widely expressed throughout the body. It has been found in vascular smooth muscle cells and is more abundant in vascular smooth muscle cells of pulmonary arteries isolated from PH patients [60]. The role of PDE2 in the treatment of PH has received little attention to date; however it has been shown that the PDE2 inhibitor, erythro-9-(2-hydroxy-3-nonyl) adenine can dose-dependently reduce acute hypoxic pulmonary vasoconstriction in isolated perfused rat lungs [32]. In addition, we have recently shown that the selective PDE2 inhibitor BAY 60-7550 reduces pulmonary hypertension and right ventricular hypertrophy caused by chronic hypoxia in mice [8].

PDE3

PDE3 expression is increased in chronically hypoxic rats [60] and the PDE3 inhibitor, milrinone attenuates pulmonary artery pressure in rats with PH and congestive heart failure [33]. However, it is likely that the effects are more due to involvement of cAMP than cGMP as PDE3 hydrolyses cAMP at a rate of tenfold more than cGMP [39]. In addition, cGMP inhibits PDE3, thus PDE3 is termed a cGMP-inhibited PDE [7]. This cGMP-mediated PDE3 inhibition may help to explain why there is added benefit of treatment with iloprost (a prostacyclin analogue which reduces PH by up-regulation of cAMP) and sildenafil [93]. Indeed, this cross-talk between cyclic nucleotides and PDE isoforms (discussed in [98]) could be the basis of improved outcomes observed when sildenafil is added to epoprostenol infusion [79].

Other PDEs

In addition to PDE5, PDE6 and PDE9 are also cGMP-specific isozymes. PDE6 has been identified predominantly in the retina and the pineal gland, but recently expression has been shown in human lungs, and interestingly, up-regulated expression was found in fibrotic lungs [65]. Thus a role for PDE6 in PH should not yet be ruled out. PDE9 is a more recently discovered isozyme [19], and as yet little is known about this protein, other than that it has the highest affinity for cGMP [7]. There is evidence to suggest that both PDE6 and PDE9 can be inhibited by PDE5 inhibitors, giving rise to the possibility that effects of PDE5 inhibitors are due, in part, to other PDEs [39]. PDE1, PDE2, PDE3, PDE10 and PDE11 all possess dual-specificity with cAMP [7]. Since the elevation of both cGMP (via PDE5 inhibitors and sGC stimulators) and cAMP (via prostacyclin-based therapies) appears to be helpful in the treatment of PH, PDEs with specificity for both cyclic nucleotides could be potentially superior treatment strategies, depending on their expression and activity in the pulmonary circulation. Further research on these PDEs in the coming years may prove additional benefit over PDE5 inhibition. Due to their recent discovery there is limited knowledge on the contribution of PDE10 and PDE11 to PH. Using the monocrotaline model of PH in rats, Tian and colleagues have shed more light into the role of these PDEs. They found that lung expression of PDE10 is up-regulated in this model of PH, whilst PDE11 expression is unchanged. Furthermore, treatment with papaverine, an inhibitor of PDE10, reduced right ventricular systolic pressure and pulmonary vascular resistance. Notably, this appeared to be largely a cAMP-mediated response [83].

Summary

PH remains a progressive, fatal disease and current treatments only slow an often inexorable decline. PDE5 inhibitors are a first-line treatment for PH, but they have limited benefit when given alone. Perhaps one reason for this is that PDE5 inhibitors target only one aspect of the cGMP pathway. Emerging evidence suggests that combination therapy may offer a superior approach to therapeutically augmenting cGMP signalling for the treatment of PH. Increasing cGMP synthesis whilst simultaneously preventing cGMP breakdown is a viable option for new therapeutic intervention; in addition, facilitating natriuretic peptide signalling may offer a more pulmonary-selective approach. By investigating combination therapies of existing drugs that target the cGMP pathway at various points, the treatment of PH could become more successful in the near future.

References

1. Adnot S, Andrivet P, Chabrier PE, Piquet J, Plas P, Braquet P, et al. Atrial natriuretic factor in chronic obstructive lung disease with pulmonary hypertension. Physiological correlates and response to peptide infusion. J Clin Invest. 1989;83(3):986–93.
2. Ahluwalia A, MacAllister RJ, Hobbs AJ. Vascular actions of natriuretic peptides. Cyclic GMP-dependent and -independent mechanisms. Basic Res Cardiol. 2004;99(2):83–9.
3. Andrew PJ, Mayer B. Enzymatic function of nitric oxide synthases. Cardiovasc Res. 1999;43(3):521–31.
4. Baliga RS, MacAllister RJ, Hobbs AJ. New perspectives for the treatment of pulmonary hypertension. Br J Pharmacol. 2011;163(1):125–40.
5. Baliga RS, Milsom AB, Ghosh SM, Trinder SL, Macallister RJ, Ahluwalia A, et al. Dietary nitrate ameliorates pulmonary hypertension: cytoprotective role for endothelial nitric oxide synthase and xanthine oxidoreductase. Circulation. 2012;125(23):2922–32.
6. Baliga RS, Zhao L, Madhani M, Lopez-Torondel B, Visintin C, Selwood D, et al. Synergy between natriuretic peptides and phosphodiesterase 5 inhibitors ameliorates pulmonary arterial hypertension. Am J Respir Crit Care Med. 2008;178(8):861–9.
7. Bender AT, Beavo JA. Cyclic nucleotide phosphodiesterases: molecular regulation to clinical use. Pharmacol Rev. 2006;58(3):488–520.

8. Bubb KJ, Trinder S, Baliga R, MacAllister RJ, Hobbs AJ. Validation Of Phosphodiesterase 2 As A Novel Therapeutic Target In Pulmonary Hypertension Am J Respir Crit Care Med 187: Meeting Abstracts, 2013, A4623-A4623.
9. Cargill RI, Lipworth BJ. Acute effects of ANP and BNP on hypoxic pulmonary vasoconstriction in humans. Br J Clin Pharmacol. 1995;40(6):585–90.
10. Chusho H, Tamura N, Ogawa Y, Yasoda A, Suda M, Miyazawa T, et al. Dwarfism and early death in mice lacking C-type natriuretic peptide. Proc Natl Acad Sci U S A. 2001;98(7): 4016–21.
11. Cook S, Vollenweider P, Menard B, Egli M, Nicod P, Scherrer U. Increased eNO and pulmonary iNOS expression in eNOS null mice. Eur Respir J. 2003;21(5):770–3.
12. Corbin JD, Beasley A, Blount MA, Francis SH. High lung PDE5: a strong basis for treating pulmonary hypertension with PDE5 inhibitors. Biochem Biophys Res Commun. 2005; 334(3):930–8.
13. Crosswhite P, Sun Z. Inhibition of phosphodiesterase-1 attenuates cold-induced pulmonary hypertension. Hypertension. 2013;61(3):585–92.
14. Cunnington C, Van Assche T, Shirodaria C, Kylintireas I, Lindsay AC, Lee JM, et al. Systemic and vascular oxidation limits the efficacy of oral tetrahydrobiopterin treatment in patients with coronary artery disease. Circulation. 2012;125(11):1356–66.
15. Dumitrascu R, Weissmann N, Ghofrani HA, Dony E, Beuerlein K, Schmidt H, et al. Activation of soluble guanylate cyclase reverses experimental pulmonary hypertension and vascular remodeling. Circulation. 2006;113(2):286–95.
16. Evgenov OV, Busch CJ, Evgenov NV, Liu R, Petersen B, Falkowski GE, et al. Inhibition of phosphodiesterase 1 augments the pulmonary vasodilator response to inhaled nitric oxide in awake lambs with acute pulmonary hypertension. Am J Physiol Lung Cell Mol Physiol. 2006;290(4):L723–9.
17. Evgenov OV, Kohane DS, Bloch KD, Stasch JP, Volpato GP, Bellas E, et al. Inhaled agonists of soluble guanylate cyclase induce selective pulmonary vasodilation. Am J Respir Crit Care Med. 2007;176(11):1138–45.
18. Fagan KA, Fouty BW, Tyler RC, Morris Jr KG, Hepler LK, Sato K, et al. The pulmonary circulation of homozygous or heterozygous eNOS-null mice is hyperresponsive to mild hypoxia. J Clin Invest. 1999;103(2):291–9.
19. Fisher DA, Smith JF, Pillar JS, St Denis SH, Cheng JB. Isolation and characterization of PDE9A, a novel human cGMP-specific phosphodiesterase. J Biol Chem. 1998;273(25): 15559–64.
20. Forstermann U. Nitric oxide and oxidative stress in vascular disease. Pflugers Arch. 2010; 459(6):923–39.
21. Francis SH, Busch JL, Corbin JD, Sibley D. cGMP-dependent protein kinases and cGMP phosphodiesterases in nitric oxide and cGMP action. Pharmacol Rev. 2010;62(3):525–63.
22. Friebe A, Koesling D. Regulation of nitric oxide-sensitive guanylyl cyclase. Circ Res. 2003;93(2):96–105.
23. Galiè N, Müller K, Scalise AV, Grünig E. PATENT PLUS: a blinded, randomised and extension study of riociguat plus sildenafil in PAH. Eur Respir J. 2015 Feb 5. pii: ERJ-01059-2014. [Epub ahead of print]
24. Galie N, et al. Updated treatment algorithm of pulmonary arterial hypertension. J Am Coll Cardiol. 2013;62:D60–72.
25. Galie N, Ghofrani HA, Torbicki A, Barst RJ, Rubin LJ, Badesch D, et al. Sildenafil citrate therapy for pulmonary arterial hypertension. N Engl J Med. 2005;353(20):2148–57.
26. Ghofrani HA, Galie N, Grimminger F, Humbert M, Keogh A, Langleben D, et al. Riociguat for the treatment of pulmonary arterial hypertension: a randomised, double-blind, placebo-controlled study (PATENT-1). Chest. 2012;142(4_MeetingAbstracts):1027A.
27. Ghofrani HA, Galiè N, Grimminger F, Grünig E, Humbert M, Jing ZC, Keogh AM, Langleben D, Kilama MO, Fritsch A, Neuser D, Rubin LJ, PATENT-1 Study Group. Riociguat for the treatment of pulmonary arterial hypertension. N Engl J Med. 2013;369(4):330–40.

28. Ghofrani HA, D'Armini AM, Grimminger F, Hoeper MM, Jansa P, Kim NH, Mayer E, Simonneau G, Wilkins MR, Fritsch A, Neuser D, Weimann G, Wang C, CHEST-1 Study Group. Riociguat for the treatment of chronic thromboembolic pulmonary hypertension. N Engl J Med. 2013;369(4):319–29.
29. Giaid A, Saleh D. Reduced expression of endothelial nitric oxide synthase in the lungs of patients with pulmonary hypertension. N Engl J Med. 1995;333(4):214–21.
30. Goyal P, Kiran U, Chauhan S, Juneja R, Choudhary M. Efficacy of nitroglycerin inhalation in reducing pulmonary arterial hypertension in children with congenital heart disease. Br J Anaesth. 2006;97(2):208–14.
31. Hampl V, Tristani-Firouzi M, Hutsell TC, Archer SL. Nebulized nitric oxide/nucleophile adduct reduces chronic pulmonary hypertension. Cardiovasc Res. 1996;31(1):55–62.
32. Haynes Jr J, Killilea DW, Peterson PD, Thompson WJ. Erythro-9-(2-hydroxy-3-nonyl)adenine inhibits cyclic-3′,5′-guanosine monophosphate-stimulated phosphodiesterase to reverse hypoxic pulmonary vasoconstriction in the perfused rat lung. J Pharmacol Exp Ther. 1996; 276(2):752–7.
33. Hentschel T, Yin N, Riad A, Habbazettl H, Weimann J, Koster A, et al. Inhalation of the phosphodiesterase-3 inhibitor milrinone attenuates pulmonary hypertension in a rat model of congestive heart failure. Anesthesiology. 2007;106(1):124–31.
34. Itoh T, Nagaya N, Murakami S, Fujii T, Iwase T, Ishibashi-Ueda H, et al. C-type natriuretic peptide ameliorates monocrotaline-induced pulmonary hypertension in rats. Am J Respir Crit Care Med. 2004;170(11):1204–11.
35. Jin H, Yang RH, Chen YF, Jackson RM, Oparil S. Atrial natriuretic peptide attenuates the development of pulmonary hypertension in rats adapted to chronic hypoxia. J Clin Invest. 1990;85(1):115–20.
36. Jin H, Yang RH, Oparil S. Cicletanine blunts the pulmonary pressor response to acute hypoxia in rats. Am J Med Sci. 1992;304(1):14–9.
37. Kapil V, Webb AJ, Ahluwalia A. Inorganic nitrate and the cardiovascular system. Heart. 2010;96(21):1703–9.
38. Kass DA, Champion HC, Beavo JA. Phosphodiesterase type 5: expanding roles in cardiovascular regulation. Circ Res. 2007;101(11):1084–95.
39. Keravis T, Lugnier C. Cyclic nucleotide phosphodiesterase (PDE) isozymes as targets of the intracellular signalling network: benefits of PDE inhibitors in various diseases and perspectives for future therapeutic developments. Br J Pharmacol. 2012;165(5):1288–305.
40. Kishimoto I, Dubois SK, Garbers DL. The heart communicates with the kidney exclusively through the guanylyl cyclase-A receptor: acute handling of sodium and water in response to volume expansion. Proc Natl Acad Sci U S A. 1996;93(12):6215–9.
41. Klinger JR, Arnal F, Warburton RR, Ou LC, Hill NS. Downregulation of pulmonary atrial natriuretic peptide receptors in rats exposed to chronic hypoxia. J Appl Physiol. 1994; 77(3):1309–16.
42. Klinger JR, Petit RD, Warburton RR, Wrenn DS, Arnal F, Hill NS. Neutral endopeptidase inhibition attenuates development of hypoxic pulmonary hypertension in rats. J Appl Physiol. 1993;75(4):1615–23.
43. Klinger JR, Thaker S, Houtchens J, Preston IR, Hill NS, Farber HW. Pulmonary hemodynamic responses to brain natriuretic peptide and sildenafil in patients with pulmonary arterial hypertension. Chest. 2006;129(2):417–25.
44. Klinger JR, Warburton RR, Pietras L, Hill NS. Brain natriuretic peptide inhibits hypoxic pulmonary hypertension in rats. J Appl Physiol. 1998;84(5):1646–52.
45. Klinger JR, Warburton RR, Pietras LA, Smithies O, Swift R, Hill NS. Genetic disruption of atrial natriuretic peptide causes pulmonary hypertension in normoxic and hypoxic mice. Am J Physiol. 1999;276(5 Pt 1):L868–74.
46. Landmesser U, Dikalov S, Price SR, McCann L, Fukai T, Holland SM, et al. Oxidation of tetrahydrobiopterin leads to uncoupling of endothelial cell nitric oxide synthase in hypertension. J Clin Invest. 2003;111(8):1201–9.

47. Lang M, Kojonazarov B, Tian X, Kalymbetov A, Weissmann N, Grimminger F, et al. The soluble guanylate cyclase stimulator riociguat ameliorates pulmonary hypertension induced by hypoxia and SU5416 in rats. PLoS One. 2012;7(8):e43433.
48. Le Cras TD, Xue C, Rengasamy A, Johns RA. Chronic hypoxia upregulates endothelial and inducible NO synthase gene and protein expression in rat lung. Am J Physiol. 1996;270(1 Pt 1):L164–70.
49. Li H, Oparil S, Meng QC, Elton TS, Chen YF. Selective downregulation of ANP-clearance-receptor gene expression in lung of rats adapted to hypoxia. Am J Physiol. 1995;268(2 Pt 1):L328–35.
50. Lincoln TM, Dey N, Sellak H. Invited review: cGMP-dependent protein kinase signaling mechanisms in smooth muscle: from the regulation of tone to gene expression. J Appl Physiol. 2001;91(3):1421–30.
51. Maack T. Receptors of atrial natriuretic factor. Annu Rev Physiol. 1992;54:11–27.
52. Mangiafico S, Costello-Boerrigter LC, Andersen IA, Cataliotti A, Burnett Jr JC. Neutral endopeptidase inhibition and the natriuretic peptide system: an evolving strategy in cardiovascular therapeutics. Eur Heart J. 2013;34(12):886–93.
53. Mason NA, Springall DR, Burke M, Pollock J, Mikhail G, Yacoub MH, et al. High expression of endothelial nitric oxide synthase in plexiform lesions of pulmonary hypertension. J Pathol. 1998;185(3):313–8.
54. Mehta S, Stewart DJ, Langleben D, Levy RD. Short-term pulmonary vasodilation with L-arginine in pulmonary hypertension. Circulation. 1995;92(6):1539–45.
55. Michelakis ED. The role of the NO axis and its therapeutic implications in pulmonary arterial hypertension. Heart Fail Rev. 2003;8(1):5–21.
56. Misono KS, Philo JS, Arakawa T, Ogata CM, Qiu Y, Ogawa H, et al. Structure, signaling mechanism and regulation of the natriuretic peptide receptor guanylate cyclase. FEBS J. 2011;278(11):1818–29.
57. Mitani Y, Maruyama K, Sakurai M. Prolonged administration of L-arginine ameliorates chronic pulmonary hypertension and pulmonary vascular remodeling in rats. Circulation. 1997;96(2):689–97.
58. Morris CR, Morris Jr SM, Hagar W, Van Warmerdam J, Claster S, Kepka-Lenhart D, Machado L, Kuypers FA, Vichinsky EP. Arginine therapy: a new treatment for pulmonary hypertension in sickle cell disease? Am J Respir Crit Care Med. 2003;168(1):63–9.
59. Murata T, Sato K, Hori M, Ozaki H, Karaki H. Decreased endothelial nitric-oxide synthase (eNOS) activity resulting from abnormal interaction between eNOS and its regulatory proteins in hypoxia-induced pulmonary hypertension. J Biol Chem. 2002;277(46):44085–92.
60. Murray F, MacLean MR, Pyne NJ. Increased expression of the cGMP-inhibited cAMP-specific (PDE3) and cGMP binding cGMP-specific (PDE5) phosphodiesterases in models of pulmonary hypertension. Br J Pharmacol. 2002;137(8):1187–94.
61. Murthy KK, Thibault G, Garcia R, Gutkowska J, Genest J, Cantin M. Degradation of atrial natriuretic factor in the rat. Biochem J. 1986;240(2):461–9.
62. Nagaya N, Nishikimi T, Uematsu M, Satoh T, Kyotani S, Sakamaki F, et al. Plasma brain natriuretic peptide as a prognostic indicator in patients with primary pulmonary hypertension. Circulation. 2000;102(8):865–70.
63. Nagaya N, Uematsu M, Oya H, Sato N, Sakamaki F, Kyotani S, Ueno K, Nakanishi N, Yamagishi M, Miyatake K. Short-term oral administration of L-arginine improves hemodynamics and exercise capacity in patients with precapillary pulmonary hypertension. Am J Respir Crit Care Med. 2001;163(4):887–91.
64. Nandi M, Miller A, Stidwill R, Jacques TS, Lam AA, Haworth S, et al. Pulmonary hypertension in a GTP-cyclohydrolase 1-deficient mouse. Circulation. 2005;111(16):2086–90.
65. Nikolova S, Guenther A, Savai R, Weissmann N, Ghofrani HA, Konigshoff M, et al. Phosphodiesterase 6 subunits are expressed and altered in idiopathic pulmonary fibrosis. Respir Res. 2010;11:146.
66. Palmer RM, Ashton DS, Moncada S. Vascular endothelial cells synthesize nitric oxide from L-arginine. Nature. 1988;333(6174):664–6.

67. Potter LR, Abbey-Hosch S, Dickey DM. Natriuretic peptides, their receptors, and cyclic guanosine monophosphate-dependent signaling functions. Endocr Rev. 2006;27(1):47–72.
68. Preston IR, Hill NS, Gambardella LS, Warburton RR, Klinger JR. Synergistic effects of ANP and sildenafil on cGMP levels and amelioration of acute hypoxic pulmonary hypertension. Exp Biol Med (Maywood). 2004;229(9):920–5.
69. Priviero FB, Webb RC. Heme-dependent and independent soluble guanylate cyclase activators and vasodilation. J Cardiovasc Pharmacol. 2010;56(3):229–33.
70. Reffelmann T, Kloner RA. Therapeutic potential of phosphodiesterase 5 inhibition for cardiovascular disease. Circulation. 2003;108(2):239–44.
71. Resta TC, Gonzales RJ, Dail WG, Sanders TC, Walker BR. Selective upregulation of arterial endothelial nitric oxide synthase in pulmonary hypertension. Am J Physiol. 1997;272(2 Pt 2):H806–13.
72. Rybalkin SD, Yan C, Bornfeldt KE, Beavo JA. Cyclic GMP phosphodiesterases and regulation of smooth muscle function. Circ Res. 2003;93(4):280–91.
73. Saadjian A, Philip-Joet F, Paganelli F, Arnaud A, Levy S. Long-term effects of cicletanine on secondary pulmonary hypertension. J Cardiovasc Pharmacol. 1998;31(3):364–71.
74. Schermuly RT, Kreisselmeier KP, Ghofrani HA, Yilmaz H, Butrous G, Ermert L, et al. Chronic sildenafil treatment inhibits monocrotaline-induced pulmonary hypertension in rats. Am J Respir Crit Care Med. 2004;169(1):39–45.
75. Schermuly RT, Pullamsetti SS, Kwapiszewska G, Dumitrascu R, Tian X, Weissmann N, et al. Phosphodiesterase 1 upregulation in pulmonary arterial hypertension: target for reverse-remodeling therapy. Circulation. 2007;115(17):2331–9.
76. Sebkhi A, Strange JW, Phillips SC, Wharton J, Wilkins MR. Phosphodiesterase type 5 as a target for the treatment of hypoxia-induced pulmonary hypertension. Circulation. 2003; 107(25):3230–5.
77. Shaul PW, Yuhanna IS, German Z, Chen Z, Steinhorn RH, Morin 3rd FC. Pulmonary endothelial NO synthase gene expression is decreased in fetal lambs with pulmonary hypertension. Am J Physiol. 1997;272(5 Pt 1):L1005–12.
78. Shekerdemian LS, Ravn HB, Penny DJ. Intravenous sildenafil lowers pulmonary vascular resistance in a model of neonatal pulmonary hypertension. Am J Respir Crit Care Med. 2002;165(8):1098–102.
79. Simonneau G, Rubin LJ, Galiè N, Barst RJ, Fleming TR, Frost AE, Engel PJ, Kramer MR, Burgess G, Collings L, Cossons N, Sitbon O, Badesch DB, PACES Study Group. Addition of sildenafil to long-term intravenous epoprostenol therapy in patients with pulmonary arterial hypertension: a randomized trial. Ann Intern Med. 2008;149(8):521–30.
80. Stasch JP, Pacher P, Evgenov OV. Soluble guanylate cyclase as an emerging therapeutic target in cardiopulmonary disease. Circulation. 2011;123(20):2263–73.
81. Steiner MK, Preston IR, Klinger JR, Hill NS. Pulmonary hypertension: inhaled nitric oxide, sildenafil and natriuretic peptides. Curr Opin Pharmacol. 2005;5(3):245–50.
82. Steudel W, Scherrer-Crosbie M, Bloch KD, Weimann J, Huang PL, Jones RC, et al. Sustained pulmonary hypertension and right ventricular hypertrophy after chronic hypoxia in mice with congenital deficiency of nitric oxide synthase 3. J Clin Invest. 1998;101(11):2468–77.
83. Tian X, Vroom C, Ghofrani HA, Weissmann N, Bieniek E, Grimminger F, et al. Phosphodiesterase 10A upregulation contributes to pulmonary vascular remodeling. PLoS One. 2011;6(4):e18136.
84. Tsai EJ, Kass DA. Cyclic GMP signaling in cardiovascular pathophysiology and therapeutics. Pharmacol Ther. 2009;122(3):216–38.
85. Tyler RC, Muramatsu M, Abman SH, Stelzner TJ, Rodman DM, Bloch KD, et al. Variable expression of endothelial NO synthase in three forms of rat pulmonary hypertension. Am J Physiol. 1999;276(2 Pt 1):L297–303.
86. van Faassen EE, Bahrami S, Feelisch M, Hogg N, Kelm M, Kim-Shapiro DB, et al. Nitrite as regulator of hypoxic signaling in mammalian physiology. Med Res Rev. 2009;29(5): 683–741.

87. Vanderford PA, Wong J, Chang R, Keefer LK, Soifer SJ, Fineman JR. Diethylamine/nitric oxide (NO) adduct, an NO donor, produces potent pulmonary and systemic vasodilation in intact newborn lambs. J Cardiovasc Pharmacol. 1994;23(1):113–9.
88. Veale CA, Alford VC, Aharony D, Banville DL, Bialecki RA, Brown FJ, et al. The discovery of non-basic atrial natriuretic peptide clearance receptor antagonists. Part 1. Bioorg Med Chem Lett. 2000;10(17):1949–52.
89. Verhaar MC, Westerweel PE, van Zonneveld AJ, Rabelink TJ. Free radical production by dysfunctional eNOS. Heart. 2004;90(5):494–5.
90. Vermeersch P, Buys E, Pokreisz P, Marsboom G, Ichinose F, Sips P, et al. Soluble guanylate cyclase-alpha1 deficiency selectively inhibits the pulmonary vasodilator response to nitric oxide and increases the pulmonary vascular remodeling response to chronic hypoxia. Circulation. 2007;116(8):936–43.
91. Weimann J, Ullrich R, Hromi J, Fujino Y, Clark MW, Bloch KD, et al. Sildenafil is a pulmonary vasodilator in awake lambs with acute pulmonary hypertension. Anesthesiology. 2000; 92(6):1702–12.
92. Wharton J, Strange JW, Moller GM, Growcott EJ, Ren X, Franklyn AP, et al. Antiproliferative effects of phosphodiesterase type 5 inhibition in human pulmonary artery cells. Am J Respir Crit Care Med. 2005;172(1):105–13.
93. Wilkens H, Guth A, Konig J, Forestier N, Cremers B, Hennen B, et al. Effect of inhaled iloprost plus oral sildenafil in patients with primary pulmonary hypertension. Circulation. 2001;104(11):1218–22.
94. Wu C, Wu F, Pan J, Morser J, Wu Q. Furin-mediated processing of Pro-C-type natriuretic peptide. J Biol Chem. 2003;278(28):25847–52.
95. Xue C, Johns RA. Endothelial nitric oxide synthase in the lungs of patients with pulmonary hypertension. N Engl J Med. 1995;333(24):1642–4.
96. Yan W, Wu F, Morser J, Wu Q. Corin, a transmembrane cardiac serine protease, acts as a pro-atrial natriuretic peptide-converting enzyme. Proc Natl Acad Sci U S A. 2000;97(15): 8525–9.
97. Yandle TG, Richards AM, Nicholls MG, Cuneo R, Espiner EA, Livesey JH. Metabolic clearance rate and plasma half life of alpha-human atrial natriuretic peptide in man. Life Sci. 1986;38(20):1827–33.
98. Zaccolo M, Movsesian MA. cAMP and cGMP signaling cross-talk: role of phosphodiesterases and implications for cardiac pathophysiology. Circ Res. 2007;100(11):1569–78.
99. Zhao L, Long L, Morrell NW, Wilkins MR. NPR-A-Deficient mice show increased susceptibility to hypoxia-induced pulmonary hypertension. Circulation. 1999;99(5):605–7.
100. Zhao L, Mason NA, Morrell NW, Kojonazarov B, Sadykov A, Maripov A, et al. Sildenafil inhibits hypoxia-induced pulmonary hypertension. Circulation. 2001;104(4):424–8.
101. Zhao L, Mason NA, Strange JW, Walker H, Wilkins MR. Beneficial effects of phosphodiesterase 5 inhibition in pulmonary hypertension are influenced by natriuretic Peptide activity. Circulation. 2003;107(2):234–7.
102. Zhao YY, Zhao YD, Mirza MK, Huang JH, Potula HH, Vogel SM, et al. Persistent eNOS activation secondary to caveolin-1 deficiency induces pulmonary hypertension in mice and humans through PKG nitration. J Clin Invest. 2009;119(7):2009–18.

Chapter 16
Combination Therapy for the Treatment of Pulmonary Arterial Hypertension

Andrew T. Levinson and James R. Klinger

Abstract A variety of medical therapies are presently available for the treatment of pulmonary arterial hypertension (PAH). Unfortunately, none are curative and most patients will experience progression of their disease despite treatment. Presently available medications target four different cellular signaling pathways that have been implicated in the pathogenesis of PAH. It is unclear to what extent each pathway contributes to the progression of pulmonary hypertension in individual patients and little data are available to guide practitioners in drug selection. The multiplicity of altered cell signaling pathways in PAH provides a strong rationale for the use of more than one drug to treat PAH, but the paucity of properly controlled data makes it difficult to determine if combination therapy provides superior efficacy compared to single agents. Recent data derived from studies in which a second drug is added to a therapy already being used by the patient and recently published studies of up-front combination therapy in treatment-naïve patients suggest that combination therapy may be more efficacious than treatment with a single drug. These findings support the hypothesis that multiple drugs may be necessary to achieve optimal benefit and may alter the therapeutic approach to PAH. This chapter discusses the rationale for combination therapy and reviews the findings of recently completed "add-on" and "up-front" combination studies that provide the basis for using this approach to treat PAH.

Keywords Pulmonary arterial hypertension • Pulmonary hypertension treatment • Combination therapy • Medical therapy for pulmonary hypertension

A.T. Levinson, M.D., M.P.H. • J.R. Klinger, M.D. (✉)
Division of Pulmonary, Sleep and Critical Care Medicine, Rhode Island Hospital, Alpert Medical School of Brown University, 593 Eddy Street, Providence, RI 02903, USA
e-mail: James_Klinger@brown.edu

J.R. Klinger, R.P. Frantz (eds.), *Diagnosis and Management of Pulmonary Hypertension*, Respiratory Medicine 12, DOI 10.1007/978-1-4939-2636-7_16

Abbreviations

6MWD	6-min walk distance
ANP	Atrial natriuretic peptide
BNP	Brain natriuretic peptide
cAMP	Cyclic adenosine monophosphate
cGMP	Cyclic guanosine monophosphate
CTEPH	Chronic thromboembolic pulmonary hypertension
ERA	Endothelin receptor antagonist
ET-1	Endothelin-1
ET_A	Endothelin receptor A
ET_B	Endothelin receptor B
LV	Left ventricle
mPAP	Mean pulmonary artery pressure
NO	Nitric oxide
PAH	Pulmonary arterial hypertension
PAP	Pulmonary artery pressure
PDE	Phosphodiesterase
PDE5	Phosphodiesterase type 5
PGI_2	Prostacyclin
PH	Pulmonary hypertension
PVR	Pulmonary vascular resistance
RV	Right ventricle
RVSP	Right ventricular systolic pressure
TPR	Total pulmonary resistance
WHO	World Health Organization

Introduction

Pulmonary arterial hypertension (PAH) is a pulmonary vasculopathy characterized by proliferation and hypertrophy of pulmonary arterial endothelial and smooth muscle cells. As the disease progresses, pulmonary vascular resistance (PVR) rises and the right ventricle (RV) becomes unable to compensate for the increase in afterload. These changes lead to right ventricular failure and eventually the inability to maintain adequate cardiac output. In the absence of treatment, 50 % of patients progress to right heart failure and death within 3 years of diagnosis. Proper diagnosis of PAH requires accurate assessment of pressures in the pulmonary arterial (PA) and pulmonary venous bed, a technique that is best accomplished by right-heart catheterization. The finding of elevated pulmonary artery pressure (PAP) and normal left-sided filling pressure in the proper clinical scenario (see Chap. 2) confirms the diagnosis of PAH [1]. Once a diagnosis of PAH is made, a variety of noninvasive techniques are often used to follow disease progression and response to therapy. These include

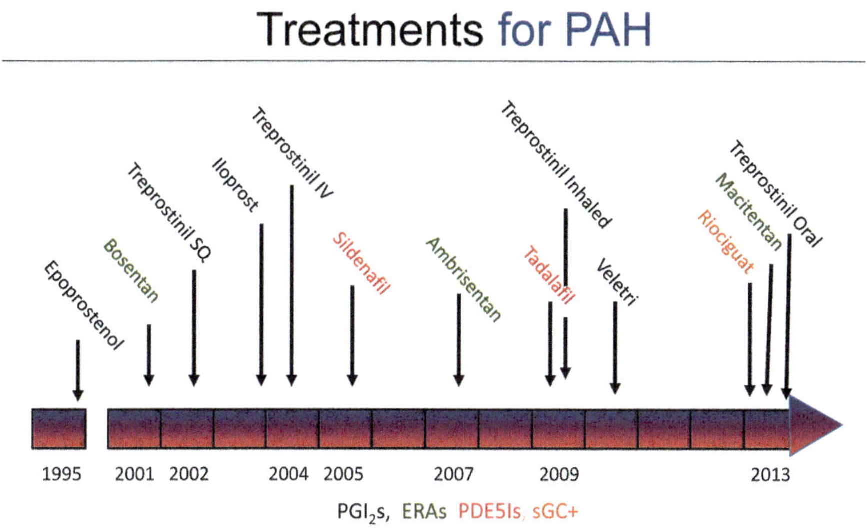

Fig. 16.1 Timeline of drugs approved for treatment of pulmonary arterial hypertension in the USA. *PGI2* prostaglandins, *ERAs* endothelial receptor antagonists, *PDE5Is* phosphodiesterase type-5 inhibitors, *sGC+* soluble guanylate cyclase stimulator

WHO functional class, 6-min walk distance (6MWD), plasma brain natriuretic peptide (BNP) levels, and transthoracic echocardiography to assess RV size and function as well as estimate PA systolic pressure. Right-heart catheterization is often repeated at 1–2-year intervals to confirm the results of noninvasive testing or sooner if clinical deterioration occurs.

Over a dozen medicines have been developed and approved for the treatment of PAH in the last 20 years (Fig. 16.1). Few studies have been undertaken to determine their relative efficacy in reducing PAP, improving functional capacity, or extending survival, making it difficult to determine which medications are best suited for individual patients. Updated guidelines for the treatment of PAH have recently been published by the American College of Chest Physicians and by the WHO fifth international meeting on PAH [2, 3]. These guidelines recommend that patients who present with advanced disease (WHO functional class IV) be treated with a continuous intravenous infusion of prostacyclin, but that those who present with more moderate disease (WHO functional class II or III) be treated initially with one of several orally active agents. Those who respond favorably are carefully monitored for disease progression. Those who do not respond, or who worsen on their original therapy, should be treated with other medications. Although it has not been determined whether it is better to switch a patient with an unsatisfactory response from one agent to another or to add additional therapy to the medication already being used, the most common approach has been the sequential addition of new medications. This approach worked fairly well when only a handful of medications were available to treat PAH, but with the increasing number of approved agents, it has become difficult to determine which drugs should be used together and in what sequence they should be added.

Medications Presently Available for Treatment of PAH

There are currently four classes of medications approved for the treatment of PAH. The first of these are the prostacyclin analogues. Prostacyclin (PGI_2) was discovered by Sir John Vane in the late 1970s [4] and is a member of the prostaglandin family of peptides and is synthesized in platelets and vascular endothelial cells. It has potent vasodilatory effects on vascular smooth muscle and anti-aggregation effects on platelets. The expression of prostacyclin synthase, the major enzyme involved in the synthesis of prostacyclins, is decreased in the lungs of PAH patients as is the ratio of circulating PGI_2 to thromboxane, suggesting a state of relative PGI_2 deficiency [5, 6]. Intravenous prostacyclin was found to be a potent pulmonary vasodilator and its ability to improve functional capacity and pulmonary hemodynamics in patients with PAH led to its development as pharmaceutical agent. In 1995, the synthetic PGI_2, epoprostenol, became the first FDA-approved treatment for PAH. The need for continuous intravenous infusion via central venous access makes epoprostenol a challenging therapy for most patients and its risk of catheter-related infection has led to the development of alternative prostacyclin therapies for PAH. Treprostinil is a prostacyclin derivative that is stable at room temperature and has a considerably longer half-life than epoprostenol. It was designed for continuous subcutaneous infusion, thereby obviating the need for a central venous catheter. This approach was found to be effective, but is associated with significant pain at the site of infusion making it difficult for some patients to continue treatment. Since its initial release in 2001, treprostinil has been approved for intravenous, inhaled, and oral administration. Iloprost is another prostacyclin derivative that is approved in the USA as an inhalational therapy for treating PAH, although its shorter half-life compared to treprostinil has resulted in the need for more frequent treatments. All three prostanoids have been shown to be efficacious at improving pulmonary hemodynamics, 6MWD, and/or WHO functional class in PAH, although the efficacy data for inhaled and oral prostacyclin therapy do not appear to be as robust as for intravenous or subcutaneous infusion [7–10].

Increased expression of endothelin-1 (ET-1), a potent vasoconstrictor and smooth muscle mitogen, has also been implicated in the pathogenesis of PAH. ET-1 is expressed at high levels in the pulmonary vascular lesions of PAH patients [11]. Plasma ET-1 levels are increased in patients with PAH compared to controls and correlate with the severity of PH [12, 13]. The biologic activity of ET-1 is mediated by endothelin receptor A and endothelin receptor B (ET_A and ET_B). Both nonselective endothelin receptor antagonists (ERAs) and antagonists selective for ET_A have been developed for the treatment of PAH and have been shown to improve pulmonary hemodynamics and 6MWD and to delay time to clinical worsening [14, 15].

The secondary messenger cGMP plays important roles in modulating pulmonary hypertensive and right ventricular hypertrophic responses. Intracellular cGMP levels are increased by activation of soluble and particulate guanylate cyclases in response to nitric oxide (NO) and the natriuretic peptides, respectively. A considerable body of evidence has accumulated to suggest that decreased bioavailability of NO contributes to the pathogenesis of PAH (for review, see Klinger et al. [16]).

Circulating levels of atrial and brain natriuretic peptide (ANP and BNP) are increased in patients with PAH, but the ratio of urinary cyclic GMP/BNP is markedly decreased suggesting downregulation of the particulate guanylate cyclase, natriuretic peptide receptor-A [17]. cGMP levels are also regulated by the activity of a family of phosphodiesterases (PDE) that are primarily responsible for its degradation. PDE type-5 (PDE5) is the primary enzyme responsible for degradation of cyclic GMP in the lung. Its activity has been shown to be increased in animal models of PH [18]. Drugs that inhibit PDE5 such as sildenafil and tadalafil have been shown to be effective at lowering PVR and improving 6MWD in patients with PAH [19, 20] and have been approved for treatment. Other drugs, such as inhaled NO or the recently approved soluble guanylate cyclase stimulator, riociguat that stimulate the synthesis of cGMP, have also been found to be effective treatments for PAH [21].

Rationale for Combination Therapy

There are two major reasons that are most often cited for combining different therapies in the treatment of PAH. The first is that numerous mechanisms contribute to the pathogenesis of PAH and therefore multiple signaling pathways need to be targeted simultaneously. The second is that there are potential interactions between the known classes of PAH-specific medications that could provide additive or synergistic effects when used together. For example, many of the beneficial effects of prostacyclins on the pulmonary circulation are mediated by intracellular cAMP levels. Cyclic GMP acts as a substrate for some of the same phosphodiesterases that metabolize cyclic AMP and elevation of intracellular cGMP by PDE-5 inhibitors may slow the metabolism of cAMP. Indeed, studies have shown that PDE inhibitors that increase intracellular levels of cGMP in the RV of rats with monocrotaline-induced pulmonary hypertension also result in an increase in cAMP levels that increase right ventricular contractility [22]. Thus, combining prostacyclin therapy with a PDE5 inhibitor may result in better elevation of both cyclic nucleotide levels and potentially increase their clinical efficacy. Similarly, NO and the natriuretic peptides have been shown to suppress synthesis of endothelin, likely via elevation of intracellular cyclic GMP levels [23, 24]. Thus, a combination of a PDE5 inhibitor and an ERA may be more effective at blunting the effects of endothelin than either agent alone.

Clinical Trials of Combination Therapy

The pharmacologic approach to treating PAH has evolved considerably over the last two decades as new medications have been developed. When the number of drugs available for treating PAH was limited, it was common practice to start a patient on a single agent and then add additional therapy if the patient failed to improve. Rather than switching patients from one agent to another, physicians preferred to simply add a second class of drug that targeted a different biologic pathway and continue the original therapy that the patient was taking. This approach developed for several reasons. First, when a PAH patient does not improve on a given therapy, it is difficult to exclude the possibility that the treatment is still having some beneficial effect and that the patient's disease will not worsen if the drug is removed. Second, the several months that most medications need to be effective would result in patients essentially starting over if they were switched from one drug to another. Finally, a variety of animal studies began to demonstrate the additive effects of some pulmonary vasodilator agents when used in combination to blunt the development of experimental pulmonary hypertension [25].

The evolution of clinical practice to use multiple drugs in combination for the treatment of PAH led to the organization of numerous clinical trials to examine the efficacy of combination therapy (Table 16.1). Unfortunately, few studies have examined the efficacy of combination therapy for PAH in a properly controlled randomized clinical trial. In order to evaluate the difference in efficacy between two drugs versus one drug, patients need to be randomized to one of the three arms: (1) drug A + placebo, (2) drug B + placebo, or (3) drug A + drug B (Fig. 16.2). Due to the large number of treatment-naïve patients needed for this approach, this type of study protocol has not been used until very recently. Instead, the vast majority of clinical trials evaluating combination therapy in PAH have used a protocol where patients who are clinically stable on drug A are randomized to drug A + drug B or drug A + placebo (Fig. 16.2). The limitation of this "add-on" approach is that the beneficial effect in the combination therapy group may result from drug B simply being superior to drug A rather than any additive or synergistic effects between the two drugs. In other words, the effect may have been the same if the patients were switched to drug B from drug A instead of adding drug B to drug A.

There is also a problem with selection bias in "add-on"-type trials. Patients may be more likely to be recruited into an "add-on" study if they had an unsatisfactory response to their initial therapy and this may increase the likelihood that they respond to the new drug. Such selection bias is shown in Fig. 16.3. If some PAH patients are more responsive to one class of PAH medication than the other drug classes, then monotherapy would select out those patients who do not respond to the initial medication. When a new medication is added to the failed background therapy, patients who improve may simply be responding to the new medication and not the combination of the original and newly added agent (Fig. 16.3a). If, however, the great majority of PAH patients have similar responses to all of the three major drug classes, then it is unlikely that the beneficial effect of adding a new medication to the old is due to the new medication alone. In this scenario, the beneficial treatment is likely to be due to the additive or synergistic effect of the two medications working together (Fig. 16.3b). Despite these limitations, a considerable body of data has been produced using add-on studies to examine the effect of combination therapies in PAH.

Table 16.1 Summary of major clinical trials of combination therapy

Study	Number enrolled	Study design	Treatment groups	Patient population	Primary outcomes	Results
Phosphodiesterase inhibitors and prostacyclin analogues						
Ghofrani, H.A. et al. (2002) Ann Intern Med 136: 515–522.	30	Randomized, controlled open-label trial	12.5 mg sildenafil, 50 mg sildenafil, 12.5 mg sildenafil + iloprost, 50 mg sildenafil + iloprost	Severe PAH or CTEPH	Maximum reduction of pulmonary vascular resistance (PVR), increase in cardiac index (CI) followed over 2 h	Iloprost + sildenafil more effective then sildenafil alone at reducing PVR and increasing CI
Ghofrani, H.A. et al. (2003) J Am Coll Cardiol 42: 158–164.	14	Prospective non-randomized observational study	Patients who deteriorated on iloprost were given sildenafil + iloprost	Severe PPH, PAH	6MWD over 12 months	Increase in 6MWD
Simonneau, G. et al. (2008) Ann Intern Med 149: 521–530.	267	Double-blind placebo-controlled parallel group study	Patients being treated with epoprostenol randomized to sildenafil or placebo	Class I–IV PAH	6MWD, mean PA pressure, cardiac output, time to clinical worsening over 16 weeks	Improvement in 6MWD, mean PA pressure, and cardiac output and time to clinical worsening
Endothelin receptor antagonists and prostacyclin analogues						
Hoeper, M.M. et al. (2006) Eur Respir J 28: 691–694.	40	Multicenter randomized, open-label, controlled trial	Patients on bosentan randomized bosentan + inhaled iloprost or bosentan + placebo	Class III PPH	6MWD over 12 weeks	No change in 6MWD
Humbert, M. et al. (2004) Eur Respir J 24: 353–359.	33	Double-blind placebo-controlled prospective study	Patients starting epoprostenol randomized to bosentan or placebo in a 2:1 ratio	Class III or IV PAH	TPR, 6MWD, dyspnea score, NYHA functional class over 16 weeks	No change in TPR, dyspnea, 6MWD, NYHA class

(continued)

Table 16.1 (continued)

Study	Number enrolled	Study design	Treatment groups	Patient population	Primary outcomes	Results
Mclaughlin, V. et al. (2006) Am J Respir Crit Care Med 174: 1257–1263.	67	Double-blind randomized multicenter trial	Patients stable on bosentan randomized to bosentan + iloprost or bosentan + placebo	Class III or IV PPH and PAH	6MWD, change in NYHA class over 12 weeks	Increase in 6MWD and improvement in NYHA class
Mclaughlin, V.V. et al. (2010) J Am Coll Cardiol 55: 1915–1922	235	Randomized placebo-controlled multicenter study	Patients receiving a stable dose of sildenafil or bosentan randomized to treprostinil or placebo	Class III or IV PAH	6MWD over 12 weeks	Significant improvement in 6MWD
Seyfarth, H.J. et al. (2005) Chest 128: 709–713.	16	Prospective non-randomized open-label study	Patients on a background of beraprost or iloprost randomized to add bosentan or placebo	Class II–IV PAH or CTEPH	RV function index, 6MWD followed from 6 to 22 months	Improvement in RV function index and 6MWD
Prostacyclins and endothelin receptor antagonists and/or phosphodiesterase-5 inhibitors						
Tapson, V.F. et al, (2012) Chest 142:1383–1390.	350	Double blind, placebo controlled	Patients on an ERA, PDE-5 inhibitor, or both, randomized to oral treprostinil initiated at an initial dose of 1 mg bid, or placebo	Severe PAH	Change in 6MWD from baseline to week 16	No change in 6MWD
Tapson, V.F. et al, (2013) Chest in press.	310	Double blind, placebo controlled	Patients on an ERA, PDE-5 inhibitor, or both, randomized to oral treprostinil initiated at an initial dose of 0.25 mg bid, or placebo	Severe PAH	Change in 6MWD from baseline to week 16	No change in 6MWD

Phosphodiesterase-5 inhibitors and endothelin receptor antagonists						
Hoeper, M.M. et al. (2004) Eur Respir J 24: 1007–1010.	9	Prospective non-randomized observational study	Patients on bosentan with clinical deterioration or no improvement were given sildenafil + bosentan	Class III or IV PAH	6MWD over 12 weeks	Improvement in 6MWD and CPET
Publication pending.	500	Randomized, double-blind, placebo-controlled trial	Treatment-naïve patients randomized to tadalafil 40 mg + placebo, ambrisentan 10 mg + placebo, or tadalafil 10 mg + ambrisentan 10 mg	Class III or IV	Time to clinical worsening	Time to clinical worsening was significantly longer in patients given tadalafil + ambrisentan compared to either drug alone

PAH pulmonary arterial hypertension, *CTPEH* chronic thromboembolic hypertension, *PPH* primary pulmonary hypertension, *6MWD* 6-min walk distance, *CPET* cardiopulmonary exercise testing, *TPR* total pulmonary resistance, *RV function* right ventricular function, *PA* pulmonary artery, *ERA* endothelin-receptor antagonist, *PDE-5 inhibitor* phosphodiesterase-5 inhibitor

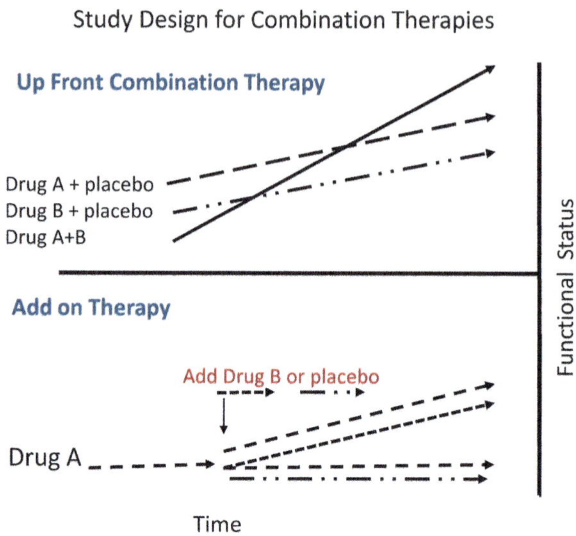

Fig. 16.2 Proper testing of the efficacy of combination of two therapies requires three arms. One tests the efficacy of the first drug alone, the second arm tests the efficacy of the other agent alone, and the third arm tests the efficacy of the two drugs together (up-front combination therapy). In order to blind the patient and investigators a placebo for each drug is required. Studies that add either a second drug or placebo after patients have already been treated with another agent (add-on therapy) cannot determine if any improvement is due to the combination of the two medications or the second medication alone. See text for discussion

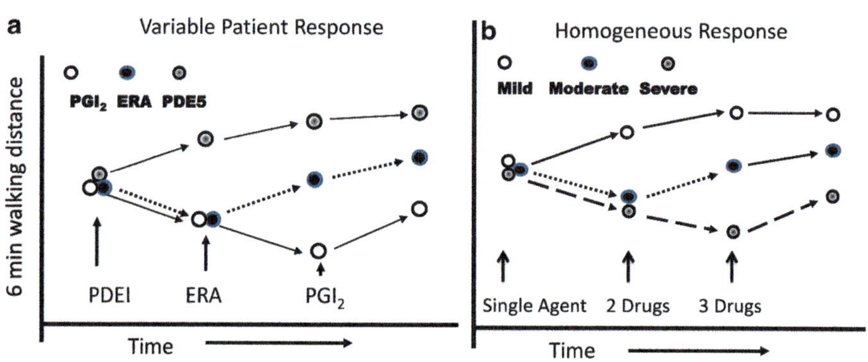

Fig. 16.3 Patient response to multiple therapies may be affected by how varied the underlying pathogenesis is in the treatment group. (**a**) If the study population consists of a mix of patients with different underlying mechanisms for their disease such that some are more likely to respond to one class of medication than the other, then clinical improvement observed after addition of a new therapy may be due to the new therapy alone. In this scenario, the benefit of multiple medications derives from increasing the odds that the patients will receive a medication that they are capable of responding to rather than any synergistic effects of the medicines used. (**b**) If all patients studied have the same pathogenic mechanism for their disease and are expected to respond similarly to each medication, then clinical improvement observed after addition of a new therapy to the old is more likely to be the result of the combined effect of the medications. In this example, patients with mild disease may only need one drug to improve while those with more severe disease require the additive or synergistic effects of multiple medications. *PDEI* phosphodiesterase inhibitor, *ERA* endothelin receptor antagonist, *PGI*^{2} prostacyclin

Phosphodiesterase Inhibitors and Prostacyclin Analogues

The effect of elevating intracellular cAMP via prostanoid administration and cGMP via inhibition of PDE5 has been examined in animal models of pulmonary hypertension. In an early study of rats by Itoh et al. [25], both sildenafil and the prostacyclin derivative beraprost were shown to blunt the development of monocrotaline-induced pulmonary hypertension, but the combination of sildenafil plus beraprost caused a significantly greater attenuation in right ventricular systolic pressure, right ventricular hypertrophy, and pulmonary vascular remodeling. In addition, none of the animals treated with the combination of sildenafil and beraprost died during the 6 weeks of study, whereas one died in the sildenafil-alone group and two died in the beraprost-alone group. Similarly, the combination of sildenafil and beraprost was found to be more effective than beraprost alone at acutely improving pulmonary hemodynamics in a small group of patients with PAH [26]. Patients were given beraprost on day 1 and the combination of sildenafil and beraprost on day 2. The reduction in mean PA pressure was 2-fold greater and the decrease in PVR was 1.6-fold greater with the combination of sildenafil plus beraprost than with beraprost alone, although there was no significant difference in cardiac output or right atrial pressure. At the same time, sildenafil was shown to enhance the acute pulmonary vasodilator effect of the inhaled prostacyclin derivative, iloprost in 30 patients with PAH or chronic thromboembolic pulmonary hypertension (CTEPH) [27]. In that study, patients were randomized to receive 12.5 or 50 mg of sildenafil either alone or in combination with inhaled iloprost. Sildenafil produced decreases in mean PA pressure and PVR that were similar to inhaled iloprost alone, but the effect was greater when both drugs were used together and sustained for a longer period of time.

Sildenafil has also been shown to improve functional capacity when added to a background of prostacyclin therapy. In one study, of 14 patients who had deteriorated on inhaled iloprost over an average of 18 months after initially improving during the first 3 months of therapy, the addition of sildenafil to their regular iloprost treatments increased 6MWD approximately 100 m and the improvement in walking distance was sustained for up to 12 months when both therapies were continued together [28].

Perhaps the most robust data to suggest that PDE5 inhibitors and prostacyclin have additive effects come from the Pulmonary Arterial Hypertension Combination Study of Epoprostenol and Sildenafil (PACES) [29]. This double-blind, placebo-controlled, parallel group study is the largest study to examine the effect of any add-on therapy in PAH. The study randomized 267 patients who were on a stable dose of intravenous epoprostenol for at least 3 months to receive either placebo or sildenafil in addition to their regular epoprostenol infusion. The primary outcome was placebo-corrected change from baseline in 6MWD. Secondary endpoints included time to clinical worsening, change in mean PA pressure, and change in Borg Dyspnea Scale. After 16 weeks, there was a placebo-corrected increase of 28.8 m in the group that received sildenafil (Fig. 16.4). Patients who received sildenafil also had greater decrease in mean PA pressure, improved cardiac output, and

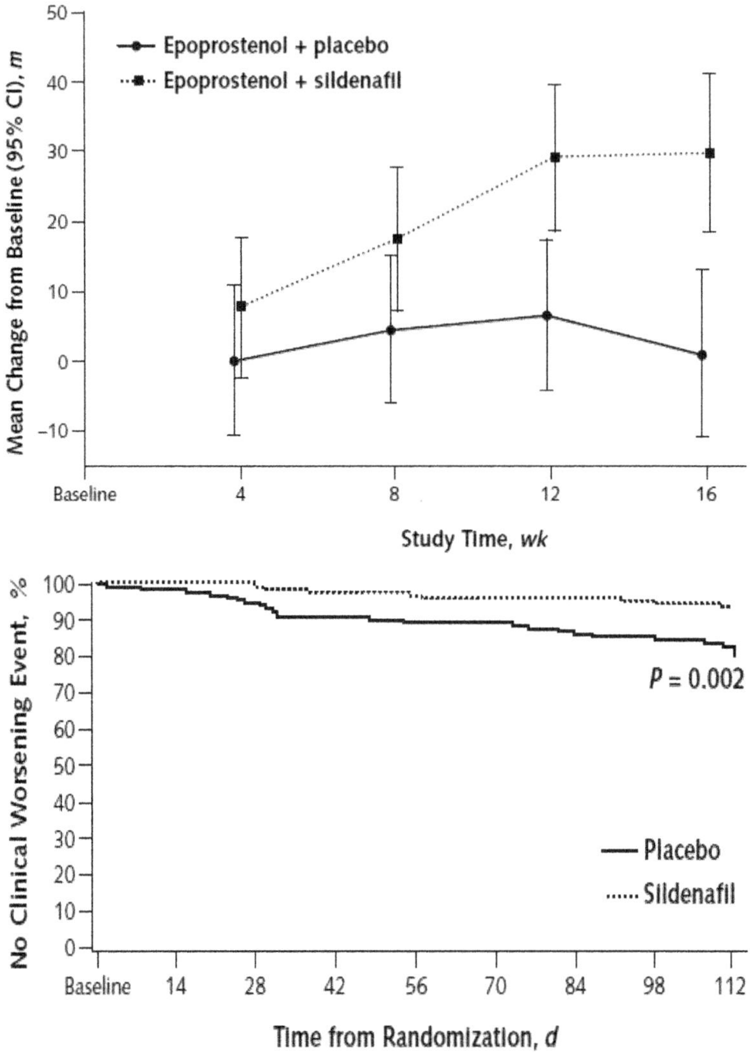

Fig. 16.4 (*Upper panel*) Improvement in 6-min walk distance after adding sildenafil or placebo to pulmonary arterial hypertension patients who were on background therapy with continuous epoprostenol infusion. (*Lower panel*) Time to clinical worsening in the same study cohort as the above panel (from Simonneau G et al. Ann Intern Med 2009;149:521–530)

longer time to clinical worsening than those given placebo (Fig. 16.4). This landmark study greatly advanced the concept of combination therapy in PAH for several reasons. First, it was the largest randomized, double-blind placebo-controlled study to evaluate the effect of adding one therapy to another. Second, there were consistent improvements in both the primary and secondary outcome variables. Finally, the improvement in the outcome variables was similar in scope to that achieved in treatment-naïve patients, but occurred in patients who had been on continuous intravenous infusion of epoprostenol for an average of 1 year at the time of randomization. Prior to the PACES study, patients on chronic epoprostenol infusion were felt to be on maximum medical therapy. The demonstration that even patients on long-term treatment with what is considered to be the most efficacious therapy for PAH could experience significant improvement by the addition of an oral agent strongly suggested that combination therapy is more efficacious than treatment with a single agent. Long-term follow-up of the PACES cohort demonstrated at 3 years that 66 % of patients were known to be alive, 24 % known to be deceased, and 10 % lost to follow-up. Maintenance or improvement in 6-min walk was present in 59 %, 44 %, and 33 % at 1, 2, and 3 years, respectively [30]. Together, the above studies demonstrate that patients who have either deteriorated or who are no longer responding to therapy with inhaled or intravenous prostanoids may improve with the addition of a PDEI. Conversely, failure to improve after such additional therapy is concerning, and should promote consideration of evaluation for lung transplantation.

Prostacyclins and Endothelin Receptor Antagonists

Several studies have examined the effect of adding an ERA to a prostacyclin derivative. One of the first was the BREATHE-2 study that randomized 33 patients with PAH to bosentan or placebo 48 h after starting therapy with intravenous epoprostenol [31]. The primary outcome was change in total pulmonary resistance (TPR) from baseline to week 16. Secondary outcomes included change in 6MWD, dyspnea scores, and NYHA functional class. There was a trend toward a greater reduction in TPR in the group that received combination therapy compared to the epoprostenol + placebo group, but the difference was not statistically significant. There was also no statistically significant difference in 6MWD, dyspnea scores, and NYHA functional class between the two groups. Part of the reason the study failed to find significant differences may have been due to the relatively small number of patients studied. On the other hand, two patients in the bosentan + epoprostenol group died while receiving treatment and a third patient died after being withdrawn from the study for worsening PAH, whereas there were no deaths in the epoprostenol + placebo group.

Another small study examined the effect of adding bosentan to beraprost or inhaled or intravenous iloprost in 16 patients with PAH or CTEPH who had shown no improvement in RV function index, 6MWD, or NYHA class after a year of prostanoid treatment [32]. Patients were then given bosentan in addition to their prostanoid therapy and were found to have a significant improvement in 6MWD and RV function index after 6 months of the combined therapies. The improvement over prostanoid therapy alone was sustained for up to 22 months and there was an improvement in NYHA class in 9 of the 16 patients.

The effect of adding inhaled iloprost to patients who had been treated with bosentan alone was evaluated in two separate studies conducted during the same period. The STEP study (Safety and pilot efficacy Trial in combination with bosentan for Evaluation in Pulmonary arterial hypertension) was a multicenter, double-blinded study of 67 PAH patients in NYHA functional class III or IV who were randomized to iloprost or placebo after at least 16 weeks of treatment with bosentan alone [33]. After 12 weeks of add-on therapy, the difference in placebo-adjusted 6MWD from baseline (the primary study endpoint) was an increase of 30 m in the bosentan + iloprost group and an increase of 4 m in bosentan + placebo group. The placebo-corrected difference of 26 m did not quite reach statistical significance ($p = 0.051$). However there was a significant improvement in NYHA functional class, reduction in mean PA pressure, and delay in time to clinical worsening in the bosentan plus iloprost group compared to bosentan plus placebo [33]. The other study, known as the COMBI Trial (Combination Therapy of Bosentan and aerosolized Iloprost in Idiopathic Pulmonary Arterial Hypertension), was a 12-week, phase IV, open-label, randomized, controlled multicenter study conducted in Germany that randomized IPAH patients who were functional class III to bosentan plus inhaled iloprost or bosentan plus placebo [34]. The primary study endpoint was the change in 6MWD after 12 weeks. Secondary endpoints included changes in functional class and clinical worsening. The trial was terminated early after enrolling 40 patients when an interim analysis showed futility of the combination therapy with a mean decrease in 6MWD of only 9 m in the iloprost group compared to a 1 m mean increase in the placebo group ($p = 0.49$). No statistically significant differences were seen between the bosentan plus iloprost or bosentan plus placebo groups.

The largest and most recent study to examine the effect of combining prostacyclin and an ERA comes from the TRIUMPH study (Treprostinil Sodium Inhalation Used in the Management of Pulmonary Arterial Hypertension) in which 235 patients with WHO functional class III or IV PAH who were clinically stable on a background therapy of either bosentan (70 %) or sildenafil monotherapy (30 %) were randomized to receive 12 weeks of inhaled treprostinil or placebo four times daily [10]. The primary endpoint was changed from baseline in 6MWD. Secondary endpoints included time to clinical worsening, Borg Dyspnea Scale, and change in NYHA functional class. There was a statistically significant increase in 6MWD of 19 m in the group treated with inhaled treprostinil, but no differences were seen in most of the secondary endpoints, including time to clinical worsening, Borg Dyspnea Scale, and NYHA functional class.

Two recent randomized placebo-controlled multicenter international trials have examined the effect of giving an oral prostacyclin to patients with PAH who are already taking an ERA or PDE5 inhibitor or who are already on combination therapy with an ERA and a PDE5 inhibitor. In the first study, FREEDOM-C, 350 patients with PAH on stable background therapy with an ERA and/or a PDE5 inhibitor were randomized to receive either oral treprostinil or placebo bid [8]. All patients were in a steady clinical state on background therapy of their PDE5 inhibitor and/or ERA. At the beginning of the 16-week study patients in the treatment group were started at a dose of 1 mg bid of treprostinil. Treatment doses were titrated up to a maximum of 16 mg bid over the 16-week study period based on tolerance of the study drug side effects and clinical symptoms. The primary endpoint was placebo-corrected change in 6MWD at the end of the 16-week study period. Secondary endpoints included time to clinical worsening, Borg Dyspnea Scale, and decrease in WHO functional class. The study found no statistically significant improvement in 6MWD or in most of the secondary endpoints [8]. There was a high discontinuation rate of the study drug that the authors hypothesized could have been caused by too high of a starting dose or by increasing the dose of study drug in too great of an increment. In a subsequent study by the same authors, the FREEDOM-C2 study, an additional 310 patients were enrolled using the same study design and primary outcome criteria [35]; however, the starting dosage of oral treprostinil was reduced to 0.25 mg BID. As in the prior study, no difference in the primary outcome of 6MWD at 16 weeks was found [35].

Phosphodiesterase-5 Inhibitors and Endothelin Receptor Antagonists

Perhaps the most attractive combination therapy from the patient perspective is the use of a PDE5 inhibitor in conjunction with an ERA. Both drugs can be administered orally and are available in a once-a-day dose, allowing patients the benefit of combination therapy without needing to take numerous medications. Until recently, only a few studies had examined the combined effects of these classes of drug. In a small non-randomized observational study, 9 of 58 patients with functional class III or IV PAH who were treated initially with bosentan alone failed to improve or had a decline in their 6MWD and cardiopulmonary exercise testing after 3 months of therapy [36]. These patients were subsequently given 25–50 mg of sildenafil in addition to bosentan. After 3 months of combined therapy, the 6MWD increased from 277 to 392 m ($p=0.007$) and the improvement was sustained over an average of 9 months of follow-up. Benza et al. published similar results in abstract form using a somewhat different design [37]. In their study, 16/100 (16 %) treatment-naïve PAH patients treated with bosentan alone reached a predetermined 6MWD goal of >360 m by week 16. Six other patients withdrew from the study. The remaining 78 were given sildenafil 20 mg tid in addition to bosentan. Twelve weeks later, 15/78 patients treated with the combination of bosentan and sildenafil were able to achieve a 6MWD >380 m. Although it is possible that the improvement in 6MWD between weeks 16 and 28 was due to a delayed effect of bosentan alone, previous studies have suggested that the maximum effect of bosentan on 6MWD is achieved within the first 3–4 months of therapy [14]. More information on the efficacy of combining an ERA and PDE5 inhibitor may be determined by the results of the recently completed trial called COMPASS 2 in which patients with PAH who were clinically stable on monotherapy with sildenafil were randomized to receive bosentan or placebo. This phase IV, prospective, randomized, double-blind, placebo-controlled, study examined the effect of adding bosentan on the time to first morbidity or mortality event. Although the observed risk reduction of 17 % observed with bosentan versus placebo did not reach statistical significance, ($p=0.25$), there was a 22 m improvement in 6MWD at week 16 ($p=0.01$) [38].

As discussed previously, none of the studies of any of the drug combinations discussed to this point properly examined the effects of combination versus monotherapy because they did not employ a treatment protocol that compared the combination of drugs to either drug alone. Thus, it is not possible to determine if any of the beneficial effects observed in the above "add-on" studies were due to the combination of the background therapy plus the new medication or to the new medication alone. Recently, the AMBITION study (A Randomized, Multicenter Study of First-Line Ambrisentan and Tadalafil Combination Therapy in Subjects With Pulmonary Arterial Hypertension) compared the efficacy of up-front combination therapy with a PDE5 inhibitor and an ERA to up-front therapy with a PDE5 inhibitor or ERA alone [39]. This phase IV prospective clinical trial randomized 500 patients to receive (1) tadalafil plus ambrisentan placebo, (2) ambrisentan plus tadalafil placebo, or (3) tadalafil plus ambrisentan in a 1:1:2 randomization scheme. Study drug was increased to doses of 10 mg ambrisentan and 40 mg tadalafil. The primary endpoint was time to first clinical failure event, defined as time from randomization to the first occurrence of death, hospitalization for worsening PAH, disease progression, or unsatisfactory long-term clinical response. The treatment effect observed was a 50 % reduction in the primary endpoint in the group treated with the combination of ambrisentan and tadalafil [40]. Statistically significant improvements versus the pooled monotherapy arm were also seen in median change from baseline to week 24 in 6MWD (49.0 m vs. 23.8 m; $p<0.0001$), N-terminal pro-B-type natriuretic peptide (NT-proBNP) (−67.4 % vs. −49.7 %; $p<0.0001$), and percentage of patients with satisfactory clinical response at week 24 (39 % vs. 29 %; $p=0.026$), although there was no difference between treatment groups in the change in WHO functional class [40].

This study has provided the strongest data thus far to suggest that combination therapy is more efficacious than treatment with a single agent for patients with PAH. It is interesting to speculate what mechanism is responsible for the better performance of tadalafil and ambrisentan when used together compared to either drug alone. cGMP has been shown to inhibit endothelin release in cultured endothelial cells and it is possible that inhibition of PDE5 by tadalafil reduces pulmonary vascular endothelin levels, thereby making ambrisentan more effective. Alternatively, cGMP may be a more effective pulmonary vasodilator when the endothelin receptor A is blocked by ambrisentan. Alternatively, it is possible that some patients are more responsive to PDE5 inhibitors and that others are more responsive to ERAs and that the use of both drugs together simply resulted in more patients having a favorable response.

ATPAHSS (A Clinical Trial of Ambrisentan and Tadalafil in Pulmonary Arterial Hypertension Associated With Systemic Sclerosis) is a similar randomized, double-blind, parallel group study that randomized patients with PAH secondary to systemic sclerosis to the same three groups as in AMBITION [41]. The primary endpoint is the effect of the various medications on right ventricular mass as assessed by cardiac MRI and *pulmonary* vascular PVR by right-heart catheterization. Secondary endpoints are similar to those in AMBITION. The study has completed enrollment and results should be available in 2015.

The hypothesis that the initial treatment of PAH with a combination of medications is more efficacious than monotherapy is also supported by the results of a recently published observational study of up-front triple combination therapy in patients with newly diagnosed severe PAH. In this retrospective analysis, 18 consecutive patients who met the criteria of severe PAH at the time of diagnosis were treated with a combination of epoprostenol, bosentan, and sildenafil and demonstrated a 3-year survival of 100 %, although one patient required lung transplantation after 3 months [42]. This remarkable report, in a set of patients with a very high predicted mortality, raises the provocative possibility that up-front triple therapy may be more effective than the traditional sequential therapy. Further clinical trials of this approach seem appropriate erring on the side of more up-front therapy and possibly withdrawal of medications if patients become highly stable.

Summary and Conclusions

Combining presently available therapies to treat PAH has scientific rationale and is supported by preclinical studies in animal models of PH and by the results of recently completed clinical trials. Using more than a single agent up front increases the odds of a patient being treated with a drug to which they will respond and provides the possibility of an additive or synergistic effect of the two medications. Several placebo-controlled trials have shown improvement in functional capacity, hemodynamic measurements, and time to clinical worsening in patients given a new PAH medication after failing to respond or deteriorating on their original therapy. In these trials, it is not known if the benefit observed was the result of the combined effects of the new therapy and the old or if similar results would have been obtained by simply switching from their initial therapy to the new one. Recently released findings from the AMBITION study strongly suggest that the combination of PDE5 inhibitor and ERA is more efficacious for the treatment of PAH than either drug alone. If future studies are able to better determine which patients are more likely to respond to different drug classes, the use of multiple drugs as initial therapy may not be necessary. Until that time however, the use of combination therapy appears to have significant advantages over monotherapy and should be strongly considered both for PAH patients who have failed to improve with monotherapy and as initial therapy in patients with newly diagnosed PAH.

References

1. Simonneau G, Robbins IM, Beghetti M, et al. Updated clinical classification of pulmonary hypertension. J Am Coll Cardiol. 2009;54:S43–54.
2. Taichman DB, Ornelas J, Chung L, Klinger JR, Lewis S, Mandel J, Palevsky HI, Rich S, Sood N, Rosenzweig EB, Trow TK, Yung R, Elliott CG, Badesch DB. Pharmacologic therapy for pulmonary arterial hypertension in adults: CHEST guideline and expert panel report. Chest. 2014;146(2):449–75.
3. Galiè N, Corris PA, Frost A, Girgis RE, Granton J, Jing ZC, Klepetko W, McGoon MD, McLaughlin VV, Preston IR, Rubin LJ, Sandoval J, Seeger W, Keogh A. Updated treatment algorithm of pulmonary arterial hypertension. J Am Coll Cardiol. 2013;62(25 Suppl):D60–72.
4. Moncada S, Gryglewski R, Bunting S, et al. An enzyme isolated from arteries transforms prostaglandin endoperoxides to an unstable substance that inhibits platelet aggregation. Nature. 1976;263:663–5.
5. Tuder RM, Cool CD, Geraci MW, et al. Prostacyclin synthase expression is decreased in lungs from patients with severe pulmonary hypertension. Am J Respir Crit Care Med. 1999;159: 1925–32.
6. Christman BW, McPherson CD, Newman JH, et al. An imbalance between the excretion of thromboxane and prostacyclin metabolites in pulmonary hypertension. N Engl J Med. 1992;327:70–5.
7. Barst RJ, Rubin LJ, Long WA, et al. A comparison of continuous intravenous epoprostenol (prostacyclin) with conventional therapy for primary pulmonary hypertension. The Primary Pulmonary Hypertension Study Group. N Engl J Med. 1996;334:296–302.
8. Tapson VF, Torres F, Kermeen F, Keogh AM, Allen RP, Frantz RP, Badesch DB, Frost AE, Shapiro SM, Laliberte K, Sigman J, Arneson C, Galiè N. Oral treprostinil for the treatment of pulmonary arterial hypertension in patients on background endothelin receptor antagonist and/or phosphodiesterase type 5 inhibitor therapy (the FREEDOM-C study): a randomized controlled trial. Chest. 2012;142(6):1383–90.
9. Simonneau G, Barst RJ, Galie N, Naeije R, Rich S, Bourge RC, Keogh A, Oudiz R, Frost A, Blackburn SD, Crow JW, Rubin LJ, Treprostinil Study Group. Continuous subcutaneous infusion of treprostinil, a prostacyclin analogue, in patients with pulmonary arterial hypertension: a double-blind, randomized, placebo-controlled trial. Am J Respir Crit Care Med. 2002; 165(6):800–4.
10. McLaughlin VV, Benza RL, Rubin LJ, et al. Addition of inhaled treprostinil to oral therapy for pulmonary arterial hypertension: a randomized controlled clinical trial. J Am Coll Cardiol. 2010;55:1915–22.
11. Giaid A, Yanagisawa M, Langleben D, et al. Expression of endothelin-1 in the lungs of patients with pulmonary hypertension. N Engl J Med. 1993;328:1732–9.
12. Stewart DJ, Levy RD, Cernacek P, et al. Increased plasma endothelin-1 in pulmonary hypertension: marker or mediator of disease? Ann Intern Med. 1991;114:464–9.
13. Rubens C, Ewert R, Halank M, et al. Big endothelin-1 and endothelin-1 plasma levels are correlated with the severity of primary pulmonary hypertension. Chest. 2001;120:1562–9.
14. Rubin LJ, Badesch DB, Barst RJ, et al. Bosentan therapy for pulmonary arterial hypertension. N Engl J Med. 2002;346:896–903.
15. Galie N, Olschewski H, Oudiz RJ, et al. Ambrisentan for the treatment of pulmonary arterial hypertension: results of the ambrisentan in pulmonary arterial hypertension, randomized, double-blind, placebo-controlled, multicenter, efficacy (ARIES) study 1 and 2. Circulation. 2008;117:3010–9.
16. Klinger JR, Abman SH, Gladwin MT. Nitric oxide deficiency and endothelial dysfunction in pulmonary arterial hypertension. Am J Respir Crit Care Med. 2013;188(6):639–46.
17. Charloux A, Chaouat A, Piquard F, et al. Renal hyporesponsiveness to brain natriuretic peptide: both generation and renal activity of cGMP are decreased in patients with pulmonary hypertension. Peptides. 2006;27:2993–9.

18. Hanson KA, Ziegler JW, Rybalkin SD, et al. Chronic pulmonary hypertension increases fetal lung cGMP phosphodiesterase activity. Am J Physiol. 1998;275:L931–41.
19. Galie N, Ghofrani HA, Torbicki A, et al. Sildenafil citrate therapy for pulmonary arterial hypertension. N Engl J Med. 2005;353:2148–57.
20. Galie N, Brundage BH, Ghofrani HA, et al. Tadalafil therapy for pulmonary arterial hypertension. Circulation. 2009;119:2894–903.
21. Ghofrani HA, Galiè N, Grimminger F, Grünig E, Humbert M, Jing ZC, Keogh AM, Langleben D, Kilama MO, Fritsch A, Neuser D, Rubin LJ, PATENT-1 Study Group. Riociguat for the treatment of pulmonary arterial hypertension. N Engl J Med. 2013;369(4):330–40.
22. Nagendran J, Archer SL, Soliman D, et al. Phosphodiesterase type 5 is highly expressed in the hypertrophied human right ventricle, and acute inhibition of phosphodiesterase type 5 improves contractility. Circulation. 2007;116:238–48.
23. Emori T, Hirata Y, Imai T, et al. Cellular mechanism of natriuretic peptides-induced inhibition of endothelin-1 biosynthesis in rat endothelial cells. Endocrinology. 1993;133:2474–80.
24. Boulanger C, Luscher TF. Release of endothelin from the porcine aorta. Inhibition by endothelium-derived nitric oxide. J Clin Invest. 1990;85:587–90.
25. Itoh T, Nagaya N, Fujii T, et al. A combination of oral sildenafil and beraprost ameliorates pulmonary hypertension in rats. Am J Respir Crit Care Med. 2004;169:34–8.
26. Ikeda D, Tsujino I, Ohira H, et al. Addition of oral sildenafil to beraprost is a safe and effective therapeutic option for patients with pulmonary hypertension. J Cardiovasc Pharmacol. 2005;45:286–9.
27. Ghofrani HA, Wiedemann R, Rose F, et al. Combination therapy with oral sildenafil and inhaled iloprost for severe pulmonary hypertension. Ann Intern Med. 2002;136:515–22.
28. Ghofrani HA, Rose F, Schermuly RT, et al. Oral sildenafil as long-term adjunct therapy to inhaled iloprost in severe pulmonary arterial hypertension. J Am Coll Cardiol. 2003;42: 158–64.
29. Simonneau G, Rubin LJ, Galie N, et al. Addition of sildenafil to long-term intravenous epoprostenol therapy in patients with pulmonary arterial hypertension: a randomized trial. Ann Intern Med. 2008;149:521–30.
30. Simonneau G, Rubin LJ, Galiè N, Barst RJ, Fleming TR, Frost A, Engel P, Kramer MR, Serdarevic-Pehar M, Layton GR, Sitbon O, Badesch DB, PACES Study Group. Long-term sildenafil added to intravenous epoprostenol in patients with pulmonary arterial hypertension. J Heart Lung Transplant. 2014;33(7):689–97.
31. Humbert M, Barst RJ, Robbins IM, et al. Combination of bosentan with epoprostenol in pulmonary arterial hypertension: BREATHE-2. Eur Respir J. 2004;24:353–9.
32. Seyfarth HJ, Pankau H, Hammerschmidt S, et al. Bosentan improves exercise tolerance and Tei index in patients with pulmonary hypertension and prostanoid therapy. Chest. 2005; 128:709–13.
33. McLaughlin VV, Oudiz RJ, Frost A, et al. Randomized study of adding inhaled iloprost to existing bosentan in pulmonary arterial hypertension. Am J Respir Crit Care Med. 2006;174:1257–63.
34. Hoeper MM, Leuchte H, Halank M, et al. Combining inhaled iloprost with bosentan in patients with idiopathic pulmonary arterial hypertension. Eur Respir J. 2006;28:691–4.
35. Tapson VF, Jing ZC, Xu KF, et al. Oral treprostinil for the treatment of pulmonary arterial hypertension in patients on background endothelin receptor antagonist and/or phosphodiesterase type 5 inhibitor therapy (The FREEDOM-C2 Study): a randomized controlled trial. Chest. 2013;144(3):952–8.
36. Hoeper MM, Faulenbach C, Golpon H, et al. Combination therapy with bosentan and sildenafil in idiopathic pulmonary arterial hypertension. Eur Respir J. 2004;24:1007–10.
37. Benza RL, Gupta H, Soto FJ, Park MH, Torres F, Frey N, Murali S. Safety and efficacy of bosentan in combination with sildenafil in PAH patients who experience inadequate clinical response to monotherapy: The COMPASS-3 Study. Chest. 2010;138:840.

38. http://www.thepharmaletter.com/article/actelion-says-compass-2-bosentan-study-fails-primary-endpoint
39. Abstract (#2916) European Respiratory Society International Congress, 2014.
40. http://www.gilead.com/news/press-releases/2014/9/firstline-combination-of-ambrisentan-and-tadalafil-reduces-risk-of-clinical-failure-compared-to-monotherapy-in-pulmonary-arterial-hypertension-outcomes-study#sthash.9Qj0LxBX.dpuf.
41. Clinicaltrials.gov
42. Sitbon O, Jaïs X, Savale L, Cottin V, Bergot E, Macari EA, Bouvaist H, Dauphin C, Picard F, Bulifon S, Montani D, Humbert M, Simonneau G. Upfront triple combination therapy in pulmonary arterial hypertension: a pilot study. Eur Respir J. 2014;43(6):1691–7.

Chapter 17
Investigative Therapies in Pulmonary Arterial Hypertension

Karen A. Fagan

Abstract Pulmonary arterial hypertension (PAH) remains a serious, life threatening disease of unclear etiology. Despite the rapid development of numerous drugs to treat the disease, no cure is presently available. New treatments for PAH that are able to reverse the abnormal pulmonary vascular remodeling that is responsible for much of this disease are badly needed. To accomplish this goal, novel therapies that target many of the dysfunctional pathways that have been identified in PAH will need to be developed. This chapter reviews many of the known alterations in gene expressions, vasoconstriction, inflammation, metabolism, and cellular proliferation that have been identified in the pathogenesis of PAH. Potential pharmacologic targets arising from these abnormalities are reviewed along with data, where available, from animal studies and small clinical trials that have attempted to treat pulmonary vascular disease through manipulation of these pathways.

Keywords Pulmonary arterial hypertension • Investigational therapy • Gene therapy • Cell therapy • Bone morphogenic protein receptor 2

Abbreviations

5HT	Serotonin
ACE	Angiotensinogen-converting enzyme
ALK-1	Activin like kinase 1
AT III	Angiotensin III
AT-1	Angiotensinogen receptor-1
AT-2	Angiotensinogen receptor-2
BMPR2	Bone morphogenetic protein receptor 2
CML	Chronic myelogenous leukemia
COPD	Chronic obstructive lung disease

K.A. Fagan, M.D. (✉)
Pulmonary Diseases and Critical Care Medicine, Division of Pulmonary and Critical Care, Pulmonary Hypertension Center, University of South Alabama, Mastin Professional Building, 2451 Fillingim Street, Mobile, AL 36617, USA
e-mail: kfagan@usouthal.edu

J.R. Klinger, R.P. Frantz (eds.), *Diagnosis and Management of Pulmonary Hypertension*, Respiratory Medicine 12, DOI 10.1007/978-1-4939-2636-7_17

DCA	Dichloroacetate
DHEA	Dehydroepiandrosterone
EIF2AK4	Eukaryotic translation initiation factor 2 alpha kinase 4
eNOS	Endothelial nitric oxide synthase
EPCs	Endothelial progenitor cells
HDAC	Histone deacetylase
HIF1α	Hypoxia inducible factor 1α
IL-1	Interleukin-1
IL-13	Interleukin-13
IL-6	Interleukin-6
KCNK3	Potassium channel subfamily K member 3
Kv	Voltage-gated potassium channels
miRNA	MicroRNA
MSC	Mesenchymal stems cells
NFAT-1	Nuclear factor of activated T-cells 1
NO	Nitric oxide
PAH	Pulmonary arterial hypertension
PASMC	Pulmonary artery smooth muscle cells
PDGF	Platelet-derived growth factor
PGI2	Prostacyclin
PH	Pulmonary hypertension
PPAR γ/β	Peroxisome proliferator-activated receptors γ/β
RAAS	Renin–angiotensin–aldosterone system
RV	Right ventricle
SERCA 2a	Sarcoendoplasmic reticulum calcium transport ATPase 2a
siRNA	Small interfering RNA
SOD2	Superoxide dismutase 2
TGF β	Transforming growth factor β
TKI	Tyrosine kinase inhibitor
TRPC	Transient receptor potential channels
TXA2	Thromboxane
VEGF	Vascular endothelial growth factor receptor
VEGFr	Vascular endothelial growth factor receptor
VIP	Vasoactive intestinal peptide

Introduction

Despite the availability of multiple therapies specifically approved by regulatory agencies for the treatment of pulmonary arterial hypertension (PAH), the diagnosis remains indicative of a progressive, life-limiting process resulting in substantial morbidity and mortality. Identification of treatments aimed to normalize life expectancy in these patients is a significant priority and to date no single therapy for PAH can achieve this goal. This is not at all surprising given the multifactorial nature of the pathogenesis of PAH and the clinical heterogeneity of patients classified as World Health Organization Group 1 PAH. Future effective treatments for PAH may ultimately rely on identification and development of multi-targeted strategies that go well beyond our current therapeutic targets. It is impossible to summarize all the potential therapies that are being evaluated for PAH. Focusing on important pathologic processes in PAH and investigative therapies related therein may provide an important approach to identify integrative, complementary, pluripotent therapies for future consideration [1].

Potential Therapeutic Targets for PAH

The pathophysiology of PAH is complex with many potential targets that have been identified through various studies including genomic approaches, clinical investigations, and preclinical animal studies. There are equally numerous ways to categorize these targets. For purposes of this review, selected targets for future treatments will be considered. Additionally, most current and future treatments are aimed at reversing the abnormal structure and function of the pulmonary circulation. Enhancing right ventricle (RV) function is also an important consideration in improving patient functional status and outcome.

Genetic and Epigenetic Targets

Identification of bone morphogenetic protein receptor 2 (BMPR2) mutations as a cause of familial PAH in 2000 heralded over 14 years of research devoted to understanding how the wide variety of mutations cause PAH. Haploinsufficiency, dominant negative effects, and abnormal signaling through downstream pathways have all been associated with PAH. Because of these variable effects of the BMPR2 mutation, the approach to restoring normal gene expression and function of BMPR2 is daunting. What is clear is that developing ways to increase expression of the normal BMPR2 allele may result in substantial benefit. Gene therapy via adenoviral gene transfer in animal studies has demonstrated benefit of increasing expression of the normal BMPR2 [2]. However, gene therapy in humans with PAH is significantly in the future. Alternative strategies, aimed at increasing BMPR2 expression and activity, have led to several new lines of clinical investigation. Recently, FK506 (tacrolimus) has been identified as a potential potent inducer of BMPR2 activity. Its effect on BMPR2 is only partially explained by inhibition of calcineurin and nuclear factor of activated T-cells 1 (NFAT-1) signaling. Tacrolimus was also able to improve endothelial cell function in cells derived from PAH patients as well as decrease pulmonary hypertension (PH) in hypoxic mice with BMPR2 haploinsufficiency and rats with monocrotaline and vascular endothelial growth factor receptor (VEGFr)/hypoxia-induced PAH [3].

Other targets aimed to increase BMPR2 expression and activity by acting as molecular chaperones and increasing transcription have been proposed. Ataluren increases ribosomal transcription of genes with stop codon mutations [4] and has been tested in several genetic diseases with mixed results. Ongoing trials in patients with cystic fibrosis are taking place now [5] and may point to a possible option in PAH patients with specific BMPR2 mutations in the future. Some mutations of BMPR2 are associated with protein folding abnormalities that do not allow BMPR2 trafficking out of the endoplasmic reticulum and several different chaperones to move the mis-folded protein to the cell surface have been studied [6].

While mutations in BMPR2 are most commonly associated with PAH, other genes such as activin-like kinase 1 (ALK-1), endoglin, potassium channel subfamily K member 3 (KCNK3), eukaryotic translation initiation factor 2 alpha kinase 4 (EIF2AK4), and voltage-gated potassium channels (Kv's) that are mutated or abnormally expressed in PAH may also benefit from the approaches above. Additionally, abnormal activity of BMPR2 signaling may also alter the expression of endogenous regulators of the lung circulation. One such example is apelin, a peptide that is implicated in endothelial and smooth muscle proliferation and vasodilation, which is reduced by mutations in BMPR2 that disrupt peroxisome proliferator-activated receptors γ/β (PPAR γ/β) signaling, thus providing some rationale for the therapeutic potential of PPAR agonists in PAH [7–9]. PPAR agonists are also associated with attenuation of PH in animal models by modulating the levels of other vasoactive mediators such as endothelin-1 and VEGF [10].

Other epigenetic changes are also found in PAH patients. One area of increasing interest is the role of micro RNAs (miRNAs) and small interfering RNAs (siRNAs) to regulate gene expression in PAH. Transfection of RNA containing vectors to enhance or inhibit gene expression has been proposed as potential future therapies as increasing evidence supports the role of miRNA and siRNA in PAH. A recent review highlighted many of the RNAs implicated in PAH with additional RNA targets reported every year [11].

DNA modifications such as increased methylation lead to changes in expression of the gene. An example is the methylation of superoxide dismutase 2 (SOD2) by methyltransferases resulting in decreased SOD expression, changes in redox state and increased expression of pro-proliferative signals such as hypoxia inducible factor 1α (HIF1α) [12, 13]. Modification of histones by acetylation in PAH has also been proposed as an important epigenetic phenomenon. Inhibition of de-acetylation by inhibitors of histone deacetylase (HDAC) causes changes in gene expression that result in inactivation of some genes and activation of others. In PAH, studies in pulmonary artery smooth muscle cells (PASMCs) and several animal models of PH have demonstrated a decrease in PASMC proliferation and inflammation associated with targeted inhibitors of HDAC [14]. Inhibitors of HDAC have also been used in studies looking at RV function in models of PAH with mixed results. In left ventricular hypertrophy, inhibitors of HDAC were beneficial, whereas in studies of different models of PAH and with different HDAC inhibitors, effects on the RV were beneficial (in compensated RV hypertrophy and monocrotaline-induced PH) but were associated with RV failure in others [15, 16].

Manipulating the expression of genes implicated in PAH is a promising area of active investigation. Hopefully, restoration of more normal gene expression and ultimately more normal cell signaling will restore normal pulmonary vascular and RV function and improve the life expectancy in PAH patients.

Vasoconstriction and Vasoactive Targets

Enhanced pulmonary vasoconstrictive responses to a wide variety of stimuli have been identified in PAH. Indeed, all currently available PAH treatments directly target vasoconstrictive pathways.

Vasoconstriction of vascular smooth muscle requires an influx of calcium in order to activate the contractile machinery. Calcium can be released from intracellular stores or imported from the extracellular environment. Transient receptor potential channels (TRPC) regulate the release of calcium from intracellular stores. Increased activity of TRPC 6 has been identified in PAH patients and is associated with a single-nucleotide polymorphism [17]. Increased expression of TRPC 6 was also associated with enhanced proliferation of PASMCs [18]. Loss of TRPC 4 channel activity in rats is associated with improved survival in models of PAH [19]. The sarcoendoplasmic reticulum calcium transport ATPase 2a (SERCA 2a), a channel that regulates release of calcium from the sarcoplasmic reticulum, has also been implicated in PAH [20]. Modulating the influx of calcium has been a target of PAH therapies by directly inhibiting the entry of calcium through T- or L-type channels using calcium channel blockers. However, the clinical effectiveness of these alone has been modest at best and more selective regulators of calcium entry such as the channels above may provide important treatment targets [21].

Calcium influx occurs when the smooth muscle cell is depolarized. In PAH, several voltage-gated potassium channels (Kv) have been implicated. Down regulation of several potassium channels, most notable Kv1.2 and 1.5 are associated with membrane depolarization and calcium influx. Maneuvers that increase Kv expression and function (by gene transfer, dichloroacetate, etc.) reduce experimental PH by causing cellular hyperpolarization [22]. Recently, the KCNK3 gene that encodes potassium channel subfamily number 3 has been identified as a cause of heritable PAH in several families. Mutations in this channel lead to a channelopathy characterized by loss of potassium channel function and hyperpolarization of smooth muscle cells [23]. This finding definitively links abnormal potassium channel function to PAH and restoring normal channel function is a viable strategy for future consideration.

Vasoconstriction can also be achieved by a variety of vasoactive molecules that interact with cell surface receptors and cause vasoconstriction through a variety of intracellular signaling processes. Current treatments including endothelin-1 receptor blockade or increasing levels of prostacyclin-generated cAMP and nitric oxide-generated cGMP \take advantage of this strategy to lessen or enhance downstream signals respectively. There are many other molecules that modulate vasoconstriction including vasoactive intestinal peptide (VIP), thromboxane (TXA2), angiotensin III (AT III), apelin, serotonin (5HT), etc. all of which may cause pulmonary vasoconstriction through several different pathways. VIP inhibits vasoconstriction and also acts to vasodilate the circulation. Decreased VIP expression results in worse PH in animal models, and treatment with exogenous VIP attenuates this effect [24]. However, despite positive results from early clinical trials, VIP administration in PAH patients did not result in measureable improvements [25]. 5HT has long been associated with PAH and interference with the serotonin transporter has been demonstrated to decrease PH in animal models [26]. Terguride, is a 5HT transporter inhibitor, that was not found to be effective in the treatment of PAH in a preliminary phase IIa study [27], but continues to be investigated in combination with other drugs. Apelin, as described above is decreased in PAH due to mutations in BMPR2. It has many effects on the pulmonary circulation and dilates the lung circulation of animals with PH possibly through its effects on altering expression of endothelial nitric oxide synthase (eNOS) to increase nitric oxide (NO) production. Apelin administration has been associated with decreased PH in animal models [28].

Activation of Rho kinase in PAH leads to sustained contraction in PASMCs through "Ca sensitization" of the contractile apparatus, namely increased levels of phosphorylated myosin light chain [29, 30]. Inhibitors of Rho kinase, both direct and indirect, result in substantial reversal of vasoconstriction and vascular remodeling in several animal models of PH [31–36]. Several small scale human clinical trials of acute administration of the direct Rho kinase inhibitor fasudil in PAH patients demonstrated acute pulmonary vasodilatory effects [37–40]. Long-term clinical trials of direct Rho kinase inhibitors have not yet been carried out. Indirect inhibitors of Rho kinase, such as dehydroepiandrosterone (DHEA), are attractive candidate drugs that have been associated with attenuation and reversal of PH in animal models [41] and improved exercise capacity in patients with chronic obstructive lung disease (COPD) associated PH [42].

Identification, testing and production of specific inhibitors of the above mentioned agents (many of which are implicated in PAH), are daunting. A strategy that identifies important intracellular signaling hubs common to several important players in the pathogenesis of PAH may prove more effective than targeting pathways individually.

Inflammation and Inflammatory Mediator Targets

Inflammation that sets in motion a series of events that promote vascular dysfunction and remodeling has long been hypothesized to be an important contributor to the development of PAH [43]. The association of PAH with autoimmune and inflammatory diseases is a significant part of this hypothesis. However, immunosuppressive therapies have had limited effectiveness in the treatment of PAH. The pro-inflammatory cytokines, interleukin-1 (IL-1) and -6 (IL-6), are increased in PAH patients and inhibition of these is associated with decreased PH in animal models. IL-13 and signaling via transforming growth factor β (TGF β) is additionally associated with schistosomiasis-related PAH [44]. Several animal studies and case reports have found that inhibition of IL-6 is associated with decreased PH [45]. The anti-IL-6 monoclonal antibody has been associated with decreased pulmonary vascular disease in a patient with PAH associated with connective tissue disease and may represent a future therapeutic option for some PAH patients [46]. Cell-mediated immune functions have also been implicated in PAH and may represent important therapeutic targets. Patients with human HIV and athymic rats are more susceptible to PH suggesting an important role of T-cells and chronic inflammation in PAH [47, 48]. Given the relationship to autoimmune diseases, B-cell activation may play a role in PAH suggesting the potential option for anti-B-lymphocyte antigen CD20 treatment in the future. Several case reports suggest that rituximab may be helpful in patients with PAH associated with connective tissue disease [49, 50].

Vascular Cell Proliferation and Vessel Remodeling Targets

Excessive proliferation of cells in the walls of the pulmonary arteries and formation of the plexiform lesion is a hallmark of severe PAH. Events leading to the alteration of the normal vascular structure likely are multifactorial involving biochemical and mechanical forces that promote cell proliferation and angiogenesis. Many molecules known to be important in PAH such as NO, 5HT, TXB2, Rho kinase, and prostacyclin (PGI2). have direct effects on vascular tone, but also contribute to the proliferative phenotype. Thus, manipulation of these agents may help to decrease or reverse pulmonary vascular remodeling in addition to decreasing pulmonary vascular tone.

More direct approaches to address vascular remodeling target specific growth factor pathways and the extracellular matrix. Several important growth factors have been implicated in PAH. Platelet derived growth factor (PDGF) has been implicated in the proliferation of pulmonary vascular cells. Imatinib, a tyrosine kinase inhibitor (TKI) that inhibits the PDGF receptor, has been the most widely studied tyrosine kinase inhibitor in PAH. Imatinib was originally developed to inhibit the pro-oncogenic tyrosine kinase Bcr-abl in chronic myelogenous leukemia (CML). Given its ability to inhibit PDGF receptor and proto-oncogene c-Kit, imatinib was proposed as a potential regulator of PAH-related vascular proliferation [51, 52]. Despite initial excitement in animal models, case reports and small clinical trials [53, 54], imatinib failed to achieve regulatory approval after a large-scale clinical trial identified important concerns regarding the risk to benefit ratio of the treatment [55]. Other TKIs that target PDGF have also had some encouraging preclinical success, but may have limited clinical usefulness owing to other less beneficial effects. For example, dasitinib, a TKI with broader inhibitory properties than imatinib, also approved for treatment of CML, has been associated with the development of PAH [56].

Other potential targets are TKIs targeting epidermal growth factor receptor (erlotinib, gefitinib) and multi-kinase inhibitors (sorafenib, sunitinib), but as was seen with imatinib, significant limitations to their use lie in unacceptable adverse events and side effects and limited efficacy in animal models [57, 58]. Given these contradictory clinical effects and substantial adverse events, the future of TKIs in PAH is uncertain [59].

Modulation of extracellular matrix in PAH may also be a potential target for future treatments. Increased activity of elastases located in the pulmonary vascular wall allows for degradation of the extracellular matrix and, by inducing expression of other molecules such as tenacin and fibronectin, promotes cell proliferation and vascular remodeling [60]. Elafin, an inhibitor of serine protease, decreases and reverses severe PH in animal models [61, 62] and will likely undergo clinical testing in the near future.

Metabolic Targets

Derangements in the energy metabolism of pulmonary artery cells in PAH are being characterized. Examination of the RV and lungs of patients and animals with experimentally induced PH demonstrate a wide array of changes in expression of genes engaged in metabolic processes [63, 64]. Several mitochondrial abnormalities have been found in pulmonary vascular cells and the RV that lead to anaerobic metabolism (glycolysis) instead of aerobic metabolism through activation of pyruvate dehydrogenase kinase. This glycolytic state then leads to decreased intracellular reactive oxygen species generation, increased HIF1α expression and activity, and ultimately activation of vasoconstrictive and proliferative signaling by decreasing Kv channel expression and activity [65]. Dichloroacetate (DCA), an inhibitor of mitochondrial pyruvate dehydrogenase has demonstrated reversal or reduction of PH in animal models [66–69] and is undergoing clinical testing in PAH patients. Oxidation of fatty acids also contributes to this glycolytic shift, and several inhibitors of fatty acid oxidation, trimetazidine and ranolazine, have demonstrated potential efficacy in animal models of PAH by reversing the shift toward glycolysis [70, 71] Ranolazine is currently being evaluated in PAH patients at a single clinical center.

Neurohormonal Targets

Much of the morbidity and mortality of PAH patients lies in the adaptation and function of the RV to the increased demands of downstream resistance. Clearly, developing effective treatments to decrease the resistance due to vasoconstriction and remodeling is the ultimate RV "specific" treatment. Short of this, improving adaptation of the RV is an important therapeutic consideration. Many of the proposed PAH treatments above additionally involve adaptations that are seen in the

RV as well as pulmonary vasculature. Recently, attention to the neurohormonal activation in PAH patients has received increasing attention. The sympathetic nervous system and renin–angiotensin–aldosterone system (RAAS) are activated in PAH [72] and represent potential targets for treatment.

Sympathetic tone is increased in patients with PAH and adrenergic receptor expression is also reported as increased in the RV of patients with PAH right ventricles [73, 74]. Activation of this system was considered adaptive to sustain cardiac output by increasing contractility, heart rate, and systemic blood pressure, and thus, manipulation of adrenergic receptors was considered unsafe in PAH patients. However, sympathetic activation has been associated with increased mortality in PAH patients [75] which has led to a number of studies of selective β-receptor blockade in PAH. In several preclinical models of PAH, the α1/β1/β2-adrenergic receptor antagonist carvedilol and β1-selective receptor antagonist bisoprolol are associated with improved RV function [76–78]. A retrospective review of PAH patients revealed no difference in clinical outcomes in patients who received β-blockers compared to those who did not [79, 80] suggesting that the safety of β-blockade in PAH patients should be reconsidered [72].

Activation of RAAS is also found in patients with PAH [72, 81]. Several case series of patients with PAH hinted at efficacy of angiotensinogen converting enzyme (ACE) inhibition [82], but concerns regarding the potential for hypotension limited further investigations. More recently, approaches aimed at selective targeting of the angiotensin (AT) pathway have identified the potential therapeutic value of targeting AT receptor-1 (AT1) (using the AT-1 antagonist losartan) while keeping ACE and AT-2 function (both with purported vasodilatory effects) and signaling intact [81]. Additional support of this approach is demonstrated by the use of ACE-2 agonists to decrease pulmonary artery pressure and RV hypertrophy and dysfunction in animal models of PAH [83–85].

Aldosterone antagonism is a mainstay of left ventricular failure treatment [86], but its role in RV failure is less well understood. However, increased levels of aldosterone are found in PAH patients [87] and treatment with aldosterone antagonists is included in several recent treatment guidelines. Evidence for this recommendation is increasingly apparent as demonstrated in recent studies that identified that upregulation of aldosterone is associated with increased ET-1 and decreased NO availability which is reversed by aldosterone antagonists in animal models of PAH [88, 89]. Review of the ARIES data of the selective ET-1, a receptor antagonist ambrisentan in PAH, suggests a complimentary benefit when combined with the aldosterone antagonist spironolactone [90].

Lung Cell-Targeted and Cell-Based Therapeutic Targets

Therapies designed to repair and remodel the pulmonary arteries in PAH may be best approached using strategies to deliver pharmacologic agents and genes directly to the abnormal lung circulation or to repopulate the pulmonary vasculature with cells that have normal phenotypes and behaviors. Targeting molecules to the lung circulation can be achieved by a number of mechanisms including the use of chaperones, exploiting lung-specific cell surface receptors, targeting lung-specific gene expression and identification of lung-specific signaling pathways. Numerous examples of this strategy are being investigated including use of specific lung endothelial cell surface receptors, peptides that chaperone molecules to abnormal pulmonary endothelium, and RNAs that target lung-specific gene expression. By using lung-targeted approaches, the limitations of systemic delivery of therapeutics and potential systemic side effects may be limited [91].

Cell-based strategies to deliver molecules to the lung circulation or act as therapeutics directly are an attractive approach in PAH. Repair and reversal of vascular changes in PAH through delivery of pluripotent mesenchymal stems cells (MSCs) or endothelial progenitor cells (EPCs) that repopulate the vessel wall and potentially carry genes to promote repair is one potential approach [92, 93]. In PAH patients, alterations in the numbers of circulating EPCs have been observed [94]. EPCs alone or carrying specific genes, such as eNOS, have prevented and reversed PAH in several animal models of PAH [95]. Autologous EPCs in a small trial of PAH patients resulted in improvement in exercise capacity and hemodynamics [96]. A trial of autologous EPCs overexpressing eNOS in PAH patients is underway.

Summary

Identification of new treatments that will normalize life expectancy for patient with PAH will certainly be a complex and challenging endeavor is likely to involve the targeting of multiple pathways. It is unlikely, that any single agent exists that is capable of completely reversing or preventing disease progression in PAH, but careful assessment of the molecular underpinnings of PAH, followed by the rational development of complementary multi-targeted approaches, may represent the best hope for the future.

References

1. Morrell NW, Archer SL, Defelice A, Evans S, Fiszman M, Martin T, Saulnier M, Rabinovitch M, Schermuly R, Stewart D, Truebel H, Walker G, Stenmark KR. Anticipated classes of new medications and molecular targets for pulmonary arterial hypertension. Pulm Circ. 2013;3: 226–44.
2. Reynolds AM, Holmes MD, Danilov SM, Reynolds PN. Targeted gene delivery of BMPR2 attenuates pulmonary hypertension. Eur Respir J. 2012;39:329–43.
3. Spiekerkoetter E, Tian X, Cai J, Hopper RK, Sudheendra D, Li CG, El-Bizri N, Sawada H, Haghighat R, Chan R, Haghighat L, de Jesus Perez V, Wang L, Reddy S, Zhao M, Bernstein D, Solow-Cordero DE, Beachy PA, Wandless TJ, Ten Dijke P, Rabinovitch M. FK506 activates BMPR2, rescues endothelial dysfunction, and reverses pulmonary hypertension. J Clin Invest. 2013;123:3600–13.

4. Peltz SW, Morsy M, Welch EM, Jacobson A. Ataluren as an agent for therapeutic nonsense suppression. Annu Rev Med. 2013;64:407–25.
5. Kerem E, Konstan MW, De Boeck K, Accurso FJ, Sermet-Gaudelus I, Wilschanski M, Elborn JS, Melotti P, Bronsveld I, Fajac I, Malfroot A, Rosenbluth DB, Walker PA, McColley SA, Knoop C, Quattrucci S, Rietschel E, Zeitlin PL, Barth J, Elfring GL, Welch EM, Branstrom A, Spiegel RJ, Peltz SW, Ajayi T, Rowe SM. Ataluren for the treatment of nonsense-mutation cystic fibrosis: a randomised, double-blind, placebo-controlled phase 3 trial. Lancet Respir Med. 2014;2:539–47.
6. Frump AL, Lowery JW, Hamid R, Austin ED, de Caestecker M. Abnormal trafficking of endogenously expressed BMPR2 mutant allelic products in patients with heritable pulmonary arterial hypertension. PLoS One. 2013;8:e80319.
7. Poirier O, Ciumas M, Eyries M, Montagne K, Nadaud S, Soubrier F. Inhibition of apelin expression by BMP signaling in endothelial cells. Am J Physiol Cell Physiol. 2012;303: C1139–45.
8. Alastalo TP, Li M, Perez Vde J, Pham D, Sawada H, Wang JK, Koskenvuo M, Wang L, Freeman BA, Chang HY, Rabinovitch M. Disruption of PPARgamma/beta-catenin-mediated regulation of apelin impairs BMP-induced mouse and human pulmonary arterial EC survival. J Clin Invest. 2011;121:3735–46.
9. Hansmann G, de Jesus Perez VA, Alastalo TP, Alvira CM, Guignabert C, Bekker JM, Schellong S, Urashima T, Wang L, Morrell NW, Rabinovitch M. An antiproliferative BMP-2/ PPARgamma/apoE axis in human and murine SMCs and its role in pulmonary hypertension. J Clin Invest. 2008;118:1846–57.
10. Kim EK, Lee JH, Oh YM, Lee YS, Lee SD. Rosiglitazone attenuates hypoxia-induced pulmonary arterial hypertension in rats. Respirology (Carlton, Vic). 2010;15:659–68.
11. Yuan K, Orcholski M, Tian X, Liao X, de Jesus Perez VA. MicroRNAs: promising therapeutic targets for the treatment of pulmonary arterial hypertension. Expert Opin Ther Targets. 2013;17:557–64.
12. Archer SL, Marsboom G, Kim GH, Zhang HJ, Toth PT, Svensson EC, Dyck JR, Gomberg-Maitland M, Thebaud B, Husain AN, Cipriani N, Rehman J. Epigenetic attenuation of mitochondrial superoxide dismutase 2 in pulmonary arterial hypertension: a basis for excessive cell proliferation and a new therapeutic target. Circulation. 2010;121:2661–71.
13. Kim GH, Ryan JJ, Marsboom G, Archer SL. Epigenetic mechanisms of pulmonary hypertension. Pulm Circ. 2011;1:347–56.
14. Saco TV, Parthasarathy PT, Cho Y, Lockey RF, Kolliputi N. Role of epigenetics in pulmonary hypertension. Am J Physiol Cell Physiol. 2014;306:C1101–5.
15. Bogaard HJ, Mizuno S, Hussaini AA, Toldo S, Abbate A, Kraskauskas D, Kasper M, Natarajan R, Voelkel NF. Suppression of histone deacetylases worsens right ventricular dysfunction after pulmonary artery banding in rats. Am J Respir Crit Care Med. 2011;183:1402–10.
16. Cho YK, Eom GH, Kee HJ, Kim HS, Choi WY, Nam KI, Ma JS, Kook H. Sodium valproate, a histone deacetylase inhibitor, but not captopril, prevents right ventricular hypertrophy in rats. Circ J. 2010;74:760–70.
17. Yu Y, Keller SH, Remillard CV, Safrina O, Nicholson A, Zhang SL, Jiang W, Vangala N, Landsberg JW, Wang JY, Thistlethwaite PA, Channick RN, Robbins IM, Loyd JE, Ghofrani HA, Grimminger F, Schermuly RT, Cahalan MD, Rubin LJ, Yuan JX. A functional single-nucleotide polymorphism in the TRPC6 gene promoter associated with idiopathic pulmonary arterial hypertension. Circulation. 2009;119:2313–22.
18. Yu Y, Fantozzi I, Remillard CV, Landsberg JW, Kunichika N, Platoshyn O, Tigno DD, Thistlethwaite PA, Rubin LJ, Yuan JX. Enhanced expression of transient receptor potential channels in idiopathic pulmonary arterial hypertension. Proc Natl Acad Sci U S A. 2004; 101:13861–6.
19. Alzoubi A, Almalouf P, Toba M, O'Neill K, Qian X, Francis M, Taylor MS, Alexeyev M, McMurtry IF, Oka M, Stevens T. TRPC4 inactivation confers a survival benefit in severe pulmonary arterial hypertension. Am J Pathol. 2013;183:1779–88.

20. Makanga M, Dewachter C, Maruyama H, Vuckovic A, Rondelet B, Naeije R, Dewachter L. Downregulated bone morphogenetic protein signaling in nitrofen-induced congenital diaphragmatic hernia. Pediatr Surg Int. 2013;29:823–34.
21. Kuhr FK, Smith KA, Song MY, Levitan I, Yuan JX. New mechanisms of pulmonary arterial hypertension: role of Ca(2)(+) signaling. Am J Physiol Heart Circ Physiol. 2012;302: H1546–62.
22. Park WS, Firth AL, Han J, Ko EA. Patho-, physiological roles of voltage-dependent K+ channels in pulmonary arterial smooth muscle cells. J Smooth Muscle Res. 2010;46:89–105.
23. Ma L, Roman-Campos D, Austin ED, Eyries M, Sampson KS, Soubrier F, Germain M, Tregouet DA, Borczuk A, Rosenzweig EB, Girerd B, Montani D, Humbert M, Loyd JE, Kass RS, Chung WK. A novel channelopathy in pulmonary arterial hypertension. N Engl J Med. 2013;369:351–61.
24. Said SI, Hamidi SA. Pharmacogenomics in pulmonary arterial hypertension: toward a mechanistic, target-based approach to therapy. Pulm Circ. 2011;1:383–8.
25. Galiè N, Boonstra A, Ewert R, et al. Effects of inhaled aviptadil (vasoactive intestinal peptide) in patients with pulmonary arterial hypertension (PAH). Am J Respir Crit Care Med. 2010;181:A2516.
26. Dumitrascu R, Kulcke C, Konigshoff M, Kouri F, Yang X, Morrell N, Ghofrani HA, Weissmann N, Reiter R, Seeger W, Grimminger F, Eickelberg O, Schermuly RT, Pullamsetti SS. Terguride ameliorates monocrotaline-induced pulmonary hypertension in rats. Eur Respir J. 2011;37: 1104–18.
27. Ghofrani HA, Al-Hiti H, Vonk Noordegraaf A, et al. Proof-of-concept study to investigate the efficacy, hemodynamics and tolerability of terguride vs. placebo in subjects with pulmonary arterial hypertension: results of a double blind, randomised, prospective phase IIa study. Am J Respir Crit Care Med. 2012;185:A2496.
28. Andersen CU, Hilberg O, Mellemkjaer S, Nielsen-Kudsk JE, Simonsen U. Apelin and pulmonary hypertension. Pulm Circ. 2011;1:334–46.
29. McMurtry IF, Abe K, Ota H, Fagan KA, Oka M. Rho kinase-mediated vasoconstriction in pulmonary hypertension. Adv Exp Med Biol. 2010;661:299–308.
30. Oka M, Fagan KA, Jones PL, McMurtry IF. Therapeutic potential of RhoA/Rho kinase inhibitors in pulmonary hypertension. Br J Pharmacol. 2008;155:444–54.
31. Fagan KA, Oka M, Bauer NR, Gebb SA, Ivy DD, Morris KG, McMurtry IF. Attenuation of acute hypoxic pulmonary vasoconstriction and hypoxic pulmonary hypertension in mice by inhibition of Rho-kinase. Am J Physiol Lung Cell Mol Physiol. 2004;287:L656–64.
32. Nagaoka T, Fagan KA, Gebb SA, Morris KG, Suzuki T, Shimokawa H, McMurtry IF, Oka M. Inhaled Rho kinase inhibitors are potent and selective vasodilators in rat pulmonary hypertension. Am J Respir Crit Care Med. 2005;171:494–9.
33. Nagaoka T, Gebb SA, Karoor V, Homma N, Morris KG, McMurtry IF, Oka M. Involvement of RhoA/Rho kinase signaling in pulmonary hypertension of the fawn-hooded rat. J Appl Physiol (Bethesda, Md: 1985). 2006;100:996–1002.
34. Nagaoka T, Morio Y, Casanova N, Bauer N, Gebb S, McMurtry I, Oka M. Rho/Rho kinase signaling mediates increased basal pulmonary vascular tone in chronically hypoxic rats. Am J Physiol Lung Cell Mol Physiol. 2004;287:L665–72.
35. Oka M, Homma N, McMurtry IF. Rho kinase-mediated vasoconstriction in rat models of pulmonary hypertension. Methods Enzymol. 2008;439:191–204.
36. Oka M, Homma N, Taraseviciene-Stewart L, Morris KG, Kraskauskas D, Burns N, Voelkel NF, McMurtry IF. Rho kinase-mediated vasoconstriction is important in severe occlusive pulmonary arterial hypertension in rats. Circ Res. 2007;100:923–9.
37. Fujita H, Fukumoto Y, Saji K, Sugimura K, Demachi J, Nawata J, Shimokawa H. Acute vasodilator effects of inhaled fasudil, a specific Rho-kinase inhibitor, in patients with pulmonary arterial hypertension. Heart Vessels. 2010;25:144–9.
38. Fukumoto Y, Matoba T, Ito A, Tanaka H, Kishi T, Hayashidani S, Abe K, Takeshita A, Shimokawa H. Acute vasodilator effects of a Rho-kinase inhibitor, fasudil, in patients with severe pulmonary hypertension. Heart (British Cardiac Society). 2005;91:391–2.

39. Fukumoto Y, Yamada N, Matsubara H, Mizoguchi M, Uchino K, Yao A, Kihara Y, Kawano M, Watanabe H, Takeda Y, Adachi T, Osanai S, Tanabe N, Inoue T, Kubo A, Ota Y, Fukuda K, Nakano T, Shimokawa H. Double-blind, placebo-controlled clinical trial with a rho-kinase inhibitor in pulmonary arterial hypertension. Circ J. 2013;77:2619–25.
40. Ishikura K, Yamada N, Ito M, Ota S, Nakamura M, Isaka N, Nakano T. Beneficial acute effects of rho-kinase inhibitor in patients with pulmonary arterial hypertension. Circ J. 2006;70: 174–8.
41. Alzoubi A, Toba M, Abe K, O'Neill KD, Rocic P, Fagan KA, McMurtry IF, Oka M. Dehydroepiandrosterone restores right ventricular structure and function in rats with severe pulmonary arterial hypertension. Am J Physiol Heart Circ Physiol. 2013;304:H1708–18.
42. Dumas de La Roque E, Savineau JP, Metivier AC, Billes MA, Kraemer JP, Doutreleau S, Jougon J, Marthan R, Moore N, Fayon M, Baulieu EE, Dromer C. Dehydroepiandrosterone (DHEA) improves pulmonary hypertension in chronic obstructive pulmonary disease (COPD): a pilot study. Ann Endocrinol. 2012;73:20–5.
43. El Chami H, Hassoun PM. Immune and inflammatory mechanisms in pulmonary arterial hypertension. Prog Cardiovasc Dis. 2012;55:218–28.
44. Graham BB, Chabon J, Gebreab L, Poole J, Debella E, Davis L, Tanaka T, Sanders L, Dropcho N, Bandeira A, Vandivier RW, Champion HC, Butrous G, Wang XJ, Wynn TA, Tuder RM. Transforming growth factor-beta signaling promotes pulmonary hypertension caused by Schistosoma mansoni. Circulation. 2013;128:1354–64.
45. Groth A, Vrugt B, Brock M, Speich R, Ulrich S, Huber LC. Inflammatory cytokines in pulmonary hypertension. Respir Res. 2014;15:47.
46. Furuya Y, Satoh T, Kuwana M. Interleukin-6 as a potential therapeutic target for pulmonary arterial hypertension. Int J Rheumatol. 2010;2010:720305.
47. Taraseviciene-Stewart L, Nicolls MR, Kraskauskas D, Scerbavicius R, Burns N, Cool C, Wood K, Parr JE, Boackle SA, Voelkel NF. Absence of T cells confers increased pulmonary arterial hypertension and vascular remodeling. Am J Respir Crit Care Med. 2007;175:1280–9.
48. Tcherakian C, Couderc LJ, Humbert M, Godot V, Sitbon O, Devillier P. Inflammatory mechanisms in HIV-associated pulmonary arterial hypertension. Semin Respir Crit Care Med. 2013;34:645–53.
49. Hennigan S, Channick RN, Silverman GJ. Rituximab treatment of pulmonary arterial hypertension associated with systemic lupus erythematosus: a case report. Lupus. 2008;17:754–6.
50. Padilla-Ibarra J, Sanchez-Ortiz A, Sandoval-Castro C, Ramos-Remus C. Rituximab treatment for pulmonary arterial hypertension in adult-onset Still's disease. Clin Exp Rheumatol. 2013;31:657–8.
51. Perros F, Montani D, Dorfmuller P, Durand-Gasselin I, Tcherakian C, Le Pavec J, Mazmanian M, Fadel E, Mussot S, Mercier O, Herve P, Emilie D, Eddahibi S, Simonneau G, Souza R, Humbert M. Platelet-derived growth factor expression and function in idiopathic pulmonary arterial hypertension. Am J Respir Crit Care Med. 2008;178:81–8.
52. Nakamura K, Akagi S, Ogawa A, Kusano KF, Matsubara H, Miura D, Fuke S, Nishii N, Nagase S, Kohno K, Morita H, Oto T, Yamanaka R, Otsuka F, Miura A, Yutani C, Ohe T, Ito H. Pro-apoptotic effects of imatinib on PDGF-stimulated pulmonary artery smooth muscle cells from patients with idiopathic pulmonary arterial hypertension. Int J Cardiol. 2012;159: 100–6.
53. Schermuly RT, Dony E, Ghofrani HA, Pullamsetti S, Savai R, Roth M, Sydykov A, Lai YJ, Weissmann N, Seeger W, Grimminger F. Reversal of experimental pulmonary hypertension by PDGF inhibition. J Clin Invest. 2005;115:2811–21.
54. Ghofrani HA, Seeger W, Grimminger F. Imatinib for the treatment of pulmonary arterial hypertension. N Engl J Med. 2005;353:1412–3.
55. Hoeper MM, Barst RJ, Bourge RC, Feldman J, Frost AE, Galie N, Gomez-Sanchez MA, Grimminger F, Grunig E, Hassoun PM, Morrell NW, Peacock AJ, Satoh T, Simonneau G, Tapson VF, Torres F, Lawrence D, Quinn DA, Ghofrani HA. Imatinib mesylate as add-on therapy for pulmonary arterial hypertension: results of the randomized IMPRES study. Circulation. 2013;127:1128–38.

56. Montani D, Bergot E, Gunther S, Savale L, Bergeron A, Bourdin A, Bouvaist H, Canuet M, Pison C, Macro M, Poubeau P, Girerd B, Natali D, Guignabert C, Perros F, O'Callaghan DS, Jais X, Tubert-Bitter P, Zalcman G, Sitbon O, Simonneau G, Humbert M. Pulmonary arterial hypertension in patients treated by dasatinib. Circulation. 2012;125:2128–37.
57. Dahal BK, Cornitescu T, Tretyn A, Pullamsetti SS, Kosanovic D, Dumitrascu R, Ghofrani HA, Weissmann N, Voswinckel R, Banat GA, Seeger W, Grimminger F, Schermuly RT. Role of epidermal growth factor inhibition in experimental pulmonary hypertension. Am J Respir Crit Care Med. 2010;181:158–67.
58. Gomberg-Maitland M, Maitland ML, Barst RJ, Sugeng L, Coslet S, Perrino TJ, Bond L, Lacouture ME, Archer SL, Ratain MJ. A dosing/cross-development study of the multikinase inhibitor sorafenib in patients with pulmonary arterial hypertension. Clin Pharmacol Ther. 2010;87:303–10.
59. Godinas L, Guignabert C, Seferian A, Perros F, Bergot E, Sibille Y, Humbert M, Montani D. Tyrosine kinase inhibitors in pulmonary arterial hypertension: a double-edge sword? Semin Respir Crit Care Med. 2013;34:714–24.
60. Cowan KN, Jones PL, Rabinovitch M. Elastase and matrix metalloproteinase inhibitors induce regression, and tenascin-C antisense prevents progression, of vascular disease. J Clin Invest. 2000;105:21–34.
61. Kim YM, Haghighat L, Spiekerkoetter E, Sawada H, Alvira CM, Wang L, Acharya S, Rodriguez-Colon G, Orton A, Zhao M, Rabinovitch M. Neutrophil elastase is produced by pulmonary artery smooth muscle cells and is linked to neointimal lesions. Am J Pathol. 2011;179:1560–72.
62. Zaidi SH, You XM, Ciura S, Husain M, Rabinovitch M. Overexpression of the serine elastase inhibitor elafin protects transgenic mice from hypoxic pulmonary hypertension. Circulation. 2002;105:516–21.
63. Gomez-Arroyo J, Mizuno S, Szczepanek K, Van Tassell B, Natarajan R, dos Remedios CG, Drake JI, Farkas L, Kraskauskas D, Wijesinghe DS, Chalfant CE, Bigbee J, Abbate A, Lesnefsky EJ, Bogaard HJ, Voelkel NF. Metabolic gene remodeling and mitochondrial dysfunction in failing right ventricular hypertrophy secondary to pulmonary arterial hypertension. Circ Heart Fail. 2013;6:136–44.
64. Fessel JP, Hamid R, Wittmann BM, Robinson LJ, Blackwell T, Tada Y, Tanabe N, Tatsumi K, Hemnes AR, West JD. Metabolomic analysis of bone morphogenetic protein receptor type 2 mutations in human pulmonary endothelium reveals widespread metabolic reprogramming. Pulm Circ. 2012;2:201–13.
65. Archer SL, Fang YH, Ryan JJ, Piao L. Metabolism and bioenergetics in the right ventricle and pulmonary vasculature in pulmonary hypertension. Pulm Circ. 2013;3:144–52.
66. Guignabert C, Tu L, Izikki M, Dewachter L, Zadigue P, Humbert M, Adnot S, Fadel E, Eddahibi S. Dichloroacetate treatment partially regresses established pulmonary hypertension in mice with SM22alpha-targeted overexpression of the serotonin transporter. FASEB J. 2009;23:4135–47.
67. Li B, Yan J, Shen Y, Liu Y, Ma Z. Dichloroacetate prevents but not reverses the formation of neointimal lesions in a rat model of severe pulmonary arterial hypertension. Mol Med Rep. 2014;10:2144–52.
68. McMurtry MS, Bonnet S, Wu X, Dyck JR, Haromy A, Hashimoto K, Michelakis ED. Dichloroacetate prevents and reverses pulmonary hypertension by inducing pulmonary artery smooth muscle cell apoptosis. Circ Res. 2004;95:830–40.
69. Piao L, Sidhu VK, Fang YH, Ryan JJ, Parikh KS, Hong Z, Toth PT, Morrow E, Kutty S, Lopaschuk GD, Archer SL. FOXO1-mediated upregulation of pyruvate dehydrogenase kinase-4 (PDK4) decreases glucose oxidation and impairs right ventricular function in pulmonary hypertension: therapeutic benefits of dichloroacetate. J Mol Med (Berlin, Germany). 2013;91:333–46.
70. Fang YH, Piao L, Hong Z, Toth PT, Marsboom G, Bache-Wiig P, Rehman J, Archer SL. Therapeutic inhibition of fatty acid oxidation in right ventricular hypertrophy: exploiting Randle's cycle. J Mol Med (Berlin, Germany). 2012;90:31–43.

71. Sutendra G, Bonnet S, Rochefort G, Haromy A, Folmes KD, Lopaschuk GD, Dyck JR, Michelakis ED. Fatty acid oxidation and malonyl-CoA decarboxylase in the vascular remodeling of pulmonary hypertension. Sci Transl Med. 2010;2:4458.
72. de Man FS, Handoko ML, Guignabert C, Bogaard HJ, Vonk-Noordegraaf A. Neurohormonal axis in patients with pulmonary arterial hypertension: friend or foe? Am J Respir Crit Care Med. 2013;187:14–9.
73. Mak S, Witte KK, Al-Hesayen A, Granton JJ, Parker JD. Cardiac sympathetic activation in patients with pulmonary arterial hypertension. Am J Physiol Regul Integr Comp Physiol. 2012;302:R1153–7.
74. Bristow MR, Minobe W, Rasmussen R, Larrabee P, Skerl L, Klein JW, Anderson FL, Murray J, Mestroni L, Karwande SV, et al. Beta-adrenergic neuroeffector abnormalities in the failing human heart are produced by local rather than systemic mechanisms. J Clin Invest. 1992;89:803–15.
75. Ciarka A, Doan V, Velez-Roa S, Naeije R, van de Borne P. Prognostic significance of sympathetic nervous system activation in pulmonary arterial hypertension. Am J Respir Crit Care Med. 2010;181:1269–75.
76. Bogaard HJ, Natarajan R, Mizuno S, Abbate A, Chang PJ, Chau VQ, Hoke NN, Kraskauskas D, Kasper M, Salloum FN, Voelkel NF. Adrenergic receptor blockade reverses right heart remodeling and dysfunction in pulmonary hypertensive rats. Am J Respir Crit Care Med. 2010;182:652–60.
77. de Man FS, Handoko ML, van Ballegoij JJ, Schalij I, Bogaards SJ, Postmus PE, van der Velden J, Westerhof N, Paulus WJ, Vonk-Noordegraaf A. Bisoprolol delays progression towards right heart failure in experimental pulmonary hypertension. Circ Heart Fail. 2012;5:97–105.
78. Drake JI, Gomez-Arroyo J, Dumur CI, Kraskauskas D, Natarajan R, Bogaard HJ, Fawcett P, Voelkel NF. Chronic carvedilol treatment partially reverses the right ventricular failure transcriptional profile in experimental pulmonary hypertension. Physiol Genomics. 2013;45:449–61.
79. So PP, Davies RA, Chandy G, Stewart D, Beanlands RS, Haddad H, Pugliese C, Mielniczuk LM. Usefulness of beta-blocker therapy and outcomes in patients with pulmonary arterial hypertension. Am J Cardiol. 2012;109:1504–9.
80. Thenappan T, Roy SS, Duval S, Glassner-Kolmin C, Gomberg-Maitland M. Beta-blocker therapy is not associated with adverse outcomes in patients with pulmonary arterial hypertension: a propensity score analysis. Circulation. 2014. doi:10.1161/CIRCHEARTFAILURE.114.001429.
81. de Man FS, Tu L, Handoko ML, Rain S, Ruiter G, Francois C, Schalij I, Dorfmuller P, Simonneau G, Fadel E, Perros F, Boonstra A, Postmus PE, van der Velden J, Vonk-Noordegraaf A, Humbert M, Eddahibi S, Guignabert C. Dysregulated renin-angiotensin-aldosterone system contributes to pulmonary arterial hypertension. Am J Respir Crit Care Med. 2012;186:780–9.
82. Alpert MA, Pressly TA, Mukerji V, Lambert CR, Mukerji B. Short- and long-term hemodynamic effects of captopril in patients with pulmonary hypertension and selected connective tissue disease. Chest. 1992;102:1407–12.
83. Hampl V, Herget J, Bíbová J, Baňasová A, Husková Z, Vaňourková Z, Jíchová Š, Kujal P, Vernerová Z, Sadowski J, Červenka L. Intrapulmonary activation of the angiotensin-converting enzyme type 2/angiotensin 1-7/G-protein-coupled Mas receptor axis attenuates pulmonary hypertension in Ren-2 transgenic rats exposed to chronic hypoxia. Physiol Res. 2015;64:25–38.
84. Li G, Liu Y, Zhu Y, Liu A, Xu Y, Li X, Li Z, Su J, Sun L. ACE2 activation confers endothelial protection and attenuates neointimal lesions in prevention of severe pulmonary arterial hypertension in rats. Lung. 2013;191:327–36.
85. Shenoy V, Ferreira AJ, Qi Y, Fraga-Silva RA, Diez-Freire C, Dooies A, Jun JY, Sriramula S, Mariappan N, Pourang D, Venugopal CS, Francis J, Reudelhuber T, Santos RA, Patel JM, Raizada MK, Katovich MJ. The angiotensin-converting enzyme 2/angiogenesis-(1-7)/Mas axis confers cardiopulmonary protection against lung fibrosis and pulmonary hypertension. Am J Respir Crit Care Med. 2010;182:1065–72.

86. D'Elia E, Krum H. Mineralcorticoid antagonists in heart failure. Heart Fail Clin. 2014;10:559–64.
87. Maron BA, Opotowsky AR, Landzberg MJ, Loscalzo J, Waxman AB, Leopold JA. Plasma aldosterone levels are elevated in patients with pulmonary arterial hypertension in the absence of left ventricular heart failure: a pilot study. Eur J Heart Fail. 2013;15:277–83.
88. Maron BA, Zhang YY, White K, Chan SY, Handy DE, Mahoney CE, Loscalzo J, Leopold JA. Aldosterone inactivates the endothelin-B receptor via a cysteinyl thiol redox switch to decrease pulmonary endothelial nitric oxide levels and modulate pulmonary arterial hypertension. Circulation. 2012;126:963–74.
89. Maron BA, Leopold JA. The role of the renin-angiotensin-aldosterone system in the pathobiology of pulmonary arterial hypertension (2013 Grover Conference series). Pulm Circ. 2014;4:200–10.
90. Maron BA, Waxman AB, Opotowsky AR, Gillies H, Blair C, Aghamohammadzadeh R, Loscalzo J, Leopold JA. Effectiveness of spironolactone plus ambrisentan for treatment of pulmonary arterial hypertension (from the [ARIES] study 1 and 2 trials). Am J Cardiol. 2013;112:720–5.
91. Urakami T, Jarvinen TA, Toba M, Sawada J, Ambalavanan N, Mann D, McMurtry I, Oka M, Ruoslahti E, Komatsu M. Peptide-directed highly selective targeting of pulmonary arterial hypertension. Am J Pathol. 2011;178:2489–95.
92. Suen CM, Mei SH, Kugathasan L, Stewart DJ. Targeted delivery of genes to endothelial cells and cell- and gene-based therapy in pulmonary vascular diseases. Compr Physiol. 2013;3: 1749–79.
93. Yang JX, Pan YY, Zhao YY, Wang XX. Endothelial progenitor cell-based therapy for pulmonary arterial hypertension. Cell Transplant. 2013;22:1325–36.
94. Asosingh K, Aldred MA, Vasanji A, Drazba J, Sharp J, Farver C, Comhair SA, Xu W, Licina L, Huang L, Anand-Apte B, Yoder MC, Tuder RM, Erzurum SC. Circulating angiogenic precursors in idiopathic pulmonary arterial hypertension. Am J Pathol. 2008;172:615–27.
95. Zhao YD, Courtman DW, Deng Y, Kugathasan L, Zhang Q, Stewart DJ. Rescue of monocrotaline-induced pulmonary arterial hypertension using bone marrow-derived endothelial-like progenitor cells: efficacy of combined cell and eNOS gene therapy in established disease. Circ Res. 2005;96:442–50.
96. Wang XX, Zhang FR, Shang YP, Zhu JH, Xie XD, Tao QM, Zhu JH, Chen JZ. Transplantation of autologous endothelial progenitor cells may be beneficial in patients with idiopathic pulmonary arterial hypertension: a pilot randomized controlled trial. J Am Coll Cardiol. 2007;49: 1566–71.

Chapter 18
Pulmonary Hypertension in Critically Ill Patients

Hooman D. Poor, Corey E. Ventetuolo, and Todd M. Bull

Abstract Pulmonary hypertension (PH) in critically ill patients requiring the intensive care unit (ICU) is a complex and challenging disorder. Whether the elevations of pulmonary arterial pressures are acute or preexisting, significant PH in the setting of acute illness can lead to rapid deterioration of right ventricular (RV) function, precipitating hemodynamic collapse and death. Outcomes of patients with PH who require the ICU are quite poor. In patients with underlying pulmonary arterial hypertension (PAH) or inoperable chronic thromboembolic PH (CTEPH) who are admitted to the ICU, mortality rates between 30 and 41 % have been reported. Given their fragile hemodynamic status, understanding the pathogenesis of RV failure secondary to PH is critical for RV rescue and successful treatment of these patients. In this chapter, we will discuss the pathophysiology of RV failure and management of PH and RV failure in the ICU.

Keywords Pulmonary hypertension • Pulmonary arterial pressures • Right ventricular (RV) function • Pulmonary arterial hypertension • RV dysfunction

Introduction

Pulmonary hypertension (PH) in critically ill patients requiring the intensive care unit (ICU) is a complex and challenging disorder. Whether the elevations of pulmonary arterial pressures are acute or preexisting, significant PH in the setting of acute

H.D. Poor, M.D.
Division of Pulmonary, Critical Care and Sleep, Mount Sinai Hospital, New York, NY, USA

C.E. Ventetuolo, M.D., M.S.
Division of Pulmonary, Sleep and Critical Care Medicine, Rhode Island Hospital, Alpert Medical School of Brown University, Providence, RI, USA

T.M. Bull, M.D. (✉)
Division of Pulmonary Sciences and Critical Care Medicine and Cardiology, The University of Colorado, Denver, CO, USA

12505 E. 16th Avenue, 3rd Floor, Aurora, CO 80045, USA
e-mail: Todd.Bull@ucdenver.edu

J.R. Klinger, R.P. Frantz (eds.), *Diagnosis and Management of Pulmonary Hypertension*, Respiratory Medicine 12, DOI 10.1007/978-1-4939-2636-7_18

illness can lead to rapid deterioration of right ventricular (RV) function, precipitating hemodynamic collapse and death. Outcomes of patients with PH who require the ICU are quite poor. In patients with underlying pulmonary arterial hypertension (PAH) or inoperable chronic thromboembolic PH (CTEPH) who are admitted to the ICU, mortality rates between 30 and 41 % have been reported [1–3]. Given their fragile hemodynamic status, understanding the pathogenesis of RV failure secondary to PH is critical for RV rescue and successful treatment of these patients. In this chapter, we will discuss the pathophysiology of RV failureand management of PH and RV failure in the ICU.

Normal Structure and Function of the RV

The RV should not be viewed as simply a smaller and weaker version of the left ventricle (LV). The two ventricles are embryologically, morphologically, and functionally distinct [4, 5]. Although the RV contains helical fibers, unlike the LV, it lacks circumferential constrictor fibers and must therefore rely on longitudinal shortening. This results in a bellows-like contraction beginning near the apex of the heart and moving in a wave toward the outflow tract [6].

The low pressure and high capacitance of the pulmonary vasculature give rise to pressure–volume relationships for the RV that differ markedly from the pressure–volume relationships for the LV. Under normal loading conditions, the RV has only brief periods of isovolumic contraction and relaxation and has sustained ejection during pressure rise and fall. This circuit structure makes for a highly efficient right heart pump. Myocardial energy expenditure in the RV is approximately one-fifth that of the LV despite similar cardiac outputs (COs). This is due primarily to the much lower RV afterload. Increases in RV afterload significantly change this dynamic and lead to the development of prolonged periods of isovolumic contraction and relaxation, ultimately resulting in a decline in RV performance [6, 7] (Fig. 18.1).

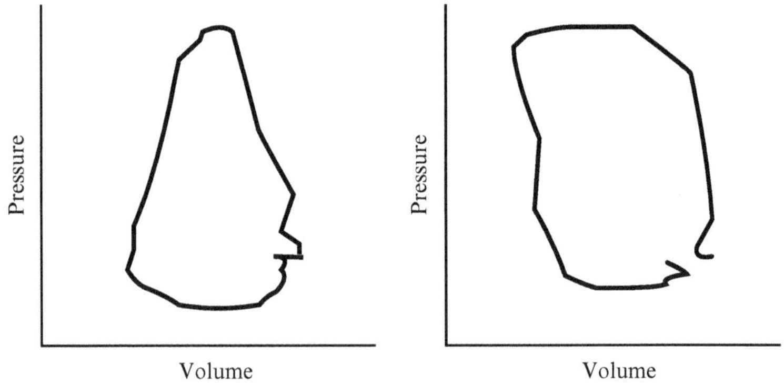

Fig. 18.1 Right ventricular pressure–volume curve from normal subject (**a**) and from patient with increased right ventricular afterload (**b**). Adapted from Redington et al. [7]

Coronary perfusion also differs between the two ventricles. Myocardial perfusion in the LV occurs predominantly during diastole, when intra-myocardial tissue pressure falls below aortic root pressure. Because RV intra-myocardial tissue pressure remains below aortic root pressure throughout the cardiac cycle under normal loading conditions, the RV receives continuous coronary flow from the right coronary artery (RCA) [8, 9].

Last, the RV and LV cannot be viewed as isolated chambers because they share the same visceral cavity (the pericardium), common myofibers, and the interventricular septum. As a result of this ventricular interdependence and the contractile relationships noted above, RV systolic function depends significantly on the LV and changes in the condition of one ventricle can significantly impact the function of the other. Importantly, since both ventricles share myofibers in the septum, LV systolic function augments RV pressure generation and RV systolic performance [10, 11]. With these normal anatomical and physiologic characteristics in mind, the pathophysiologic derangements that occur in the ICU setting may be better understood.

Pathophysiology of RV Failure

Right ventricular failure can be defined as low CO and systemic hypoperfusion despite high RV filling pressures [12]. Because the RV is very sensitive to increases in afterload, rapid elevations in RV afterload decrease RV ejection fraction and induce RV dilatation [13]. In contrast, when RV afterload rises more gradually, adaptive RV myocardial hypertrophy may occur, reducing wall stress to maintain adequate stroke volume [14–18]. In the acute setting, a pressure-overloaded RV dilates and RV end-diastolic volumes and pressures rise, increasing RV wall stress and placing the RV on the descending portion of the Frank-Starling curve [19]. The Laplace relation, which states that wall stress is inversely proportional to the thickness of the wall, helps explain why the thinner RV free wall experiences a greater rise in wall tension with incremental elevations in RV pressure compared with the thicker LV free wall [8].

Higher wall stress in the RV increases myocardial oxygen demand and oxygen consumption [20, 21]. As RV wall tension increases, RCA blood flow, normally continuous during both systole and diastole, occurs only during diastole, causing a further decrease in oxygen delivery to the RV [9, 22]. The combination of increased myocardial oxygen demand and decreased oxygen supply leads to RV ischemia and decreased RV contractility [20, 23]. Right ventricular function is further compromised when the tricuspid valve annulus widens in the setting of RV dilatation, with failure of the tricuspid valve leaflets to coapt properly and worsening tricuspid regurgitation [24]. These changes result in a perpetuating cycle of increasing wall stress, worsening ischemia, tricuspid regurgitation, and unfavorable loading conditions that ultimately lead to RV failure [25] (Fig. 18.2).

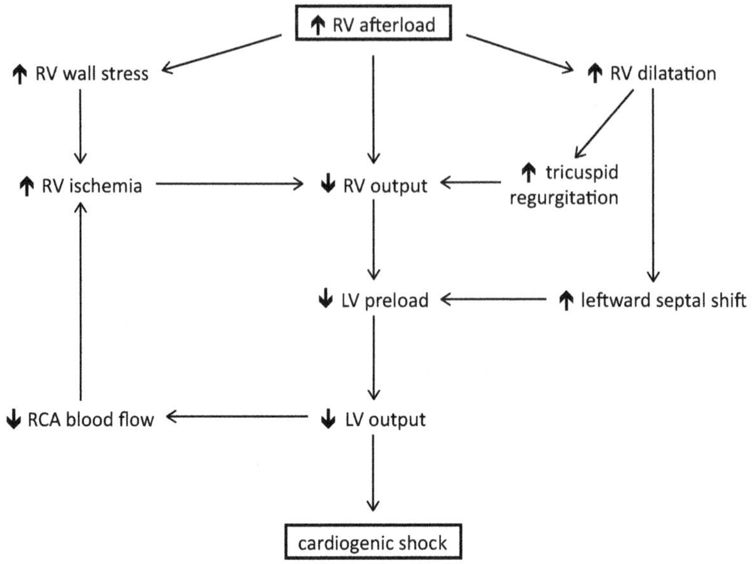

Fig. 18.2 Pathogenesis of right ventricular failure secondary to increased right ventricular afterload. *RV* right ventricle, *LV* left ventricle, *RCA* right coronary artery

Because the RV and LV share the space provided by the pericardium, increases in RV size are at the expense of LV volume. With RV dilatation, the interventricular septum undergoes leftward displacement, impinging upon the LV cavity. The septum's encroachment on the LV impairs LV filling, and the distortion in LV geometry causes a decline in LV systolic performance [26–30]. In addition, the LV is only able to pump the stroke volume received from the right heart, which steadily declines in the failing RV. The resultant decrease in LV stroke volume and CO leads to a fall in RCA blood flow and an exacerbation of RV ischemia, fueling the RV failure cascade (Fig. 18.2).

Acute RV failure from rapid increases in RV afterload can occur in the setting of massive pulmonary embolism (PE). In patients without prior cardiopulmonary disease, good correlation has been observed between hemodynamics and the degree of angiographic obstruction from PE [31–33]. Mean pulmonary artery (PA) pressures of greater than 20 mmHg occur when there is greater than 25–30 % obstruction of the pulmonary vascular bed. When more than 50 % of the pulmonary vascular bed is occluded acutely, patients with are unable to generate mean PA pressures of greater than 40 mmHg, presumably the maximum pressure a normal RV can generate. Thus, when pulmonary vascular obstruction exceeds 50 %, the inability of the RV to generate higher pressures leads to a decrease in CO and the initiation of the RV failure cascade [31, 34]. Mean PA pressures of greater than 40 mmHg suggest that the RV has hypertrophied from chronic increases in afterload such as those caused by underlying cardiopulmonary disease [17]. Patients with poor cardiopulmonary status, manifest a greater deterioration in hemodynamics with a lesser degree of pulmonary vascular obstruction [35]. In patients with PAH, venous stasis, a sedentary lifestyle, dilated right heart chambers, and sluggish pulmonary blood flow together increase the risk for intrapulmonary thrombosis and thromboembolism.

RV failure can also occur in the absence of increased afterload, as seen in RV infarction. RV infarction results in both decreased RV systolic performance from profound depression of RV free wall contraction as well as RV diastolic dysfunction from ischemia [36, 37]. The culprit vessel for RV infarction is usually the RCA and significant RV infarction nearly always occurs in the setting of acute transmural inferior-posterior LV infarction [38]. When the RCA lesion is proximal to the right atrial (RA) branches, RA ischemia can impair RA function, further worsening right-sided hemodynamics [30, 36, 39]. With RV dilatation and decreased RV output, an RV failure cascade similar to that described above can occur. In the absence of preexisting pulmonary vascular disease or significant LV dysfunction, RV systolic and PA pressures do not rise. As LV septal contraction augments RV systolic pressure, concomitant LV infarction, particularly if the septum is involved, may result in further hemodynamic compromise [36, 40]. The short-term prognosis of patients with RV infarction is poor, owing to a higher incidence of cardiogenic shock, ventricular arrhythmias, and high-grade atrioventricular block. The increase in short-term mortality appears to be related to the actual presence of RV infarction and not total myocardial infarct size [41–46]. On the other hand, for patients who survive the acute period, the long-term prognosis is quite favorable even without successful coronary intervention, as RV function is able to return to near normal both at rest and with exercise [47, 48]. This dramatic improvement in RV function in the absence of reperfusion in survivors may be due to transient RV ischemia and myocardial stunning in the acute period, not true RV infarction [49–51]. The RV is less susceptible to true infarction for several reasons. First, its smaller mass and lower afterload result in lesser oxygen demand; Second, it receives coronary perfusion continuously throughout both diastole and systole; Finally, it has more extensive collateral flow from the left to the right coronary arteries. In fact, chronic RV failure attributable solely to RV infarction is a very rare occurrence [9, 51–53].

Triggers for RV Failure

A patient with preexisting pulmonary vascular and RV dysfunction can deteriorate rapidly when challenged by various insults. The prompt identification of contributing or inciting factors is therefore critical in the successful management of these patients [19]. A broad differential diagnosis should be considered because clinical worsening in these patients may be due to a variety of multisystem derangements and etiologies.

A rigorous search for potential sources of infection should be conducted when patients with PH become acutely ill. In a patient with chronic RV dysfunction and venous congestion, reduced bowel perfusion can impair the function of the intestinal barrier, leading to translocation of bacteria and/or release of endotoxin [54].

Patients with chronic PAH who have indwelling central venous catheters for the administration of vasoactive therapies are at increased risk for developing catheter-related skin and soft tissue infections as well as bacteremia [19]. Chronic PAH therapies, specifically prostacyclins, may also have immunosuppressive effects [55–58]. Pneumonia is particularly problematic in patients with pulmonary vascular disease because the resultant shunt with hypoxia can lead to vasoconstriction and further elevation in pulmonary vascular resistance (PVR).

The hemodynamic perturbations in sepsis can cause profound deterioration in patients with severe PH and RV failure. The increase in capillary leak and venous capacitance observed in sepsis results in decreased venous return and lower RV filling pressures, a condition poorly tolerated by a failing RV. The failing RV relies heavily on elevated end diastolic pressures to maintain cardiac output and is sensitive to abrupt changes in loading conditions [59]. Systemic hypotension from sepsis-induced peripheral vasodilation can result in decreased RCA blood flow, exacerbating RV ischemia and compromising RV function. Even in the absence of preexisting pulmonary vascular disease, sepsis has been shown to cause RV myocardial dysfunction directly through cytokine-mediated myocardial depression, as well as indirectly via hypoxic pulmonary vasoconstriction from associated lung injury [60–63]. As discussed later in the text, the addition of vasopressors and inotropes are fraught with their own difficulties in this hemodynamically fragile patient population. Irrespective of the site of infection, the development of sepsis can be devastating and must be managed aggressively, as described below. For these reasons, when infection is suspected, clinicians should have a low threshold to promptly administer antibiotics.

Acute respiratory distress syndrome (ARDS) can lead to the development of RV dysfunction, primarily via increases in RV afterload [64–70]. A variety of factors contribute to pulmonary vascular dysfunction in ARDS, namely, pulmonary vasoconstriction from hypercapnia and hypoxia, and increased intra-thoracic pressures secondary to mechanical ventilation and high positive end-expiratory pressures [70, 71]. Thrombosis also contributes to the increased RV afterload as postmortem studies have demonstrated thromboemboli in 95 % of patients with ARDS [65, 72]. A sub-study from a large clinical trial of ARDS found that 73 % of patients with ARDS had pulmonary vascular dysfunction, as evidenced by an increase in the transpulmonary gradient (TPG) and pulmonary vascular resistance index. The presence of pulmonary vascular dysfunction was independently associated with increased mortality in a dose-dependent fashion, such that increasing TPG was associated with higher mortality [64]. Although the mortality rates of patients with chronic PH who develop ARDS have not been well studied, it seems likely that PH patients may be particularly susceptible to poor outcomes in the setting of ARDS.

Atrial tachyarrhythmias may contribute to hemodynamic compromise in critically ill patients with pulmonary vascular disease. In a cohort of 231 patients with PAH or inoperable CTEPH, the annual incidence of new-onset supraventricular tachycardia was 2.8 %, most commonly due to atrial fibrillation or atrial flutter [73]. Because patients with PH may already have impaired LV filling, these tachyarrhythmias are poorly tolerated and can lead to clinical decompensation. In addition, the loss of atrial contractions may be deleterious in the setting of a noncompliant RV [25, 74]. The maintenance or restoration of sinus rhythm may be helpful in the management strategy discussed below, although data supporting this approach are lacking.

Other factors that may contribute to RV failure in the setting of PH include anemia, hypoxemia, hypercapnia, acidosis, PE, and metabolic abnormalities [24]. Iatrogenic causes include the abrupt withdrawal of pulmonary vasodilators leading to rebound PH, the administration of medications with negative inotropic properties such as β-blockers and certain calcium channel blockers, and the use of positive pressure ventilation, especially with high mean airway pressures and volumes [19]. In a study of 46 patients with PAH or inoperable CTEPH admitted to the ICU, 19 patients had an identifiable trigger for RV decompensation, of which 11 had infection, 3 had unplanned modification or withdrawal of pulmonary vasodilator therapy, 1 had unplanned withdrawal of diuretics, 3 had cardiac arrhythmias, and 1 had unplanned pregnancy [1].

Monitoring in the ICU

Close monitoring of patients with PH and RV failure is critical and may incorporate a mix of noninvasive and invasive modalities. The use of cardiac biomarkers may help in risk assessment because natriuretic peptides are secreted in the setting of right atrial and RV myocardial stretching and cardiac troponin is released during myocardial necrosis from RV ischemia [75]. Elevations in troponin and natriuretic peptides are associated with worse outcomes in chronic PH and acute pulmonary embolism [21, 75–82]. In a prospective cohort study examining 46 patients with PAH or inoperable CTEPH high brain natriuretic peptide levels on admission to the ICU were associated with increased mortality, although no statistical link was found between troponin levels and survival [1].

Echocardiography is a noninvasive modality that plays a central role in the management of patients with PH by providing information about RV function and geometry. In addition, it can help elucidate possible precipitating factors of RV failure, including LV dysfunction and valvular disease. Common echocardiographic signs of RV failure include RV dilatation with associated loss of its typical triangular shape and paradoxical motion of the interventricular septum during systole [83]. In chronic PAH, echocardiographic predictors of poor outcomes include RA enlargement, pericardial effusion, low tricuspid annular plane systolic excursion, and septal displacement, although their ability to discriminate between patients who do well and those who deteriorate in the acute care setting remains unclear [84–86].

The presence of a large pericardial effusion in critically ill patients with pulmonary vascular disease and/or RV failure can be alarming, particularly in the setting of decreased cardiac output or hypotension. The question of "silent tamponade" often arises because elevated RVEDP may prevent the normal echocardiographic findings of RV collapse during inspiration. However, drainage of pericardial effusions in PAH patients traditionally has not been advised due to high reported mortality rates following pericardiocentesis or the placement of a pericardial window [87]. Acute RV decompensation following removal of pericardial fluid likely occurs because of a sudden increase in RV transmural pressure. Under normal conditions the RV is well suited to accommodate this relative increase in RV filling pressure, but in the acutely or chronically overloaded RV, filling pressures have often reached extremely high levels and any further increase may result in a fall in RV contractility. In fact, pericardial effusion in chronic RV failure is often caused by high RVEDP that impedes drainage of pericardial fluid [87]. Gradual removal of fluid may obviate this concern. A more recent single center experience with pericardiocentesis in PAH found low procedural mortality, suggesting that in highly experienced hands there may be a role for this procedure if tamponade is suspected [88]. However, extreme caution is advised.

For patients with PH presenting in shock, it is imperative to obtain adequate central venous access and to perform frequent and blood pressure monitoring. Pulmonary artery catheterization (PAC) may help to differentia maldistributive from cardiogenic shock as well as guide ICU therapy. For example, the measurement of PA oxygen saturation, a marker of the adequacy of oxygen delivery for the body's oxygen demand, may determine the need for inotropes [83].

The use of PAC in critically ill patients without PH has declined over time because multiple studies have shown that outcomes are not improved with its use [89–92]. However, no studies have been carried out in the acute setting for the "pulmonary vascular" population and obtaining and following pulmonary hemodynamics may be important during acute illness for certain PH patients [90]. As the RV is usually severely dilated in advanced PAH, it is advisable to use fluoroscopy to guide the PA catheter into place in order to avoid excessive ectopy and arrhythmias. It is important to note that the PA diastolic pressure cannot be substituted for the pulmonary capillary wedge pressure in patients with PAH due to the presence of a significant TPG. An accurate pulmonary capillary wedge pressure can be difficult to obtain in patients with PAH but is a critical value and requires due diligence, as the approach to management differs markedly in PAH as compared to pulmonary venous hypertension.

Management

General management goals for patients with PH and RV failure include optimization of RV preload, maintenance of adequate mean systemic arterial pressure, enhancement of RV contractility, and reduction of RV afterload, while treating any potentially reversible causes for the acute decompensation [90]. Unfortunately, PH in the ICU setting has not been robustly studied, and consensus guidelines are lacking. Management strategies therefore rely heavily on the guidance of experienced PH specialists.

Volume Management

Optimizing preload in patients with RV failure is complex because both hypovolemia and hypervolemia can have detrimental effects on CO. In most but not all cases of RV failure, the dilated and stretched RV is operating on the flat portion of the Frank-Starling curve. Volume expansion in this scenario often does not augment CO and can instead exacerbate RV dilatation, increase RV wall tension, worsen tricuspid regurgitation, and displace the inter-ventricular septum toward the LV. These adverse effects on RV function and LV filling contribute to reducing CO and worsening clinical status. The goal, therefore, should be to maintain a negative fluid balance with the use of diuretics and, if necessary, hemofiltration, to decrease the volume load on the distended and failing RV without compromising preload. Adjustments in the rate and amount of volume removal should be made according to hemodynamic response [12, 93–97]. In the case of clear intravascular volume depletion, a conservative strategy of holding diuretics, encouraging oral hydration (if applicable), or judiciously using small fluid boluses is preferred.

Vasopressors

Mean systemic arterial pressure must be maintained to minimize RV ischemia. Increased RV wall stress leads to RCA hypoperfusion as PVR approaches SVR or as SVR falls in mixed shock states (i.e., vasodilatory shock with concomitant RV failure). If PVR exceeds SVR, RCA perfusion will occur only during diastole, exacerbating RV ischemia. With the use of vasopressors, SVR can be increased, leading to augmentation of mean systemic arterial pressure, lowering of the PVR/SVR ratio, and, ultimately, improvement in RV myocardial perfusion [9, 90, 98]. In addition, the use of vasopressors increases LV afterload, helping to normalize distorted LV geometry from a leftward-bowed septum [25]. In choosing a vasopressor agent, it is important to be aware of each drug's effect on PVR because increases in PVR may contribute to clinical decompensation.

Norepinephrine causes vasoconstriction through the α_1 receptor and has limited inotropic properties from β_1 receptor stimulation [99]. It has been shown to improve RV performance and PA/RV coupling in animal models of acute PH and RV dysfunction by way of β_1 effects on contractility [20, 100, 101]. In a study of ten patients with septic shock, PH, and RV dysfunction, norepinephrine increased SVR and improved the RV oxygen supply/demand ratio but also caused an increase in PVR and failed to improve RV ejection fraction [102]. Evidence for the use of norepinephrine in critically ill patients with PH comes from a large randomized trial of ICU patients with shock, in which norepinephrine use, as compared to dopamine use, was associated with decreased mortality at 28 days in the prespecified subgroup of patients with cardiogenic shock and with a decreased rate of arrhythmias in all patients [103].

Phenylephrine, an α_1 receptor agonist with no β_1 receptor activity, improves RCA perfusion in RV failure, but this benefit is offset by its elevation of PVR and lack of β_1-mediated enhancement of contractility [98, 100, 104]. In addition, reflex bradycardia secondary to phenylephrine may have detrimental effects in the setting of RV failure [105].

Epinephrine, a potent α and β receptor agonist that causes vasoconstriction and increased inotropy, increased CO without altering the PVR/SVR ratio in hypoxic newborn piglets [106]. A small study in patients with RV dysfunction from severe septic shock showed that epinephrine increased RV contractility [107]. The use of epinephrine has not been well studied in patients with PH, however. For these reasons, norepinephrine is a more favorable choice for patients with PH in the ICU than either phenylephrine or epinephrine.

Vasopressin causes vasoconstriction by acting upon V1 receptors on vascular smooth muscle cells and also increases vascular responsiveness to catecholamines [99]. Low doses of vasopressin cause pulmonary vasodilation through endothelium-mediated nitric oxide (NO) production in animals, although high doses cause vasoconstriction through an endothelium-independent mechanism [108]. Vasopressin's effect on the pulmonary vasculature has been inconsistent in human studies [105]. At higher infusion rates, vasopressin may have direct myocardial depressive effects and causes coronary vasoconstriction [109, 110]. Although low-dose (i.e., 0.01–0.03 U min^{-1}) vasopressin may be effective in managing patients with RV failure, higher doses should be used with caution.

Inotropes

Dopamine activates dopaminergic receptors at doses less than 5 μg kg^{-1} min^{-1}, β_1 receptors at doses between 5 and 10 μg kg^{-1} min^{-1}, and α_1 receptors at doses greater than 10 μg kg^{-1} min^{-1}, although actual plasma dopamine levels for a given infusion rate may vary unpredictably in critically ill patients [99, 111]. In a large animal model of hypoxia-induced PH, dopamine did not increase PVR at doses up to 10 μg kg^{-1} min^{-1} [112]. In fact, in patients with PH secondary to left heart disease, dopamine in doses ranging from 2 to 16 μg kg^{-1} min^{-1} increased CO and heart rate but did not significantly change PVR [113]. Similarly, in a small study of patients with PH and septic shock, dopamine improved CO without increasing PVR but failed to improve RV ejection fraction [102]. As discussed above, although the routine use of dopamine in the critical care setting is not supported by current data, in low doses it may be a reasonable option in patients with PH and RV failure. Aggravation of tachycardia can be a limitation.

Dobutamine has inotropic effects through β_1 receptor stimulation and a variable degree of vasodilatory effects through the β_2 receptor [99]. In an animal model of PH, dobutamine at doses of 5–10 μg kg^{-1} min^{-1} restored CO and arterial pressure without affecting PA resistance or elastance, improving PA/RV coupling [20]. Doses up to 10 μg kg^{-1} min^{-1} in patients with left heart failure result in improved myocardial contractility, reduced PVR and SVR, and less tachycardia when compared with dopamine [114]. Dobutamine has been shown to improve hemodynamics in patients with PH at liver transplantation and after severe RV infarction [97, 115]. However, it has significant β_2-mediated systemic vasodilatory properties and thus, it is important to avoid high doses, anticipate possible systemic hypotension, and be prepared to add systemic vasopressors if systemic hypotension occurs [90].

Milrinone, a selective phosphodiesterase-3 inhibitor, that acts via delaying metabolism of intracellular cAMP has positive inotropic effects and direct-acting vasodilatory properties on the pulmonary circulation [99]. In animal models of both acute and chronic PH, milrinone improved RV function and decreased PVR [116, 117]. In patients with pulmonary vascular dysfunction in the setting of LV failure, post-ventricular assist, or cardiac transplantation, milrinone has been shown to reduce pulmonary pressures and improve RV function and is often the agent of choice in these settings [118–120]. Systemic hypotension often limits the use of milrinone in the treatment of patients with PAH and hemodynamic instability, but it may be effective in patients with PH associated with LV dysfunction. Dopamine, dobutamine, and milrinone therapies are all capable of inducing cardiac tachyarrhythmias that are poorly tolerated in patients with PH and may be a limiting factor in their use in some patients. A few case series suggest that inhaled milrinone may be useful in PH because it minimizes systemic hypotension by delivering the drug directly to the pulmonary vasculature [121–124].

Levosimendan, a novel drug that enhances myocardial contractility by sensitizing troponin C to calcium while also acting as a pulmonary vasodilator, is a promising agent for patients with PH and RV failure but has not yet been thoroughly investigated in this patient population [125–129]. Irrespective of the specific agent, inotropes should generally be considered when there is evidence of inadequate oxygen delivery and/or in the case of volume overload not successfully managed with diuretics alone. It is especially important to avoid "supra-normalization" of oxygen delivery in these patients because this strategy not only is associated with worse outcomes in the general ICU population but may also increase PA pressures and worsen cardiac function in patients with pulmonary vascular disease [130, 131].

Pulmonary Vasodilators

Because increased RV afterload plays a central role in RV failure associated with PH, the use of pulmonary vasodilators to unload the RV is critical. The ability of even a severely dilated and overloaded RV to return to normal size and function is illustrated by the restoration of RV function after pulmonary thromboendarterectomy for CTEPH and lung transplantation in patients with PH [132–134].

Inhaled NO is a potent pulmonary vasodilator with minimal systemic vasodilatory effects because it is rapidly inactivated by hemoglobin within the pulmonary capillaries. Because of its short half-life, continuous administration through a face mask, a nasal cannula, or, a ventilator circuit is required [135]. In patients with chronic PAH, NO reduces PVR and improves CO without a drop in SVR [136–138]. In 26 patients admitted to the ICU with acute RV failure, NO administration resulted in a greater than 20 % increase in CO and/or decrease in PVR in half of the patients [139]. With prolonged use at high concentrations, methemoglobinemia may develop, necessitating periodic surveillance of methemoglobin levels and routine assessment for cyanosis [140]. Nitrogen dioxide (NO_2) will accumulate when NO is delivered with high FiO_2 and needs to be monitored continuously in the ventilator circuit. Care must be taken in the discontinuation of NO because abrupt withdrawal has been associated with rebound PH and hemodynamic collapse [141–143]. After prolonged use, complete discontinuation of even low-dose inhaled NO may necessitate bridging therapy with another targeted pulmonary vasodilator.

Prostacyclins, including epoprostenol, treprostinil, and iloprost, are potent, short-acting agents that cause pulmonary vasodilation and inhibit platelet aggregation. In chronic PAH, these medications improve exercise capacity, hemodynamics, and, in the case of continuous infusion epoprostenol, survival [144–149]. In the critical care setting, prostacyclins have been mainly studied in patients with PH after cardiac surgery or transplantation, where they have been shown to reduce PVR and improve RV function [150–156]. The use of intravenous prostacyclins and up-titration of their dose in the ICU is usually limited by systemic hypotension and other systemic adverse effects including nausea, flushing, headache, and diarrhea [55]. Prostacyclins should be avoided in patients with significant left heart dysfunction and elevated pulmonary venous pressures because their use in this setting can generate further increases in left-sided filling pressures, leading to the development of pulmonary edema, pleural effusions and/or the deterioration of LV function [157].

Importantly, vasodilation of the pulmonary vasculature by systemic prostacyclin or prostacyclin analogues is nonselective and can exacerbate ventilation-perfusion mismatch, leading to worsened gas exchange and hypoxemia. These effects may be particularly problematic in patients with intrinsic lung disease and hypoxic PH. This phenomenon maybe circumvented with the use of inhaled preparations whereby pulmonary blood flow to well-ventilated regions in the lung is increased, thereby decreasing intra pulmonary shunt [158]. The inhaled prostacyclins iloprost and treprostinil are approved for outpatient use with specific devices (the I-neb Adaptive Aerosol Delivery device and the Optineb-ir, respectively). Iloprost is increasingly being used “off-label” in the postoperative and ICU setting with an ultrasonic nebulizer, although dosing and drug absorption are not standardized. Drug delivery and pharmacokinetics using alternative systems (i.e., conventional nebulizers and ventilator circuits) have also not been studied. Finally, abrupt discontinuation of prostacyclin infusions in chronically treated patients should be avoided because this may precipitate severe rebound PAH and even death [159]. Patients with PAH on chronic prostacyclin therapies who develop vasodilatory or mixed shock may require dose reductions during their acute illness, so as to not exacerbate systemic hypotension and/or create (relative) high-output failure, but this should be done under the guidance of a PH specialist.

The endothelin receptor antagonists and phosphodiesterase-5 (PDE5) inhibitors are proven oral medications for the management of chronic PAH, but they have not been investigated in critically ill patients with RV failure [160–163]. An intravenous formulation of the PDE5 inhibitor sildenafil has recently become available and may prove useful in the acute setting, although future studies in this patient population are needed [164]. By increasing downstream cyclic guanosine monophosphate signaling, PDE5 inhibitors reduce PVR and may also augment RV function by exerting a milrinone-like effect through inhibition of phosphodiesterase-3 [165–168]. With a rapid onset of action and a relatively prolonged half-life of 3–4 h, intravenous sildenafil must be used cautiously in critically ill patients to avoid systemic hypotension and exacerbation of ventilation-perfusion mismatch [164, 169]. Anecdotally, intravenous dosing should be approximately one third to one half that of the anticipated oral sildenafil dose.

Supportive Care

Maintaining peripheral oxygen saturations greater than 90 % in PAH; this is critically important in the acute setting, to prevent or reverse any contributing hypoxic pulmonary vasoconstriction [170]. Oxygen inhalation has been shown to reduce PVR and improve CO in patients with PH [171, 172]. Hypercapnia and acidemia worsen hypoxic pulmonary vasoconstriction and RV contractility and should be avoided [173, 174]. Although no studies have been performed to determine the optimal hemoglobin level for patients with PH and RV failure, many experts recommend maintaining a hemoglobin level of greater than 10 g dL^{-1} to optimize oxygen-carrying capacity and minimize RV ischemia [25]. Volume status should be monitored carefully and diuretics adjusted appropriately with transfusion. As mentioned previously, patients with PH and RV failure are intolerant of electrolyte disturbances, metabolic derangements, and vagal stimuli, and care must be taken to normalize these imbalances if present.

Mechanical Ventilation

Endotracheal intubation of patients with PH and RV failure should be avoided when at all possible. If intubation is necessary, etomidate is generally the preferred induction sedative because it has minimal effects on SVR, PVR, and cardiac contractility. Propofol should be avoided given its propensity to cause systemic hypotension. Systemic vasopressors should be readily available or started preemptively to maintain SVR and counteract peri-intubation hypotension, which, if occurs in a patient with severe PH and RV failure, can be catastrophic and result in cardiac arrest [175, 176].

Because elevated intrathoracic pressures decrease RV and LV preload and increase PVR, ventilator strategies that use high inflation lung volumes and pressures should be avoided to prevent these detrimental effects [90, 177]. High positive end-expiratory pressures may, in theory, increase pulmonary vascular resistance and should be avoided, as should atelectasis or reduced lung volumes. In general, ventilation strategies should aim to keep lung volumes close to Functional Residual Capacity (FRC) while maintaining adequate oxygenation and ventilation while avoiding high peak inspiratory or end expiratory pressures.

Mechanical Support

When conventional support for the RV is ineffective in severe cases of PH and RV failure, mechanical support, including RV-assist devices and venoarterial extracorporeal membrane oxygenation (VA-ECMO), may be considered. The use of intra-aortic balloon counterpulsation in isolated RV failure has been reported, and improves CO by augmenting coronary blood flow [178, 179]. Although RV-assist devices are effective in primary RV dysfunction or RV failure secondary to LV failure, thus far, they have not been shown to be successful in patients with significantly elevated PVR. In this setting, the increase in pulmonary blood flow, particularly if pulsatile, gives rise to markedly elevated pulmonary vascular pressures, which can damage the pulmonary microcirculation and lead to intraparenchymal pulmonary hemorrhage, hemoptysis, and death [180, 181].

VA-ECMO has been used successfully in patients with massive PE, in patients with PH and RV failure as a bridge to lung transplantation, and in patients with CTEPH as a bridge to or for complications arising after pulmonary thromboendarterectomy [182–189]. By unloading the RV and providing additional blood flow to the systemic circulation, VA-ECMO improves the hemodynamics of patients with PH and RV failure. In addition, it can help reverse hypoxic pulmonary vasoconstriction by performing gas exchange and has been successfully used in awake, spontaneously breathing patients (a number of whom had PAH) as a bridge to lung transplantation [190]. VA-ECMO is not without potentially serious complications, however, and may include bleeding, infection, thromboembolism, and neurologic sequelae [180]. More recently, pumpless lung-assist devices have been developed and used in patients with PAH as a bridge to lung transplantation, connecting the PA to the left atrium with a low-resistance membrane oxygenator. With the blood flow through the circuit powered by the patient's own RV, these devices unload the RV and enhance LV filling in a manner similar to balloon atrioseptostomy; however, in contrast to septostomy, these devices improve instead of impair gas exchange [191, 192].

Cardiopulmonary Resuscitation

Cardiopulmonary resuscitation (CPR) in patients with PH and RV failure is largely unsuccessful. In a retrospective, multicenter study, 132 patients with PAH had circulatory arrest and implementation of CPR, of which only 8 patients (6 %) survived for more than 90 days. In addition, seven of these eight surviving patients had correctable causes of their cardiopulmonary arrest, including vasovagal reactions, digitalis toxicity, and pericardial tamponade [193]. One explanation for the lack of efficacy of CPR in this patient population is that high PVR makes it unlikely that chest compressions will achieve adequate pulmonary blood flow and LV filling. In addition, the use of epinephrine during CPR causes even further increases in PVR [194]. In light of the poor outcomes of CPR in patients with severe PH and RV failure, having timely discussions about the possibility of "Do Not Resuscitate" orders with these patients and their families is crucial, particularly in patients in whom a reversible cause for decompensation cannot be determined.

Conclusion

Patients with PH and RV failure who require ICU admission are at significant risk for worsening morbidity and mortality. In the setting of PH, RV failure can be triggered by various factors, giving rise to a vicious cycle of worsening RV function, profound shock, and death. Given their tenuous hemodynamics, these patients must be monitored closely with indicators of end-organ perfusion, cardiac biomarkers, echocardiography, and, in select situations, PAC. Management goals include optimizing RV preload with diuretics or hemofiltration, maintaining mean systemic arterial pressure with systemic vasopressors, augmenting RV contractility with inotropes, decreasing RV afterload with selective pulmonary vasodilators, and reversing any identifiable inciting factors. In severe cases, VA-ECMO or other forms of mechanical support may be considered. Although there have been marked advances in therapeutic strategies for PAH over the last several decades, acute care of patients with pulmonary vascular and RV dysfunction remains largely unstudied and guided by clinical expertise.

References

1. Sztrymf B, et al. Prognostic factors of acute heart failure in patients with pulmonary arterial hypertension. Eur Respir J. 2010;35(6):1286–93.
2. Kurzyna M, et al. Characteristics and prognosis of patients with decompensated right ventricular failure during the course of pulmonary hypertension. Kardiol Pol. 2008;66(10): 1033–9. discussion 1040–1.
3. Huynh TN, et al. Prognostic factors and outcomes of patients with pulmonary hypertension admitted to the intensive care unit. J Crit Care. 2012;27(6):739e7–13.

4. Greyson CR. Pathophysiology of right ventricular failure. Crit Care Med. 2008;36(1 Suppl):S57–65.
5. Zaffran S, et al. Right ventricular myocardium derives from the anterior heart field. Circ Res. 2004;95(3):261–8.
6. Sheehan F, Redington A. The right ventricle: anatomy, physiology and clinical imaging. Heart. 2008;94(11):1510–5.
7. Redington AN, et al. Changes in the pressure-volume relation of the right ventricle when its loading conditions are modified. Br Heart J. 1990;63(1):45–9.
8. Greyson CR. The right ventricle and pulmonary circulation: basic concepts. Rev Esp Cardiol. 2010;63(1):81–95.
9. Lowensohn HS, et al. Phasic right coronary artery blood flow in conscious dogs with normal and elevated right ventricular pressures. Circ Res. 1976;39(6):760–6.
10. Damiano Jr RJ, et al. Significant left ventricular contribution to right ventricular systolic function. Am J Physiol. 1991;261(5 Pt 2):H1514–24.
11. Hoffman D, et al. Left-to-right ventricular interaction with a noncontracting right ventricle. J Thorac Cardiovasc Surg. 1994;107(6):1496–502.
12. Layish DT, Tapson VF. Pharmacologic hemodynamic support in massive pulmonary embolism. Chest. 1997;111(1):218–24.
13. Brent BN, et al. Physiologic correlates of right ventricular ejection fraction in chronic obstructive pulmonary disease: a combined radionuclide and hemodynamic study. Am J Cardiol. 1982;50(2):255–62.
14. Sharma S, et al. Dynamic changes of gene expression in hypoxia-induced right ventricular hypertrophy. Am J Physiol Heart Circ Physiol. 2004;286(3):H1185–92.
15. Simon MA. Right ventricular adaptation to pressure overload. Curr Opin Crit Care. 2010; 16(3):237–43.
16. Baandrup JD, et al. Pressure load: the main factor for altered gene expression in right ventricular hypertrophy in chronic hypoxic rats. PLoS One. 2011;6(1):e15859.
17. Badano LP, et al. Right ventricle in pulmonary arterial hypertension: haemodynamics, structural changes, imaging, and proposal of a study protocol aimed to assess remodelling and treatment effects. Eur J Echocardiogr. 2010;11(1):27–37.
18. Dias CA, et al. Reversible pulmonary trunk banding. II. An experimental model for rapid pulmonary ventricular hypertrophy. J Thorac Cardiovasc Surg. 2002;124(5):999–1006.
19. Matthews JC, McLaughlin V. Acute right ventricular failure in the setting of acute pulmonary embolism or chronic pulmonary hypertension: a detailed review of the pathophysiology, diagnosis, and management. Curr Cardiol Rev. 2008;4(1):49–59.
20. Kerbaul F, et al. Effects of norepinephrine and dobutamine on pressure load-induced right ventricular failure. Crit Care Med. 2004;32(4):1035–40.
21. Torbicki A, et al. Detectable serum cardiac troponin T as a marker of poor prognosis among patients with chronic precapillary pulmonary hypertension. Circulation. 2003;108(7):844–8.
22. Gibbons Kroeker CA, et al. Compression induced by RV pressure overload decreases regional coronary blood flow in anesthetized dogs. Am J Physiol Heart Circ Physiol. 2006;290(6): H2432–8.
23. Chin KM, Kim NH, Rubin LJ. The right ventricle in pulmonary hypertension. Coron Artery Dis. 2005;16(1):13–8.
24. Chemla D, et al. Haemodynamic evaluation of pulmonary hypertension. Eur Respir J. 2002;20(5):1314–31.
25. Hoeper MM, Granton J. Intensive care unit management of patients with severe pulmonary hypertension and right heart failure. Am J Respir Crit Care Med. 2011;184(10):1114–24.
26. Gan CT, et al. Impaired left ventricular filling due to right-to-left ventricular interaction in patients with pulmonary arterial hypertension. Am J Physiol Heart Circ Physiol. 2006;290(4):H1528–33.
27. Mahmud E, et al. Correlation of left ventricular diastolic filling characteristics with right ventricular overload and pulmonary artery pressure in chronic thromboembolic pulmonary hypertension. J Am Coll Cardiol. 2002;40(2):318–24.

28. Stojnic BB, et al. Left ventricular filling characteristics in pulmonary hypertension: a new mode of ventricular interaction. Br Heart J. 1992;68(1):16–20.
29. Marcus JT, et al. Interventricular mechanical asynchrony in pulmonary arterial hypertension: left-to-right delay in peak shortening is related to right ventricular overload and left ventricular underfilling. J Am Coll Cardiol. 2008;51(7):750–7.
30. Brookes C, et al. Acute right ventricular dilatation in response to ischemia significantly impairs left ventricular systolic performance. Circulation. 1999;100(7):761–7.
31. McIntyre KM, Sasahara AA. The hemodynamic response to pulmonary embolism in patients without prior cardiopulmonary disease. Am J Cardiol. 1971;28(3):288–94.
32. McIntyre KM, Sasahara AA. Hemodynamic alterations related to extent of lung scan perfusion defect in pulmonary embolism. J Nucl Med. 1971;12(4):166–70.
33. Azarian R, et al. Lung perfusion scans and hemodynamics in acute and chronic pulmonary embolism. J Nucl Med. 1997;38(6):980–3.
34. Wood KE. Major pulmonary embolism: review of a pathophysiologic approach to the golden hour of hemodynamically significant pulmonary embolism. Chest. 2002;121(3):877–905.
35. McIntyre KM, Sasahara AA. Determinants of right ventricular function and hemodynamics after pulmonary embolism. Chest. 1974;65(5):534–43.
36. Goldstein JA, et al. Determinants of hemodynamic compromise with severe right ventricular infarction. Circulation. 1990;82(2):359–68.
37. Toldo S, et al. Right ventricular dysfunction following acute myocardial infarction in the absence of pulmonary hypertension in the mouse. PLoS One. 2011;6(3):e18102.
38. Bowers TR, et al. Patterns of coronary compromise resulting in acute right ventricular ischemic dysfunction. Circulation. 2002;106(9):1104–9.
39. Goldstein JA, et al. Right atrial ischemia exacerbates hemodynamic compromise associated with experimental right ventricular dysfunction. J Am Coll Cardiol. 1991;18(6):1564–72.
40. Goldstein JA, et al. Importance of left ventricular function and systolic ventricular interaction to right ventricular performance during acute right heart ischemia. J Am Coll Cardiol. 1992;19(3):704–11.
41. Zehender M, et al. Right ventricular infarction as an independent predictor of prognosis after acute inferior myocardial infarction. N Engl J Med. 1993;328(14):981–8.
42. Bowers TR, et al. Effect of reperfusion on biventricular function and survival after right ventricular infarction. N Engl J Med. 1998;338(14):933–40.
43. Bueno H, et al. In-hospital outcome of elderly patients with acute inferior myocardial infarction and right ventricular involvement. Circulation. 1997;96(2):436–41.
44. Mehta SR, et al. Impact of right ventricular involvement on mortality and morbidity in patients with inferior myocardial infarction. J Am Coll Cardiol. 2001;37(1):37–43.
45. Gumina RJ, et al. Strong predictive value of TIMI risk score analysis for in-hospital and long-term survival of patients with right ventricular infarction. Eur Heart J. 2002;23(21): 1678–83.
46. Shiraki H, et al. Acute impact of right ventricular infarction on early hemodynamic course after inferior myocardial infarction. Circ J. 2010;74(1):148–55.
47. Lim ST, et al. Right ventricular performance at rest and during stress with chronic proximal occlusion of the right coronary artery. Am J Cardiol. 2003;92(10):1203–6.
48. Dell'Italia LJ, et al. Hemodynamically important right ventricular infarction: follow-up evaluation of right ventricular systolic function at rest and during exercise with radionuclide ventriculography and respiratory gas exchange. Circulation. 1987;75(5):996–1003.
49. Ramzy IS, et al. Right ventricular stunning in inferior myocardial infarction. Int J Cardiol. 2009;136(3):294–9.
50. Ketikoglou DG, et al. Echocardiographic evaluation of spontaneous recovery of right ventricular systolic and diastolic function in patients with acute right ventricular infarction associated with posterior wall left ventricular infarction. Am J Cardiol. 2004;93(7):911–3.
51. Goldstein JA. Acute right ventricular infarction: insights for the interventional era. Curr Probl Cardiol. 2012;37(12):533–57.

52. Kusachi S, et al. Right and left ventricular oxygen metabolism in open-chest dogs. Am J Physiol. 1982;243(5):H761–6.
53. Haupt HM, Hutchins GM, Moore GW. Right ventricular infarction: role of the moderator band artery in determining infarct size. Circulation. 1983;67(6):1268–72.
54. Krack A, et al. The importance of the gastrointestinal system in the pathogenesis of heart failure. Eur Heart J. 2005;26(22):2368–74.
55. Papierniak ES, Lowenthal DT, Mubarak K. Pulmonary arterial hypertension: classification and therapy with a focus on prostaglandin analogs. Am J Ther. 2012;19(4):300–14.
56. Oudiz RJ, et al. Micrococcus-associated central venous catheter infection in patients with pulmonary arterial hypertension. Chest. 2004;126(1):90–4.
57. Rich JD, et al. The effect of diluent pH on bloodstream infection rates in patients receiving IV treprostinil for pulmonary arterial hypertension. Chest. 2012;141(1):36–42.
58. Kallen AJ, et al. Bloodstream infections in patients given treatment with intravenous prostanoids. Infect Control Hosp Epidemiol. 2008;29(4):342–9.
59. Zanotti Cavazzoni SL, Dellinger RP. Hemodynamic optimization of sepsis-induced tissue hypoperfusion. Crit Care. 2006;10 Suppl 3:S2.
60. Sharma AC. Sepsis-induced myocardial dysfunction. Shock. 2007;28(3):265–9.
61. Court O, et al. Clinical review: Myocardial depression in sepsis and septic shock. Crit Care. 2002;6(6):500–8.
62. Kimchi A, et al. Right ventricular performance in septic shock: a combined radionuclide and hemodynamic study. J Am Coll Cardiol. 1984;4(5):945–51.
63. Parker MM, et al. Right ventricular dysfunction and dilatation, similar to left ventricular changes, characterize the cardiac depression of septic shock in humans. Chest. 1990;97(1): 126–31.
64. Bull TM, et al. Pulmonary vascular dysfunction is associated with poor outcomes in patients with acute lung injury. Am J Respir Crit Care Med. 2010;182(9):1123–8.
65. Zapol WM, Snider MT. Pulmonary hypertension in severe acute respiratory failure. N Engl J Med. 1977;296(9):476–80.
66. Sibbald WJ, et al. Biventricular function in the adult respiratory distress syndrome. Chest. 1983;84(2):126–34.
67. Schulman DS, Matthay RA. The right ventricle in pulmonary disease. Cardiol Clin. 1992;10(1):111–35.
68. Vieillard-Baron A, et al. Acute cor pulmonale in acute respiratory distress syndrome submitted to protective ventilation: incidence, clinical implications, and prognosis. Crit Care Med. 2001;29(8):1551–5.
69. Vieillard-Baron A, et al. Echo-Doppler demonstration of acute cor pulmonale at the bedside in the medical intensive care unit. Am J Respir Crit Care Med. 2002;166(10):1310–9.
70. Vieillard-Baron A, Jardin F. Why protect the right ventricle in patients with acute respiratory distress syndrome? Curr Opin Crit Care. 2003;9(1):15–21.
71. Jardin F, et al. Relation between transpulmonary pressure and right ventricular isovolumetric pressure change during respiratory support. Cathet Cardiovasc Diagn. 1989;16(4):215–20.
72. Tomashefski Jr JF, et al. The pulmonary vascular lesions of the adult respiratory distress syndrome. Am J Pathol. 1983;112(1):112–26.
73. Tongers J, et al. Incidence and clinical relevance of supraventricular tachyarrhythmias in pulmonary hypertension. Am Heart J. 2007;153(1):127–32.
74. Goldstein JA, et al. Hemodynamic importance of systolic ventricular interaction, augmented right atrial contractility and atrioventricular synchrony in acute right ventricular dysfunction. J Am Coll Cardiol. 1990;16(1):181–9.
75. Henzler T, et al. Pulmonary embolism: CT signs and cardiac biomarkers for predicting right ventricular dysfunction. Eur Respir J. 2012;39(4):919–26.
76. Fijalkowska A, et al. Serum N-terminal brain natriuretic peptide as a prognostic parameter in patients with pulmonary hypertension. Chest. 2006;129(5):1313–21.

77. Mauritz GJ, et al. Usefulness of serial N-terminal pro-B-type natriuretic peptide measurements for determining prognosis in patients with pulmonary arterial hypertension. Am J Cardiol. 2011;108(11):1645–50.
78. Leuchte HH, et al. Clinical significance of brain natriuretic peptide in primary pulmonary hypertension. J Am Coll Cardiol. 2004;43(5):764–70.
79. Nagaya N, et al. Plasma brain natriuretic peptide as a prognostic indicator in patients with primary pulmonary hypertension. Circulation. 2000;102(8):865–70.
80. Mehta NJ, Jani K, Khan IA. Clinical usefulness and prognostic value of elevated cardiac troponin I levels in acute pulmonary embolism. Am Heart J. 2003;145(5):821–5.
81. La Vecchia L, et al. Increased cardiac troponin I on admission predicts in-hospital mortality in acute pulmonary embolism. Heart. 2004;90(6):633–7.
82. Lega JC, et al. Natriuretic peptides and troponins in pulmonary embolism: a meta-analysis. Thorax. 2009;64(10):869–75.
83. Gayat E, Mebazaa A. Pulmonary hypertension in critical care. Curr Opin Crit Care. 2011;17(5):439–48.
84. Ghio S, et al. Prognostic relevance of the echocardiographic assessment of right ventricular function in patients with idiopathic pulmonary arterial hypertension. Int J Cardiol. 2010;140(3):272–8.
85. Lopez-Candales A, et al. Apical systolic eccentricity index: a better marker of right ventricular compromise in pulmonary hypertension. Echocardiography. 2010;27(5):534–8.
86. Raymond RJ, et al. Echocardiographic predictors of adverse outcomes in primary pulmonary hypertension. J Am Coll Cardiol. 2002;39(7):1214–9.
87. Hemnes AR, Gaine SP, Wiener CM. Poor outcomes associated with drainage of pericardial effusions in patients with pulmonary arterial hypertension. South Med J. 2008;101(5): 490–4.
88. Fenstad ER, Le RJ, Sinak LJ, Maradit-Kremers H, et al. Pericardial effusions in pulmonary arterial hypertension: characteristics, prognosis, and role of drainage. Chest. 2013;144(5): 1530–8.
89. Hadian M, Pinsky MR. Evidence-based review of the use of the pulmonary artery catheter: impact data and complications. Crit Care. 2006;10 Suppl 3:S8.
90. Price LC, et al. Pulmonary vascular and right ventricular dysfunction in adult critical care: current and emerging options for management: a systematic literature review. Crit Care. 2010;14(5):R169.
91. Harvey S, et al. Assessment of the clinical effectiveness of pulmonary artery catheters in management of patients in intensive care (PAC-Man): a randomised controlled trial. Lancet. 2005;366(9484):472–7.
92. Sandham JD, et al. A randomized, controlled trial of the use of pulmonary-artery catheters in high-risk surgical patients. N Engl J Med. 2003;348(1):5–14.
93. Belenkie I, et al. Effects of volume loading during experimental acute pulmonary embolism. Circulation. 1989;80(1):178–88.
94. Forrest P. Anaesthesia and right ventricular failure. Anaesth Intensive Care. 2009;37(3): 370–85.
95. Ghignone M, Girling L, Prewitt RM. Volume expansion versus norepinephrine in treatment of a low cardiac output complicating an acute increase in right ventricular afterload in dogs. Anesthesiology. 1984;60(2):132–5.
96. Mebazaa A, et al. Acute right ventricular failure—from pathophysiology to new treatments. Intensive Care Med. 2004;30(2):185–96.
97. Ferrario M, et al. Hemodynamics of volume loading compared with dobutamine in severe right ventricular infarction. Am J Cardiol. 1994;74(4):329–33.
98. Vlahakes GJ, Turley K, Hoffman JI. The pathophysiology of failure in acute right ventricular hypertension: hemodynamic and biochemical correlations. Circulation. 1981;63(1):87–95.
99. Hollenberg SM. Vasoactive drugs in circulatory shock. Am J Respir Crit Care Med. 2011;183(7):847–55.

100. Hirsch LJ, et al. Norepinephrine and phenylephrine effects on right ventricular function in experimental canine pulmonary embolism. Chest. 1991;100(3):796–801.
101. Ducas J, et al. Treatment of canine pulmonary hypertension: effects of norepinephrine and isoproterenol on pulmonary vascular pressure-flow characteristics. Circulation. 1987;75(1): 235–42.
102. Schreuder WO, et al. Effect of dopamine vs. norepinephrine on hemodynamics in septic shock. Emphasis on right ventricular performance. Chest. 1989;95(6):1282–8.
103. De Backer D, et al. Comparison of dopamine and norepinephrine in the treatment of shock. N Engl J Med. 2010;362(9):779–89.
104. Rich S, Gubin S, Hart K. The effects of phenylephrine on right ventricular performance in patients with pulmonary hypertension. Chest. 1990;98(5):1102–6.
105. Zamanian RT, et al. Management strategies for patients with pulmonary hypertension in the intensive care unit. Crit Care Med. 2007;35(9):2037–50.
106. Cheung PY, Barrington KJ. The effects of dopamine and epinephrine on hemodynamics and oxygen metabolism in hypoxic anesthetized piglets. Crit Care. 2001;5(3):158–66.
107. Le Tulzo Y, et al. Effects of epinephrine on right ventricular function in patients with severe septic shock and right ventricular failure: a preliminary descriptive study. Intensive Care Med. 1997;23(6):664–70.
108. Evora PR, Pearson PJ, Schaff HV. Arginine vasopressin induces endothelium-dependent vasodilatation of the pulmonary artery. V1-receptor-mediated production of nitric oxide. Chest. 1993;103(4):1241–5.
109. Leather HA, et al. Effects of vasopressin on right ventricular function in an experimental model of acute pulmonary hypertension. Crit Care Med. 2002;30(11):2548–52.
110. Indrambarya T, et al. Low-dose vasopressin infusion results in increased mortality and cardiac dysfunction following ischemia-reperfusion injury in mice. Crit Care. 2009;13(3):R98.
111. Juste RN, et al. Dopamine clearance in critically ill patients. Intensive Care Med. 1998;24(11):1217–20.
112. Lejeune P, et al. Effects of dopamine and dobutamine on hyperoxic and hypoxic pulmonary vascular tone in dogs. Am Rev Respir Dis. 1987;136(1):29–35.
113. Holloway EL, Polumbo RA, Harrison DC. Acute circulatory effects of dopamine in patients with pulmonary hypertension. Br Heart J. 1975;37(5):482–5.
114. Leier CV, et al. Comparative systemic and regional hemodynamic effects of dopamine and dobutamine in patients with cardiomyopathic heart failure. Circulation. 1978;58(3 Pt 1):466–75.
115. Acosta F, et al. Effects of dobutamine on right ventricular function and pulmonary circulation in pulmonary hypertension during liver transplantation. Transplant Proc. 2005;37(9): 3869–70.
116. Chen EP, et al. Milrinone improves pulmonary hemodynamics and right ventricular function in chronic pulmonary hypertension. Ann Thorac Surg. 1997;63(3):814–21.
117. Deb B, Bradford K, Pearl RG. Additive effects of inhaled nitric oxide and intravenous milrinone in experimental pulmonary hypertension. Crit Care Med. 2000;28(3):795–9.
118. Oztekin I, et al. Effects of low-dose milrinone on weaning from cardiopulmonary bypass and after in patients with mitral stenosis and pulmonary hypertension. Yakugaku Zasshi. 2007;127(2):375–83.
119. Kihara S, et al. Effects of milrinone for right ventricular failure after left ventricular assist device implantation. Heart Vessels. 2002;16(2):69–71.
120. Eichhorn EJ, et al. Differential effects of milrinone and dobutamine on right ventricular preload, afterload and systolic performance in congestive heart failure secondary to ischemic or idiopathic dilated cardiomyopathy. Am J Cardiol. 1987;60(16):1329–33.
121. Singh R, et al. Inhaled nitroglycerin versus inhaled milrinone in children with congenital heart disease suffering from pulmonary artery hypertension. J Cardiothorac Vasc Anesth. 2010;24(5):797–801.
122. Sablotzki A, et al. Selective pulmonary vasodilation with inhaled aerosolized milrinone in heart transplant candidates. Can J Anaesth. 2005;52(10):1076–82.

123. Wang H, et al. Comparison of inhaled and intravenous milrinone in patients with pulmonary hypertension undergoing mitral valve surgery. Adv Ther. 2009;26(4):462–8.
124. Haraldsson sA, Kieler-Jensen N, Ricksten SE. The additive pulmonary vasodilatory effects of inhaled prostacyclin and inhaled milrinone in postcardiac surgical patients with pulmonary hypertension. Anesth Analg. 2001;93(6):1439–45. table of contents.
125. Kerbaul F, et al. Effects of levosimendan versus dobutamine on pressure load-induced right ventricular failure. Crit Care Med. 2006;34(11):2814–9.
126. Kleber FX, et al. Repetitive dosing of intravenous levosimendan improves pulmonary hemodynamics in patients with pulmonary hypertension: results of a pilot study. J Clin Pharmacol. 2009;49(1):109–15.
127. Kerbaul F, et al. Effects of levosimendan on acute pulmonary embolism-induced right ventricular failure. Crit Care Med. 2007;35(8):1948–54.
128. Missant C, et al. Levosimendan improves right ventriculovascular coupling in a porcine model of right ventricular dysfunction. Crit Care Med. 2007;35(3):707–15.
129. Yontar OC, Yalta K, Yilmaz MB. Superiority of levosimendan over dobutamine in right ventricle failure. Crit Care Med. 2010;38(1):342–3. author reply 343–4.
130. Hayes MA, et al. Elevation of systemic oxygen delivery in the treatment of critically ill patients. N Engl J Med. 1994;330(24):1717–22.
131. Gattinoni L, et al. A trial of goal-oriented hemodynamic therapy in critically ill patients. SvO2 Collaborative Group. N Engl J Med. 1995;333(16):1025–32.
132. Kramer MR, et al. Recovery of the right ventricle after single-lung transplantation in pulmonary hypertension. Am J Cardiol. 1994;73(7):494–500.
133. Reesink HJ, et al. Reverse right ventricular remodeling after pulmonary endarterectomy in patients with chronic thromboembolic pulmonary hypertension: utility of magnetic resonance imaging to demonstrate restoration of the right ventricle. J Thorac Cardiovasc Surg. 2007;133(1):58–64.
134. D'Armini AM, et al. Reverse right ventricular remodeling after pulmonary endarterectomy. J Thorac Cardiovasc Surg. 2007;133(1):162–8.
135. Griffiths MJ, Evans TW. Inhaled nitric oxide therapy in adults. N Engl J Med. 2005; 353(25):2683–95.
136. Pepke-Zaba J, et al. Inhaled nitric oxide as a cause of selective pulmonary vasodilatation in pulmonary hypertension. Lancet. 1991;338(8776):1173–4.
137. Vizza CD, et al. Acute hemodynamic effects of inhaled nitric oxide, dobutamine and a combination of the two in patients with mild to moderate secondary pulmonary hypertension. Crit Care. 2001;5(6):355–61.
138. Cockrill BA, et al. Comparison of the effects of nitric oxide, nitroprusside, and nifedipine on hemodynamics and right ventricular contractility in patients with chronic pulmonary hypertension. Chest. 2001;119(1):128–36.
139. Bhorade S, et al. Response to inhaled nitric oxide in patients with acute right heart syndrome. Am J Respir Crit Care Med. 1999;159(2):571–9.
140. Weinberger B, et al. The toxicology of inhaled nitric oxide. Toxicol Sci. 2001;59(1):5–16.
141. Christenson J, et al. The incidence and pathogenesis of cardiopulmonary deterioration after abrupt withdrawal of inhaled nitric oxide. Am J Respir Crit Care Med. 2000;161(5):1443–9.
142. Cueto E, et al. Life-threatening effects of discontinuing inhaled nitric oxide in children. Acta Paediatr. 1997;86(12):1337–9.
143. Lavoie A, et al. Life-threatening effects of discontinuing inhaled nitric oxide in severe respiratory failure. Am J Respir Crit Care Med. 1996;153(6 Pt 1):1985–7.
144. Olschewski H, et al. Inhaled iloprost for severe pulmonary hypertension. N Engl J Med. 2002;347(5):322–9.
145. Simonneau G, et al. Continuous subcutaneous infusion of treprostinil, a prostacyclin analogue, in patients with pulmonary arterial hypertension: a double-blind, randomized, placebo-controlled trial. Am J Respir Crit Care Med. 2002;165(6):800–4.
146. Benza RL, et al. Long-term effects of inhaled treprostinil in patients with pulmonary arterial hypertension: the Treprostinil Sodium Inhalation Used in the Management of Pulmonary

Arterial Hypertension (TRIUMPH) study open-label extension. J Heart Lung Transplant. 2011;30(12):1327–33.
147. Hoeper MM, et al. A comparison of the acute hemodynamic effects of inhaled nitric oxide and aerosolized iloprost in primary pulmonary hypertension. German PPH study group. J Am Coll Cardiol. 2000;35(1):176–82.
148. Humbert M, Sitbon O, Simonneau G. Treatment of pulmonary arterial hypertension. N Engl J Med. 2004;351(14):1425–36.
149. Barst RJ, et al. A comparison of continuous intravenous epoprostenol (prostacyclin) with conventional therapy for primary pulmonary hypertension. N Engl J Med. 1996;334(5): 296–301.
150. Ocal A, et al. Efficiency of prostacyclin in the treatment of protamine-mediated right ventricular failure and acute pulmonary hypertension. Tohoku J Exp Med. 2005;207(1):51–8.
151. Schmid ER, et al. Inhaled nitric oxide versus intravenous vasodilators in severe pulmonary hypertension after cardiac surgery. Anesth Analg. 1999;89(5):1108–15.
152. Elliott CG, Palevsky HI. Treatment with epoprostenol of pulmonary arterial hypertension following mitral valve replacement for mitral stenosis. Thorax. 2004;59(6):536–7.
153. Lowson SM, et al. Inhaled prostacyclin for the treatment of pulmonary hypertension after cardiac surgery. Crit Care Med. 2002;30(12):2762–4.
154. De Wet CJ, et al. Inhaled prostacyclin is safe, effective, and affordable in patients with pulmonary hypertension, right heart dysfunction, and refractory hypoxemia after cardiothoracic surgery. J Thorac Cardiovasc Surg. 2004;127(4):1058–67.
155. Rex S, et al. Inhaled iloprost to control pulmonary artery hypertension in patients undergoing mitral valve surgery: a prospective, randomized-controlled trial. Acta Anaesthesiol Scand. 2008;52(1):65–72.
156. Yurtseven N, et al. A comparison of the acute hemodynamic effects of inhaled nitroglycerin and iloprost in patients with pulmonary hypertension undergoing mitral valve surgery. Ann Thorac Cardiovasc Surg. 2006;12(5):319–23.
157. Califf RM, et al. A randomized controlled trial of epoprostenol therapy for severe congestive heart failure: the Flolan International Randomized Survival Trial (FIRST). Am Heart J. 1997;134(1):44–54.
158. Walmrath D, et al. Effects of inhaled versus intravenous vasodilators in experimental pulmonary hypertension. Eur Respir J. 1997;10(5):1084–92.
159. Badesch DB, et al. Medical therapy for pulmonary arterial hypertension: updated ACCP evidence-based clinical practice guidelines. Chest. 2007;131(6):1917–28.
160. Galie N, et al. Tadalafil therapy for pulmonary arterial hypertension. Circulation. 2009;119(22):2894–903.
161. Galie N, et al. Sildenafil citrate therapy for pulmonary arterial hypertension. N Engl J Med. 2005;353(20):2148–57.
162. Rubin LJ, et al. Bosentan therapy for pulmonary arterial hypertension. N Engl J Med. 2002;346(12):896–903.
163. Galie N, et al. Ambrisentan for the treatment of pulmonary arterial hypertension: results of the ambrisentan in pulmonary arterial hypertension, randomized, double-blind, placebo-controlled, multicenter, efficacy (ARIES) study 1 and 2. Circulation. 2008;117(23):3010–9.
164. Vachiery JL, et al. Safety, tolerability and pharmacokinetics of an intravenous bolus of sildenafil in patients with pulmonary arterial hypertension. Br J Clin Pharmacol. 2011; 71(2):289–92.
165. Preston IR, et al. Acute and chronic effects of sildenafil in patients with pulmonary arterial hypertension. Respir Med. 2005;99(12):1501–10.
166. Michelakis E, et al. Oral sildenafil is an effective and specific pulmonary vasodilator in patients with pulmonary arterial hypertension: comparison with inhaled nitric oxide. Circulation. 2002;105(20):2398–403.
167. Nagendran J, et al. Phosphodiesterase type 5 is highly expressed in the hypertrophied human right ventricle, and acute inhibition of phosphodiesterase type 5 improves contractility. Circulation. 2007;116(3):238–48.

168. Archer SL, Michelakis ED. Phosphodiesterase type 5 inhibitors for pulmonary arterial hypertension. N Engl J Med. 2009;361(19):1864–71.
169. Cornet AD, et al. Sildenafil attenuates pulmonary arterial pressure but does not improve oxygenation during ARDS. Intensive Care Med. 2010;36(5):758–64.
170. McLaughlin VV, et al. ACCF/AHA 2009 expert consensus document on pulmonary hypertension: a report of the American College of Cardiology Foundation Task Force on Expert Consensus Documents and the American Heart Association: developed in collaboration with the American College of Chest Physicians, American Thoracic Society, Inc., and the Pulmonary Hypertension Association. Circulation. 2009;119(16):2250–94.
171. Moloney ED, Evans TW. Pathophysiology and pharmacological treatment of pulmonary hypertension in acute respiratory distress syndrome. Eur Respir J. 2003;21(4):720–7.
172. Roberts DH, et al. Oxygen therapy improves cardiac index and pulmonary vascular resistance in patients with pulmonary hypertension. Chest. 2001;120(5):1547–55.
173. Balanos GM, et al. Human pulmonary vascular response to 4 h of hypercapnia and hypocapnia measured using Doppler echocardiography. J Appl Physiol. 2003;94(4):1543–51.
174. Mekontso Dessap A, et al. Impact of acute hypercapnia and augmented positive end-expiratory pressure on right ventricle function in severe acute respiratory distress syndrome. Intensive Care Med. 2009;35(11):1850–8.
175. Pritts CD, Pearl RG. Anesthesia for patients with pulmonary hypertension. Curr Opin Anaesthesiol. 2010;23(3):411–6.
176. Gordon C, Collard CD, Pan W. Intraoperative management of pulmonary hypertension and associated right heart failure. Curr Opin Anaesthesiol. 2010;23(1):49–56.
177. Feihl F, Broccard AF. Interactions between respiration and systemic hemodynamics. Part II: practical implications in critical care. Intensive Care Med. 2009;35(2):198–205.
178. Darrah WC, et al. Intraaortic balloon counterpulsation improves right ventricular failure resulting from pressure overload. Ann Thorac Surg. 1997;64(6):1718–23. discussion 1723–4.
179. Arafa OE, et al. Intraaortic balloon pumping for predominantly right ventricular failure after heart transplantation. Ann Thorac Surg. 2000;70(5):1587–93.
180. Keogh AM, et al. Interventional and surgical modalities of treatment in pulmonary hypertension. J Am Coll Cardiol. 2009;54(1 Suppl):S67–77.
181. Berman M, et al. Life-threatening right ventricular failure in pulmonary hypertension: RVAD or ECMO? J Heart Lung Transplant. 2008;27(10):1188–9.
182. Maggio P, et al. Extracorporeal life support for massive pulmonary embolism. J Trauma. 2007;62(3):570–6.
183. Kolvekar SK, et al. Extracorporeal membrane oxygenator for pulmonary embolism. Ann Thorac Surg. 1997;64(3):883–4.
184. Deehring R, et al. Extracorporeal membrane oxygenation as a bridge to surgical embolectomy in acute fulminant pulmonary embolism. Am J Emerg Med. 2006;24(7):879–80.
185. Olsson KM, et al. Extracorporeal membrane oxygenation in nonintubated patients as bridge to lung transplantation. Am J Transplant. 2010;10(9):2173–8.
186. de Perrot M, et al. Impact of extracorporeal life support on outcome in patients with idiopathic pulmonary arterial hypertension awaiting lung transplantation. J Heart Lung Transplant. 2011;30(9):997–1002.
187. Gregoric ID, et al. Extracorporeal membrane oxygenation as a bridge to emergency heart-lung transplantation in a patient with idiopathic pulmonary arterial hypertension. J Heart Lung Transplant. 2008;27(4):466–8.
188. Berman M, et al. Successful extracorporeal membrane oxygenation support after pulmonary thromboendarterectomy. Ann Thorac Surg. 2008;86(4):1261–7.
189. Mydin M, et al. Extracorporeal membrane oxygenation as a bridge to pulmonary endarterectomy. Ann Thorac Surg. 2011;92(5):e101–3.
190. Fuehner T, et al. Extracorporeal membrane oxygenation in awake patients as bridge to lung transplantation. Am J Respir Crit Care Med. 2012;185(7):763–8.

191. Strueber M, et al. Bridge to thoracic organ transplantation in patients with pulmonary arterial hypertension using a pumpless lung assist device. Am J Transplant. 2009;9(4):853–7.
192. Schmid C, et al. Bridge to lung transplantation through a pulmonary artery to left atrial oxygenator circuit. Ann Thorac Surg. 2008;85(4):1202–5.
193. Hoeper MM, et al. Outcome after cardiopulmonary resuscitation in patients with pulmonary arterial hypertension. Am J Respir Crit Care Med. 2002;165(3):341–4.
194. Smith AM, et al. The role of vasopressin in cardiorespiratory arrest and pulmonary hypertension. QJM. 2006;99(3):127–33.

Chapter 19
Perioperative Management of Pulmonary Hypertension

Yuliya B. Goldsmith, Natalia Ivascu, Dana McGlothlin, Paul M. Heerdt, and Evelyn M. Horn

Abstract Any form of pulmonary hypertension (PH) uniformly increases the perioperative risks of both cardiac and noncardiac surgery. Specific perioperative management of PH patients is dependent upon the etiology and severity of disease as well as the planned operation. A detailed understanding of right ventricular (RV) physiology and the impact of chronic as well as acute-on-chronic PH is paramount to decisions on selection for surgery, preoperative preparation, anesthetic plan and postoperative care. The highest risk PH patients should be referred to PH centers where a multidisciplinary approach to patient care can be planned and where expertise exists in using a multitude of inhaled and systemic pulmonary vasodilators, as well as pharmacological and emergent mechanical interventions for right ventricular failure. This chapter is intended to be a guide for all physicians managing the perioperative care of patients with pulmonary hypertension, with an emphasis on noncardiac surgery.

Keywords Pulmonary hypertension • Perioperative management • Anesthesia • High-risk surgery • Right ventricle • Pulmonary vascular resistance

Y.B. Goldsmith • E.M. Horn, M.D. (✉)
Department of Medicine, Weill Cornell Medical College, New York, NY, USA

Perkin Heart Failure Center, Division of Cardiology, Weill Cornell Medical Center, 520 East 70th Street, Starr 443, New York, NY 10021, USA
e-mail: horneve@med.cornell.edu

N. Ivascu
Department of Anesthesiology, Weill Cornell Medical College, New York, NY, USA

D. McGlothlin
Department of Cardiology, Kaiser San Francisco Medical Center, San Francisco, CA, USA

P.M. Heerdt
Department of Anesthesiology, Weill Cornell Medical College, New York, NY, USA

Department of Pharmacology, Weill Cornell Medical College, New York, NY, USA

J.R. Klinger, R.P. Frantz (eds.), *Diagnosis and Management of Pulmonary Hypertension*, Respiratory Medicine 12, DOI 10.1007/978-1-4939-2636-7_19

Abbreviations

BiPAP	Bi-level positive airway pressure
CI	Cardiac index
CPAP	Continuous positive airway pressure
DVT	Deep venous thrombosis
ERA	Endothelin receptor antagonists
ES	Eisenmenger's Syndrome
HFpEF	Heart failure with preserved ejection fraction
HPV	Hypoxic pulmonary vasoconstriction
ILD	Interstitial lung disease
iNO	Inhaled nitric oxide
LAP	Left atrial pressure
LV	Left ventricle, left ventricular
LVEDP	Left ventricular end-diastolic pressure
mPAP	Mean pulmonary artery pressure
PA	Pulmonary artery
PAH	Pulmonary arterial hypertension WHO Group 1 PH
PASP	Pulmonary artery systolic pressure
PCWP	Pulmonary capillary wedge pressure
PDG	Pulmonary diastolic gradient
PDE5-I	Phosphodiesterase 5 inhibitors
PE	Pulmonary embolism
PEEP	Positive end-expiratory pressure
PH	Pulmonary hypertension
Ppm	Parts per million
PPV	Pulse-pressure variation
PV	Pressure–volume (relationship)
PVR	Pulmonary vascular resistance
RAP	Right atrial pressure
RHC	Right heart catheterization
RV	Right ventricle, right ventricular
RVH	Right ventricular hypertrophy
SVR	Systemic vascular resistance
TAPSE	Tricuspid annular plane systolic excursion
TEE	Transesophageal echocardiography
TPG	Transpulmonary gradient
WU	Wood Units

Introduction

Pulmonary arterial hypertension (PAH, WHO Group 1 PH) has traditionally been thought of as a rare disease and therefore of concern only to a small group of cardiovascular and pulmonary specialists. However, many patients with various comorbidities are adversely affected by pulmonary vascular disease. For example, PAH has been associated with stories of doomed Eisenmenger's Syndrome (ES) parturients facing exorbitant mortality rates [1–3]. Pulmonary venous hypertension (WHO Group 2 PH) is a known final common pathway for many untreated cardiac lesions, resulting in higher morbidity and mortality when repaired [4–9]. PH associated with respiratory insufficiency (WHO Group 3) including obesity related hypoventilation, sleep apnea, and parenchymal lung diseases is also a marker of perioperative morbidity [10]. In recent years, an increased understanding of the pathogenesis and pathophysiology of PAH as well as advances in drug therapies have greatly improved survival. Furthermore, an increased awareness of PH in general, has led to more diagnoses of various degrees of non WHO Group 1 PH in the entire population, many of whom go on to surgery. Hospital based specialists are modifying traditional management of acute disease to address coexisting chronic or acute on chronic PH and acute on chronic right ventricular dysfunction. This is particularly evident in the perioperative and peripartum populations requiring anesthesiologists, intensivists, obstetricians, pulmonologists, and cardiologists to have a comprehensive understanding in physiology and treatment of PH and the associated right ventricular dysfunction.

Six retrospective studies have analyzed the outcomes for PH patients undergoing noncardiac surgery [11–15]. The studies used a variety of methods to define PH as well as the severity of disease, so clear conclusions cannot be drawn. What is defined by these studies, however, is a very high rate of perioperative mortality (6–10 %) [12–15]. The rate of complications in all categories were also reported to be extremely elevated. In a more recent prospective international survey of 114 well characterized PAH patients undergoing surgery, Meyer et al. reported a 6.1 % major complication rate (bleeding with estimated blood loss >1 l, systemic inflammatory response or septicemia requiring catecholamine therapy, right heart failure requiring inotropic support, or death), and perioperative mortality of 3.5 % with 15 % (2/13) for emergency procedures vs. 2 % (2/101) for nonemergency procedures [16]. Note is made that some previous studies quoting higher mortality rates (specifically that of Minai et al. 18 %) included mostly patients prior to 2002, before the most PAH specific therapies were available [17]. Also, noteworthy is the fact that a 2 % mortality rate for elective surgery resulted from procedures that were mostly performed at the PH center [16].

Hemodynamics and Perioperative Physiology

The definition and classification of PH has been discussed elsewhere. For the purposes of discussing perioperative management it is useful to review the hemodynamics of PH with reference to pre- vs. post-capillary PH, cardiac output, left atrial and left ventricular end-diastolic pressures, right ventricular systolic and diastolic pressure–volume relationships, interventricular interdependence, and underlying respiratory physiology. The increased pulmonary vascular resistance (PVR) of PAH produces elevated pulmonary pressures regardless of the left atrial pressures. This "pre-capillary" PH is distinguished by the presence of a PVR ≥3.0 Wood units (WU) with normal pulmonary capillary wedge pressure (PCWP) (i.e., ≤15 mmHg) [18]. In contrast, the "post-capillary" PH will occur due to elevated left atrial filling pressures (LAP) which may be due to left ventricular, valvular abnormalities or a noncompliant left atrium. The elevated LAP is transmitted to the pulmonary veins down their origination at the pulmonary capillaries. Post-capillary PH is characterized by an elevated PCWP (>15–18 mmHg) with normal PVR, transpulmonary gradient (TPG) which is the difference between the mPAP (mean pulmonary artery pressure) and PCWP, and pulmonary diastolic gradient (PDG)—the difference between the pulmonary artery (PA) diastolic pressure and PCWP. In some, the chronic engorgement of the pulmonary vasculature produces vascular remodeling. This results in an elevated TPG, PDG, and PVR. This "mixed" PH is also referred to as "reactive" PH. Mixed PH features PCWP>15 mmHg, PVR≥2.5–3.0 WU, TPG≥12–15 mmHg, and DPG>5 [18–23]. Least common, is a fourth hemodynamic condition in which increased pulmonary blood flow produces PH with normal or minimally increased PVR or increased left heart pressures. This situation arises from systemic-to-pulmonary shunt or high cardiac output states (e.g., anemia, sepsis, portal hypertension, thyrotoxicosis, hemodialysis related large fistula, and myeloproliferative disorders) [18].

Assessment of the hemodynamic phenotype, response to pulmonary and systemic vasodilators, and inodilators should be assessed preoperatively and plans discussed between the pulmonary hypertension specialist, critical care anesthesiologist and intensivist for best recommendations for appropriate use of these agents intraoperatively and postoperatively in the critical care unit.

Perioperative Physiology

For patients suffering from PH, the primary goal throughout the perioperative period is to maintain optimal mechanical matching between the RV and pulmonary circulation. Optimal care requires a comprehensive awareness of intraoperative events that affect RV afterload, inotropy, and oxygen supply–demand relationships.

When interpreting the available data relevant to intraoperative management, it is important to consider a few basic limitations. First, given the relative rarity of PAH in the surgical population, much of the available clinical data are anecdotal and therefore biased to some degree; few clinicians are inclined to report cases in which the outcome was bad. Second, while experimental data are quite useful for demonstrating concepts, there are remarkably few studies in which a model of chronic PAH was used to study perioperative physiology. Finally, as with all studies involving RV physiology, it is important to appreciate that some methods developed for characterization of left ventricular (LV) mechanical performance may not be directly applicable to the RV. For example, as shown in Fig. 19.1, under normal circumstances, the RV pressure–volume relationship is distinctly different than that of the

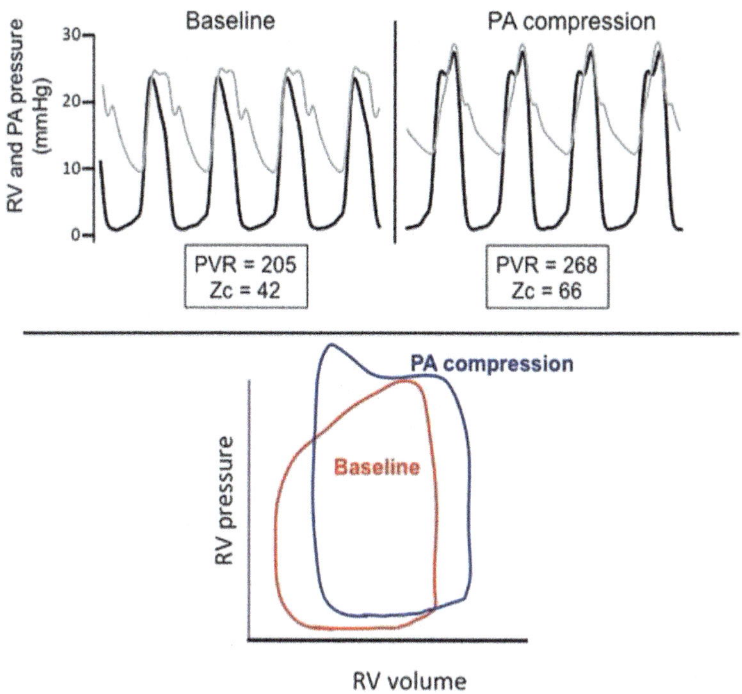

Fig. 19.1 *Top panel*. Right ventricular (RV) and pulmonary arterial (PA) pressures before and after compression of the left PA in an experimental animal (swine). Changes in both the amplitude and morphology of the pressure waveforms are evident. *Bottom panel*. Changes in the RV pressure–volume relationship produced by compression of the left PA are depicted

LV, particularly in regard to a clearly defined end-systolic point, and the period of isovolumic relaxation (of which the RV normally has little).

These differences reflect fundamental properties of each chamber in regard to the pattern of free wall contraction (the RV shows sequential shortening from the inflow to outflow tract), septal motion, the timing of peak pressure (early for the RV, late for the LV), and the contribution of inertia to maintaining flow out of the ventricle late in systole (minimal for the LV) [24, 25]. For a normal RV ejecting into a normal pulmonary circulation, these differences may complicate simple application of principles derived for characterization of LV systolic function such as the linear end-systolic pressure–volume relationship based upon automated detection of a discrete end-systolic point from pressure–volume loop analysis, and the myocardial performance index based in part upon echocardiographic assessment of isovolumic relaxation time. However, in the setting of PAH, RV free wall shortening can become more synchronous, ventricular interdependence changes, peak pressure occurs later in systole, and the inertial component of blood flow into the PA is diminished [24, 25]. As shown in Fig. 19.1, under these conditions the RV pressure–volume relationship resembles that for the LV with a more clearly defined end-systolic point and an isovolumic relaxation period.

Preoperative Evaluation

In 2007, the American College of Cardiology and the American Heart Association published the most current guidelines for perioperative cardiovascular evaluation for noncardiac surgery. This expert consensus document stratifies patients into three categories of risk factors: major, intermediate, and minor clinical predictors. Similarly the guidelines also categorize the type of surgery as high, intermediate, or low risk [26]. This type of risk calculation can be used to consider the specific perioperative risk for PH patients.

Assessing Surgical Risk with PH

For general practitioners and many cardiologists, the specifics of surgical procedures may not be known. The ACC/AHA guidelines define high-risk procedures to include emergent major operations, aortic and major vascular surgery, peripheral vascular surgery, and anticipated prolonged procedures associated with large blood loss or fluid shifts [26]. For PH patients this list must be expanded to include procedures with risk for venous embolism (air, fat, cement), elevations in venous pressures (laparoscopy, Trendelenburg positioning), reduction in pulmonary vascular volume (lung compression or resection), perioperative systemic inflammatory response, and emergency procedures (Table 19.1). Again, effective communication between the PH specialist, surgeon and anesthesiologist can determine the risks and benefits of the proposed surgery or surgical technique. This will be revisited below.

Assessing Patient Risk Factors in PH

A known history of PH will prompt an evaluation of functional status, cardiac function (especially RV function), pulmonary function and current severity of disease. Echocardiography and right heart catheterization are essential to make these assessments. Meyer et al. reviewed major risk factors as being, an elevated right atrial (RA) pressure, a 6 min walking distance <399 m at the last evaluation and need for emergency surgery [16]. The discerning physician must also identify patients with risk factors for PH who as yet may have gone undiagnosed such as patients with scleroderma spectrum of disease, obstructive sleep apnea, cardiac valvular lesions, depressed left ventricular function, heart failure with preserved ejection fraction (HFpEF) or interstitial lung disease (ILD). At a minimum, symptoms of pulmonary hypertension or RV failure should be elicited (shortness of breath, abnormal cardiac silhouette on chest radiograph, elevated jugular venous distension, etc.). Intermediate- or high-risk surgeries might prompt a screening echocardiogram.

Table 19.1 Risk factors for morbidity and mortality in noncardiac surgery

Patient factors
• History of PE [14], CAD [12], CKD [11]
• NYHA/WHO FC ≥ II [14]
• Higher ASA class [12]
• RAD on ECG [14]
• Echo parameters: RVH, RVMPI ≥ 0.75 [14]
• Hemodynamics: higher PAP [11, 12], RVSP/SBP ratio >0.66 [14]
Operative factors
• Emergency surgery [13, 14]
• Intermediate- or high-risk operations [12–14]
– Procedures with high risk for venous embolism (air, fat, cement) [79–82]
– Procedures inducing elevation in venous pressure (Trendelenburg positioning, insufflation) [88–94]
– Procedures involving reduction in lung vascular volume (lung compression or resection) [85–87]
– Procedures inducing severe systemic inflammatory response [79]
• Longer duration of anesthesia [13, 14]
• Intra-operative vasopressor use [14]

Summary of the risk factors identified from studies of patients with pulmonary hypertension undergoing noncardiac surgery

PE pulmonary embolism, *CAD* coronary artery disease, *CKD* chronic kidney disease, *NYHA* New York Heart Association, *WHO* World Health Organization, *RAD* right axis deviation, *ECG* electrocardiogram, *RVH* right ventricular hypertrophy, *RVMPI* right ventricular myocardial performance index, *PAP* pulmonary artery pressure, *SBP* systolic blood pressure, *ASA* American Surgical Association

Comorbidities such as coronary artery disease (CAD), chronic renal insufficiency, history of pulmonary embolism, NYHA functional class III/IV have been correlated with increased morbidity and mortality in cardiac surgery. Right ventricular impairment is also a predictor of worse outcome. Right axis deviation (RAD) ($p=0.02$), RV hypertrophy (RVH) ($p=0.04$), RV index of myocardial performance (RVMPI) ≥0.075 ($p=0.03$), RV systolic pressure to systemic systolic blood pressure ratio ≥2/3 ($p=0.01$) all predict increased postoperative mortality [14].

Evaluation

The preoperative evaluation of a patient with pulmonary hypertension should seek out indications of right ventricular dysfunction to determine areas for potential optimization or disqualification for surgery due to unacceptable risk. This section will review common preoperative testing modalities to highlight their utility in diagnosing right ventricular insufficiency.

History and Physical

The evaluation begins with the history and physical examination. The most common complaints among PH patients, albeit nonspecific, are dyspnea and generalized fatigue [27]. Angina, pre-syncope, and syncope are indications of advanced PAH and may portend a poor prognosis [27, 28]. Physical signs of elevated RV pressure include jugular venous distension, right ventricular S3 gallop, hepatomegaly, ascites, and peripheral edema. By contrast, pulmonary crackles indicate left-sided heart failure or primary lung disease and not PAH.

Echocardiography

Transthoracic echocardiography (TTE) is easy to obtain and an excellent screening tool to estimate pulmonary arterial pressures as well as evaluate cardiac function. A complete assessment of ventricular and valvular pathology provides invaluable data to determine advancement of disease as well as etiology. By measuring the tricuspid regurgitant jet velocity, the PA systolic pressure (PASP) can be estimated. There is limited accuracy of this measurement in PH patients compared to catheterization, but it is useful as a screening tool [29]. Right ventricular dilation and contractility vary depending on severity and chronicity of disease. Objective measurements of RV function include tricuspid annular plane systolic excursion (TAPSE), RV fractional area change, and RV myocardial performance index, and possible use of mid and late systolic RV outflow Doppler notching to assess RV-PA coupling [30, 31]. Patent foramen ovale can be discovered by injection of agitated saline contrast, as well as intracardiac or intrapulmonary shunts, which may have clinical significance in the operative setting.

The elevated RV pressure during systole results in paradoxical ventricular septal flattening, pathognomonic for PH. Similar septal flattening during diastole marks RV volume overload, typically from RV failure with or without severe tricuspid regurgitation. Analysis of the blood flow through the mitral valve and pulmonary veins, as well as tissue Doppler velocities can determine LV filling patterns and identify elevations in left atrial pressure. Of note this technique is limited to patients in normal sinus rhythm. Left atrial size and function are useful to assess for the WHO 2 PH patient.

TTE may be used to suggest the possibility of HFpEF; however, cardiac catheterization is generally used to confirm the diagnosis. Reduced LV systolic function, severe left sided valvular lesions and left atrial enlargement in the presence of PH suggest a post-capillary etiology. Low grade diastolic dysfunction observed on echocardiography may still be attributable to pre-capillary PH and is not uncommon in PAH, parenchymal lung disease or CTEPH, when LV filling is impaired by altered RV function. It is not surprising that markers of significant RV dysfunction (right atrial enlargement, reduced TAPSE, increased interventricular septal flattening) are associated with poor overall prognosis in PAH patients and can probably be extrapolated to expect poor perioperative outcomes as well [31–33].

Heart Catheterization and Preoperative Optimization

Right heart catheterization (RHC) should be considered for PH patients undergoing intermediate- to high-risk operations or patients with moderate or severe PH by history, noninvasive screening, or with related comorbidities (e.g., obesity, sleep apnea, scleroderma, or risk factors for HFpEF such as atrial fibrillation and LAE). Left heart catheterization should also be performed in patients with coexisting left heart disease because of discrepancies between PCWP and left ventricular end-diastolic pressure (LVEDP) that could lead to misclassification of PH and have significant implications in treatment paradigms [34].

Ideally, RHC should be performed well in advance of surgery to allow for an adequate period of optimization for elective and semi-elective surgery. In all other cases, attempts should be made to lower PVR and enhance RV function prior to surgery. Routine vasoreactivity testing is performed during diagnostic RHC to determine candidates for vasodilator therapy [35, 36]. Although inhaled nitric oxide (iNO) is the drug of choice for testing due to lack of systemic effects and ease of administration, intravenous adenosine, epoprostenol, sildenafil, and inhaled iloprost can also be tried. Pre-capillary PH patients may benefit from advancing targeted pulmonary vasodilator therapy. When surgery cannot be delayed, phosphodiesterase 5 inhibitors (PDE5-I) such as sildenafil 20–40 mg three times daily, can provide acute vasodilatory effects and augmentation of right ventricular inotropy [37]. In those with high-risk hemodynamics (high right atrial pressure (RAP), low cardiac index (CI)), initiation of parenteral prostanoids should be considered prior to surgery. Furthermore, this same vasoactive testing is likewise useful in the perioperative period to guide intraoperative and postoperative management, such as the use of iNO, inhaled prostacyclins, and less commonly continuous epoprostenol. Patients with parenchymal lung disease and a component of hypoxic pulmonary vasoconstriction may also experience an improvement in PA pressures via an iNO mediated improvement in V/Q matching. Post-capillary PH patients may not benefit at all from pulmonary vasodilator therapy and moreover treatment may worsen pulmonary edema formation. In these patients, perioperative treatment should focus on diuresis and control of systemic hypertension. Some of the sickest WHO group 2 PH patients may need preoperative inodilators for low output states with aggressive up titration of the systemic vasodilators. WHO group 2 PH patients who have an increase in their PCWP in response to pulmonary vasodilators are at risk for developing worsening pulmonary vascular congestion and an increase in the driving force of left atrial hypertension with use of pulmonary vasodilators. Abnormal pulmonary function should be optimized with treatments such as oxygen, continuous positive airway pressure (CPAP), bronchodilators, antibiotics, and steroids where appropriate. Physical therapy and weight loss in obese patients may be beneficial although usually require a long-term plan [38, 39].

Optimal hemodynamic stability would include: mean arterial pressure (MAP) $\geq$ 60 mmHg, systolic BP $\geq$ 85 mmHg, oxygen saturation > 92 %, RAP < 12, mPAP < 35 (if feasible), PVR/SVR < 0.5 (if feasible), PCW 8–12 (some WHO 2 PH < 18), and CI $\geq$ 2.2 L/min/m^2.

Dyspnea at rest, syncope, hemodynamic findings of severe RV failure (low CI, high RAP >15 mmHg), metabolic acidosis, and marked hypoxemia are all signs of advanced, unstable disease and serious consideration should be given to cancelling or postponing the surgery until/unless improvement and stabilization or pulmonary hypertension can be achieved [37].

Planning for Surgery

Preoperative coordination of care among the multidisciplinary team is crucial for best outcomes. Ideally, all patients except those with the lowest risk PH and lowest risk procedures should be operated on in a tertiary care center, where a multidisciplinary team of specialists experienced in managing patients with PH is available. The multidisciplinary team for preoperative management of PH patients includes anesthesiologist, cardiologists, intensivists and pulmonologists, surgeons, and experienced allied health-care members including respiratory therapists, pharmacy (availability of medications and a pharmacist with experience in administration of PH therapies), as well as nurse managers (systemic prostacyclin administration requires staff training and often is approved only in certain units). Meticulous advanced planning and discussion amongst team members must take place to transition from oral to IV/inhaled therapies where prolonged surgery/intubation/extended NPO periods are expected. Generally, chronic PAH therapies, including PDE5-I (sildenafil, tadalafil), endothelin receptor anatagonists (ERAs) (bosentan, ambrisentan, macitentan), and prostanoids (inhaled, intravenous, subcutaneous, oral) should be continued throughout the perioperative period, with appropriate substitutions as above when necessary (intravenous for oral PDE5-I, intravenous for subcutaneous prostacyclin infusion, etc., depending on the surgery and interference of subcutaneous site,). If inhaled prostacyclin analogues cannot be continued due to intubation appropriate substitution should be planned with iNO, intermittent nebulized prostacyclin, continuous inhaled epoprostenol, vs. occasional conversion to IV prostanoids (there are no significant bleeding complications with IV prostanoids, despite platelet inhibition) [37]. Oral therapies should be resumed as soon as possible after procedure, keeping in mind that compromised absorption can result in low drug levels and rebound PH. Coumadin can usually be discontinued with judicious decision regarding heparin bridging depending on risk/benefit of bleeding vs. clotting (such as hypercoagulable states, pulmonary embolism (PE), or mechanical valves). In high-risk situations (such as major orthopedic surgeries), retrievable preoperative IVC filter placement may be considered [40]. Careful perioperative deep venous thrombosis (DVT) prophylaxis should be instituted and early ambulation is essential for both DVT/PE prevention and avoiding deconditioning.

Meetings with the patient and family must take place preoperatively and include some discussion of modes of anesthesia, need for invasive monitoring, and their role during the recovery period.

Intraoperative Management

The primary physiological concept is to maintain optimal right ventricular-pulmonary arterial coupling and promote adequate left sided filling and systemic perfusion. Thus, all interventions that affect RV preload, RV inotropy, RV afterload including pulmonary vascular resistance, large pulmonary artery capacitance or impedance, thoracic pressures, and oxygen supply and demand relationship need to be taken into consideration.

Right Ventricular Afterload

Pulmonary vascular disease leads to an increase in RV afterload that impedes RV ejection and thereby leads to increased RV wall stress, RV diastolic overload, RV dilation, and in the more chronic state, RVH. In contrast to the LV, the thinner walled RV is subjected to greater wall tension for the same degree of increase in end diastolic volume; this leads to an increase in RV myocardial oxygen demand and consumption.

Although often described simply as PVR (the *steady-state*, mean pressure/mean flow relationship largely dictated by small vessels), the true interaction between the RV and the pulmonary circulation is pulsatile and *dynamic*. Accordingly, the concept of input impedance has been applied as a means to summarize the resistive, elastic, and reflective components of afterload, and provide for some discrimination between the relative contributions of small vessels (steady state resistance) and large elastic ones ("characteristic" impedance) [25]. However, assessment of input impedance requires simultaneous measurement of pressure and flow, and generally involves analysis in the "frequency domain," i.e., mathematical resolution of pressure and flow waves into their individual frequency components and then defining their ratio at set frequencies along a spectrum. Not surprisingly, the complexity of both measuring and interpreting input impedance spectra has limited clinical utility. Nonetheless, there has been general acceptance of "lumped parameter" models such as the Windkessel to help conceptualize the static and dynamic contributions to afterload. Essentially adaptations of electrical circuits, these models incorporate a resistor (PVR), a capacitor (vascular compliance), and an inductor (characteristic impedance) to represent the basic physiological components dictating input impedance. While alternative methods for calculating characteristic impedance as a measure of large vessel load from more conventional "time-domain" measures (PA pressure, PA diameter, and stroke volume) have been described [41], from a clinical perspective, prognostic significance has focused more upon compliance (calculated as stroke volume/pulse pressure) and its reciprocal relationship with PVR [42–45]. Data suggest that early in the course of PAH, a relatively small rise in PVR will be accompanied by a larger relative decline in compliance, while later in the disease course, the fall in compliance elicited by increased PVR will diminish since the vascular wall approaches maximum stiffness [41]. Functionally, an acute change in compliance will lessen the ability of large elastic vessels to "absorb" pressure waves reflected from more distal potions of the circulation. This effect can be directly observed in the RV and proximal PA pressure waveform as the timing of peak pressure achievement moves from early to late in systole. This "late phase load" produced by summation of reflective pressure components parallels the systolic augmentation described for systemic vessels and contributes to a widened PA pulse pressure. This is particularly relevant to acute insults that may occur during surgery and affect RV pulsatile load, and importantly, may be underestimated by PA catheter tracings where pressure is measured more distal in the circulation. For example, compliance and PVR may be altered by events such as the addition of positive end-expiratory pressure (PEEP) to mechanical ventilation (Fig. 19.2), a change to prone or Trendelenburg positions, pneumoperitoneum during a laparoscopic procedure (Fig. 19.3), venous emboli (including air emboli or particulate matter, i.e., from orthopedic procedures), and any direct compression or displacement of the large PA branches.

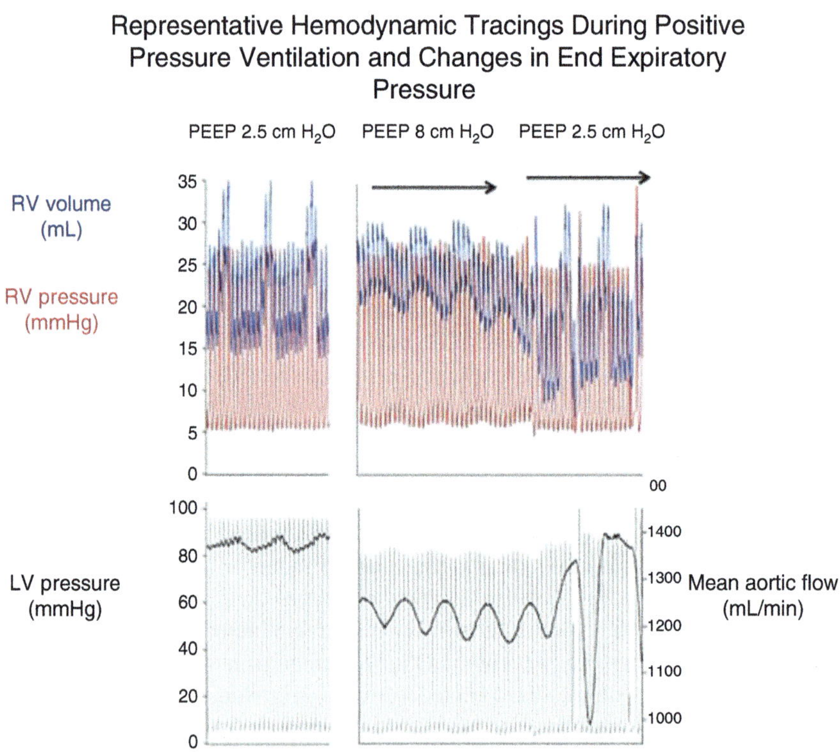

Fig. 19.2 Representative tracings of right (RV) and left (LV) ventricular pressures along with RV volume and aortic blood flow during positive pressure ventilation and variations in positive end-expiratory pressure (PEEP) in an experimental animal (dog). Marked respiratory variation in RV volume and aortic flow is evident, particularly with increased levels of PEEP

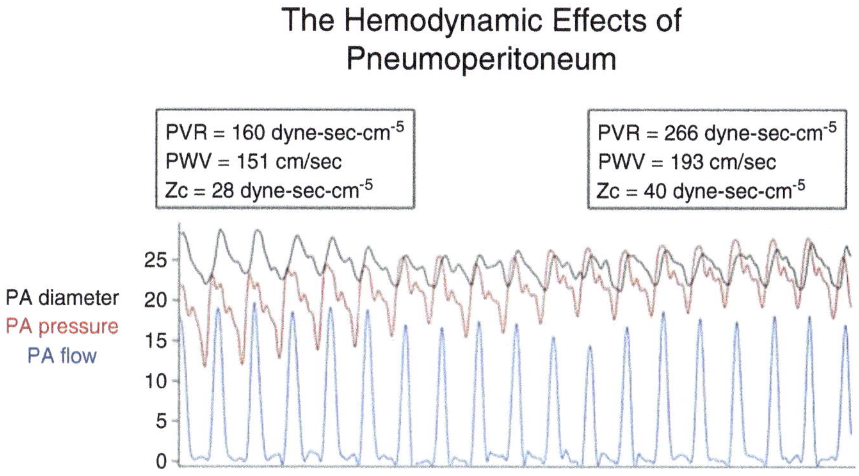

Fig. 19.3 The representative effect of inducing pneumoperitoneum and increasing positive end-expiratory pressure (PEEP) on pulmonary arterial (PA) pressure, diameter, flow, pulse wave velocity (PWV), and characteristic impedance (Zc). The data indicate an acute increase in right ventricular afterload in terms of effects on both pulmonary vascular resistance (PVR, primary determined by small vessels) and characteristic impedance (Zc, primarily determined by large vessels). In addition, the increase in pulse wave velocity (PWV) suggests that pressure waves will be reflected from the distal pulmonary circulation more rapidly, potentially contributing to increased afterload

Changes in Myocardial Supply and Demand

Under normal circumstances the RV intramyocardial pressure is lower than the aortic root pressure and the RV coronary perfusion occurs throughout the cardiac cycle. In PH, due to the elevated RV intramyocardial pressure, coronary flow occurs predominantly during diastole, which further worsens the mismatch between oxygen demand and supply promoting RV ischemia and diminished RV contractility [46, 47]. Low RV oxygen supply is associated with a shift away from aerobic glucose and fatty acid oxidation to the less efficient RV glycolytic pathways [25].

Systemic vasodilatation and hypotension with anesthesia (see Sect. "Choice of Anesthetics") leads to a relative increase in the PVR/SVR ratios, and hypotension induced RV ischemia in the setting of increased oxygen demands [48].

Intraoperative manipulation of the heart and/or great vessels may further contribute to the hypotension.

Interventricular Dependence

The combination of elevated PVR/reduced RV compliance and systemic hypotension may promote RV ischemia resulting in the "lethal combination" of RV dilatation, interventricular septal bulging into the left ventricle, and insufficient left ventricular filling, with resulting progressive decline in CO and further systemic hypotension [49]. Management should be focused on RV unloading with pulmonary vasodilators, optimizing intravascular fluid balance, and maintaining adequate systemic pressure. Combination of RV inotropes and systemic pressors may be needed [50]. Dobutamine may be a preferred RV inotrope in this situation due to less systemic vasodilation as compared to milrinone which may cause further LV unloading and septal displacement; vasopressin may be a good option to maintain systemic pressure although there is some institutional bias as well with the choice of systemic pressors and catecholamine sparing. Ongoing monitoring of arterial pressure, central venous pressure, cardiac output, central venous oxygen saturation, arterial blood gases, and lactate levels are necessary, ideally supplemented by transesophageal echocardiography (TEE) guided assessment of RV/LV filling.

General Anesthetic Management

Preparation

Decision making regarding choice of anesthesia in a PH patient depends on the type of planned surgery, PH severity, comorbidities, and patient's preference. While conscious sedation may result in less anesthetic related problems in a non-PH patient, even mild hypoxia and hypercarbia (frequently associated with conscious sedation) can cause pulmonary vasoconstriction and lead to sudden decompensation in a PH patient. Also, any baseline comorbidity predisposing to hypoxia (sleep apnea, obesity, lung disease) may be an additional indication for a protected airway. Thus, elective intubation and general anesthesia are frequently preferable. Also, any procedures associated with high risk of pulmonary emboli (such as orthopedic procedures) may require intubation, general anesthesia, and invasive hemodynamic monitoring in a PH patient, as to avoid emergent intubation should hemodynamic instability or suboptimal oxygenation be precipitated.

Particular care should be taken to de-air all lines and syringes, as even a small amount of air can cause hemodynamic decompensation in a PH patient [51]; there is also a high risk of passage of air to systemic circulation via PFO. Hypothermia should be avoided as it inhibits physiologic hypoxic pulmonary vasoconstriction (HPV) and may result in worsened VQ mismatch, which may have considerable effect in procedures requiring reduction of lung volume [52].

Airway and Optimal Ventilator Strategies

With any type of non-general anesthesia, airway patency needs to be insured, and an airway access should be planned should ventilation become compromised. With any means of anesthetic administration (face mask, laryngeal airway, or ET) supplemental oxygen must be administered for its direct pulmonary vasodilating effects [53].

With general anesthesia, carefully planning the induction is critical, as uncontrolled ventilation with possibility of hypoxia, and sympathetic stimuli from laryngoscopy can result in acute rise in PVR. Use of 100 % oxygen by mask prior to induction and optimizing depth of anesthesia prior to laryngoscopy and intubation can minimize this effect. In patient with difficult airway, OSA or intrinsic lung disease and poor functional reserve capacity, "awake intubation" with fiberoptic bronchoscopy may be preferable to avoid a period of poor ventilation with regular induction and intubation. Use of systemic pressors to protect against any acute vagal mediated vasodilatory response is often suggested.

After securing airway, ventilator management in PH is focused on use of higher FiO_2, with mild hyperventilation (goal PCO_2 of 35 % or less) and maintenance of lung volumes at normal functional residual capacity (Table 19.2) [54–56]. There is a U-shape relationship between lung volumes and PVR during mechanical ventilation, with PVR being the lowest at functional residual capacity. At low lung volumes, resulting hypercapnia and hypoxia will cause hypoxic vasoconstriction and an increase in PVR, while hyperinflation and high PEEP (preferably <10 mmHg) will result in an undesirable compression of the intra-alveolar vessels which can also lead to increase in PVR [56, 57].

Table 19.2 Perioperative ventilatory conditions to avoid and promote

Avoid pulmonary vasoconstrictors
• Hypoxemia
• Inspiratory pressure >30 mmHg
• High PEEP (>15 mmHg)
• Hypercapnia
• Acidosis
Promote pulmonary vasodilation
• Improve oxygenation (e.g., FiO_2 1.0)
• Permissive hypocapnia (pCO_2 ≤30–35 mmHg)
• Alkalosis (pH N 7.4)
• Optimal ventilatory volume

This table summarizes the conditions to avoid or promote during mechanical ventilation in patients with pulmonary hypertension
PEEP positive end-expiratory pressure, *FiO_2* fraction of inspired oxygen

Choice of Anesthetics

All anesthetic techniques have been safely employed in PH patients with appropriate judgment and monitoring. However, two anesthetic effects are of special significance when choosing an agent for a PH patient: avoiding direct myocardial depression and unfavorable effects on autonomic tone.

Many anesthetics are known to have myocardial depressant effects [58–62], by the means of directly affecting calcium cycling by myocytes, or the sensitivity of the contractile proteins to calcium, as well as their indirect effect on the autonomic nervous system. Direct myocardial depression is dose dependent. Propofol causes direct myocardial depression but only at relatively high concentrations and can still be used with caution [55, 57]. Studies showed that with frequently used inhaled anesthetics such as isoflurane, sevoflurane, and desflurane, depression of LV systolic function is offset by a decrease in systemic afterload. However, due to a smaller effect on decreasing RV afterload, there is a resulting disparity of LV and RV workload [60–62]. Ketamine has a modest myocardial depressant effect and with optimal ventilation and acid-base balance it may have pulmonary vasodilating properties [63, 64]. However, ketamine may also cause pulmonary vasoconstriction by the means of sympathetic stimulation [51]. With neuraxial (spinal, epidural) anesthesia, blockade of sympathetic nerves can precipitate hypotension. In addition high spinal or epidural anesthesia could result in cardiac sympathetic blockade, with unopposed parasympathetic stimulation from the cranial region [65]. Such an acute shift in autonomic balance in PH patient may result in profound hypotension and severe hemodynamic compromise [65]. In general, gradual epidural dosing or low spinal techniques are safe.

Intraoperative Pharmacological and Inhalation Therapy

Volume Status

Baseline hemodynamics, including "average" resting CVP, PA sat, and CO/CI are very useful at guiding intraoperative and postoperative fluid management [66]. For a normotensive patient, the goal should be to maintain the lowest baseline CVP. Whereas volume resuscitation is often guided by pulse-pressure variation (PPV), this is not feasible in PH patients. With the failing RV, PPV does not predict volume responsiveness and PPV due to increased RV afterload may erroneously suggest volume responsiveness [67, 68]. Although recent studies question the adequacy of both static (CVP) and dynamic (PPV) indices of preload assessment in PH, clinical experience suggests that targeting a CVP of 8–12 mmHg may have utility in managing systemic hypotension.

Pressors and Inotropes

Pressors of choice for the PAH patient include norepinephrine and vasopressin. While many institutions use phenylephrine and it is effective in increasing the coronary artery driving pressure it is less favorable for RV hemodynamics and relative PVR/SVR ratios [69, 70]. With more significant RV dysfunction, vasopressors with inotropic properties, such as norepinephrine and epinephrine, may be preferable. In experimental models, vasopressin was demonstrated to stimulate nitric oxide release and was vasodilating in pulmonary circulation, while causing peripheral vasoconstriction via V1 receptor stimulation [71], providing in vitro rationale for it as a preferable choice. Although there is no definitive clinical trial showing its superiority to catecholamines, there is some clinical experience [72], and applicability of the lessons of vasodilatory shock [73, 74]. For RV inotropy, especially with underfilled LV, dobutamine may be preferable to milrinone due to less arterial vasodilation [75]. For the WHO group 2 patient, milrinone or dobutamine are appropriate, with pressor support with norepinephrine or vasopressin as indicated.

Pulmonary Vasodilators

For WHO Group 1 patients, continuation of chronic pulmonary vasodilators through surgery is essential. Specifically, oral therapies should be given up to and including the day of surgery. Long-term inhaled prostacyclin therapies should be given just prior to surgery and depending on the length of the procedure, arrangements should be made for intraoperative treatments or alternative therapies such as continuous iNO, or continuous inhaled epoprostenol [76, 77]. Patients on intravenous or subcutaneous prostanoids should have lines marked "not to touch," and timely cassette changes planned in advance to avoid sudden interruption of drug delivery. Unlike usual intraoperative titratable medications, prostacyclin and remodulin are not to be titrated upward during the procedure due to risk of systemic hypotension. Inhaled pulmonary vasodilators are more suitable for acute PH management due to their pulmonary selectivity [76, 77]. Down titration of chronic PH therapies due to hypotension is also not recommended due to possibility of abrupt worsening of PVR; rather, pressors should be used as needed for systemic hypotension. Inhaled pulmonary vasodilators have the added benefit of selectively reaching well-ventilated lung areas and diminishing VQ mismatch in patients with intrinsic lung disease. For patients with WHO 2 PH, PO/IV sildenafil may be considered for perioperative PH management, though are unproven (with caution due to possibility of precipitating pulmonary edema), while diuresis and systemic vasodilator remains the mainstay of treatment.

Immediate Postoperative Period

For patients undergoing general anesthesia for major procedures associated with large fluid shifts, it is generally advisable to delay extubation until optimal hemodynamics are accomplished with diuresis vs. volume repletion as needed (with arterial line and CVP vs. pulmonary artery catheter monitoring). Care should be taken to prevent sympathetic activation with meticulous pain management. Avoidance of hypothermia and shivering aids in maintaining optimal oxygenation and PVR. Aggressive pulmonary toilet is necessary for excessive secretions. Patients with OSA may benefit from postoperative bi-level positive airway pressure (BiPAP) or CPAP to augment ventilation, and their home mask should be made readily available.

Special Considerations

Certain types of surgical procedures may require particularly careful management in PH patients.

Orthopedics

Orthopedic procedures in PH patients may require general anesthesia, as described above [78]. Joint replacement and hip fracture repair are the highest risk orthopedic procedures in PH patients. While hip surgery in the setting of fracture is an urgent and necessary procedure, joint replacement is an elective surgery that, in PH patients, is associated with a high morbidity and mortality due to high potential for pulmonary embolization, and risk and benefits of it have to be carefully considered [79]. The surgical technique of reaming the bone results in extremely high intramedullary pressure that causes bone fragments, marrow, fat, and inflammatory mediators to pass into the bloodstream [79, 80] with exacerbation of PH hemodynamics and systemic vasodilation. If bone cement is used to stabilize the prosthesis, the exothermic reaction of the compound during cementing causes it to expand within intramedullary space, and may results in pressures as high as 5,000 mmHg [81], increasing the potential for particularly large emboli [82]. Multiple pulmonary emboli, even with overall small embolic load, cause a release of pro-inflammatory mediators and result in significant increase in PVR with a possibility of acute RV failure [79, 83].

Preemptive inotropic support needs to be instituted for patients with baseline RV failure [80, 84], and systemic hypotension needs to be aggressively treated with vasopressors.

Thoracic Surgery

Single lung ventilation for lung biopsy or resection may represent a significant risk for PH patients, due to intentional collapse of the operative lung. As the tidal volume is shifted to the ventilated, non-operative lung, hypoxic pulmonary vasoconstriction (HPV) will lead to redistribution of flow away from non-ventilated lung; in PH patients the effects of flow redistribution may result in an acute rise in PA pressure [85, 86]; iNO or inhaled prostacyclins may aid in optimizing blood flow in the aerated lung thus preventing V/Q mismatch [87]. In this situation, limiting IV pulmonary vasodilators may be beneficial (with dose-appropriate inhaled agent substitution) to minimize HPV inhibition and avoid systemic hypoxia. Even when normal dual lung ventilation is resumed, PA pressure may remain elevated from baseline despite increase in therapies, especially if lung resection took place [86]. In addition, epidural analgesia frequently used in postoperative pain management for thoracic procedures, may cause systemic hypotension by suppressing sympathetic tone, and provoke LV underfilling [51]. Manipulation of the pulmonary artery such as compression and displacement of the large PA branches increases cumulative RV afterload as mentioned above.

Laparoscopy

Insufflation of the abdomen with carbon dioxide during laparoscopy causes diaphragmatic displacement, with resulting need for increased inspiratory pressures and PEEP to prevent atelectasis and maintain ventilation. This may result in a progressive rise of PVR as well as direct PA compression with decreased compliance, increased pulse wave velocity, and an abrupt increase in the pulsatile component of RV afterload (Fig. 19.3) [88].

Prolonged steep Trendelenburg positioning (up to 45°) required for robotic-assisted lower abdominal procedures, such as prostatectomy or hysterectomy, can cause further increases in RV afterload [89–94]. Even in otherwise healthy patients, there is a two to threefold increase in LV and RV filling pressures with resulting PH (as defined by mPAP >35 mmHg) in 75 % of these patients; in otherwise healthy patients there is a corresponding increase in MAP, and overall stable hemodynamics with unchanged CO, and no evidence of RV pressure overload despite 65 % increase of RV stroke work index. [92, 93] It is expected that in PH patients such hemodynamic alterations can be detrimental, although this technique has not been specifically studied in the PH population. Even when pneumoperitoneum is reversed, the PA pressure may not return to baseline for some time due to factors such as atelectasis and subcutaneous emphysema, with gradual CO_2 reabsorption resulting in postoperative hypercarbia [90–94].

Obstetrics

Pregnancy and delivery are known to be associated with high morbidity and mortality in PH patients, especially in the postpartum period with mortality rates available from small case series reported to be 30–70 % [1–3, 15, 95]. Traditionally, avoidance of pregnancy or early termination are strongly recommended. In the last decade, due to careful pregnancy and peripartum care, mortality in IPAH patients has declined to 17 % but in congenital heart disease associated PH and other PH cases, mortality remains as high as 28–33 % [95].

In IPAH, invasive hemodynamic monitoring is frequently necessary in peripartum period to guide therapy [96]. The vaginal route with assisted second stage delivery is preferred (unless there are obstetric indications for a Cesarean section) due to less fluid shifts, and lower incidence of bleeding and infection, although some institutions will prefer scheduled C sections with availability of the most experienced multidisciplinary team. Epidural anesthesia (with slow cautious administration to minimize risk of hypotension) prevents sympathetic activation due to pain. Dobutamine may be used for inotropic RV support, and pressors (preferably vasopressin) can be used as necessary. Availability of backup cardiothoracic surgical team support for emergency ECMO for the sickest patients as a bridge to recovery should be considered. Knowledge that the hemodynamic insult is often at its maximum at 72 h after delivery necessitates the ongoing care of the multidisciplinary team beyond the delivery phase.

Liver Surgery

Anything but mild porto-pulmonary hypertension (PPH) represents a challenge in the setting of liver transplant. Moderate-to-severe PPH (MPAP$\geq$35) is diagnosed in up to 10 % of patients referred for liver transplant [97, 98], and has been associated with high complication rates and perioperative mortality [99–101]. Multiple studies in recent years have demonstrated that treatment with pulmonary vasodilators may control and improve the degree of PPH, and reduce perioperative risk [102, 103]. While a significant degree of PPH is considered a contraindication to liver transplant, survival in the absence of transplant is as low as 38 % in 3 years, and 28 % in 5 years, while transplantation can be curative [104–106]. Prostacyclin analogues have been successfully used both preoperatively to reduce the PAP, and intra- and postoperatively to control residual PH [98, 107]. ERAs and PDE5-Is, and various drug combinations have been used preoperatively with some success [108–111]. In these studies, liver transplant was undertaken when MPAP of <35 was accomplished. Epoprostenol was continued throughout surgery and into posttransplant period; some of the patients eventually did not require pulmonary vasodilators [108]. Careful preoperative assessment of RV function with echocardiography, and intraoperative TEE are helpful to assess the RV response to increase in CO and PVR that occur with reperfusion, and to preempt and treat resulting acute RV failure. In many ways, the hemodynamics of liver transplant parallel that of the postpartum woman in the autotransfusion of a high capacitance low resistance circuit into the central volume with an acute rise in the right atrial pressure and potential load on a borderline RV.

Unrecognized PPH can lead to poor clinical outcomes of procedures designed to manage complications of portal hypertension, such as transjugular intrahepatic portosystemic shunt (TIPS). The creation of TIPS causes diversion of the portal flow into the systemic circulation, therefore reducing the incidence of variceal bleeding and refractory ascites; it also causes increase in cardiac index, and rise in PVR, PA pressure, and RAP. One month after TIPS, pulmonary pressure remains elevated.

Currently, absolute contraindications to TIPS include congestive heart failure, severe tricuspid regurgitation, and severe pulmonary hypertension (mean pulmonary pressure >45 mmHg). Whether patients with milder pulmonary hypertension can receive a TIPS safely is unclear [112]. It is important to keep in mind that prevalence of PPH in advanced cirrhosis patients with cirrhosis complications such as refractory ascites may be as high as 16 % [113]; careful pre-procedural screening for significant PPH is essential in preventing TIPS-induced abrupt increase in PVR and RV failure.

Postoperative Management

The postoperative deaths frequently occur in the first few days after surgery, and are frequently sudden, necessitating extended ICU monitoring for PH patients. The hemodynamic deterioration and deaths are attributed to increased sympathetic tone, fluid shifts, worsening pulmonary vasoconstriction (due to hypoxia, hypothermia, acidosis), and pulmonary embolism.

The most feared postoperative complication is RV failure due to PH exacerbation, with resulting LV underfilling, systemic hypotension, and arrhythmias [114–116].

Atrial tachyarrhythmias are usually managed with digoxin and amiodarone; use of beta blockers and calcium channel blockers may occasionally be appropriate (with extreme caution due to negative inotropy); electrical cardioversion is usually reserved for hemodynamically unstable patients, but if catecholamines are markedly elevated and filling pressures are high, recurrences are high.

Any noncardiac complications that increase RV workload (such as infection, anemia, and acidemia) need to be rapidly treated. Acidemia, in particular, increases PVR, while mild alkalosis may be beneficial (Goal pCO_2 is ≤30–35 mmHg, and goal pH ≥7.4) [117, 118]. Normothermia has to be maintained [52]. Both hypovolemia (bleeding) and volume overload are poorly tolerated in PH patients, as hypertrophied RV requires optimal preload, and excessive volume may precipitate worsening RV failure and septal shift, compromising LV filling. Diuretic use can be guided by CVP (aiming at "best baseline" preoperative CVP, vs. CVP 5–10 for borderline blood pressure, to ensure adequate filling); ultrafiltration can be used for diuretic resistance. PEEP has to be taken in to consideration in hypotensive intubated patients with CVP ≤10 mmHg; if lifting patients legs results in increased MAP, fluids are indicated; if CVP ≥15 and/or leg rising does not lead to increase in MAP, diuretics are likely needed. Vasopressors and inotropes are used as needed to maintain systemic blood pressure.

While iNO is optimal for the early postoperative period to decrease PVR, it has a potential for formation of toxic metabolites with prolonged use, and is expensive. Weaning to 5 parts per million (ppm) and bridging transition with inhaled prostacyclin derivatives to prevent rebound PH in weaning of the last 3–4 ppm is usually recommended; IV/PO sildenafil used for additional pulmonary vasodilatation may be helpful in the weaning process and in the highest risk patients, nasally delivered iNO and slower down titration to allow extubation is also feasible. Inhaled milrinone has also been used [119, 120]. The calcium sensitizer levosimendan (available in Europe) showed some promise in optimizing PH hemodynamics in small studies [121] but is not routinely used or available. IV prostanoids may be initiated in the postoperative period in patients with severe PH who are candidates for chronic PH therapies and ideally should have been instituted preoperatively. In patients with WHO group 2 PH, combined systemic and pulmonary vasodilators such as sodium nitroprusside, nitroglycerin, milrinone, nesiritide (and perhaps levosimendan) are beneficial; pulmonary vasodilators can worsen LV failure and pulmonary venous congestion, and precipitate further V/Q mismatch in underlying lung disease.

The multidisciplinary approach is equally essential in the postoperative period as it is in the preoperative and intraoperative settings. Early ambulation and physical therapy, as well as nutritional support for prevention of postoperative complications are routine. Well trained and coordinated multidisciplinary teams have the ability to optimize outcomes and lower mortality in high-risk PH patients. Further studies of anesthesia and surgery in PH patients will help in understanding of the preoperative risks and complications, and refine current treatment strategies.

References

1. Weber RK, Buda AJ, Levene DL. General anesthesia in Eisenmenger's syndrome. CMAJ. 1977;117(12):1413–4.
2. Kahn ML. Eisenmenger's syndrome in pregnancy. N Engl J Med. 1993;329:887.
3. Roberts NV, Keast PJ. Pulmonary hypertension and pregnancy—a lethal combination. Anaesth Intensive Care. 1990;18:366–74.
4. Bernstein AD, Parsonnet V. Bedside estimation of risk as an aid for decision-making in cardiac surgery. Ann Thorac Surg. 2000;69(3):823–8.
5. Denault A, Deschamps A, Tardif JC, Lambert J, Perrault L. Pulmonary hypertension in cardiac surgery. Curr Cardiol Rev. 2010;6(1):1–14.
6. Malouf JF, Enriquez-Sarano M, Pellikka PA, Oh JK, Bailey KR, Chandrasekaran K, et al. Severe pulmonary hypertension in patients with severe aortic valve stenosis: clinical profile and prognostic implications. J Am Coll Cardiol. 2002;40:789–95.
7. Reich LD, Bodian AC, Krol M, et al. Intraoperative hemodynamic predictors of mortality, stroke, and myocardial infarction after coronary artery bypass surgery. Anesth Analg. 1999;89:814.
8. Tremblay NA, Hardy JF, Perrault J, Carrier M. A simple classification of the risk in cardiac surgery: the first decade. Can J Anaesth. 1993;40(2):103–11.
9. Tuman KJ, McCarthy RJ, March RJ, Najafi H, Ivankovich AD. Morbidity and duration of ICU stay after cardiac surgery. A model for preoperative risk assessment. Chest. 1992;102: 36–44.
10. Leone N, Courbon D, Thomas F, Bean K, Jégo B, Leynaert B, et al. Lung function impairment and metabolic syndrome. The critical role of abdominal obesity. Am J Respir Crit Care Med. 2009;179:509–16.
11. Kaw R, Pasupuleti V, Deshpande A, Hamieh T, Walker E, Minai OA. Pulmonary hypertension: an important predictor of outcomes in patients undergoing non-cardiac surgery. Respir Med. 2011;105(4):619–24.

12. Lai HC, Wang KY, Lee WL, Ting CT, Liu TJ. Severe pulmonary hypertension complicates postoperative outcome of non-cardiac surgery. Br J Anaesth. 2007;99:184–90.
13. Price LC, Montani D, Jaïs X, Dick JR, Simonneau G, Sitbon O, et al. Noncardiothoracic nonobstetric surgery in mild-to-moderate pulmonary hypertension. Eur Respir J. 2010;35: 1294–302.
14. Ramakrishna G, Sprung J, Ravi BS, Chandrasekaran K, McGoon MD. Impact of pulmonary hypertension on the outcomes of noncardiac surgery: predictors of perioperative morbidity and mortality. J Am Coll Cardiol. 2005;45(10):1691–9.
15. Ammash NM, Connolly HM, Abel MD, Warnes CA. Noncardiac surgery in Eisenmenger syndrome. J Am Coll Cardiol. 1999;33:222–7.
16. Meyer S, McLaughlin VV, Seyfarth HJ, Bull TM, Vizza CD, Gomberg-Maitland M, et al. Outcomes of noncardiac, nonobstetric surgery in patients with PAH: an international prospective survey. Eur Respir J. 2013;41:1302–7.
17. Minai OA, Venkateshiah SB, Arroliga AC. Surgical intervention in patients with moderate to severe pulmonary arterial hypertension. Conn Med. 2006;70(4):239–43.
18. Chatterjee K, De Marco T, Alpert JS. Pulmonary hypertension: hemodynamic diagnosis and management. Arch Intern Med. 2002;162:1925–33.
19. Oudiz RJ. Pulmonary hypertension associated with left-sided heart disease. Clin Chest Med. 2007;28(1):233–41, x. Review.
20. Capomolla S, Febo O, Guazzotti G, Gnemmi M, Mortara A, Riccardi G, et al. Invasive and non-invasive determinants of pulmonary hypertension in patients with chronic heart failure. J Heart Lung Transplant. 2000;19:426–38.
21. Drazner MH, Hamilton MA, Fonarow G, Creaser J, Flavell C, Stevenson LW. Relationship between right and left-sided filling pressures in 1000 patients with advanced heart failure. J Heart Lung Transplant. 1999;18(11):1126–32.
22. Drazner MH, Prasad A, Ayers C, Markham DW, Hastings J, Bhella PS, et al. The relationship of right- and left-sided filling pressures in patients with heart failure and a preserved ejection fraction. Circ Heart Fail. 2010;3(2):202–6.
23. Enriquez-Sarano M, Rossi A, Seward JB, Bailey KR, Tajik AJ. Determinants of pulmonary hypertension in left ventricular dysfunction. J Am Coll Cardiol. 1997;29(1):153–9.
24. Haddad F, Hunt SA, Rosenthal DN, Murphy DJ. Contemporary reviews in cardiovascular medicine: right ventricular function in cardiovascular disease, Part I: anatomy, physiology, aging, and functional assessment of the right ventricle. Circulation. 2008;117:1436–48.
25. Bellofiore A, Chesler NC. Methods for measuring right ventricular function and hemodynamic coupling with the pulmonary vasculature. Ann Biomed Eng. 2013;41(7):1384–98.
26. Fleisher LA, Beckman JA, Brown KA, Calkins H, Chaikof E, Fleischmann KE, et al. ACC/AHA 2007 guidelines on perioperative cardiovascular evaluation and care for noncardiac surgery. A report of the American College of Cardiology/American Heart Association Task Force on Practice Guidelines (Writing Committee to Revise the 2002 Guidelines on Perioperative Cardiovascular Evaluation for Noncardiac Surgery). Circulation. 2007;116(17): e418–99.
27. Mikhail GW, Gibbs JSR, Yacoub MH. Pulmonary and systemic arterial pressure changes during syncope in primary pulmonary hypertension. Circulation. 2001;104(11):1326–7.
28. McLaughlin VV, Archer SL, Badesch DB, Barst RJ, Farber HW, Lindner JR, et al. for the American College of Cardiology Foundation Task Force on Expert Consensus Documents and the American Heart Association. ACCF/AHA 2009 expert consensus document on pulmonary hypertension developed in collaboration with the American College of Chest Physicians, American Thoracic Society, and the Pulmonary Hypertension Association. Circulation. 2009;119:2250–94.
29. Raymond RJ, Hinderliter AL, Willis PW, Ralph D, Caldwell EJ, Williams W, et al. Echocardiographic predictors of adverse outcomes in primary pulmonary hypertension. J Am Coll Cardiol. 2002;39(7):1214–9.
30. Rudski LG, Lai WW, Afilalo J, Hua L, Handschumacher MD, Chandrasekaran K, et al. Guidelines for the echocardiographic assessment of the right heart in adults: a report from the

American Society of Echocardiography. Endorsed by the European Association of Echocardiography, a registered branch of the European Society of Cardiology, and the Canadian Society of Echocardiography. J Am Soc Echocardiogr. 2010;23:685–713.

31. Roberts JD, Forfia PR. Diagnosis and assessment of pulmonary vascular disease by Doppler echocardiography. Pulm Circ. 2011;1(2):160–81.
32. McLaughlin VV, Presberg KW, Doyle RL, Abman SH, McCrory DC, Fortin T, et al. Prognosis of pulmonary arterial hypertension: ACCP evidence-based clinical practice guidelines. Chest. 2004;126(1 Suppl):78S–92.
33. Yeo TC, Dujardin KS, Tei C, Mahoney DW, McGoon MD, Seward JB. Value of a Doppler-derived index combining systolic and diastolic time intervals in predicting outcome in primary pulmonary hypertension. Am J Cardiol. 1998;81(9):1157–61.
34. Halpern SD, Taichman DB. Misclassification of pulmonary hypertension due to reliance on pulmonary capillary wedge pressure rather than left ventricular end-diastolic pressure. Chest. 2009;136(1):37–43.
35. Badesch DB, Champion HC, Sanchez MA, Hoeper MM, Loyd JE, Manes A, et al. Diagnosis and assessment of pulmonary arterial hypertension. J Am Coll Cardiol. 2009;54(1 Suppl):S55–66.
36. Rich GF, Murphy Jr GD, Roos CM, Johns RA. Inhaled nitric oxide. Selective pulmonary vasodilation in cardiac surgical patients. Anesthesiology. 1993;78(6):1028–35.
37. McGlothlin D, Ivascu N, Heerdt PM. Anesthesia and pulmonary hypertension. Prog Cardiovasc Dis. 2012;55(2):199–217.
38. Poirier P, Alpert MA, Fleisher LA, Thompson PD, Sugerman HJ, Burke LE, et al. Cardiovascular evaluation and management of severely obese patients undergoing surgery: a science advisory from the American Heart Association. Circulation. 2009;120:86–95.
39. Mereles D, Ehlken N, Kreuscher S, Ghofrani S, Hoeper MM, Halank M, et al. Exercise and respiratory training improve exercise capacity and quality of life in patients with severe chronic pulmonary hypertension. Circulation. 2006;114:1482–9.
40. Strauss EJ, Egol KA, Alaia M, Hansen D, Bashar M, Steiger D. The use of retrievable inferior vena cava filters in orthopaedic patients. J Bone Joint Surg Br. 2008;90-B:662–7.
41. Saouti N, Westerhof N, Postmus PE, Vonk-Noordegraaf A. The arterial load in pulmonary hypertension. Eur Respir Rev. 2010;19(117):197–203.
42. Kussmaul WG, Noordergraaf A, Laskey WK. Right ventricular-pulmonary arterial interactions. Ann Biomed Eng. 1992;20(1):63–80.
43. Mahapatra S, Nishimura RA, Sorajja P, Cha S, McGoon MD. Relationship of pulmonary arterial capacitance and mortality in idiopathic pulmonary arterial hypertension. J Am Coll Cardiol. 2006;47(4):799–803.
44. Dupont M, Mullens W, Skouri HN, Abrahams Z, Wu Y, Taylor DO, et al. Prognostic role of pulmonary arterial capacitance in advanced heart failure. Circ Heart Fail. 2012;5(6):778–85.
45. Lankhaar JW, Westerhof N, Faes TJ, et al. Quantification of right ventricular afterload in patients with and without pulmonary hypertension. Am J Physiol Heart Circ Physiol. 2006;291:H1731–7.
46. van Wolferen SA, Marcus JT, Westerhof N, Spreeuwenberg MD, Marques KM, Bronzwaer JG, et al. Right coronary artery flow impairment in patients with pulmonary hypertension. Eur Heart J. 2008;29(1):120–7.
47. Gómez A, Bialostozky D, Zajarias A, Santos E, Palomar A, Martínez ML, et al. Right ventricular ischemia in patients with primary pulmonary hypertension. J Am Coll Cardiol. 2001;38(4):1137–42.
48. Vlahakes GJ, Turley K, Hoffman JI. The pathophysiology of failure in acute right ventricular hypertension: hemodynamic and biochemical correlations. Circulation. 1981;63:87–95.
49. Hsia HH, Haddad F. Pulmonary hypertension: a stage for ventricular interdependence? J Am Coll Cardiol. 2012;59(24):2203–5.

50. Lahm T, McCaslin CA, Wozniak TC, Ghumman W, Fadl YY, Obeidat OS, et al. Medical and surgical treatment of acute right ventricular failure. J Am Coll Cardiol. 2010;56(18):1435–46.
51. Strumpher J, Jacobsohn E. Pulmonary hypertension and right ventricular dysfunction: physiology and perioperative management. J Cardiothorac Vasc Anesth. 2011;25(4):687–704.
52. Benumof JL, Wahrenbrock EA. Dependency of hypoxic pulmonary vasoconstriction on temperature. J Appl Physiol Respir Environ Exerc Physiol. 1977;42(1):56–8.
53. Teo YW, Greenhalgh DL. Update on anaesthetic approach to pulmonary hypertension. Eur J Anaesthesiol. 2010;27(4):317–23.
54. Subramaniam K, Yared JP. Management of pulmonary hypertension in the operating room. Semin Cardiothorac Vasc Anesth. 2007;11(2):119–36.
55. Fischer LG, Van Aken H, Bürkle H. Management of pulmonary hypertension: physiological and pharmacological considerations for anesthesiologists. Anesth Analg. 2003;96(6):1603–16.
56. Kiely DG, Cargill RI, Lipworth BJ. Effects of hypercapnia on hemodynamic, inotropic, lusitropic, and electrophysiologic indices in humans. Chest. 1996;109(5):1215–21.
57. Bovill JG. Intravenous anesthesia for the patient with left ventricular dysfunction. Semin Cardiothorac Vasc Anesth. 2006;10(1):43–8.
58. Bovill JG. Inhalation anaesthesia: from diethyl ether to xenon. Handb Exp Pharmacol. 2008;182:121–42.
59. Sprung J, Ogletree-Hughes ML, Moravec CS. The effects of etomidate on the contractility of failing and nonfailing human heart muscle. Anesth Analg. 2000;91(1):68–75.
60. Kerbaul F, Rondelet B, Motte S, Fesler P, Hubloue I, Ewalenko P. Isoflurane and desflurane impair right ventricular-pulmonary arterial coupling in dogs. Anesthesiology. 2004;101(6):1357–62.
61. Heerdt PM, Gandhi CD, Dickstein ML. Disparity of isoflurane effects on left and right ventricular afterload and hydraulic power generation in swine. Anesth Analg. 1998;87(3):511–21.
62. Kerbaul F, Bellezza M, Mekkaoui C, Feier H, Guidon C, Gouvernet J, et al. Sevoflurane alters right ventricular performance but not pulmonary vascular resistance in acutely instrumented anesthetized pigs. J Cardiothorac Vasc Anesth. 2006;20(2):209–16.
63. Maxwell BG, Jackson E. Role of ketamine in the management of pulmonary hypertension and right ventricular failure. J Cardiothorac Vasc Anesth. 2012;26(3):e24–5. author reply e25–6.
64. Kaye AD, Banister RE, Fox CJ, Ibrahim IN, Nossaman BD. Analysis of ketamine responses in the pulmonary vascular bed of the cat. Crit Care Med. 2000;28(4):1077–82.
65. Missant C, Rex S, Claus P, Derde S, Wouters PF. Thoracic epidural anaesthesia disrupts the protective mechanism of homeometric autoregulation during right ventricular pressure overload by cardiac sympathetic blockade: a randomised controlled animal study. Eur J Anaesthesiol. 2011;28(7):535–43.
66. Richard C, Monnet X, Teboul JL. Pulmonary artery catheter monitoring in 2011. Curr Opin Crit Care. 2011;17(3):296–302.
67. Daudel F, Tüller D, Krähenbühl S, Jakob SM, Takala J. Pulse pressure variation and volume responsiveness during acutely increased pulmonary artery pressure: an experimental study. Crit Care. 2010;14:R122.
68. Wyler von Ballmoos M, Takala J, Roeck M, Porta F, Tueller D, Ganter CC. Pulse-pressure variation and hemodynamic response in patients with elevated pulmonary artery pressure: a clinical study. Crit Care. 2010;14:111.
69. Rich S, Gubin S, Hart K. The effects of phenylephrine on right ventricular performance in patients with pulmonary hypertension. Chest. 1990;98(5):1102–6.
70. Kwak YL, Lee CS, Park YH, Hong YW. The effect of phenylephrine and norepinephrine in patients with chronic pulmonary hypertension. Anaesthesia. 2002;57:9–14.

71. Evora PR, Pearson PJ, Schaff HV. Arginine vasopressin induces endothelium-dependent vasodilatation of the pulmonary artery. V1-receptor-mediated production of nitric oxide. Chest. 1993;103(4):1241–5.
72. Price LC, Forrest P, Sodhi V, Adamson DL, Nelson-Piercy C, Lucey M, et al. Use of vasopressin after Caesarean section in idiopathic pulmonary arterial hypertension. Br J Anaesth. 2007;99(4):552–5.
73. Landry DW, Levin HR, Gallant EM, Seo S, D'Alessandro D, Oz MC, et al. Vasopressin pressor hypersensitivity in vasodilatory septic shock. Crit Care Med. 1997;25(8):1279–82.
74. Tayama E, Ueda T, Shojima T, Akasu K, Oda T, Fukunaga S, et al. Arginine vasopressin is an ideal drug after cardiac surgery for the management of low systemic vascular resistant hypotension concomitant with pulmonary hypertension. Interact Cardiovasc Thorac Surg. 2007;6(6):715–9.
75. Overgaard CB, Džavík V. Contemporary reviews in cardiovascular medicine. Inotropes and vasopressors. Review of physiology and clinical use in cardiovascular disease. Circulation. 2008;118:1047–56.
76. Hoeper MM, Granton J. Intensive care unit management of patients with severe pulmonary hypertension and right heart failure. Am J Respir Crit Care Med. 2011;184(10):1114–24.
77. Antoniou T, Prokakis C, Athanasopoulos G, Thanopoulos A, Rellia P, Zarkalis D. Inhaled nitric oxide plus Iloprost in the setting of post-left assist device right heart dysfunction. Ann Thorac Surg. 2012;94(3):792–8.
78. Memtsoudis SG, Ma Y, Chiu YL, Walz JM, Voswinckel R, Mazumdar M. Perioperative mortality in patients with pulmonary hypertension undergoing major joint replacement. Anesth Analg. 2010;111(5):1110–6.
79. Donaldson AJ, Thomson HE, Harper NJ, Kenny NW. Bone cement implantation syndrome. Br J Anaesth. 2009;102(1):12–22.
80. Memtsoudis SG, Rosenberger P, Walz JM. Critical care issues in the patient after major joint replacement. J Intensive Care Med. 2007;22(2):92–104.
81. McCaskie AW, Barnes MR, Lin E, Harper WM, Gregg PJ. Cement pressurisation during hip replacement. J Bone Joint Surg Br. 1997;79(3):379–84.
82. Lafont ND, Kostucki WM, Marchand PH, Michaux MN, Boogaerts JG. Embolism detected by transoesophageal echocardiography during hip arthroplasty. Can J Anaesth. 1994;41(9): 850–3.
83. Bombardieri AM, Memtsoudis SG, Go G, Ma Y, Sculco T, Sharrock N. Pulmonary circulatory changes after bilateral total knee arthroplasty during regional anesthesia. J Clin Anesth. 2013;25(1):4–8.
84. Colucci WS, Wright RF, Jaski BE, Fifer MA, Braunwald E. Milrinone and dobutamine in severe heart failure: differing hemodynamic effects and individual patient responsiveness. Circulation. 1986;73(3 Pt 2):III175–83.
85. Park BJ, Heerdt PM. Minimally invasive surgical techniques in the treatment of lung cancer. Minerva Chir. 2009;64(6):573–88.
86. Heerdt PM. Cardiovascular adaptation to lung resection. Thoracic anesthesia. 3rd ed. Philadelphia, PA: Churchill Livingstone Inc.; 2003. p. 423–35.
87. Rocca GD, Passariello M, Coccia C, Costa MG, Di Marco P, Venuta F, et al. Inhaled nitric oxide administration during one-lung ventilation in patients undergoing thoracic surgery. J Cardiothorac Vasc Anesth. 2001;15(2):218–23.
88. Alfonsi P, Vieillard-Baron A, Coggia M, Guignard B, Goeau-Brissonniere O, Jardin F, et al. Cardiac function during intraperitoneal CO_2 insufflation for aortic surgery: a transesophageal echocardiographic study. Anesth Analg. 2006;102(5):1304–10.
89. Joris JL, Noirot DP, Legrand MJ, Jacquet NJ, Lamy ML. Hemodynamic changes during laparoscopic cholecystectomy. Anesth Analg. 1993;76(5):1067–71.
90. Safran D, Sgambati S, Orlando III R. Laparoscopy in high-risk cardiac patients. Surg Gynecol Obstet. 1993;176(6):548–54.
91. Murthy T, Gupta P. Laparoscopic cholecystectomy with pulmonary hypertension: anaesthetic challenges—a case report. Indian J Anaesth. 2008;52(2):217–20.

92. Samper O, Guillen V. Severe pulmonary hypertension: implications for anesthesia in laparoscopic surgery. Rev Esp Anestesiol Reanim. 2008;55(7):438–41.
93. Harris SN, Ballantyne GH, Luther MA, Perrino Jr AC. Alterations of cardiovascular performance during laparoscopic colectomy: a combined hemodynamic and echocardiographic analysis. Anesth Analg. 1996;83(3):482–7.
94. Lestar M, Gunnarsson L, Lagerstrand L, Wiklund P, Odeberg-Wernerman S. Hemodynamic perturbations during robot-assisted laparoscopic radical prostatectomy in 45 degrees Trendelenburg position. Anesth Analg. 2011;113(5):1069–75.
95. Bédard E, Dimopoulos K, Gatzoulis MA. Has there been any progress made on pregnancy outcomes among women with pulmonary arterial hypertension? Eur Heart J. 2009;30(3): 256–65.
96. Zwicke DL, Buggy BP. Pregnancy and pulmonary arterial hypertension: successful management of 37 consecutive patients. Chest. 2008;134(4_MeetingAbstracts):s64002.
97. Swanson KL, Wiesner RH, Nyberg SL, Rosen CB, Krowka MJ. Survival in portopulmonary hypertension: Mayo Clinic experience categorized by treatment subgroups. Am J Transplant. 2008;8:244–2453.
98. Kuo PC, Plotkin JS, Gaine S, Schroeder RA, Rustgi VK, Rubin LJ, et al. Portopulmonary hypertension and the liver transplant candidate. Transplantation. 1999;67:1087–93.
99. Krowka MJ, Mandell MS, Ramsay MA, Kawut SM, Fallon MB, Manzarbeitia C. Hepatopulmonary syndrome and portopulmonary hypertension: a report of the multicenter liver transplant database. Liver Transpl. 2004;10:174–82.
100. Hadengue A, Benhayoun MK, Lebrec D, Benhamou JP. Pulmonary hypertension complicating portal hypertension: prevalence and relation to splanchnic hemodynamics. Gastroenterology. 1991;100:520–8.
101. Talwalkar JA, Swanson KL, Krowka MJ, Andrews JC, Kamath PS. Prevalence of spontaneous portosystemic shunts in patients with portopulmonary hypertension and effect on treatment. Gastroenterology. 2011;141:1673–9.
102. Raevens S, De Pauw M, Reyntjens K, Geerts A, Verhelst X, Berrevoet F, et al. Oral vasodilator therapy in patients with moderate to severe portopulmonary hypertension as a bridge to liver transplant. Eur J Gastroenterol Hepatol. 2013;25(4):495–502.
103. Chua R, Keogh A, Miyashita M. Novel use of sildenafil in the treatment of portopulmonary hypertension. J Heart Lung Transplant. 2005;24:498–500.
104. Kawut SM, Taichman DB, Ahya VN, Kaplan S, Archer-Chicko CL, Kimmel SE, et al. Hemodynamics and survival in patients with portopulmonary hypertension. Liver Transpl. 2005;11:1107–11.
105. Losay J, Piot D, Bougaran J, Ozier Y, Devictor D, Houssin D, et al. Early liver transplantation is crucial in children with liver disease and pulmonary artery hypertension. J Hepatol. 1998;28:337–42.
106. Schott R, Chaouat A, Launoy A, Pottecher T, Weitzenblum E. Improvement of pulmonary hypertension after liver transplantation. Chest. 1999;115(6):1748–9.
107. Tan HP, Markowitz JS, Montgomery RA, Merritt WT, Klein AS, Thuluvath PJ, et al. Liver transplantation in patients with severe portopulmonary hypertension treated with preoperative chronic intravenous epoprostenol. Liver Transpl. 2001;7:745–9.
108. Sussman N, Kaza V, Barshes N, Stribling R, Goss J, O'Mahony C, et al. Successful liver transplantation following medical management of portopulmonary hypertension: a single-center series. Am J Transplant. 2006;6:2177–82.
109. Ashfaq M, Chinnakotla S, Rogers L, Ausloos K, Saadeh S, Klintmalm GB, et al. The impact of treatment of portopulmonary hypertension on survival following liver transplantation. Am J Transplant. 2007;7:1258–64.
110. Makisalo H, Koivusalo A, Vakkuri A, Hockerstedt K. Sildenafil for portopulmonary hypertension in a patient undergoing liver transplantation. Liver Transpl. 2004;10:945–50.
111. Hoeper MM, Krowka MJ, Strassburg CP. Portopulmonary hypertension and hepatopulmonary syndrome. Lancet. 2004;363:1461–8.

112. Huonker M, Schumacher YO, Ochs A, Sorichter S, Keul J, Rössle M. Cardiac function and haemodynamics in alcoholic cirrhosis and effects of the transjugular intrahepatic portosystemic stent shunt. Gut. 1999;44:743–8.
113. Benjaminov FS, Prentice M, Sniderman KW, Siu S, Liu P, Wong F. Portopulmonary hypertension in decompensated cirrhosis with refractory ascites. Gut. 2003;52(9):1355–62.
114. Rodriguez RM, Pearl RG. Pulmonary hypertension and major surgery. Anesth Analg. 1998;87(4):812–5.
115. Roessler P, Lambert TF. Anaesthesia for caesarean section in the presence of primary pulmonary hypertension. Anaesth Intensive Care. 1986;14(3):317–20.
116. Burrows FA, Klinck JR, Rabinovitch M, Bohn DJ. Pulmonary hypertension in children: perioperative management. Can Anaesth Soc J. 1986;33(5):606–28.
117. Forrest P. Anaesthesia and right ventricular failure. Anaesth Intensive Care. 2009;37(3): 370–85.
118. Fullerton DA, McIntyre Jr RC, Kirson LE, St Cyr JA, Whitman GJ, Grover FL. Impact of respiratory acid-base status in patients with pulmonary hypertension. Ann Thorac Surg. 1996;61(2):696–701.
119. Lamarche Y, Perrault LP, Maltais S, Tétreault K, Lambert J, Denault AY. Preliminary experience with inhaled milrinone in cardiac surgery. Eur J Cardiothorac Surg. 2007;31(6): 1081–7.
120. Lowson SM. Inhaled alternatives to nitric oxide. Crit Care Med. 2005;33(3 Suppl):S188–95. Review.
121. Ebade AA, Khalil MA, Mohamed AK. Levosimendan is superior to dobutamine as an inodilator in the treatment of pulmonary hypertension for children undergoing cardiac surgery. J Anesth. 2013;27(3):334–9.

ERRATUM TO

Echocardiography

Paul Forfia and Hayan Al Maluli

J.R. Klinger, R.P. Frantz (eds.), *Diagnosis and Management of Pulmonary Hypertension*, Respiratory Medicine 12, DOI 10.1007/978-1-4939-2636-7_9

DOI 10.1007/978-1-4939-2636-7_20

In Chapter 9 (Echocardiography) "Hayan Al Maluli" was not listed among the authors

---

The online version of the original chapter can be found at http://dx.doi.org/10.1007/978-1-4939-2636-7_9

J.R. Klinger, R.P. Frantz (eds.), *Diagnosis and Management of Pulmonary Hypertension*, Respiratory Medicine 12, DOI 10.1007/978-1-4939-2636-7_20

Index

A

Acceleration time (AcT), 212
Acidosis, 419, 457
Activin-like kinase 1 (ALK-1), 400
Acute respiratory distress syndrome (ARDS), 418
Adjunct therapy
  anticoagulation
    aminorex, 308
    APAH subgroup, 309
    autopsy lung specimens, 308
    heparin and warfarin treatment, 309
    plexogenic arteriopathy, 308
    prothrombotic abnormalities, 307
    rivaroxaban, 310
    SSc-APAH, 309
    thrombotic arteriopathy, 307–308
    ventilation-perfusion (V/Q) scan, 309
    warfarin therapy, 308–309
  digoxin therapy, 304–306
  diuretics, 312
  oxygen therapy, 310–311
Ambrisentan, 346–347
Aminorex, 7, 27, 178, 308
Aminorexfumarate, 22, 26
Anaerobic threshold (AT), 269–270, 275
Anemia, 148, 170, 189, 352, 419
Anticoagulation
  aminorex, 308
  APAH subgroup, 309
  autopsy lung specimens, 308
  heparin and warfarin treatment, 309
  plexogenic arteriopathy, 308
  prothrombotic abnormalities, 307
  rivaroxaban, 310
  SSc-APAH, 309
  thrombotic arteriopathy, 307–308
  ventilation-perfusion (V/Q) scan, 309
  warfarin therapy, 308–309
Arterial blood gas (ABG) analysis, 186
Atrial tachyarrhythmias, 418–419, 457

B

Benfluorex, 26
Bland-Altman analyses, 281–283
Bone morphogenetic protein receptor 2 (BMPR2) mutations, 24–26, 39–41, 47, 48, 399–400
Bosentan
  BENEFiT, 345
  BREATHE-4, 345
  BREATHE-5, 345
  BREATHE-1 trial, 343–344
  dual ERA and ERB antagonist, 343
  FDA approval, 343
  P450 enzyme system, 344
  WHO functional class, 343
Bosentan Effects in iNopErable Forms of chronic Thromboembolic pulmonary hypertension (BENEFiT), 345
Bosentan randomized trial of endothelin antagonist therapy (BREATHE-1) trial, 343–344

C

Calcium channel blockers (CCB), 258, 313–314
Cardiac catheterization, 149, 245

J.R. Klinger, R.P. Frantz (eds.), *Diagnosis and Management of Pulmonary Hypertension*, Respiratory Medicine 12, DOI 10.1007/978-1-4939-2636-7

Cardiac glycosides, 85, 304, 305
Cardiopulmonary exercise testing (CPET)
  cardiac output (Qt)
    Fick principle, 286
    pressure-flow relationships, 288–289
    pulmonary arterial pressure, 287
    pulmonary vascular resistance, 288
    stroke volume, 287
    VO_2max, 286–287
  eiPAH (*see* Exercise induced pulmonary arterial hypertension (eiPAH))
  Harvard Fatigue Lab, 267–268
  iCPET
    Bland-Altman analyses, 281–283
    COPD, 279–280, 294–295
    cycle ergometer, 278
    diagnostic algorithms, 289–291
    HFrEF, 294
    ITP swing, 284
    maximum exercise, 280–281
    mPAP and PCWP, 280
    mPAP/Q slope, 280–281
    PCWP measurements, 278–279, 281, 283, 285–286
    pleural pressure swings, 279
    pulmonary arterial hypertension, 294
    respirophasic change, 285
    ultrasound-guided internal jugular approach, 278
    variables, 285–286
  niCPET
    AT, 269–270
    arterial O_2 desaturation, 271–272
    branch-point threshold values, 274–275
    changing sensitivity, 275–276
    diagnostic algorithm, 277–278
    EOV, 273–275
    gas exchange, 269–270
    noninvasive algorithm's sensitivity, 276
    OUES, 272–273
    $PETCO_2$, 272
    variables, 268–269
    VAT, 269–270
    ventilatory reserve, 270
    VE/VCO_2, 270–271, 275
    VO_2max, 269
Cardiopulmonary resuscitation (CPR), 427
Catheter whip artifact, 246
Caveolin-1 (*cav-1*), 41–42, 359
CCB therapy. *See* Calcium channel blockers (CCB)
Chest X-ray (CXR), 184–185, 232–233
Chronic heart failure (CHF)
  definitions, PH, 96
  evaluation of, 103, 104, 106
  HFpEF, 102–103
  HFrEF, 95
    CHAMPION study, 98, 100
    continued diuresis, 96
    hemodynamic parameters, 97–100
    hypoxemia, 102
    LVAD device implementation, 97
    mixed pulmonary hypertension, 95–96
    nitroprusside administration, 98, 100
    PCWP, 98, 101
    PHHFrEF, 102
    pulmonary artery pressure, 97
    pulmonary vasodilators, 98
    pulmonary venous pressure, 97
    sleep disordered breathing, 101–102
Chronic lung disease (CLD)
  COPD
    1-month randomized cross-over study, 108
    oxygen therapy, 107
    PH mechanisms, 106–108
    prostaglandin E1, 108
    prostanoid administration, 109
    short-term prostacyclin infusion, 108
    single-dose study, 108
    vasodilators, 107
  cystic fibrosis, 109–110
  evaluation of, PH, 103, 105–106
  interstitial lung disease, 109
  phenotypes and implications, 106, 107
  sleep-disordered breathing, 110
Chronic obstructive pulmonary disease (COPD), 294–295, 310
  chronic lung disease
    1-month randomized cross-over study, 108
    oxygen therapy, 107
    PH mechanisms, 106–108
    prostaglandin E1, 108
    prostanoid administration, 109
    short-term prostacyclin infusion, 108
    single-dose study, 108
    vasodilators, 107
  hypoxic pulmonary hypertension, 69, 73–75, 78, 80, 83
Chronic RV dysfunction and venous congestion, 417
Chronic thromboembolic pulmonary hypertension (CTEPH), 23, 25, 343
  clinical presentation, 120
  coronary artery bypass/valve surgery, 130
  DE, 214–215, 219
  endarterectomy, 130

epidemiology, 116–118
evaluation
bi-plane angiogram, 123
chest X-ray, 121
contrast echocardiography, 122
conventional pulmonary angiography, 123–124
CT angiography, 122, 124–128
DLco, 120–121
endarterectomized tissue, 124, 125
hypoxemia, 121
MRA, 127, 128
transthoracic echocardiography, 121–122
V/Q scanning, 122–123
hemodynamic measurements, 128–129
medical therapy
bosentan, 132, 134
epoprostenol, 133
ERA, 131
inoperable CTEPH, 132
intravenous prostacyclin, 134
operable CTEPH, 135
PA pressure, 133
PDE-5 inhibitors, 131
prostacyclin analogs, 131
riociguat, 133
sGC, 131
sildenafil, 132–133
treprostinil, 133
predisposing factors and pathophysiology, 118–119
PTE surgery, 116, 118, 131, 133, 135, 136
PTPA, 135–136
Cicletanine, 360
Combination therapy
ERA
medications, 380
and PGI2, 382–384
rationale, 381
timeline of drugs, 379
PDE5I
and ERA, 382, 385, 391–393
medications, 381
and PGI2, 382, 383, 387–389
rationale, 381
timeline of drugs, 379
PGI2
and ERA, 382, 384, 389–391
medications, 380
and PDE5I, 382, 384
rationale, 381
timeline of drugs, 379
selection bias, 382, 386
SGC
medications, 380
rationale, 381
timeline of drugs, 379
testing, 382, 386
Combined pulmonary fibrosis and emphysema (CPFE), 68
Computed tomographic (CT) angiography, 122, 124–128
Congenital defects, 171–172
Congenital heart disease (CHD), 28–29, 192, 311
Connective tissue diseases (CTD), 27–28, 109, 157, 173, 178, 179, 180, 189, 268
Constrictive pericarditis (CP), 247, 255–256
Continuous wave Doppler method, 210, 211
Contrast echocardiography, 122
Coronary angiography, 239, 243, 245
Cor pulmonale, 74–75
Cyclic guanosine monophosphate (CGMP)
metabolism
PDE1, 368
PDE2, 369
PDE3, 369
PDE5, 365–366, 369
PDE6, 369
PDE9, 369
PDE5A, 366
PDE5A1, 366
PDE5A2, 366
PDE5A3, 366
PDE10 and PDE11, 369–370
PDE5 inhibitors, 366–368
PDE isozymes, 364–365
PDE proteins, 365
synthesis
BH_4 deficiency, 359
BH_4 supplementation, 359
cicletanine, 360
endothelial dysfunction, 359
endothelial NO synthase, 357
endothelium-dependent dilators, 358
eNOS, 358–359
natriuretic peptides, 362–364
NO-donor therapy, 360
NOS isoforms, 357
soluble guanylate cyclase (GC), 361–362
vascular synthesis, 356–357
ventilation/perfusion *(V/Q)*, 360
Cystic fibrosis, 109–110

D
Dexfenfluramine, 26
Diastolic pressure gradient (DPG), 235, 250–251, 253
Diastolic pulmonary artery pressure (dPAP), 236
Dichloroacetate (DCA), 401, 404
Digoxin therapy, 85, 304–306
Doppler echocardiography (DE)
  PH pathophysiology, 220
  RV
    AcT, 212
    afterload, 209
    CTEPH, 214–215, 219
    exercise, 219
    IVC, 210–211
    PAH, 213–214
    PASP, 210–212, 219
    PE, 215–216
    PH_{PVD}, 217–218
    pulmonary circulation unit, 203–204
    PVH, 217–218
    PVR, 212–213
    size, shape, septal position, 207–209
    SPS, 216
    systolic function measurement, 204–206

E
Echocardiography. *See* Doppler echocardiography (DE)
Eisenmenger syndrome (ES), 28, 216
Electrocardiogram (ECG), 76, 127, 185, 234, 311
Endarterectomy, 127, 130, 132
Endothelin-1 (ET-1), 12, 41, 44, 380
Endothelin receptor A (ETA), 342–343
Endothelin receptor antagonists (ERA), 131
  adverse effects, 351–352
  ambrisentan, 346–347
  bosentan
    BENEFiT, 345
    BREATHE-4, 345
    BREATHE-5, 345
    BREATHE-1 trial, 343–344
    dual ERA and ERB antagonist, 343
    FDA approval, 343
    P450 enzyme system, 344
    WHO functional class, 343
  combination approach, 351
  CTEPH, 343
  ETA and ETB receptors, 342–343
  IPAH, 343
  macitentan, 347
  medications, 380
  vs. PAH therapy, 350
  and PGI2, 382–384
  rationale, 381
  SERAPHIN, 348–350
  timeline of drugs, 379
Endothelin receptor B (ETB), 342–343
Epigenetic targets, 400
Epinephrine, 422, 427, 453
Eukaryotic translation initiation factor 2 alpha kinase 4 (EIF2AK4), 400
Exercise induced pulmonary arterial hypertension (eiPAH)
  elevated ventilatory equivalent, 292
  exercise-induced HFpEF, 293
  incremental exercise, 290–291
  mixed eiPH, 293
  mPAP and PV, 292
  representative plateau pattern, 291–292
  representative "take-off" pattern, 291–292
  VO_2max, 291
Exercise oscillatory ventilation (EOV), 273–275

F
Femoral vein, 242–244
Fenfluramine, 26, 27, 178
Fick method, 254
Functional residual capacity (FRC), 230, 426, 451

G
Genetic targets, 399–400
Guanosine triphosphate (GTP), 356
Guanylate cyclases (GCs), 356

H
Heart failure with preserved ejection fraction (HFpEF), 102–103
Heart failure with reduced ejection fraction (HFrEF)
  CHAMPION study, 98, 100
  diuresis, 96
  hemodynamic parameters, 97–100
  hypoxemia, 102
  LVAD device implementation, 97
  mixed pulmonary hypertension, 95–96
  nitroprusside administration, 98, 100
  PCWP, 98, 101
  PHHFrEF, 102
  pulmonary artery pressure, 97
  pulmonary vasodilators, 98
  pulmonary venous pressure, 97
  sleep disordered breathing, 101–102

Hemodynamic perturbations, 190, 260, 418
Heparin, 309
Hereditary hemorrhagic telangiectasia (HHT), 40–41
High-altitude pulmonary edema (HAPE), 68, 71
Histone deacetylase (HDAC), 400
Human herpesvirus 8 (HHV-8), 50–51
5-Hydroxytryptamine (5-HT), 44–45
Hypercapnia, 76, 106, 418, 419, 425
Hypoxemia, 419
  CTEPH, 121
  left heart disease, 102, 103
Hypoxia-inducible factor (HIF), 72, 85
Hypoxia inducible factor 1α (HIF1α), 400
Hypoxic pulmonary hypertension
  clinical presentation, 75–76
  diagnosis
    brain natriuretic peptide levels determination, 77
    CT imaging, 77–78
    echocardiography, 78
    electrocardiogram, 76
    hemodynamic assessment, 78–79
    6 min walk testing, 77
    pulmonary function testing, 76–77
    RHC, 78
  epidemiology, 68–69
  pathogenesis
    cor pulmonale, 74–75
    histologic features, 69–70
    HPV, 71–72
    hypoxic pulmonary vascular remodeling, 72–74
    PH and RV dysfunction, 70
    vascular remodeling, 69
  prognostic implications, 75–76
  treatment
    cardiac glycosides, 85
    hormonal therapies/nonhormonal strategies, 86
    iNOS inhibitors, 86
    intravenous iron, 85
    loop diuretics, 80
    mesenchymal stem cell exosomes, 86
    oxygen therapy, 79
    polysomnography, 80
    pulmonary rehabilitation, 79
    pulmonary vasodilators (*see* Pulmonary vasodilators)
    smoking cessation, 79
Hypoxic pulmonary vascular remodeling, 72–73, 85
Hypoxic pulmonary vasoconstriction (HPV), 71–72, 231, 425

I

Idiopathic pulmonary arterial hypertension (IPAH), 127, 176–178, 213, 343
Idiopathic pulmonary fibrosis (IPF), 68, 76, 83
Iloprost, 331–332, 387, 390, 424
Inducible nitric oxide synthase (iNOS), 74, 86
Inferior vena cava (IVC), 77, 210
Inflammation and inflammatory mediator targets, 402–403
Inotropes, 422–423
Internal jugular (IJ) vein, 242–244
Interstitial lung disease, 109, 156, 442
Intraoperative management
  anesthetic management
    airway and optimal ventilator strategies, 451
    desflurane, 452
    isoflurane, 452
    ketamine, 452
    LV systolic function, 452
    neuraxial anesthesia, 452
    preparation, 450
    propofol, 452
    sevoflurane, 452
    spinal/epidural anesthesia, 452
  immediate postoperative period, 453–454
  interventricular dependence, 450
  myocardial supply and demand, 449
  pharmacological and inhalation therapy
    pressors and inotropes, 453
    pulmonary vasodilators, 453
    volume status, 452
  RV afterload, 447–449
  surgical procedures
    laparoscopy, 455
    liver surgery, 456–457
    obstetrics, 455–456
    orthopedics, 454
    thoracic surgery, 454–455
Invasive cardiopulmonary exercise test (iCPET)
  Bland-Altman analyses, 281–283
  COPD, 279–280, 294–295
  cycle ergometer, 278
  diagnostic algorithms, 289–291
  HFrEF, 294
  ITP swing, 284
  maximum exercise, 280–281
  mPAP and PCWP, 280
  mPAP/Q slope, 280–281
  PCWP measurements, 278–279, 281, 283, 285–286
  pleural pressure swings, 279
  pulmonary arterial hypertension, 294

Invasive cardiopulmonary exercise test (iCPET) (*cont.*)
- respirophasic change, 285
- ultrasound-guided internal jugular approach, 278
- variables, 285–286

Investigational therapy
- cell-based therapeutic targets, 406
- epigenetic targets, 400
- genetic targets, 399–400
- inflammation and inflammatory mediator targets, 402–403
- lung circulation, 405–406
- metabolic targets, 404
- neurohormonal targets, 404–405
- potential therapeutic targets, 399
- vascular cell proliferation, 403–404
- vasoactive targets, 401–402
- vasoconstriction targets, 401
- vessel remodeling targets, 403–404

Isovolemic contraction (IVCT), 206
Isovolemic relaxation (IVRT), 206

K

Kaplan–Meier product-limit method, 326
Katayama syndrome, 147

L

Left atrial pressure (LAP), 248, 250
Left ventricular assist device (LVAD), 52, 97
Left ventricular ejection fraction (LVEF), 287
Left ventricular end-diastolic volume (LVEDV), 79, 190, 287
Left ventricular (LV) systolic failure. *See* Heart failure with reduced ejection fraction (HFrEF)
Liver function testing (LFT), 351–352

M

Macitentan, 347–350
Magnetic resonance angiography (MRA), 127–128
McArdle's disease, 270
McConnell's sign, 215, 216
Mean pulmonary artery pressure (mPAP), 98, 168, 170, 235
Mechanical ventilation, 228, 241, 311, 418, 425–426, 448, 451
Metabolic abnormalities, 419
Metabolic targets, 404
Myocardial performance index (MPI), 206, 441, 443, 444

N

Neurohormonal targets, 404–405
New York Heart Association (NYHA), 326
Nocturnal oxygen therapy trial (NOTT), 310
Noninvasive testing (niCPET)
- AT, 269–270
- arterial O_2 desaturation, 271–272
- branch-point threshold values, 274–275
- changing sensitivity, 275–276
- diagnostic algorithm, 277–278
- EOV, 273–275
- gas exchange, 269–270
- noninvasive algorithm's sensitivity, 276
- OUES, 272–273
- $PETCO_2$, 272
- variables, 268–269
- VAT, 269–270
- ventilatory reserve, 270
- VE/VCO_2, 270–271, 275
- VO_2max, 269

Norepinephrine, 421, 422, 453

O

Obstructive sleep apnea (OSA), 68, 80, 311
Ohm's law, 8, 251
O_2 uptake efficiency slope (OUES), 272–273
Oxygen therapy, 310–311

P

Pathogenesis
- BMPR2, 39–41
- caveolin-1, 41–42
- cellular proliferation and vascular remodeling
  - mitogens, 46–47
  - notch signaling, 48–49
  - TGF-β signaling, 47–48
  - tyrosine kinases, 47
  - vascular endothelial growth factor, 46
- endocrine factors, 52–53
- hypercoagulability, 51–52
- infectious diseases, 50–51
- inflammation, 49–50
- vasoactive substances and imbalance
  - endothelin-1, 44
  - nitric oxide, 42–43
  - prostacyclin, 43
  - serotonin/5-HT, 44–45
  - solute channels, 45
- whole-exome sequencing, 41

Percutaneous transluminal pulmonary angioplasty (PTPA), 135–136

Perioperative management
  hemodynamics, 439–440
  intraoperative evaluation (*see* Intraoperative management)
  physiology, 440–441
  postoperative management, 457–458
  preoperative evaluation
    history and physical examination, 444
    optimal hemodynamic stability, 445
    patient risk factors, 442–443
    RHC, 445
    surgical planning, 446
    surgical risk assessment, 442, 443
    TTE, 444
Phenylephrine, 422, 453
Phosphodiesterase-5 (PDE-5) inhibitors, 131, 357
  and ERA, 382, 385, 391–393
  medications, 381
  and PGI2, 382, 383, 387–389
  rationale, 381
  timeline of drugs, 379
Pneumonia, 418
Polysomnography (PSG), 80, 188
Portopulmonary hypertension (PoPH), 28, 51, 159, 172
Potential therapeutic targets, 399
Prostacyclin therapy
  arachidonic metabolism, 324
  clinical trials
    conventional therapy group, 326
    epoprostenol infusion, 327–329
    initial dose and titration strategy, 327–328
    6MWD, 326
    scleroderma, 327
  gastrointestinal side effects, 324
  hemodynamic measurements, 325
  hydroxyeicotetraenoic acids (HETEs), 325
  inhaled iloprost and placebo, 331–332
  inhaled treprostinil, 332
  investigational prostacyclins, 334–336
  oral prostacyclin analogs, 332–334
  parenteral prostacyclin analogs, 329–331
  thromboxane A_2 (TXA_2), 324–325
  vasodilator properties, 324
Prostaglandins (PGI2) analogues, 324
  and ERA, 382, 384, 389–391
  medications, 380
  and PDE5I, 382, 384
  rationale, 381
  timeline of drugs, 379
Pulmonary angiography, 122, 123, 126, 186, 257
Pulmonary arterial hypertension (PAH), 103, 132
  BMPR2 mutation, 24–26
  cGMP (*see* Cyclic guanosine monophosphate (CGMP))
  CHD, 28–29
  combination therapy (*see* Combination therapy)
  CTD, 27–28
  drug classes, 26–27
  echocardiography, 208, 213–214, 218
  Eisenmenger syndrome, 28
  epidemiology, 29–32
  ERA (*see* Endothelin receptor antagonists (ERA))
  investigative therapy (*see* Investigational therapy)
  left-to-right shunts, 28
  pathogenesis (*see* Pathogenesis)
  postoperative PAH, 28
  prostacyclin therapy (*see* Prostacyclin therapy)
  risk factors, 26
  schistosomiasis, 29
  Sch-PAH (*see* Schistosomiasis-associated pulmonary arterial hypertension (Sch-PAH))
Pulmonary arterial pressure
  classification, 168, 169
  clinical assessment, 190–191
  clinical history
    CTD, 178
    elements, 175
    exertional chest discomfort/syncope, 176
    heritable PAH, 178
    IPAH, 176–178
    WHO criteria, 175–176
  diagnostic testing
    ABG analysis, 186
    chest computed tomography, 187
    CXR, 184–185
    ECG, 185
    echocardiography, 181–184
    exercise testing, 188
    overnight oximetry, 188
    PFT analysis, 185–186
    PSG, 188
    RHC, 190
    serologic tests, 189
    V/Q scintigraphy, 186–187
  features, 191–192
  physical examination
    cardiovascular, 179–180
    gastrointestinal, 180
    head and neck, 179

Pulmonary arterial pressure (*cont.*)
pulmonary examination, 180
skin, muscles, and joints, 180–181
pulmonary hemodynamics
elevated PCWP, 170, 172–173
elevated PVR (*see* Pulmonary vascular resistance (PVR))
elevated Qp, 170–172
mPAP, 168, 170
Pulmonary arterial systolic pressure (PASP), 181–184
Pulmonary artery occlusion pressure (PAOP), 250–252
Pulmonary artery pressure (PAP), 75, 76, 79, 84
Pulmonary artery systolic pressure (PASP), 210–212, 219
Pulmonary capillary wedge pressure (PCWP), 98, 101, 170, 172–173, 231–232, 248–250, 278–279
Pulmonary circulation
α-adrenergic receptors, 11–12
β-adrenergic receptors, 11–12
clinical assessment, 15
endothelin system, 12–13
fluid and solute exchange, 15
hemodynamic *vs.* systemic circulation, 11
historical aspects
balloon flotation catheters, 6–7
Colombo's model, 5, 6
Erasistratus' model, 5, 6
Galen's scheme, 3–6
Harvey's methods, 5, 6
lung distribution, 10
mechanical effects, 13–15
prostanoids, 13
structure and function, 8–10
systemic and pulmonary renin-angiotensin-aldosterone activities, 13
vasoconstrictors, 12
vasodilators, 12
Pulmonary embolism (PE), 117, 118, 120, 121, 215–216, 416, 419, 446, 457
Pulmonary Embolism Thrombolysis Trial (PEITHO), 117
Pulmonary fibrosis, 75, 83, 84
Pulmonary function tests (PFTs) analysis, 185–186
Pulmonary hemodynamics
definition, 227
Doppler pulmonary flow velocity curve, 237
gravitational distribution, 229, 231
hypoxia, 231, 232
invasive evaluation (*see* Right heart catheterization (RHC))
noninvasive evaluation
chest X-ray, 232–233
clinical examination, 231–232
CT scan and angiography, 233
dPAP, 236
ECG, 234
mPAP, 235
MRI, 233–234
PCWP, 231–232
sPAP, 234–235
TTE, 234
PVR, 229, 230, 236
RV function, 237–238
systemic arteries, 228
Pulmonary hypertension (PH)
adjunct therapy (*see* Adjunct therapy)
CCB (*see* Calcium channel blockers (CCB))
circulation (*see* Pulmonary circulation)
clinical classification, 23, 25
CPET (*see* Cardiopulmonary exercise testing (CPET))
CTEPH (*see* Chronic thromboembolic pulmonary hypertension (CTEPH))
definitions, 23–25
echocardiography (*see* Doppler echocardiography (DE))
Group 1, 69
Group 2, 94, 95 (*see also* Chronic heart failure)
Group 3, 67, 68 (*see also* Chronic lung disease; Hypoxic pulmonary hypertension)
perioperative management (*see* Perioperative management)
pulmonary arterial pressure (*see* Pulmonary arterial pressure)
pulmonary hemodynamics (*see* Pulmonary hemodynamics)
RHC (*see* Right heart catheterization (RHC))
RV failure (*see* Right ventricular (RV) failure)
Pulmonary hypertension with heart failure with reduced left ventricular ejection fraction (PHHFrEF), 102
Pulmonary thromboendarterectomy (PTE), 116, 118, 131, 133, 135, 136, 215
Pulmonary vascular disease (PVD), 204
Pulmonary vascular resistance (PVR), 8–9, 71, 75, 98, 173–175, 229, 230, 236
Pulmonary vascular resistance index (PVRI), 253
Pulmonary vasodilators, 81–82, 423–425
COPD, 80, 83
out of proportion PH, 84–85
PDE5 inhibitors, 84
pulmonary fibrosis, 83

Pulmonary venous hypertension (PVH)
definition, 23, 96
echocardiographic parameters, 183
LA enlargement, 217
PH_{PVD}, 217–218

R
Restrictive cardiomyopathy (RCM), 255–256
Right atrial (RA) pressure tracings, 247–248
Right heart catheterization (RHC), 78, 190, 445
cardiac output
Fick method, 254
thermodilution method, 254–255
catheterization, 243, 245
components, 239
coronary anatomy assessment, 239
equipment selection, 245–247
exercise challenge, 257
indications, 238–239
left-sided intracardiac pressures, 255–256
mechanical ventilation, 241–242
patient preparation, 240, 241
percutaneous access sites, 242–244
pressure measurements
LAP, 248, 250
PAOP, 250–252
PA pressure and waveform, 248–249
PCWP waveform, 248–250
PVR, 251–252
PVRI, 253
RA pressure and waveform, 247–248
RV pressure and waveform, 248–249
TPG and DPG, 250–251, 253
zeroing and flushing, 247
pulmonary angiography, 257
safety, 240
sedation, 240–241
vasodilator testing, 258
volume challenge, 256–257
Right ventricular ejection time (RVET), 206
Right ventricular (RV) failure
acidosis, 419
anemia, 419
ARDS, 418
atrial tachyarrhythmias, 418–419
chronic RV dysfunction and venous congestion, 417
hemodynamic perturbations, 418
hypercapnia, 419
hypoxemia, 419
ICU monitoring, 419–420
management strategies
CPR, 427
inotropes, 422–423
mechanical support, 426
mechanical ventilation, 425–426
pulmonary vasodilators, 423–425
supportive care, 425
vasopressors, 421–422
volume management, 421
metabolic abnormalities, 419
pathophysiology, 415–417
PE, 419
pneumonia, 418
reduced bowel perfusion, 417
structure and function of, 414–415
systemic hypotension, 418
Right ventricular fractional area change (RVFAC), 205
Right ventricular outflow tract (RVOT), 212–213

S
Schistosoma mansoni, 145, 146, 149, 153
Schistosomiasis, 29, 51
Schistosomiasis-associated pulmonary arterial hypertension (Sch-PAH)
adult worms, 146
cercariae, 146
clinical presentation, 154
diagnosis
abdominal ultrasound findings, 154–155
chest radiography, 156
computed tomography, 156–157
echocardiogram, 155
6MWT, 157
periportal fibrosis, 155
right heart catheterization, 155–156
epidemiology, 148–150
hepatoesplenic form, 148
hepatointestinal form, 148
hepatopulmonary syndrome, 148
Katayama syndrome, 147
parasite life cycle, 144–146
pathogenesis
genetic determinants, 151–152
granuloma formation, 151
perivascular infiltration, 152
pharmacological blockage, 153
portosystemic anastomoses, 152
SEA, 153
vascular remodeling, 152–153
pathology, 150–151
poor sanitation, 144–145

Schistosomiasis-associated pulmonary arterial hypertension (Sch-PAH) (*cont.*)
- prognosis, 159
- serological tests, 157
- squamous cell carcinoma, 148
- Symmer's fibrosis, 146–147
- systemic circulation, 146
- treatment, 157–158

Scleroderma, 327
Selexipag, 334–335
Sildenafil *vs.* endothelin receptor antagonist for pulmonary hypertension (SERAPH), 350
6 minute walk distance (6MWD), 132–134, 326, 327, 329–334, 389–392
6 minute walk test (6MWT), 155, 157, 158, 159, 188, 351
Sleep disordered breathing
- chronic lung disease, 110
- HFrEF, 101–102
- hypoxic pulmonary hypertension, 76, 80

S. mansoni-soluble egg antigens (SEA), 153
Soluble guanylate cyclase stimulator (SGC), 131, 357
- medications, 380
- rationale, 381
- timeline of drugs, 379

Systemic to pulmonary shunts (SPS), 216
Systemic vascular resistance (SVR), 170–171
Systolic pulmonary artery pressure (sPAP), 234–235

T

Thermodilution method, 15, 234, 243, 254–255
Thromboembolic-related respiratory insufficiency (TERRI), 118
Thromboendarterectomy, 116, 128, 130, 132
Transpulmonary gradient (TPG), 98, 178, 250–251, 253, 295, 418, 440
Transthoracic echocardiography (TTE), 121–122, 234, 379, 444
Treprostinil, 133, 329, 332–336, 351, 380, 390, 391, 424
Tricuspid annular plane systolic excursion (TAPSE), 155, 182, 205, 220, 444
Two-dimensional echocardiography (2DE), 181–184

U

Upstream resistance (Rup), 130

V

Vascular cell proliferation, 14, 403–404
Vasoactive targets, 401–402
Vasoconstriction targets, 401
Vasopressin, 75, 422, 450, 453, 456
Vasopressors, 418, 421–422, 425, 427, 453, 457
Vasoreactivity testing, 155, 238, 239, 240, 258, 313, 314
Venoarterial extracorporeal membrane oxygenation (VA-ECMO), 426
Ventilation-perfusion (V/Q) scintigraphy, 122–123, 186–187
Vessel remodeling targets, 403–404

W

Warfarin therapy, 47, 308–309

Printed by Printforce, the Netherlands